OXYGEN TRANSPORT IN THE CRITICALLY ILL

Oxygen Transport in the Critically Ill

James V. Snyder, M.D.
Professor of Anesthesiology/Critical Care Medicine
University of Pittsburgh School of Medicine
Associate Director, Surgical Intensive Care Unit
Presbyterian-University Hospital
Pittsburgh, Pennsylvania

ASSOCIATE EDITOR

Michael R. Pinsky, M.D.
Associate Professor of Anesthesiology and Critical Care Medicine
Research Associate Professor of Medicine
University of Pittsburgh School of Medicine
Director of Research
Division of Anesthesiology/Critical Care Medicine at
    Presbyterian-University Hospital
Pittsburgh, Pennsylvania

YEAR BOOK MEDICAL PUBLISHERS, INC.
Chicago • London

Library of Congress Cataloging-in-Publication Data

Oxygen transport in the critically ill.

   Includes bibliographies and index.
   1. Critical care medicine.   2. Oxygen transport
(Physiology)   3. Respiratory therapy.   I. Snyder,
James V.   [DNLM: 1. Critical Care.   2. Oxygen
Consumption.   QV 312 098]
RC86.7.098   1987   616'.028   86-1591
ISBN 0-8151-7903-0

         1   2   3   4   5   6   7   8   9   CY   89   88   87   86

Cover design: Charles W. Snyder III

Sponsoring Editor: David K. Marshall/Kevin M. Kelly
Manager, Copyediting Services: Frances M. Perveiler
Production Project Manager: Max Perez
Proofroom Supervisor: Shirley E. Taylor

To Ann, Cathy, and Rob,
and Chuck, Karen, and Virginia.

Contributors

FRANK J. BRUNS, M.D.
Associate Professor of Medicine, University of
Pittsburgh School of Medicine; Associate Head,
Renal Unit, Head, Dialysis Unit, Montefiore
Hospital, Pittsburgh, Pennsylvania

MICHAEL J. BURAN, M.D.
Assistant Professor, Anesthesiology and Medicine,
University of Pittsburgh School of Medicine;
Director, Surgical Intensive Care Unit, Veterans
Administration Medical Center, Pittsburgh,
Pennsylvania

JOHN B. CONE, M.D.
Assistant Professor of Surgery, University of
Arkansas for Medical Sciences; Director,
Surgical Intensive Care Unit, and Emergency
Surgical Service, University Hospital, Little
Rock, Arkansas

JUDITH A. CULPEPPER, M.D.
Assistant Professor of Anesthesiology and
Medicine/Critical Care Medicine, University of
Pittsburgh; Codirector, Surgical Intensive Care
Unit, Medical Codirector, Respiratory Therapy,
Veterans Administration Medical Center,
Pittsburgh, Pennsylvania

JOSEPH M. DARBY, M.D.
Assistant Professor of Anesthesiology and Critical
Care Medicine, University of Pittsburgh School
of Medicine, Director, Unit 64 Intensive Care
Unit, Presbyterian-University Hospital,
Pittsburgh, Pennsylvania

RICHARD M. EDWARDS, PH.D.
Associate Senior Investigator, Smith Kline and
French Laboratories, Philadelphia, Pennsylvania

PAUL R. EISENBERG, M.D., M.P.H.
Assistant Professor of Medicine, Cardiovascular
Division, Washington University; Assistant
Director, Coronary Care Unit, Barnes Hospital,
St. Louis, Missouri

PETER F. FERSON, M.D.
Assistant Professor of Surgery, University of
Pittsburgh School of Medicine; Assistant Chief,
Surgical Service, Veterans Administration
Medical Center, Pittsburgh, Pennsylvania

JOSEPH D. FONDACARO, PH.D.
Associate Research Fellow, Department of
Pharmacology, Smith Kline and French
Laboratories, Philadelphia, Pennsylvania;
Adjunct Associate Professor, Department of
Physiology, University of Cincinnati College of
Medicine, Cincinnati, Ohio

DONALD S. FRALEY, M.D.
Associate Professor of Medicine, University of
Pittsburgh School of Medicine; Assistant Head,
Renal and Electrolyte Unit, Director, Medical
Intensive Care Unit, Montefiore Hospital,
Pittsburgh, Pennsylvania

ALISON B. FROESE, M.D., F.R.C.P. (C.)
Associate Professor of Anaesthesia and Paediatrics,
Assistant Professor of Physiology, Queen's
University; Staff Anaesthetist, Kingston General
Hospital, Kingston, Ontario, Canada

ROBERT E. FROMM, JR., M.D.
Medical Staff Fellow, Critical Care Medicine,
National Institute of Health, Bethesda, Maryland

JONATHAN M. GERRARD, M.D., C.M., PH.D.
Associate Professor, Department of Pediatrics,
University of Manitoba; Director of Research
and Clinical Investigations, Children's Hospital
of Winnipeg, Manitoba Institute of Cell Biology,
Winnipeg, Manitoba, Canada

HOWARD S. GOLDBERG, M.D.
Director of Pulmonary Research, Cedars-Sinai
Medical Center; Associate Professor of
Medicine, UCLA, Los Angeles, California

BARTLEY P. GRIFFITH, M.D.
Assistant Professor of Surgery, University of
Pittsburgh School of Medicine; Staff,
Presbyterian-University Hospital, Pittsburgh,
Pennsylvania

JEAN-GILLES GUIMOND, M.D., F.R.C.P. (C.)
Assistant Professor of Anesthesiology and Critical
Care Medicine, University of Pittsburgh School
of Medicine, Codirector, Surgical Intensive Care
Unit, Oakland Veterans Administration Medical
Center, Pittsburgh, Pennsylvania

DAVID GUR, SC.D.
Professor, Department of Radiology, University of Pittsburgh School of Medicine, Pittsburgh, Pennsylvania

JOHN D. HAIGH, M.D., F.R.C.P. (C.)
Assistant Professor of Anesthesiology, Presbyterian-University Hospital, Pittsburgh, Pennsylvania

ROBERT L. HARDESTY, M.D.
Associate Professor of Surgery, University of Pittsburgh School of Medicine; Director of Cardiothoracic Services, Presbyterian-University Hospital, Pittsburgh, Pennsylvania

J. PAUL HIEBLE, PH.D.
Research Fellow, Pharmacology, Smith Kline and French Laboratories, Philadelphia, Pennsylvania

LEWIS B. KINTER, PH.D.
Assistant Director, Pharmacology/Renal, Smith Kline and French Laboratories, Philadelphia, Pennsylvania

CHRISTINE E. LAWLESS, M.D.
Assistant Professor of Medicine, Loyola University of Chicago; Staff Cardiologist, Hines Veterans Administration Hospital, Hines, Illinois

BLANCHE LEVITT, PH.D.
Postdoctoral Fellow in Pharmacology, Smith Kline and French Laboratories, Philadelphia, Pennsylvania

JOSE M. MARQUEZ, M.D.
Assistant Professor of Anesthesiology, University of Pittsburgh; Chief of Anesthesiology, Presbyterian-University Hospital, Pittsburgh, Pennsyvlania

DOUGLAS J. MARTIN, M.D., C.M., F.R.C.P. (C.)
Assistant Professor of Anesthesiology/CCM, University of Pittsburgh; Anesthesiologist, Presbyterian-University Hospital, Pittsburgh, Pennsylvania

GEORGE M. MATUSCHAK, M.D.
Assistant Professor of Anesthesiology/CCM and Medicine, University of Pittsburgh School of Medicine; Associate Director, Surgical Intensive Care Unit, Medical Director, Respiratory Therapy, Director, Intermediate Care Unit, Presbyterian-University Hospital, Pittsburgh, Pennsylvania

LOREN D. NELSON, M.D.
Assistant Professor of Surgery and Anesthesiology, University of Miami School of Medicine; Associate Director of Surgical Intensive Care Unit, Jackson Memorial Hospital, Miami, Florida

ANDREW B. PEITZMAN, M.D.
Assistant Professor of Surgery, University of Pittsburgh School of Medicine; Director, Trauma and Emergency Services, Presbyterian-University Hospital, Pittsburgh, Pennsylvania

MICHAEL R. PINSKY, M.D.
Associate Professor of Anesthesiology and Medicine, University of Pittsburgh School of Medicine; Director of Research, Division of Anesthesiology/Critical Care Medicine, Presbyterian-University Hospital, Pittsburgh, Pennsylvania

JEAN E. RINALDO, M.D.
Associate Professor of Medicine/Anesthesiology/CCM, University of Pittsburgh School of Medicine; Director, Medical Intensive Care Unit, Presbyterian-University Hospital, Pittsburgh, Pennsylvania

ROBERT R. RUFFOLO, JR., PH.D.
Director, Cardiovascular Pharmacology, Smith Kline and French Laboratories, Philadelphia, Pennsylvania

DANIEL P. SCHUSTER, M.D.
Assistant Professor of Medicine, Washington University School of Medicine; Director, RICU/MICU, Barnes Hospital, St. Louis, Missouri

B. SIMON SLASKY, M.D.
Associate Professor of Radiology, University of Pittsburgh School of Medicine; Chief of Diagnostic Radiology, Presbyterian-University Hospital, Pittsburgh, Pennsylvania

JAMES V. SNYDER, M.D.
Professor of Anesthesiology/Critical Care Medicine, University of Pittsburgh School of Medicine; Associate Director, Surgical Intensive Care Unit, Presbyterian-University Hospital, Pittsburgh, Pennsylvania

W. NEWLON TAUXE, M.D.
Professor of Radiology, University of Pittsburgh School of Medicine; Director, Department of Nuclear Medicine, Presbyterian-University Hospital, Pittsburgh, Pennsylvania

ALFREDO TRENTO, M.D.
Assistant Professor of Surgery, University of
Pittsburgh School of Medicine; Staff,
Presbyterian-University Hospital, Pittsburgh,
Pennsylvania

BARRY F. URETSKY, M.D.
Associate Professor of Medicine, University of
Pittsburgh; Co-director, Cardiac Diagnostic
Laboratories, Presbyterian-University Hospital,
Pittsburgh, Pennsylvania

HOWARD YONAS, M.D.
Associate Professor of Neurological Surgery and
Radiology, University of Pittsburgh; Department
of Neurological Surgery, Presbyterian-University
Hospital, Pittsburgh, Pennsylvania

ROBERT L. ZEID, B.S.
Department of Pharmacology, Smith Kline and
French Laboratories, Philadelphia, Pennsylvania

Foreword

One of the central themes of critical care medicine is the direct relationship between tissue integrity and the amount of oxygen consumed by the mitochondria. In turn, mitochondrial oxygen consumption is determined by the amount of oxygen required by and the amount of oxygen delivered to those subcellular organelles. The pioneers of clinical cardiopulmonary physiology, Andre Cournand, Dickinson Richards, and Carl Wiggers, clearly understood the importance of both oxygen content and blood flow to the delivery of oxygen but their seminal studies remained unappreciated until quite recently. Part of the unwillingness to immediately accept the importance of the oxygen delivery concept probably arose from the unfortunate fragmentation of cardiopulmonary pathophysiology into cardiovascular and pulmonary compartments. A conceptual barrier was erected which, for the moment, rejected the unitary concept of oxygen delivery. One group of organ specialists claimed ownership of blood flow (the cardiologists) while the other group claimed arterial oxygen tension as its raison d'être (the chest physicians). The idea of oxygen content, as opposed to tension, was shelved along with the Van Slyke-Neill manometric apparatus. The cardiologist became obsessed with cardiac arrhythmias and ventricular function; the pulmonologist with alveolar-arterial differences and ventilation/perfusion (V/Q) ratios. This fine text celebrates the rediscovery of the importance of oxygen delivery and the unified concept of human pathophysiology embodied in critical care medicine.

More than 65 years have passed since the English physiologist, Joseph Barcroft,[1] emphasized that oxygen deficits (anoxia) could be due to reduced arterial oxyhemoglobin saturation (anoxic anoxia), a low hemoglobin concentration (anemic anoxia) or decreased blood flow (stagnant anoxia). Less than 10 years later, the German urologist Werner Forssmann[6] cautiously introduced a "well-lubricated ureteral catheter of four Charrieres thickness" into his own antecubital vein. He stopped the initial experiment because his co-workers felt the procedure too dangerous but 1 week later "performed the experiment upon myself without assistance." He "examined the position of the catheter by x-ray and observed the passage of the catheter in a mirror that was held by a nurse in front of the fluorescent screen." Forssmann invented cardiac catheterization in an effort to improve resuscitative techniques by injecting medication directly into the heart; he noted, however, that the "described method offers many new possibilities for metabolic and hemodynamic studies."

Cournand and Richards, and their many associates at Columbia University and Bellevue Hospital, were clinical cardiopulmonary physiologists who dealt with the heart and lungs as a single transport system. "Studies of the Circulation in Clinical Shock" appeared in a surgical journal in 1943.[4] The carefully documented experimental study listed 8 authors and 6 technical assistants and still serves as a model for the scientific investigation of the critically ill patient. The authors rescued Forssmann's technique of right atrial catheterization from academic oblivion and used it to obtain right atrial blood samples, which they demonstrated to represent "mixed venous blood." Oxygen consumption was calculated from expired oxygen and carbon dioxide concentrations; cardiac output was determined by the direct Fick method. Arterial and venous oxygen and carbon dioxide contents, blood volume, hemoglobin, blood lactic acid concentration, pulmonary ventilation and respiratory gas exchange, and the clearance of substances by the kidney were measured in 36 patients. The investigators were charting unexplored territory and their "methods" section required more than half of the article's 31 pages.

The studies demonstrated that traumatic shock in man was "a rapid or precipitate failure of the circulation, usually associated with inadequate return flow of blood to the heart. The chief findings were decreased cardiac output, low pressure in the right auricle, low arterial pressure, and decreased blood volume." In addition, the investigators noted "marked reduction in effective renal blood flow, out of proportion to the decrease in the systemic blood flow, with a filtration fraction either normal or low" as well as severe metabolic acidosis due to accumulation of lactic acid. Measurements of this sort were not to be repeated in critically ill patients for several decades and oxygen content is almost never measured at the present time. For reasons perhaps related to the desire for rapid publication of research findings, the elegant Van Slyke-Neill manometric technique was discarded and investigators estimated arterial oxygen content from oxygen tension and a "standard" oxyhemoglobin dissociation curve (if there ever was one). Cournand and co-workers found that oxygen delivery was 568 ml/min/M^2 in normal individuals, 243 in patients with shock associated with skeletal trauma, 388 in those with shock and blunt abdominal injury and 326 in burned patients with shock. They weighed and measured their patients so that they could present their findings in relation to body surface area. Several of their extremely ill patients demonstrated what has now been identified as the adult respiratory distress syndrome and flow limited oxen consumption. One injured patient had an oxyhemoglobin saturation of 83% while a burned individual had an oxygen delivery of 129 ml/min/M^2 and an oxygen consumption of 109 ml/min/M^2. That unfortunate person extracted 84% of his available oxygen supply but still could not maintain an adequate oxygen consumption!

Almost inexplicably, the concepts of systemic oxygen delivery and consumption lay fallow during the 25 years that followed the publication of Cournand and Richard's important studies. Part of the problem was methodologic. The 1960s were dominated by continuous electrocardiographic monitoring (the cardiologists) and repeated measurement of arterial oxygen and carbon dioxide tensions (the chest physicians). Surgeons and anesthesiologists, however, needed better techniques for intra-operative monitoring and a group of clinical scientists, most notably William Shoemaker,[9] began to make measurements of oxygen delivery in seriously ill surgical patients. Shoemaker and his associates soon demonstrated that a low oxygen delivery intra-operatively and during the post-operative period was a predictor of death. A few years later, Clement Finch, a hematologist, and Claude Lenfant, a surgeon turned pulmonary physiologist (now direc-

tor of the National Heart Lung and Blood Institute) gave oxygen transport national attention in their *Medical Progress* contribution published in the New England Journal of Medicine in February, 1972.[5] "Oxygen transport is a corporate process involving several organs," they emphasized, "each with its own regulatory system." They listed the essential components of oxygen delivery as pulmonary gas exchange, blood flow, hemoglobin concentration, and hemoglobin affinity for oxygen. Echoing Cournand and Richards, they concluded that "evaluation of available oxygen in shock thus requires the measurement of arterial oxygen content, the in vivo oxygen dissociation (including allowance for body temperature) and information concerning cardiac output. The adequacy of supply may be monitored by the mixed venous oxygen tension."

One might have thought that the matter would have been settled at that point, and perhaps it was. Every discovery, particularly the most useful and revolutionary ones, has its detractors and the notion of hemodynamic monitoring was no exception. Eugene Robin,[8] for example, has recently suggested that the use of hemodynamic monitoring to guide treatment in critically ill patients has become a cult. He took the trouble to quote Webster: "Cult: A system for the cure of disease based on dogma set forth by its promulgators . . . great and faddish devotion." Wiggers, Cournand and Richards the founders of a cult—interesting suggestion! Robin was certainly correct in suggesting the need for solid clinical trials and such a plea was made by the National Institutes of Health Consensus Conference on Critical Care[7] more than one year before the publication of his polemic. But Robin misses the point in not properly understanding the great value of measuring blood flow and oxygen delivery in individuals who are at risk of death. Admittedly, catheters have been inserted by inexperienced physicians and the derived data not properly utilized for decision-making but such maturational problems require constructive support rather than blanket condemnation.

Almost as if in answer to the call for randomized trials, William Shoemaker and his associates[10] recently presented their experience with a protocol that seeks to raise cardiac output and oxygen consumption to 50% and 30% greater than predicted normal values respectively. There were 10 deaths in the 28 patients randomized in the group where the goal of therapy was restoration to published normal values. In contrast, there was only 1 death in the 27 patients in the group where cardiac output and oxygen consumption were raised to greater than normal levels ($P <$ 0.02). The sequence of studies is most convincing. The investigators first observed that survivors of critical illness frequently had higher than normal oxygen requirements. That experience led to the design of a randomized study that confirmed the hypothesis that a therapeutic increase in oxygen consumption to levels above normal could improve survival. The value of measuring oxygen delivery in critically ill patients seems to have been demonstrated.

The general acceptance of oxygen delivery as an important variable in patient survival comes at a time when the theoretic bases for mitochondrial respiration have been placed on an even stronger footing. Britton Chance has spent years studying the mitochondrial function and the state of respiratory enzyme oxidation. Using optical methods, he and his associates demonstrated that adenosine diphosphate (ADP) regulated the generation of adenosine triphosphate (ATP) and the consumption of oxygen in isolated mitochondria.[2] The ADP/ATP ratio (phosphate potential) was an indicator of mitochondrial integrity but was not particularly useful at the bedside. He leaped at the demonstration that the inorganic phosphate/phosphocreatine ratio (Pi/PCr), which could be readily measured by magnetic resonance spectroscopy, was a good surrogate for the phosphate potential and actually installed such an instrument in a pediatric intensive care unit.[3] A plot of the Pi/PCr ratio and mitochondrial oxygen tension demonstrates that a decrease in oxygen availability leads to rapidly increasing Pi/PCr ratios. The form of the relationship is a rectangular hyperbola, a function often observed in physiologic systems. Significant decreases in mitochondrial oxygen tension have little effect on the Pi/PCr ratio until a critical point is reached. At that point, a further small reduction in oxygen tension produces a very large increase in the ratio. The rising ratio portends a failure of mitochondrial respiration and cell death. Clinically, the patient "crashes."

This text reviews the importance of the clinical and laboratory assessment of oxygen delivery. A chapter comparing the clinical methods with invasive hemodynamic methods for assessing oxygen delivery emphasizes the value and limitation of continuous skillful observation. Physicians and nurses estimate regional oxygen delivery as they palpate peripheral pulses, measure the urine output, observe the color of nailbeds and analyze the patient's mental status. These clinical observations are vital because they estimate regional flow in a way not yet possible by other means. They may not be sensitive enough, however, to predict deterioration or to monitor the effects of therapeutic intervention. Each approach supplements the other and the authors of this text carefully point out the interdependency of clinical and laboratory evaluation. The preservation of mitochondrial integrity remains a major challenge for clinicians. The lessons presented here should help all who care for the critically ill keep Pi/PCr ratios at appropriately low levels.

STEPHEN M. AYRES, M.D.
DEAN, MEDICAL COLLEGE OF VIRGINIA SCHOOL OF MEDICINE
VIRGINIA COMMONWEALTH UNIVERSITY
RICHMOND, VIRGINIA

REFERENCES

1. Barcroft J: On anoxemia. *Lancet* 1920; 2:485.
2. Chance B, Williams GR: Respiratory enzymes in oxidative phosphorylation: III. The steady state. *J Biol Chem* 1955; 217:409–428.
3. Chance B, Nioka S, Leigh JSF: Metabolic control principles: The importance of the steady state reaffirmed and quantified by ^{31}P MRS. New Horizons Conference, Phoenix, Ariz, March 1986.
4. Cournand A, Riley RL, Bradley SE, et al: Studies of the circulation in clinical shock. *Surgery* 1943; 13:964–995.
5. Finch CA, Lenfant C: Oxygen transport in man. *N Engl J Med* 1972; 286:407–415.
6. Forssmann W: The catheterization of the right heart. *Klin Wochenschr* 1929; November 2085–2087.
7. Parillo JE, Ayres SM: *Major Issues in Critical Care Medicine*. Baltimore, Williams and Wilkins Co, 1984.
8. Robin ED: The cult of the Swan-Ganz catheter. *Ann Intern Med* 1985; 103:445–449.
9. Shoemaker WC, Montgomery ES, Kaplan E, et al: Physiologic patterns in surviving and

nonsurviving shock patients. *Arch Surg* 1973;
106:630.

10. Shoemaker WC, Appel PL, Kram HB: Comparison of two monitoring methods (central venous pressure versus pulmonary artery catheter) and two protocols as therapeutic goals (normal values versus values of survivors) in a prospective randomized clinical trial of critically ill surgical patients. *Crit Care Med* 1985; 13(abst):304.

Preface

Our goal throughout this text is to present the physiologic and therapeutic complexities of critical care in paradigms that incorporate recent insights and prepare the reader for the anticipated increasing focus on regional pathophysiology and treatment. Many responses to disease and therapy cannot be adequately explained by common clinical concepts. The patient in shock with increased venous oxygen tension, for example, makes perilous the application of our accepted concepts of oxygen transport and metabolism. The validity of such concepts depends entirely on intact local vasoregulation—the appropriate regulation of flow by each tissue according to its metabolic needs. In sepsis or any systemic stress, we must consider the determinants of local oxygen transport and demand to understand the physiology and direct appropriate therapy. New tools to do this are now available, and old ones are being reinvestigated. The potential consequences of manipulating local vascular resistance are greater than they first appeared. We appreciate the local effects of low-dose dopamine, for example, but those of most agents have not been determined.

Once understood, the appropriate use of local vasoconstriction could change our clinical practice. For example, tissue hypoperfusion is usually, and usually appropriately, treated by intravascular volume administration. This might better perfuse the compromised tissue, but it also increases microvascular pressure and therefore interstitial fluid throughout the body; thus, flow that is already excessive in some beds is further increased, and an unnecessarily large demand is placed on the heart. Selective constriction of vascular beds that are perfused beyond their metabolic needs might increase not only arterial pressure and flow to other beds, but also venous return and, therefore, cardiac output. We now understand the mechanism by which arterial constriction can increase venous return. We know that coupling of flow to metabolic rate can vary widely in pathologic states. Thus, we are developing the concepts and tools to incorporate local vascular physiology into clinical thinking.

We need also to resolve semantic differences. How can physiologists claim that increasing right atrial pressure decreases venous return when clinicians routinely increase cardiac output by raising the same pressure? The physiologists' concepts of the determinants of venous return, including mean systemic pressure, become more meaningful as we establish the methodology to estimate them in patients.

The appropriate support of ventilation is a major consideration in oxygen transport in critically ill patients, because of its influence on arterial oxygen content, cardiac output, distribution of cardiac output, and systemic microvascular pressure (and, therefore, fluid shifts). Less appreciated is the positive influence of increased airway pressure to increase cardiac output, and how this can be used to clinical advantage. Riley's simplification of pulmonary physiology into shunt, dead space, and ideal alveoli has facilitated our understanding of lung function for decades but now occasionally impedes correct analysis. To optimally manage pulmonary failure we must consider the local distribution of ventilation and perfusion, which warrants a careful look at various aspects of mechanical ventilation.

Several chapters are tangential to the clinical physiology of oxygen transport. Optimal cellular metabolism is the principal goal of intensive care medicine, yet cellular physiology remains somewhat distant from practice. Available tests reflect only some of the significant intracellular changes, and these are often late. In most cases, therapy is still based on systemic or regional manifestations rather than cellular metabolism per se. However, we are on the brink of vast new insight into local physiology and biochemistry, especially from nuclear magnetic imaging. To provide a foundation for comprehending and interpreting the associated literature is one goal of the section on cellular oxygenation. The chapters on prostaglandin derivatives and cellular mechanisms in the adult respiratory distress syndrome also may be more useful as preparation for the literature than as the basis for bedside intervention.

The structure of the book is designed to encourage analysis of overall oxygen transport before assessment of individual components or focal compromise. Simplifying perceptions of the monitoring and physiology of oxygen transport have been useful to popularize the fundamentals involved in the appropriate support of the critically ill patient. However, the same simplifications cause expectations in monitoring and treatment that are not satisfied. Even when technology is managed carefully, the understanding of underlying physiology is often deficient. Thus, we come back to the fundamental need for a thorough understanding of oxygen transport and consumption, and this is where the book begins.

Throughout the volume we have tried to present a clinical perspective informed by basic physiologic concepts. In doing so, we have probed the weaknesses of conventional paradigms of pathology and modified them to incorporate recent observations. We aimed to create a timely and inclusive reference for the intensive care physicians and sophisticated support teams who care for critically ill patients.

JAMES V. SNYDER, M.D.

Acknowledgments

I am grateful to the many individuals who have contributed to this book, including the many patients whose illness has stimulated our concern and provided our education.

Central to the team care of these patients are the ICU nurses, led in our unit by Barbara McCoy and Marilyn Hravnak. The technicians in the Critical Care Medicine/ICU Laboratory, directed by Jean O'Malley, have shown invaluable expertise in providing physiologic studies and chemical analyses. Drew Hrehocik and Charles Kern have been innovative leaders of the respiratory care team. The physicians that attend patients at the University Health Center of Pittsburgh Hospitals have collaborated with the physician staff and fellows of the Critical Care Medicine Program, both facilitating and challenging our care. The Health Center administration, especially Dan Stickler and Pat Shehorn, have consistently supported us and educated us in the changing role of the ICU medical director.

My associates in intensive care have helped to develop many of the concepts I present, especially Gil Carroll (oxygen transport in sepsis), Dan Schuster (high-frequency ventilation), and Judy Culpepper (pulmonary physiology), who each collaborated on the issues of *Current Problems in Surgery* from which this text grew. Mark Ravitch invited me to write those monographs, and then encouraged their expansion. I am indebted to Peter Winter, Ake Grenvik, Mike Buran, George Matuschak, and Dan Polacek for giving me free time in which to work. Many other colleagues in the broad field of oxygen transport freely gave their thoughts and advice.

Special appreciation goes to my associate editor, Michael Pinsky. Michael has added considerable scientific depth and personal enthusiam to the CCM program as well as to this text. I have gained much from his physiologic perspective on critical illness; his use of increased airway pressure to enhance cardiac output is an example.

In the production of the manuscript, Lisa Cohn provided consistent encouragement, highly constructive critical review, and superb technical editing. Kathleen Kramer accomplished indispensable organization in addition to innumerable and extensive secretarial tasks. Charles Snyder contributed a design for the book cover.

George Mitchell, Peter Safar, and Ake Grenvik all gave me important professional direction. George Mitchell taught me most of my anesthesiology and many of the pleasures in the practice and teaching of medicine. In the late 1960s, Peter Safar attracted me with his interest in intensive care and infected me with his enthusiasm. He directed my attention to brain resuscitation and buoyed me and my dedicated preceptor, Bjorn Lind, through the initial research projects. Ake Grenvik has fathered the development of critical care medicine and has been the mainstay of the program in Pittsburgh. I have benefited from his support and dedication in our joint pursuit of a stable and rational practice for the past 15 years.

For their contribution to my personal capacity and philosophy, I thank Charles Rumble, Lawrence Scheck, and Susan St. John-Reaux. Charles and Virginia Snyder started me on the path in the first place, and taught me the personal side of the business in the course of their own long and critical illnesses. Ann Snyder taught me to sense the texture of life. She has been the difference between my effort and my success. Much of my work could have been done better, but not with a better partner.

JAMES V. SNYDER, M.D.

Contents

PART 1 —————— Oxygen Supply and Demand

1   Oxygen Transport: The Model and Reality

James V. Snyder, M.D.

The adequacy of tissue oxygenation depends on the volume of oxygen delivered to the tissues (oxygen transport) and the volume consumed by the tissues (oxygen consumption). This supply/demand balance is determined by the analysis of five factors that are readily measured and of a sixth that is not. The five measured factors are hemoglobin concentration, the percentage of hemoglobin saturated with oxygen in arterial blood (Sa_{O_2}), cardiac output (CO), oxygen consumption ($\dot{V}_{O_2}$), and the affinity of hemoglobin for oxygen (P50); the sixth factor is the distribution of perfusion. The interrelations of the first five will be discussed as a model initially, and then as effects of changes in vivo. The difficulties introduced by a pathologic distribution of perfusion will be summarized here and dealt with more fully in chapter 5, "Patterns of Hemodynamic Response," and chapter 13, "Assessment of Systemic Oxygen Transport."

THE MODEL: NORMAL STATE

Arterial oxygen content (Ca_{O_2}) is the sum of the oxygen chemically bound by hemoglobin and the oxygen physically dissolved in the plasma. The amount of chemically bound oxygen is directly related to the concentration of hemoglobin and to how saturated this hemoglobin is with oxygen. Arterial oxygen content can be described by the equation:

$$Ca_{O_2} = Hb \times 1.36 \times Sa_{O_2} + Pa_{O_2} \times 0.003 \qquad \text{(Eq. 1–1)}$$

where 1.36 is the estimate of the mean volume of oxygen that can be bound by 1 gm of normal hemoglobin when it is fully saturated ($Sa_{O_2} = 1.0$), and 0.003 is the solubility coefficient of oxygen in human plasma. Arterial blood with 15 gm/dl of hemoglobin therefore normally contains about 20 ml of oxygen per 1 dl of blood. If $Sa_{O_2} = 1.0$* when Hb = 15 gm/dl, then:

$$Ca_{O_2} = 15 \times 1.36 \times 1.0 + 100 \times .003 = 20 \text{ ml/dl} + .3 \text{ ml/dl (approximately)}$$

As this equation shows, the amount of oxygen dissolved in plasma usually does not make a significant contribution to Ca_{O_2}, and it will be ignored in most of this text. (When anemia is severe and in carbon monoxide intoxication and maximal shock, very high levels of Pa_{O_2} may be useful.)

Oxygen transport or delivery ($\dot{D}_{O_2}$) is the volume of oxygen delivered to the systemic vascular bed per minute and is a product of Ca_{O_2} and cardiac output (CO):

$$\dot{D}_{O_2} = Ca_{O_2} \times CO \qquad \text{(Eq. 1–2)}$$

If hemoglobin = 15 gm/dl, saturation is complete, and CO = 5 L/min:

$$\dot{D}_{O_2} = 20 \text{ ml } O_2/dl \times 10 \text{ dl/L} \times 5 \text{ L/min} = 1,000 \text{ ml/min}$$

Oxygen consumption ($\dot{V}_{O_2}$) is the amount of oxygen that diffuses from the capillaries into all tissues, and is usually about 250 ml/min. Since oxygen transport is normally about 1,000 ml/min, about 750 ml of oxygen returns to the right atrium in venous blood each minute. This 750 ml of oxygen is still carried in 5 L, or 50 dl, of blood each minute; each 1 dl therefore carries 750 ml/min ÷ 50 dl/min = 15 ml/dl. *The normal arterial-venous oxygen content difference ($C(a-\bar{v})_{O_2}$) is 20 − 15 = 5 (or 4 to 6) ml O_2/dl* (Fig 1–1).

Because the arterial blood was fully saturated when it contained 20 ml O_2/dl, a mixed venous oxygen content of 15 ml/dl must indicate

---

*Hemoglobin saturation is normally about 0.97 when Pa_{O_2} is 100 torr.

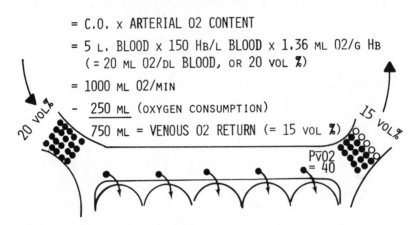

O2 TRANSPORT; NORMAL

= C.O. x ARTERIAL O2 CONTENT

= 5 L. BLOOD x 150 Hb/L BLOOD x 1.36 ML O2/G HB
(= 20 ML O2/DL BLOOD, OR 20 VOL %)

= 1000 ML O2/MIN

- 250 ML (OXYGEN CONSUMPTION)

750 ML = VENOUS O2 RETURN (= 15 VOL %)

20 VOL%

15 VOL%

$P\bar{v}O2$ = 40

FIG 1–1.
Normal oxygen transport, giving normal values for oxygen consumption and venous oxygen content. *Solid* *dots* represent oxygen in ml/dl. (From Snyder and Carroll.[21] Reproduced by permission.)

75% saturation ($S\bar{v}_{O_2}$ = .75), while an $S\bar{v}_{O_2}$ of .5 would give a mixed venous oxygen content of 10 ml/dl. All of these relationships should seem straightforward. The relation between $S\bar{v}_{O_2}$ and $P\bar{v}_{O_2}$, however, is governed by less obvious principles of physical chemistry, whereby as the tissues take up oxygen, the remaining oxygen is more readily released (at least until tissue hypoxia is severe); the reverse occurs during oxygen uptake in the lung. Hemoglobin uptake and release of oxygen is regulated in a pattern demonstrated by the familiar oxyhemoglobin dissociation curve (Fig 1–2), which specifies that normally when $S\bar{v}_{O_2}$ = .75, $P\bar{v}_{O_2}$ is about 40 torr.

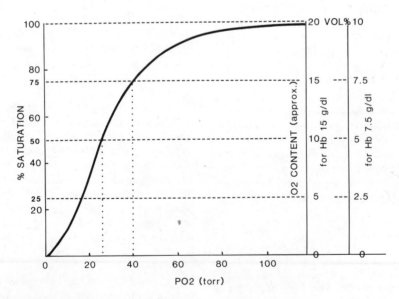

FIG 1–2.
The normal relation between oxygen saturation and partial pressure. It may be useful to add an oxygen content axis for specific levels of hemoglobin, as has been done here, to estimate the effect of a change in $C(a-\bar{v})_{O_2}$ on $P\bar{v}_{O_2}$.

CHANGING THE OXYGEN SUPPLY/DEMAND COMPONENTS

Effects in the Model

Table 1–1 presents calculations to show the effects of separately compromising each of the components of oxygen supply and demand, without compensation. The calculations not only show theoretical relations, but also serve as first approximations of real physiologic sequelae when normal compensatory mechanisms are inoperative. This tangent is worth brief pursuit: because patients with a hemoglobin value of 7.5 gm/dl (for example, in renal failure) and others with twice-normal oxygen consumption (for example, from mild shivering) often show no sign of tissue hypoxia, we may tend to underestimate the threat of those insults. Indeed, in most patients the compensatory mechanisms are adequate. However, "90% rules" do fail when applied to the remaining 10%. Those are the patients experiencing greater stress or with limited compensatory ability, for whom the physician has sensed an increased need for concern and who are therefore a constituent of the intensive care unit (ICU) population; or they are the patients who are thought to be following a routine course until they unexpectedly "crash" and require resuscitation. The physiologic basis of their failure is rarely as simple as Table 1–1 suggests, but the principle of looking at the interrelation of these components is valid. Note that an increase in $C(a-\bar{v})_{O_2}$ might reflect hypermetabolism (increased $\dot{V}_{O_2}$) or re-duced cardiac output. A normal $C(a-\bar{v})_{O_2}$ can be associated with tissue hypoxia in patients with anemia, arterial hypoxemia, or maldistributed blood flow. Furthermore, low $P\bar{v}_{O_2}$ can occur with any combination of the following: hypermetabolism, low cardiac output, low hemoglobin, low Pa_{O_2}, or low P50 (a leftward shift of the oxyhemoglobin dissociation curve). Every component must be considered when inadequate oxygen transport is suspected in a critically ill patient.

Effects In Vivo

Arterial Oxygen Content

Arterial oxygen content (Ca_{O_2}), as described in equation 1–1, is the sum of oxygen bound to hemoglobin (Hb $\times$ Sa_{O_2} $\times$ 1.36) and oxygen dissolved in plasma (Pa_{O_2} $\times$ .003).

Hemoglobin. The contribution of hemoglobin to oxygen transport is not really as linear as the model suggests. The relation between hemoglobin and oxygen transport varies with the degree and duration of anemia, with metabolic demands, and with vessel diameter. Anemia is associated with changes in blood viscosity and vessel tone, and a positive inotropic factor has been described.[8] The viscosity doubles when the hematocrit is increased from 20% to 40% at shear rates found in smaller vessels,[15] and viscosity change is greater in patients with peripheral vascular disease than in normal individuals. Anemia elicits two adaptive responses: the relative extrac-

TABLE 1–1.

Components of Normal Oxygen Supply and Demand, and Effects of Uncompensated Compromises*

			UNCOMPENSATED COMPROMISES			
OXYGEN TRANSPORT CONDITION		NORMAL	CARDIAC OUTPUT = 2.5 L/min	Hb = 7.5 gm/dl	$\dot{V}_{O_2}$ = 2×	Sa_{O_2} = .75 (Pa_{O_2} − 40)
Arterial O_2 content (Ca_{O_2}) (ml/dl)	=	20	20	10	20	15
O_2 transport (Ca_{O_2}) (ml O_2/min)	=	1,000	500	500	1,000	750
minus O_2 consumption ($\dot{V}_{O_2}$/min)	=	− 250	− 250	− 250	− 500	− 250
equals venous return (ml O_2/min)	=	750	250	250	500	500
divided by CO in dl/min	=	÷50	÷25	÷50	÷50	÷50
equals venous O_2 content ($C\bar{v}_{O_2}$) (ml/dl)	=	15	10	5	10	10
$(a-\bar{v})_{O_2}$ content ($C(a-\bar{v})_{O_2}$) (ml/dl)	=	5	10	5	10	5
Venous O_2 saturation ($S\bar{v}_{O_2}$)	=	.75	.50	.50	.50	.50
Mixed venous P_{O_2} ($P\bar{v}_{O_2}$) (torr)	=	40	27	27	27	27

*"Normal" implies the following values: Hb, 15 gm/dl; Sa_{O_2}, 1.0; cardiac output, 5 L/min; and $\dot{V}_{O_2}$, 250 ml/min. Each vertical column varies only in the component at the top. (From Snyder and Carroll.[21] Reproduced by permission.)

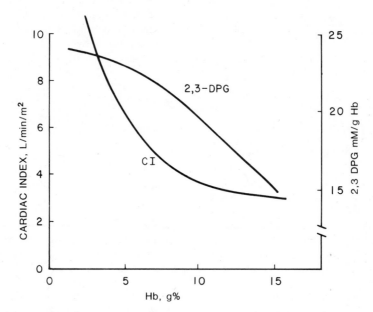

FIG 1–3.
Effect of anemia on cardiac index and 2,3-DPG. (From Finch and Lenfant.[7] Reproduced by permission of *The New* *England Journal of Medicine.* Original data from Torrance et al.[24] and Brannon et al.[3])

tion of oxygen increases when anemia is mild, and cardiac output increases (via vasodilation and perhaps an increase in inotropy) when anemia is more severe (Fig 1–3).

However, this adaptation varies with time as well as with hemoglobin concentration. For example, a moderately anemic state for 10–14 days in human subjects was associated with major basal regulatory adjustment (Table 1–2).[27] The

systemic vascular resistance (SVR) was low and the cardiac output high in acute anemia, and both returned to normal, thus lowering oxygen transport, in the chronic state. The resting $P\bar{v}_{O_2}$ was unchanged in the acute condition, then depressed. Specifically, renal blood flow was shown to decrease in the chronic phase, while the glomerular filtration rate was preserved. This suggests that the regional adaptive response to anemia is simi-

TABLE 1–2.
Oxygen Transport Dynamics in Acute Moderate Anemia and "Chronic" Adaptation*

PARAMETER	RESTING			EXERCISE		
	CONTROL	ACUTE ANEMIA	CHRONIC ANEMIA	CONTROL	ACUTE ANEMIA	CHRONIC ANEMIA
Hb (gm/dl)	15.3	10.0	9.9			
CO (ml/min · kg)	91	141	104	284	320	263
SVR (dyn/cm⁵)	1,142	685	1,128			
$P\bar{v}_{O_2}$ (torr)	40	41	35	22	22	17
$\dot{V}_{O_2}$ (ml/min · kg)	3.66	4.04	3.59	43.0	36.1	30.7
RBF (ml/min)	1,248		764			
GFR	106		104			

*The marked initial increase in flow maintains normal $P\bar{v}_{O_2}$. Adaptation (in chronic anemia) consists of return of SVR to normal and redistribution of cardiac output from organs with relatively high flows to those with greater need. Note that the calculated SVR includes the effect of blood viscosity. Most of the increase in cardiac output in acute anemia is actually attributable to the change in viscosity, and the "return of vascular resistance to normal" actually reflects greater than normal arterial tone. The $P\bar{v}_{O_2}$ of 17 torr with exercise in chronic anemia presumably reflects a better control of oxygen transport in excess of local need (enhanced vasoregulation). (Modified from Woodson et al.,[27] by permission.)

lar to but slower than the response to a decrease in cardiac output. The influence of chronic anemia—to increase the level of 2,3-diphosphoglycerate (2,3-DPG) in the red blood cell, which improves release of oxygen from the hemoglobin, increasing the pressure gradient moving oxygen to the tissues—is also shown in Figure 1–2. Experimentally, the increase in cardiac output with moderate anemia depends more on decreased blood viscosity than on metabolic regulation. Regulation by metabolic factors is seen, however, with more severe anemia.[25] Anemia played a significant role in the following case history.

CASE 1–1.—An 84-year-old man with thrombocytosis (500,000–1,000,000 platelets/mm³) had undergone left hemicolectomy for bowel torsion and repair of dehiscence 11 and 7 days respectively before he became hypotensive, obtunded, tachypneic, and oliguric; progressively acidotic; and anemic (hematocrit dropped from 37% to 30%). While observed for several hours in his room, the patient passed small amounts of bloody stool. He was transferred to the ICU for invasive monitoring, but little benefit was expected except to confirm the clinical impression of septic shock related to bowel infarction. Initial data seemed to provide that confirmation (Table 1–3).

At the time of the first analysis (see Table 1–3), arterial pH was 7.25, although many ampules of bicarbonate had been administered, and hyperventilation had decreased Pa_{CO_2} to 27 torr. Analysis was based largely on the low vascular resistance, and the data were interpreted as "high output septic shock," with the decrease in hemoglobin believed due to hemodilution from fluid resuscitation and to bleeding from gastrointestinal ischemia. Reoperation was considered futile at this stage, and a sensitive discussion of the appropriateness of limiting "extraordinary measures" was undertaken with the family. In the meantime, dopamine was increased to 20 µg/kg/min. The drop in hemoglobin to 4.2 gm/dl was initially ignored, but a minority opinion that the patient's status could be due primarily to anemia was supported by his response to transfusion of 2 units of packed RBCs. To the surprise of most, the dopamine could be decreased to 8 µg/kg/min within the first hour, and the MAP was 80 torr 90 minutes after transfusion (2:45 in Table 1–3). No evidence of sepsis was subsequently seen.

TABLE 1–3.

Cardiopulmonary Profiles of a Patient Initially Thought to be in Septic Shock, but Having Only Severe Anemia Confirmed by Response to Transfusion*

		TIME		
VARIABLE	10:30 A.M.	2:45 P.M.	3:15 A.M.	NORMAL
MAP (torr)	62	80	92	70–90
HR (beats/min)	88	90	70	60–100
WP (torr)	22	12	18	5–12
PEEP (cm H_2O)	0	10	10	0
Hb (gm/dl)	4.2	7.8	9.8	13.5–15.5
$F_{I_{O_2}}$	.6	.9	.53	NA
pHa	7.25	7.35	7.38	7.36–7.45
Pa_{CO_2} (torr)	29	24	33	36–44
Pa_{O_2} (torr)	169	169	84	NA
Sa_{O_2}	.981	.974	.958	.95
$P\bar{v}_{O_2}$ (torr)	25	30	35	35–45
CI (L/min/m²)	2.93	2.96	3.34	2.5–4.0
SVRI (Wood units)	16.2	22.7	22.7	24–30
Ca_{O_2} (ml/dl)	6.08	10.8	13.0	20
$C\bar{v}_{O_2}$ (ml/dl)	1.88	6.18	8.36	15
$C(a-\bar{v})_{O_2}$ (ml/dl)	4.19	4.63	4.64	4–6
$\dot{D}_{O_2}$ (ml/min)	368.3	654.7	897.8	800–1,000
$\dot{V}_{O_2}$ (ml/min/m²)	123.3	136.1	155.6	110–150
P50	33.3	26.7	29.0	27
Dopamine (µg/kg/min)	6.6	8.3	2.3	0

*MAP, mean arterial pressure; WP, pressure in pulmonary artery distal to balloon obstruction; PEEP, positive end-expiratory pressure; CI, cardiac index; SVRI, systemic vascular resistence index. (From Snyder and Carroll.[21] Reproduced by permission.)

Discussion.—A hyperdynamic state (in this case, relatively high cardiac output and low vascular resistance and MAP, shown in the initial cardiopulmonary profile) is characteristic of the response to sepsis if intravascular volume is adequate. However, the same changes may characterize acute moderate isovolemic anemia or severe anemia of any duration[7, 25, 27] as well as sepsis. In both anemia and sepsis the increase in cardiac output is facilitated in proportion to the reduction in blood viscosity.

As shown by the $P\bar{v}_{O_2}$ of 25 torr, which increased with blood transfusions, the metabolic acidosis was probably due to inadequate oxygen transport from low hemoglobin content rather than maldistribution of flow or other phenomena of sepsis. Deficient oxygen delivery was the most straightforward interpretation of the data at this point. It remained possible that sepsis coexisted with the anemia, but oxygen transport was still the limiting factor, even in the presence of a low-normal cardiac output and $C(a-\bar{v})_{O_2}$.

Even though arterial blood was 98% saturated, this patient would have benefited from a further increase in fraction of inspired oxygen (FI_{O_2}) and Pa_{O_2}. The usually insignificant influence (0.3 ml/dl/100 torr increase in Pa_{O_2}) on Ca_{O_2} would have been an improvement of up to 20% in this patient. The effect of the reduction in hemoglobin on viscosity should have been more than suggested by the SVRI; it is likely that the lower initial SVRI actually represents an increase in vascular tone (see section on systemic vascular resistance, in chapter 15, "Technical Problems in Data Acquisition").

The lessons learned from this case reinforce the physiology described and, more important, represent the successful pursuit of a condition that seemed unlikely to be the major threat to life. Not only was the anemia of possible clinical significance, it was also much more reversible than the more common cause of similar findings in this setting: ischemic bowel with sepsis.

While the appropriateness of transfusion in severe anemia is unquestioned, transfusion is less clearly indicated when the hemoglobin value is 10 gm/dl or higher. The doubling of viscosity that occurs with increases in hematocrit from 20% to 40% at shear rates found in smaller vessels[13] suggests that increasing hemoglobin may not be beneficial in some circumstances. It is appealing to define an optimal hematocrit level at which oxygen transport will be highest and

complications fewest. Experimentally, this optimal hematocrit was found to be lower than the physiologic hematocrit level under resting conditions, leading to the therapeutic concept that hemodilution improves the nutritive supply to the tissues and enhances acceptance of lower than normal hemoglobin levels, even in patients with impaired oxygen transport.[9] However, the optimal hematocrit level is less well defined under conditions like physical exercise, when high oxygen transport is needed, or when the vasodilatory response may be impaired. For example, oxygen delivery to resting muscle is maximal at a hematocrit of 30%, but oxygen delivery to working muscle is maximal at 52%.[9] The difference is explained in part by the fact that vasodilation is an important component of the response to anemia. When exercise has stimulated nearly maximal vasodilation, vascular conductivity can no longer change to compensate for a hematocrit-dependent increase in viscosity. It is reasonable to generalize these findings to other vasodilated states, and to infer that oxygen transport in hypoxic tissues where vasodilation is not impaired will be improved if hematocrit is increased at least to normal levels. This may be true when a high flow is sustained, but it is not true when flow is depressed. For example, clinical outcome after acute cerebral infarction was improved by hemodilution using venesection and dextran infusion.[23] Even if we could safely conclude that higher hemoglobin allows maximal oxygen transport when flow is high, and that hemodilution is better for low-flow states, clinicians are concerned with areas of high and low flow in the same patient; defining the optimal hematocrit in such cases seems practically impossible. We are therefore inclined to try to safely improve low cardiac output first, then to increase hemoglobin to nearly normal levels if $P\bar{v}_{O_2}$ is still low and hypoxia is causing tissue dysfunction.

CASE 1–2.—A 71-year-old woman became oliguric 2 days after cholecystectomy and complained of angina. MAP was 65 torr, heart rate was 110 beats per minute, and respirations were 20/min. Inspiratory rales were heard over the lower half of the lung fields posteriorly and there was an S_3 gallop. She could breathe more comfortably sitting up. ECG showed ST-segment elevation and occasional premature ventricular contractions. Electrolyte levels were normal, and Hb was 10 gm/dl. Arterial blood gas analysis revealed a pHa of 7.38, Pa_{CO_2} of 35 torr, and Pa_{O_2} of 90 torr on 70% oxygen given by face mask. A pulmonary artery catheter was inserted: the wedge pressure (WP) was 18 torr, and $P\bar{v}_{O_2}$ was 27 torr.

Discussion.—This patient had severely compromised ventricular function and inadequate perfusion of both coronary (angina, ST-segment deviation) and systemic (oliguria, $P\bar{v}_{O_2}$ of 27 torr) vascular beds. Many groups of physicians reviewing this case have usually prompted the suggestions and discussion abbreviated in Table 1–4. (The reader can review it to define his or her own position on each therapeutic option before reading further.)

A trial of simultaneous titrated administration of inotropic and vasodilating agents is usually favored as a response to this case. This course is rational but has pitfalls, which are revealed by analysis of the individual components of oxygen transport and consumption. The complete cardiopulmonary profile from case 1–2 is given in Table 1–5. Arterial oxygen content is 13 ml/dl instead of the normal 20. The compromise is due principally to a lower than normal hemoglobin value. Oxygen content (and transport) could be increased a few percentage points just by increasing $F_{I_{O_2}}$. It is surprising that the cardiac index was not clearly below normal. In fact, the systemic physiologic compromise in this patient

was *not* primarily from inadequate cardiac output, but rather indicated inability to compensate for low hemoglobin. The subtlety is that perfusion to the systemic circulation can usually be increased sufficiently to compensate for anemia, but increased myocardial work is required, and the compromised coronary vessels in this patient could not sustain the increased myocardial demand required by that compensation. The problem was compounded by a higher than normal systemic oxygen consumption from stress and increased work of breathing. Systemic oxygenation was not yet so compromised that metabolic (lactic) acidemia was present, but the $P\bar{v}_{O_2}$ of 27 torr indicates no remaining reserve in systemic oxygen transport, and coronary oxygen transport clearly was deficient.

Rarely is a simple increase in hemoglobin concentration as seriously considered by physicians as the options listed in Table 1–4. Increasing the hemoglobin concentration from 10 to 12 gm/dl might increase oxygen transport by almost 20% with a minimal increase in myocardial work. Administration of a diuretic might be required to prevent volume overload, that is, to "make room" for the RBCs. The effect of the increase in hemoglobin on flow in the compromised coronary circulation is less clear, as will be discussed in a following section. The value of

TABLE 1–4.

Arguments Relating to Therapeutic Options in Case 1–2*

OPTION	PRO	CON
Diuretic therapy	Decrease preload, decrease pulmonary edema, increase urine	Decrease in preload could decrease CO and MAP; increase in urine output is only of value if it reflects increase in perfusion
Ventilatory support	Decrease WP, decrease pulmonary edema, decrease work of breathing	May increase dysrhythmias; does nothing for basic problems
Inotropic support	Decrease WP, decrease pulmonary edema, increase renal (systemic) perfusion	Heart is irritable and ischemic already and would get worse
Nitroprusside infusion	Decrease afterload, decrease myocardial work, increase systemic perfusion	Assumes that decrease in afterload will influence the left ventricular pressure-volume relationship such that CO will increase enough to maintain arterial pressure and coronary perfusion—a risky assumption
None of the above, but tell family prognosis is very poor	No therapeutic risks taken	Nothing gained

*From Snyder and Carroll.[21] Reproduced by permission.

TABLE 1–5.

Cardiopulmonary Profile*

VARIABLE	PATIENT VALUE	NORMAL VALUES (UNITS)
Ht.	65	NA (in.)
Wt.	62	NA (kg)
BSA	1.68	NA (m^2)
Temp.	37.5	37 (°C)
F$_{IO_2}$	.7	NA
PEEP	0	0 (cm H$_2$O)
HR	110	60–100 (beats/min)
MAP	65	70–90 (torr)
WP	18	5–12 (torr)
CVP	12	0–4 (torr)
Cardiac output	3.9	NA
Pa$_{CO_2}$	38	35–45 (torr)
Pa$_{O_2}$	70	NA
Sa$_{O_2}$	.95	0.95
P$\bar{v}_{O_2}$	27	35–45 (torr)
S$\bar{v}_{O_2}$	.5	.68–.76
Hb	10	13.5–15.5 gm/dl
pHa	7.37	7.36–7.45
CI	2.31	2.5–4.5 (L/m^2)
Stroke index	21.0	35–40 (ml/m^2)
RVSWI	4.01	6–9 (gm/min/m^2)
LVSWI	13.5	35–47 (gm/min/m^2)
SVRI	22.8	24–30 (Wood units)
PVRI	3.5	2.0–3.5 (Wood units)
Art. O$_2$ content	13.1	20 (ml/dl)
Ven. O$_2$ content	6.9	15 (ml/dl)
C(a−$\bar{v}$)$_{O_2}$	6.2	3.5–5 (ml/dl)
O$_2$ transport	512	1,000 (ml/min)
O$_2$ consump./m^2	145	110–150 (ml/min/m^2)
O$_2$ extraction	.47	.22–.30
P50	27	27 (torr)
Venous admixture	.21	0.06

*The data relate to case 1–2. See discussion in text. Variables are further defined in chapter 17, "The Craft of Cardiopulmonary Profile Analysis." (From Snyder and Carroll.[21] Reproduced by permission.)

placing a pulmonary arterial catheter in this patient was to confirm and more precisely define the condition suggested clinically.

An increase in abnormal hemoglobin denotes more severe compromise than the apparent reduction in functional hemoglobin suggests, because there is no accompanying reduction in viscosity. Although high concentrations of abnormal hemoglobin are not common, like any compromise in oxygen supply/demand they may be of consequence in critically ill patients.[30] Carboxyhemoglobin (COHb) levels of 2%–5% are not uncommon in patients who smoke or have been exposed to internal combustion engines. COHb causes the obvious reduction in functional hemoglobin and in addition increases the binding between oxygen and normal hemoglobin. Nitroglycerin and nitroprusside administration may cause methemoglobinemia.[1, 32] Failure to modify the usual shunt equation when the hemoglobin concentration is abnormal results in overestimation of lung dysfunction, as detailed in chapter 17, "The Craft of Cardiopulmonary Profile Analysis."

Arterial Saturation. The contribution of arterial oxygen saturation of hemoglobin (Sa$_{O_2}$) to oxygen transport is linear. Oxygenation is usually thought to be adequate if Pa$_{O_2}$ is 60 torr, because the dissociation curve is relatively horizontal above that point. However, a Pa$_{O_2}$ of 60 torr means that arterial saturation is still about 7% less than complete if oxyhemoglobin dissociation is normal, and it represents even more desaturation if the curve is shifted to the right, for example in acidemia. Therapy to increase a usually "acceptable" Pa$_{O_2}$ might therefore be warranted when oxygen transport is borderline.

Dissolved Oxygen. Dissolved oxygen can be ignored in most circumstances, but a few exceptions merit brief description. The amount of dissolved oxygen is less than 2% of the normal arterial oxygen content, and increasing the Pa$_{O_2}$ from 100 to 500 torr increases dissolved oxygen by 400 × .003, or only 1.2 ml/dl. However, dissolved oxygen becomes increasingly important in severe anemia. For example, when hemoglobin is 3 gm/dl, bound oxygen amounts to only 3 × 1.36, or slightly more than 4 ml/dl. Increasing oxygen content by 1.2 ml/dl can be very valuable while RBCs are being secured and administered. Maintaining a high Pa$_{O_2}$ is also important after exposure to carbon monoxide, both to increase Ca$_{O_2}$ and to dislodge carbon monoxide from hemoglobin. A very high Pa$_{O_2}$ might also be of some value in shock, even if the Ca$_{O_2}$ is increased by only 5%, but this theoretical gain must be weighed against the documented toxicity of high F$_{IO_2}$ to the lung when exposure lasts more than 12 hours.

Shifts in the Oxyhemoglobin Dissociation Curve

Some familiarity with the oxyhemoglobin dissociation curve is necessary to understand both oxygen transport physiology and the influence of shifts in the curve on the adequacy of cellular oxygenation. Figure 1–2 shows a normal dissociation curve, characterized by a saturation of 50% at a P_{O_2} of about 27 torr. Note that when the hemoglobin value is known, a second vertical axis can be constructed to show oxygen *content* for any P_{O_2}.

A rightward shift—caused by hypercarbia, for example—usually results in a minimal decrease in arterial oxygen content at the same Pa_{O_2}, and if oxygen consumption is unchanged, the arterial-venous oxygen content difference will be the same: mixed-venous oxygen content will decrease exactly as much as arterial oxygen (Fig 1–4). However, because oxygen is less tightly bound to hemoglobin, the release of oxygen in systemic capillaries will occur at a higher P_{O_2}, and therefore $P\bar{v}_{O_2}$ will be higher. This seems to be a system teleologically developed to improve tissue oxygenation during cardiopulmonary embarrassment. With a rightward shift in the curve there is actually a slight *decrease* in Ca_{O_2}, owing to decreased Sa_{O_2} at the same Pa_{O_2}, but the easier release of chemically bound oxygen establishes a higher driving pressure for oxygen. It is the pressure gradient for oxygen that determines its rate of diffusion. Although it is the volume flow of oxygen in arterial blood per unit time that is responsible for maintaining the partial pressure of oxygen in capillary blood, it is the partial pressure of oxygen in capillaries that is responsible for maintaining tissue oxygenation.

Shifts of the curve to the left, such as caused by alkalosis, will increase arterial and venous oxygen contents slightly at constant partial pressures, but can cause large decreases in $P\bar{v}_{O_2}$ when $C(a-\bar{v})_{O_2}$ is constant (see Fig 1–4). The dependence of tissue oxygenation on sustaining capillary P_{O_2} above some minimum indicates that leftward shifts, causing decreases in $P\bar{v}_{O_2}$, have the potential to cause tissue dysfunction.

The relation of tissue survival to shifts in the dissociation curve has been difficult to document because many compensatory mechanisms are built into the oxygen transport system. Simply inducing a leftward shift in the curve usually will not cause tissue hypoxia, but just as for anemia, concluding that changes in the curve are not important determinants of tissue oxygenation is premature. The importance of shift in the dissociation curve can be shown by establishing some baseline compromise of oxygen transport, then increasing the affinity of hemoglobin for oxygen (decreased P50, or leftward shift in the curve). Arterial oxygen content may actually increase slightly in these experiments (if saturation is incomplete before the shift is induced), and venous content may increase also, but the $P\bar{v}_{O_2}$ decreases. For example, note the change in $P\bar{v}_{O_2}$ (to about 32 torr) when pH is increased to 7.6 and $C(a-\bar{v})_{O_2}$ is kept constant, as shown in Figure 1–4. The leftward shift ordinarily is well tolerated because the drop in $P\bar{v}_{O_2}$ usually is limited

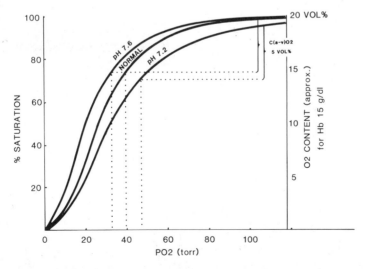

FIG 1–4.
Shifts in the oxyhemoglobin dissociation curve. When Hb is normal, Pa_{O_2} is 100 torr, and other factors are constant, $C\bar{v}_{O_2}$ remains 5 ml/dl less than Ca_{O_2}, and $P\bar{v}_{O_2}$ is about 32, 40, and 48 torr when the oxyhemoglobin dissociation curve is in the positions illustrated.

by compensatory increases in blood flow. It is likely to be consequential only in the patient or experimental subject with severely compromised oxygen supply/demand.

When the curve is shifted to the left, limited tissue oxygenation may be shown by compensatory changes in other components of the oxygen transport system (for example, an increase in regional blood flow to threatened organs) or, when compensation is inadequate, by organ dysfunction. These changes vary from organ to organ because blood flow and oxygen needs vary in different tissues. For example, a leftward shift of the curve can double blood flow to the heart and brain without changing total cardiac output.[30] The homeostatic response to the leftward shift, in this example, is dilation of the vascular beds where oxygen extraction is already high. The changes in coronary and cerebral blood flow were similar to those seen in anemia (hematocrit = 22%). In each case the change in flow appears to respond to decreased oxygen pressure in tissue.[30] As another example, hepatic dysfunction has been induced by increasing oxyhemoglobin affinity during mild hepatic ischemia.[28] Also, the mortality in a hemorrhagic shock model was increased by a leftward shift in the curve, and cerebral dysfunction and metabolic depression have resulted from the same change.[31]

As Woodson reported, comparable experiments have shown a rightward shift in the dissociation curve to improve oxygen supply when ischemia resulted in deficient oxygen delivery.[29] Inducing a rightward shift in the curve also reduced myocardial necrosis after coronary ligation in areas with reduced but still modest blood flow. As we would expect, myocardium was not preserved in areas with no or very low flow. Also, the oxygen consumption increased in hypothermic fibrillating dog hearts when they were perfused with blood 4 torr higher in P50, a result of much higher 2,3-DPG content.[29]

Watkins et al. have calculated that a shift of 2 torr in the dissociation curve position or a change of 2 torr in $P\bar{v}_{O_2}$ from the normal value is equivalent to 1.12 L of cardiac output change.[26] Their observations in critically ill patients support the importance and variability of oxyhemoglobin dissociation: they stress avoiding hypophosphatemia, prolonged acidosis, and transfusion of acid-citrate-dextrose (ACD)-preserved blood stored longer than a week, all of which diminish DPG and cause a leftward shift in the curve. In patients whose oxyhemoglobin affinity is increased from multiple transfusions of ACD-preserved blood, the curve returns toward normal more rapidly after administration of methylprednisolone sodium succinate, 30 mg/kg.[5] (Other interesting effects of high-dose methylprednisolone on oxygen transport and metabolism have been reported: cardiac output increased and SVR decreased, but also blood lactate levels significantly increased in patients with chronic obstructive pulmonary disease[6] and in patients with acute myocardial infarction.[13] The optimal appropriate use of high-dose steroids in most critically ill patients is still uncertain.[2, 20]) Alkalosis, especially respiratory, also can severely depress the P50 and thereby acutely depress tissue oxygenation. The curve shift eventually returns toward normal as alkalosis stimulates DPG production. Similarly, oxygen release to the tissues is acutely improved by increasing P_{CO_2}, until DPG production becomes depressed.[7]

It is important to recognize shift in the dissociation curve as a significant determinant of cell oxygenation in critically ill patients, in whom systemic capillary P_{O_2} may already be pathologically reduced. The easiest therapeutic method to manipulate acutely according to this thinking is mechanical ventilation. For example, we can often allow Pa_{CO_2} to rise in mechanically ventilated patients with impending or current tissue hypoxia. An increased volume of oxygen is then released at the same capillary (and mixed-venous) P_{O_2}, and all the data cited earlier suggest that borderline tissue oxygenation should be improved. Increasing Pa_{CO_2} also may increase cardiac output, via both inotropic and vasodilating effects,[4] and may decrease $\dot{V}_{O_2}$[22] by changing intracellular pH.

Studies of hypoxemia have shown that a *leftward* shift in the curve improves tissue oxygenation when Pa_{O_2} is less than 30–35 torr.[28] However, these are not good models of the hypoxemia from venous admixture that is seen in most critically ill patients. *In most patients a rightward shift is advantageous even in severe hypoxemia*, since increasing hemoglobin affinity for oxygen will not increase the oxygen content of shunted blood.[17] Apparent examples to the contrary[14] probably have other explanations.

Microcirculatory Resistance to Flow

Vascular resistance is usually expressed as the mean pressure gradient to mean flow in the vascular circuit considered: it is analogous to its electrical counterpart in Ohm's law, which relates current to potential decrease in an electrical circuit. The relation between laminar flow and pressure gradient in cylindrical tubes is well known as the Hagen-Poiseuille equation:

$$Q = \Delta P \mu r^4 / 8L \qquad \text{(Eq. 1–3)}$$

where Q is the flow, ΔP is the difference in hydrostatic pressure between two points separated by a distance L, r is the internal radius, and μ is the coefficient of viscosity. Unfortunately, blood has non-Newtonian, viscous properties, and errors in estimates of flow can be as high as 50%. When the marginal cell-free zone is taken into account, the relation between flow and pressure gradient becomes even more complex. In addition, much of what is known about the microvascular hemodynamics is based on relatively few studies in "two-dimensional" tissues such as the mesentery. Both the problems with and the need for our current simplistic conclusions have been summarized by Gow,[11] to whom credit for much of this section is due:

> [. . .] the concept of all blood vessels responding in a quantitatively similar fashion is untenable, as is the notion of any kind of 'average behavior' of a vessel in the microcirculation. Also, because blood viscosity is a function of flow rate, vessel caliber, and hematocrit, it is difficult to define the equivalent viscosity in the entire bed. On the other hand, it is often necessary, though perhaps imprecise, to make extrapolations from a few observations in single vessels to seek an average behavior so as to appreciate the manner in which changes in a vascular bed affect the circulation of the entire animal, and vice versa. It should be with these limitations in mind that changes in vascular resistance are considered.

Even in a vascular bed that has neither myogenic nor metabolic regulation of caliber, flow is not related to r^4 or to pressure gradient.[10] Factors introduced to explain this include (1) the variation in physical properties of different parts of a vascular bed, (2) the presence of collaterals that may be open or closed, (3) the rheologic behavior of blood that has a variety of properties, including pseudoplasticity, anomalous viscosity, the sigma effect, and the Fahraeus-Lindqvist effect, and (4) elastic expansion of the vessels with increasing pressure.[10]

Without pursuing these details, it is apparent that vascular beds maintain blood flow despite changes in pressure gradient, normally by varying the caliber of the arterioles in response either to change in stretch from change in arterial pressure or to metabolic factors, or both. According to Gow,[12]

> Although it is well documented . . . that reduction in shear rate leads to higher values of apparent blood viscosity in vitro . . . hypoperfusion in vivo, which reduces shear rate, does not necessarily lead to elevated blood viscosity, because normally hypoperfusion invokes autoregulatory mechanisms. There is thus an interplay of these negative feedback mechanisms with rising viscosity, which is a positive feedback effect. Under normal circumstances the gain of the negative feedback systems are high and they dominate. Any reduction of flow increases the local concentration of metabolites and leads to vasodilation, which not only restores but increases the fluidity of the blood. In abnormal situations such as regional vasoconstriction accompanying severe hemorrhage or left ventricular failure, the prolonged hypoperfusion leads to a buildup of metabolites, ultimately paralyzing the vascular muscle.

As summarized by Schmid-Schonbein, when there is a generalized or localized reduction in driving force, elastic cell-cell and cell-wall interactions interfere with the high fluidity, producing a reticulated suspension of the elastic particles with very low fluidity. The ability of RBCs to deform is reduced in patients with peripheral vascular disease compared with controls, and is less in patients with rest pain or gangrene than in those who have only intermittent claudication.[16] In the absence of adequate flow forces, the cells are not only deformed, they aggregate into typical rouleaux and networks of rouleaux.[19]

Because of the formation of elastic aggregates, blood in the microvessels has strong viscoelastic properties and hence behaves as a solid below its yield point. Thus, the blood flow in vessels parallel to main arteriovenous pathways can come to a complete stop despite a finite arteriovenous pressure gradient; that is, it behaves as a solid by "collateral blood viscidation" before clotting.[19]

Also, under conditions of local endothelial damage and thus increased microvascular wall permeability, water and some protein is lost into the interstitium. Local hemoconcentration can then occur, along with a preferential increase in high molecular weight plasma protein, leading to higher plasma viscosity and to RBC aggregation.[19] Disseminated stagnation of blood is not necessarily manifested as an increased resistance of the vascular bed, however, because shunting often occurs via collateral channels.[10] The occurrence of microvascular stagnation with no increase in resistance because of shunting collateral channels could provide the basis for explaining many of the hemodynamic patterns seen in septic shock, including the dependence of oxygen consumption on high levels of oxygen delivery (see discussion of sepsis in chapter 5, "Patterns of Hemodynamic Response").

Oxygen Consumption and Cardiac Output With Intact Vasoregulation

Oxygen consumption is relatively stable in subjects at rest, but it may vary markedly with such common ICU phenomena as respiratory distress, temperature changes, shivering, and the catabolic, anabolic, and psychic stresses of various disease processes. Oxygen consumption may therefore vary widely but still reflect only the current needs of perfused tissues. Specific causes of change in oxygen consumption are expounded further in chapter 2, "Oxygen Consumption," and chapter 11, "Cellular Oxygen Utilization."

Change in cardiac output has a linear effect on oxygen delivery, but normal vasoregulatory responses may allow reduction of oxygen delivery by 25%, the amount that is normally in excess of need, before there are signs of tissue hypoxia. However, tolerance of such a reduction in cardiac output is dependent not only on normal oxygen content and adequate release of oxygen, but also on intact vasoregulation and absence of edema. Flow to tissues normally overperfused relative to oxygen needs, such as the kidney, must be tempered, and the vessels to tissues with high baseline oxygen extraction, such as the heart and brain, must be capable of maximal dilation and not be compromised by plaque or spasm. Edema increases the distance oxygen must diffuse through the cell and, therefore, the driving pressure required (see chapter 10, "Oxygen Transport From Capillary to Cell"). Conservation of flow to vital tissues may also be in conflict with other demands, such as the need for increased oxygen by muscles of respiration, or neurohumoral dictates from the hypothalamus to dilate cutaneous vessels to lower core temperature.

Important other physiologic and pathologic variables must be considered in critically ill patients. In the classic stress response, oxygen delivery is further increased above current needs, by neural and humoral mechanisms. Because oxygen delivery is increased more than oxygen consumption, $P\bar{v}_{O_2}$ is increased. Local regulation of flow is retained, and flow remains adequate to lo-cal need, but cardiac output is proportionately redistributed in preparation for fight or flight. Thus, vasoregulation is intact, although altered in its direction and priorities. Various pathologic elements also may disturb these relations.

Distribution of Perfusion

Clinicians in intensive care are so used to manipulating cardiac output that the fundamental control of cardiac output by the tissues is often overlooked. Vessels normally dilate sufficiently to maintain flow adequate to local needs, and it is not clear that they can be dilated pharmacologically more than occurs in hypoxia. Vessels normally will also restrict flow from greatly exceeding local needs. A broad definition of normal vasoregulation allows responses by the subject to change distribution to vital systems in times of compromise. Normal vasoregulation therefore includes a wide variety of responses, from high flow, high oxygen extraction states with exercise (skeletal muscle and heart) to widely variable blood flows and oxygen extraction in stressed states, and neurohumoral control of skin and renal blood flow.[18] These, and loss of vasoregulation, are discussed further in chapter 4, "Control of Cardiac Output by the Circuit," chapter 5, "Patterns of Hemodynamic Response," and chapter 6, "Neurohumoral Regulation of Cardiovascular Function."

REFERENCES

1. Benjamin E, Iberti TJ: Methemoglobinemia and respiratory failure (letter). *Anesthesiology* 1985; 62:542–3.
2. Blaisdell FW: Controversy in shock research: Con—The role of steroids in septic shock. *Circ Shock* 1981; 8:673.
3. Brannon ES, Merrill AJ, Warren JV, et al: The cardiac output in patients with chronic anemia as measured by the technique of right atrial catheterization. *J Clin Invest* 1945; 24:332.
4. Breivik H, Grenvik A, Millen E, et al: Normalization of low arterial CO_2 tension during mechanical ventilation. *Chest* 1973; 63:525.
5. Bryan-Brown CW, Baek SM, Makabali G, et al: Consumable oxygen: Availability of oxygen in relation to oxyhemoglobin dissociation. *Crit Care Med* 1973; 1:17.
6. Farber MO, Daly RS, Strawbridge RA, et al: Steroids, hypoxemia, and oxygen transport. *Chest* 1979; 75:451.

7. Finch CA, Lenfant C: Oxygen transport in man. *N Engl J Med* 1972; 286:407.

8. Florenzano F, Diaz G, Regonesi C, et al: Left ventricular function in chronic anemia: Evidence of noncatecholamine positive inotropic factor in the serum. *Am J Cardiol* 1984; 54:638.

9. Gaehtgens P, Kreutz F: Skeletal muscle perfusion, exercise capacity, and the optimal hematocrit, in Brendel W, Zink RA (eds): *High Altitude Physiology and Medicine*. New York, Springer-Verlag, 1982, pp 123–128.

10. Gow BS: Circulatory correlates: Vascular impedance, resistance, and capacity, in Bohr DF, Somlyo AP, Sparks HV (eds): *Handbook of Physiology*. Vol 2: *The Cardiovascular System*. Bethesda, American Physiological Society, 1980, pp 353–409.

11. Gow BS: Circulatory correlates: Vascular impedance, resistance, and capacity, in Bohr DF, Somlyo AP, Sparks HV (eds): *Handbook of Physiology*. Vol 2: *The Cardiovascular System*. Bethesda, American Physiological Society, 1980, p 375.

12. Gow BS: Circulatory correlates: Vascular impedance, resistance, and capacity, in Bohr DF, Somlyo AP, Sparks HV (eds): *Handbook of Physiology*. Vol 2: *The Cardiovascular System*. Bethesda, American Physiological Society, 1980, p 377.

13. Henning RJ, Becker H, Vincent JL, et al: Use of methylprednisolone in patients following acute myocardial infarction. *Chest* 1981; 79:186.

14. Lund T, Koller M, Kofstad J: Severe hypoxemia without evidence of tissue hypoxia in adult respiratory distress syndrome. *Crit Care Med* 1984; 12:75–76.

15. Rand PW, Lacombe E, Hunt HE, et al: Viscosity of normal human blood under normothermic and hypothermic conditions. *J Appl Physiol* 1964; 19:117.

16. Reid HL, Dormandy JA, Barnes AJ, et al: Impaired red cell deformability in peripheral vascular disease. *Lancet* 1976; 1:666–669.

17. Rossoff L, Zeldin R, Hew E, et al: Changes in blood P50: Effects on oxygen delivery when arterial hypoxemia is due to shunting. *Chest* 1980; 77:142.

18. Rowell LB: Human cardiovascular adjustments to exercise and thermal stress. *Physiol Rev* 1974; 54:75.

19. Schmid-Schonbein H: Blood rheology in hemoconcentration, in Brendel W, Zink RA (eds): *High Altitude Physiology and Medicine*. New York, Springer-Verlag, 1982, pp 109–116.

20. Schumer W: Controversy in shock research: Pro—The role of steroids in septic shock. *Circ Shock* 1981; 8:667.

21. Snyder JV, Carroll GC: Tissue oxygenation: A physiologic approach to a clinical problem. *Curr Probl Surg* 1982; 19(11):650–719.

22. Springer RR, Clark DK, Lea AS, et al: Effects of changes in arterial carbon dioxide tension on oxygen consumption during cardiopulmonary bypass. *Chest* 1979; 75:549.

23. Strand T, Asplund K, Eriksson S, et al: A randomized controlled trial of hemodilution therapy in acute ischemic stroke. *Stroke* 1984; 15:980–989.

24. Torrance J, Jacobs P, Restrepo A, et al: Intraerythrocytic adaptation to anemia. *N Engl J Med* 1970; 283:165.

25. Varat MA, Adolph RJ, Fowler NO: Fundamentals of clinical cardiology. *Am Heart J* 1972; 83:415.

26. Watkins GM, Rabelo A, Plzak LF, et al: The left shifted oxyhemoglobin curve in sepsis: A preventable defect. *Ann Surg* 1974; 180:213.

27. Woodson RD, Wills RE, Lenfant C: Effect of acute and established anemia on oxygen transport at rest, submaximal and maximal work. *J Appl Physiol* 1978; 44:36.

28. Woodson RD: Physiological significance of oxygen dissociation curve shifts. *Crit Care Med* 1979; 7:368.

29. Woodson RD: Importance of 2,3-DPG in banked blood: New data in animal models, in Collins JA, Murawski K, Shafer AW (eds): *Massive Transfusion in Surgery and Trauma*. New York, Alan R Liss, Inc, 1982, pp 69–78.

30. Woodson RD, Auerbach S: Effect of increased oxygen affinity and anemia on cardiac output and its distribution. *J Appl Physiol* 1982; 53:1299.

31. Woodson RD, Fitzpatrick JH, Costello DJ, et al: Increased blood oxygen affinity decreases canine brain oxygen consumption. *J Lab Clin Med* 1982; 100:411.

32. Zurick AM, Wagner RH, Starr NJ, et al: Intravenous nitroglycerin, methemoglobinemia, and respiratory distress in a postoperative cardiac surgical patient. *Anesthesiology* 1984; 61:464.

2

Oxygen Consumption

Michael J. Buran, M.D.

The adequacy of oxygen transport must be assessed in relation to the oxygen needs of the total organism and its component organ systems: it is determined by the balance between oxygen supply and tissue oxygen demands. When the supply is adequate, oxygen consumption is usually a function of metabolic rate. When the supply is deficient, oxygen consumption is limited by the decreased availability of oxygen. Continued metabolism becomes anaerobic, and lactic acid is produced. A similar situation may result when tissue metabolic demands exceed the maximal reserves of oxygen transport. This may occur with shivering, seizure activity, or strenuous exercise. Anaerobic metabolism with decreased oxygen consumption may occur when transport is adequate if cellular metabolism is blocked. This can result from uncoupling of oxidative phosphorylation, as seen in cyanide poisoning. Anaerobic metabolism may also occur when total oxygen delivery is adequate but fails to reach local vascular beds. An example of this is the loss of autoregulation of blood flow postulated in sepsis. Thus, although oxygen transport is the most easily manipulated factor affecting oxygen consumption, it is certainly not its sole determinant.

ASSESSMENT OF OXYGEN CONSUMPTION

General Considerations

Early determinations of metabolic rate in humans were made using direct calorimetry, and such measurements were called basal metabolic rates or resting energy expenditures.[35] These are not measurements of oxygen consumption as such, although the values are directly related. Now it is much more common to measure oxygen consumption directly and convert that value into metabolic terms, such as caloric expenditures. Oxygen consumption can be measured directly or calculated using the cardiac output and the oxygen content of arterial and mixed venous blood.

Direct Measurements of Oxygen Consumption

Oxygen consumption is directly measured by analyzing the volume and composition of inspired and expired gases over a known period of time. This information is used in the following standard equation:

$$\dot{V}_{O_2} = \frac{(V_{insp} \times F_{I_{O_2}}) - (V_{exp} \times F_{E_{O_2}})}{t}$$

where $\dot{V}_{O_2}$ is the oxygen consumption, V_{insp} is the inspired volume, V_{exp} is the expired volume, $F_{I_{O_2}}$ and $F_{E_{O_2}}$ represent the fraction of inspired and expired oxygen, and t represents time.

All volumes are converted to standard temperature and pressure (V_{stpd}) by the following formula:

$$V_{stpd} = V[273/(T + 273)][(BP - P_{H_2O})/760]$$

where V is the volume, T is the temperature in degrees C, BP is the barometric pressure, and P_{H_2O} is the partial pressure of water.

V_{exp}, $F_{I_{O_2}}$, and $F_{E_{O_2}}$ are measured directly. V_{insp} can be measured directly or estimated using the Haldane transformation:

$$V_{insp} = \frac{V_{exp} \times F_{E_{N_2}}}{F_{I_{N_2}}}$$

where $F_{I_{N_2}} = 1 - F_{I_{O_2}}$ and $F_{E_{N_2}} = 1 - F_{E_{O_2}} - F_{E_{CO_2}}$. $F_{I_{N_2}}$ and $F_{E_{N_2}}$ are the fractions of nitrogen in inspired and expired gases after dehydration. Obviously, this method of measuring oxygen consumption (from this point represented by $\dot{V}_{O_2}$) depends on accurate determination of gas composition (both inspired and expired) and volume. Small errors in gas content analysis can be magnified. For example, a 1% error in F_{IO_2} determination at .21 can result in a 5% error in $\dot{V}_{O_2}$. This error is greater when F_{IO_2} is higher, as is usually the case with critically ill patients. Patients on ventilators represent a special problem, since with most standard ventilators F_{IO_2} can vary throughout the ventilatory cycle.[7] Gas volumes in the intensive care unit are usually measured with a turbine spirometer, which can be inaccurate at extremes of flow rate. Pneumotachographs are more accurate at the extremes of gas flow, but can be obstructed by secretions. Although cumbersome, the water seal spirometer is probably the most reliable device for measuring gas volumes. Finally, the modified Haldane transformation assumes the absence of gases other than O_2, CO_2, and N_2, an assumption that might not be accurate in the presence of anesthetic gases (especially nitrous oxide, which is used in high concentrations), acetone, alcohol, or ammonia. Thus, the many sources of error are potentially magnified in the critically ill patient who requires supplemental oxygen and mechanical ventilation and who may be recovering from anesthesia or suffering from ketoacidosis, alcohol intoxication, or liver failure. There are commercially available systems for performing these measurements, of which published evaluations are favorable, but the sources of error described remain potential problems.[6, 19, 33]

A second method of directly measuring $\dot{V}_{O_2}$ involves continuous breathing of a gas of known F_{IO_2} and 100% humidity in a closed system containing a CO_2 absorber. When such a system contains an accurately calibrated water seal manometer, $\dot{V}_{O_2}$ can be determined by measuring the loss of volume in the system using the following equation:

$$\dot{V}_{O_2} = \frac{\Delta V}{t \times F_{IO_2}} \text{ at STPD}$$

where ΔV is the change in volume. Unfortunately, this system still requires accurate measurement of F_{IO_2}, and attempts to use it with available mechanical ventilators have met some difficulty. Some success has been reported,[3] and a commercial version of that system is available for use in the critically ill patient (metabolic analyzer MRM 6000, Waters Instruments, Inc.,

Rochester, Minn.). One of the continuing problems is that changes in the functional residual capacity during the determination may be recorded as changes in the measured volume of the system and therefore in $\dot{V}_{O_2}$. This is a particular source of error in patients with abnormal airways and decreased lung compliance.

A third technique has recently been devised for the direct measurement of oxygen consumption in ventilated patients. A servoapparatus bleeds 100% oxygen into a mixing chamber for expired gases, under the control of an oxygen-measuring device. The same device measures F_{IO_2} and F_{EO_2} and controls the flow of oxygen into the mixing chamber to allow equalization of oxygen concentration. The volume of oxygen required to do this is directly related to the $\dot{V}_{O_2}$. This technique shows promise and has been utilized in the critical care unit.[18]

Indirect Methods

The difficulty of directly measuring oxygen consumption in the critically ill patient has resulted in the widespread use of hemodynamic and blood gas measurements to calculate $\dot{V}_{O_2}$ by the following equation:

$$\dot{V}_{O_2} = CO\ (Ca_{O_2} - C\bar{v}_{O_2})$$

where CO is the cardiac output, Ca_{O_2} is the arterial oxygen content, and $C\bar{v}_{O_2}$ is the mixed venous oxygen content.

The oxygen content of a blood specimen is calculated in the following manner:

$$Ca_{O_2} \text{ or } C\bar{v}_{O_2} = sat \times Hb \times 1.36 + P_{O_2} \times .003$$

where sat represents oxyhemoglobin saturation and Hb represents hemoglobin concentration.

As with all indirect methods, the accuracy of the measured values determines the accuracy of the final result. Difficulties with these measurements are discussed in chapter 15, "Technical Problems in Data Acquisition." Note, however, that the oxyhemoglobin saturation must be measured directly in the critically ill patient, because the calculated relation between P_{O_2} and oxyhemoglobin saturation may be altered by phosphate depletion, recent massive blood transfusion, or qualitatively abnormal hemoglobin, all of which are common in critically ill patients.

REGIONAL OXYGEN CONSUMPTION

$\dot{V}O_2$ for the intact organism may be indexed to body weight or, more commonly, to body surface area (BSA). BSA is thought by many to be the more appropriate index, since heat loss is one of the major contributors to resting energy expenditure and is proportional to BSA. Normal $\dot{V}O_2$ is within the range of 110–150 ml/min/m^2.

While systemic oxygen consumption reflects the condition of the entire organism, it conveys little information about the status of specific organ systems. Table 2–1 is a summation of data from studies[8, 17, 36] evaluating the contribution of various organ systems to basal metabolic rates, along with their relative proportions of resting blood flow.

Muscle constitutes 40% of body weight but accounts for only 16%–30% of $\dot{V}O_2$ at rest. The other organ systems listed make up less than 10% of body weight but account for 60% of resting energy utilization. Nor does resting blood flow always parallel the relationship between an organ's mass and its contribution to total $\dot{V}O_2$. For example, in resting conditions the kidneys receive roughly five times the blood flow of the coronary circulation, yet their fraction of $\dot{V}O_2$ is significantly lower.[22]

The arterial-venous oxygen content difference for the coronary circulation is 12 vol% in the resting human adult.[23] This is far greater than the normal systemic value of 3–5 vol% and implies a nearly maximal myocardial oxygen extraction at basal conditions. Because of this, the only mechanism available to accommodate acute increases in myocardial oxygen consumption is increasing coronary blood flow by coronary dila-

tion. Excessive myocardial work (i.e., increased oxygen consumption) from increased pulse rate or afterload may result in ventricular failure when coronary perfusion reserves are inadequate. This can occur when reserves are compromised by local disease (coronary atherosclerosis) or by systemic disorders, such as diastolic hypotension, anemia, or arterial hypoxemia. These conditions are all commonly encountered in the critically ill.

Intact cardiac function is required to meet any increased demands for oxygen consumption by other organ systems. For example, ventilatory muscles frequently must perform increased work in the critically ill patient. Spontaneous ventilation of normal lungs at rest accounts for 1%–3% of resting oxygen consumption. The critically ill patient with decreased pulmonary compliance or increased airway resistance may use more than 25% of his consumed oxygen to maintain spontaneous ventilation.[30] In the face of compromised oxygen delivery this can have significant consequences, as evidenced by a recent study of tamponade-induced cardiogenic shock in dogs. All of the animals died of primary respiratory arrest.[2]

The critically ill patient can thus easily enter a spiral of deteriorating cardiovascular function.[15] The patient with pulmonary edema and shock from a myocardial infarction has increased work of breathing as well as arterial hypoxemia and decreased cardiac output. The oxygen delivery demands of the straining respiratory muscles increase myocardial oxygen consumption, which cannot be supported by inadequate coronary perfusion with poorly oxygenated blood. Without supportive intervention (usually including mechanical ventilation), further myocardial ischemia will result in complete cardiopulmonary collapse.

TABLE 2–1.

Proportion of Basal $\dot{V}O_2$ and Resting Blood Flow to Major Organ Systems

ORGAN SYSTEM	% BASAL $\dot{V}O_2$*	% RESTING BLOOD FLOW†
Liver	25%–33%	10%
Brain	16%–21%	15%
Heart	9%–11%	4%
Kidney	4%–8%	23%
Muscle	16%–30%	15%

*Total > 100% reflects use of data from multiple sources.
†Derived from Mellander and Johansson.[21a]

CLINICAL CONDITIONS ASSOCIATED WITH ALTERED SYSTEMIC OXYGEN CONSUMPTION

Disturbances of Body Temperature

It is well known that $\dot{V}O_2$ varies in proportion to body temperature across the physiologic range, with a 10%–13% increase in $\dot{V}O_2$ per °C elevation above normal.[4] Likewise, $\dot{V}O_2$ can be significantly below normal without lactate production under conditions of severe hypothermia, such as that produced during cardiopulmonary bypass.[13] Studies of induced hypothermia during cardiopulmonary bypass have demonstrated an average 7% decrease in $\dot{V}O_2$ per °C decrease in body core temperature, though this may not be a truly linear relation.[16] It has been reported that $\dot{V}O_2$ can drop by 50% at 28° C and as much as 87% in profound hypothermia (18° C) in dogs.[5, 12]

Even more impressive are the transient increases in $\dot{V}O_2$ needed to raise body temperature. This occurs most commonly with the rigors of a "spiking" fever or shivering during rewarming after anesthesia-induced hypothermia. Several investigations have addressed the latter problem[26–28] and have described greater than 100% increases in $\dot{V}O_2$ with shivering during postoperative rewarming. The increased oxygen demands and associated sympathetic manifestations may be detrimental to patients with limited physiologic reserves. A significant contribution to the increased $\dot{V}O_2$ in these settings is provided by skeletal muscle in the form of shivering or rigors. These problems can be abated by administering paralyzing agents or narcotics,[27–29] by limiting heat loss, or by restoring peripheral as well as core temperature to normal before discontinuing bypass in the cardiac surgery patient.

General Anesthesia

General anesthesia decreases $\dot{V}O_2$ for many reasons.[26, 37] Loss of temperature regulation due to depression of the hypothalamus along with cutaneous vasodilation from anesthetic agents results in heat loss to the air-conditioned operating room. Paralyzing agents decrease resting muscle tone and related muscle oxygen consumption and heat generation, contributing to hypothermia. While intraoperative hypothermia may not be harmful itself, a drop in body temperature of as little as 1° C may exact a significant physiologic price during postoperative rewarming, as described earlier.[26]

The Metabolic Response to Injury

Decades ago, Cuthbertson[9] detected changes in metabolic activity associated with skeletal injury, characterized by an early decrease in $\dot{V}O_2$ (ebb or shock phase) followed by prolonged increased metabolic activity (flow phase). Using a hood canopy/spirometer system in nonintubated patients, Kinney et al.[21] demonstrated significant elevations in $\dot{V}O_2$ in patients under various degrees of physiologic stress. Increases in $\dot{V}O_2$ ranged from 10%–30% in patients with skeletal injuries to 60% in those with severe infections, and to

more than 100% in patients with large full-thickness burns. More recently, even minor trauma such as that associated with muscle biopsy has been shown to cause transient substantial increases in $\dot{V}O_2$.[10] Likewise, intensive care unit maneuvers such as chest physiotherapy have been shown to increase $\dot{V}O_2$ by 35% above that observed in the same patient during sleep.[39]

Fever, increased work of breathing, psychomotor agitation, and the need to compensate for increased heat losses (as in burns) contribute to the $\dot{V}O_2$ associated with increased resting metabolic demands. It thus appears that the "normal" $\dot{V}O_2$ of 110–150 ml/min/m^2 may be a suboptimal value in applying intermittent measurements to the evaluation of critically ill patients.

Shock

Shock is defined here as the inability of oxygen delivery to support the metabolic demands (optimal $\dot{V}O_2$) of the tissues. By definition, the $\dot{V}O_2$ of the patient in shock will be below that appropriate to his physiologic condition. Adequate resuscitation from shock is then the improvement in quantity or distribution of oxygen delivery to that point at which $\dot{V}O_2$ is appropriate.

Shoemaker et al., using a multivariate analysis of physiologic values during resuscitation from shock, discovered that a "greater than normal" $\dot{V}O_2$ (approximately 170 ml/min/m^2) in the postresuscitation period was associated with increased survival. They then showed that when this value was the physiologic end point of resuscitation, patient survival was greater than when traditional goals such as normal blood pressure were used to determine the adequacy of resuscitation.[34] Abraham, Shoemaker, and Bland have also shown that $\dot{V}O_2$ may decrease early in shock states, before the hemodynamic collapse becomes obvious.[1] In low output states, prior to the onset of "irreversible shock," one would expect $\dot{V}O_2$ to parallel oxygen transport if autoregulation were intact. In high output shock, such as from sepsis, total systemic oxygen transport appears less important than its distribution or cellular utilization. Recent reviews of this phenomenon are available elsewhere.[18, 31] Particular aspects are discussed in chapter 5, "Patterns of Hemodynamic Response," and chapter 13, "Assessment of Systemic Oxygen Transport."

Very low $\dot{V}O_2$ in shock states has been observed to correlate with nonsurvival.[1, 18, 34] This may simply indicate the severity of the shock state. Failure of resuscitation to increase $\dot{V}O_2$ has perhaps an even stronger association with poor prognosis, and may be the systemic metabolic manifestation of either diffuse cell death or widespread loss of microvascular perfusion. These have the same consequence: multiple system organ failure and ultimately death.[38]

Several researchers have investigated the relationship between $\dot{V}O_2$ and oxygen delivery in critically ill patients.[11, 20, 24, 25, 39] The consensus of their results is that increasing oxygen delivery increases $\dot{V}O_2$ at least to the normal range. Particularly in stressed patients with the adult respiratory distress syndrome,[11, 25] there is evidence that increased oxygen delivery increases $\dot{V}O_2$ well beyond the upper limits of normal. In view of the typically increased metabolic demands of critically ill patients, this is not surprising. At least one investigator found that increased serum lactic acid correlates well with the ability of increasing oxygen delivery to increase $\dot{V}O_2$, providing additional evidence for circulatory inadequacy in this situation.[14]

SUMMARY

When oxygen transport is adequate, oxygen consumption is determined by tissue metabolic demands. Several methods are available to approximate oxygen consumption in the critically ill, although none is without technical problems. The determination of systemic oxygen consumption is of little value in determining the adequacy of individual organ metabolism and may be difficult to evaluate in view of the wide range of metabolic demands seen in the various physiologic states of the critically ill patient. In the critically ill, it seems appropriate to maximize oxygen transport to support the greater than normal metabolic rates that have been observed, especially in patients being resuscitated from shock.

REFERENCES

1. Abraham E, Shoemaker WC, Bland RD, et al: Sequential cardiorespiratory patterns in septic shock. *Crit Care Med* 1983; 11:799.
2. Aubier M, Viires N, Syllic G, et al: Respiratory muscle contribution to lactic acidosis in low cardiac output. *Am Rev Respir Dis* 1982; 126:648.
3. Bartlett RH, Decheut RE, Mault JR: Measurement of metabolism in multiple organ failure. *Surgery* 1982; 92:771.
4. Beisel W, Wannemacher RW, Neufeld HA: Relation of fever to energy expenditure, in *Assessment of Energy Metabolism in Health and Disease*. Columbus, Ohio, Ross Laboratories, 1980, p 144.
5. Bigelow WG, Lindsay WK, Harrison RC, et al: Oxygen transport and utilization in dogs at low temperature. *Am J Physiol* 1950; 160:125.
6. Bohra SE, Högman B, Olsson SG, et al: A new device for continuous measurement of gas exchange during artificial ventilation. *Crit Care Med* 1980; 8:705.
7. Browning JA, Linber SE, Turney SZ, et al: The effects of a fluctuating F_{IO_2} on metabolic measurements in mechanically ventilated patients. *Crit Care Med* 1982; 10:82.
8. Brozek J, Grande F: Body composition and basal metabolism in man: Correlation analysis versus physiological approach. *Hum Biol* 1955; 27:24.
9. Cuthbertson DP: Post-shock metabolic response. *Lancet* 1942; 1:433.
10. Damask MC, Askanazi J, Weissman C, et al: Artifacts in measurement of resting energy expenditure. *Crit Care Med* 1983; 11:750.
11. Danek SJ, Lynch JP, Weg JG, et al: The dependence of oxygen uptake on oxygen delivery in the adult respiratory distress syndrome. *Am Rev Respir Dis* 1980; 122:387.
12. Fairley HB: Metabolism in hypothermia. *Br Med Bull* 1961; 17:52.
13. Fox LS, Blackstone EH, Kirklin JW, et al: Relationship of whole body oxygen consumption to perfusion flow rate during hypothermic cardiopulmonary bypass. *J Thorac Cardiovasc Surg* 1982; 83:239.
14. Gilbert GH, Haupt MT, Carlson RW: Lactate predicts the relationship between oxygen transport and oxygen consumption in patients with circulatory shock. *Crit Care Med* 1984; 12:299.
15. Goldfarb RD: Cardiac mechanical performance in circulatory shock. *Circ Shock* 1982; 9:633.
16. Harris EA, Seelye ER, Squire AW: Oxygen consumption during cardiopulmonary bypass with moderate hypothermia in man. *Br J Anaesth* 1971; 43:1113.
17. Holliday MA, Potter D, Jarrah A, et al: The relation of metabolic rate to body weight and organ size. *Pediatr Res* 1967; 1:185.
18. Houtchens BA, Westenskow DR: Oxygen con-

sumption in septic shock. *Circ Shock* 1984; 13:361.

19. Hunker FD, Brutton CW, Hunker EM et al: Metabolic and nutritional evaluation of patients supported with mechanical ventilation. *Crit Care Med* 1980; 8:628.

20. Kaufman BJ, Rackow EC, Falk JL: The relationship between oxygen delivery and consumption during fluid resuscitation of hypovolemic and septic shock. *Chest* 1984; 85:336.

21. Kinney JM, Duke JH, Long CL, et al: Tissue fuel and weight loss after injury. *J Clin Pathol* 1970; 23(suppl 4):65–72.

21a. Mellander S, Johansson B: Control of resistance, exchange, and capacitance functions in the peripheral circulation. *Pharmacol Rev* 1968; 20:117.

22. Milnor WR: Regional circulations, in Mountcastle VB (ed): *Medical Physiology*. St Louis, CV Mosby Co, 1974, p 1003.

23. Milnor WR: Regional circulations, in Mountcastle VB (ed): *Medical Physiology*. St Louis, CV Mosby Co, 1974, p 998.

24. Powers SR, Maunal R, Neclerio M, et al: Physiologic consequences of positive end expiratory pressure (PEEP) ventilation. *Ann Surg* 1973; 178:265.

25. Rhodes GR, Newell JC, Shah D, et al: Increased oxygen consumption accompanying increased oxygen delivery with hypertonic mannitol in the adult respiratory distress syndrome. *Surgery* 1978; 84:490.

26. Roc CF, Goldberg MJ, Blair CJ, et al: The influence of body temperature on early postoperative oxygen consumption. *Surgery* 1966; 60:85.

27. Rodriguez JL, Weissman C, Damask MC, et al: Physiologic requirements during rewarming: Suppression of the shivering response. *Crit Care Med* 1983; 11:490.

28. Rodriguez JL, Weissman C, Damask MC, et al: Morphine and postoperative rewarming in critically ill patients. *Circulation* 1983; 68:1238.

29. Rouby JJ, Eurin B, Glaser P, et al: Hemodynamic and metabolic effects of morphine in the critically ill. *Circulation* 1981; 64:53.

30. Roussos C, Macklen P: The respiratory muscles. *N Engl J Med* 1982; 307:786.

31. Shah DM, Newell JC, Saba TM: Defects in peripheral oxygen utilization following trauma and shock. *Arch Surg* 1981; 116:1277.

32. Shibutani K, Komatin T, Kubal K, et al: Critical level of oxygen delivery in anesthetized man. *Crit Care Med* 1983; 11:640.

33. Shimada U, Yoshiya I, Hirata T: Evaluation of a system for on-line analysis of $\dot{V}O_2$ and $\dot{V}CO_2$ for clinical applicability. *Anesthesiology* 1984; 61:311.

34. Shoemaker WC, Appel P, Bland R: Use of physiologic monitoring to predict outcome and assist in clinical decisions in critically ill postoperative patients. *Am J Surg* 1983; 146:43.

35. Snellen JW: Studies in human calorimetry, in *Assessment of Energy Metabolism in Health and Disease*. Columbus, Ohio, Ross Laboratories, 1980, pp 13–15.

36. Wade OL, Bishop JM: *Cardiac Output and Regional Blood Flow*. Oxford, Blackwell Scientific Publications, 1962.

37. Waxman K, Lazrovc S, Shoemaker WC: Physiologic responses to operation in high risk surgical patients. *Surg Gynecol Obstet* 1981; 152:633.

38. Waxman K, Shoemaker WC: Physiologic responses to massive intraoperative hemorrhage. *Arch Surg* 1982; 117:470.

39. Weissman C, Kemper M, Damask C, et al: Effect of routine intensive care interactions on metabolic rate. *Chest* 1984; 86:815.

PART 2 —————— Regulation of Oxygen Transport

3   Ventricular Pump Function

Howard S. Goldberg, M.D.

Michael R. Pinsky, M.D.

In the overall scheme of cardiovascular homeostasis the heart plays a central role in generating forward blood flow into the arterial circuit. The resultant arterial pressure (MAP) will be a function of this steady-state blood flow, as well as of arterial resistance and capacitance. Although the heart, as a muscular pump, will determine forward blood flow into the arterial tree, the distribution of this blood flow within the body will be governed primarily by vascular factors such as peripheral vasomotor tone.

The left ventricle provides the energy necessary for the circulation of blood through the systemic vessels. It behaves as a muscular hydraulic pump, converting chemical energy into mechanical energy. The mechanisms involved in these molecular energetics and the intracellular and intercellular events bearing on the conversion of chemical energy to mechanical energy are important in understanding myocardial contractility and systolic performance. However, it is not necessary to describe these processes in order to evaluate overall ventricular pump function.

The interaction of pharmacologic and autonomic changes in tone with cardiovascular function is described in greater detail in chapters 4, "Control of Cardiac Output by the Circuit;" 7, "Control of Organ Blood Flow;" and 30, "Pharmacologic Manipulation of Regional Blood Flow."

OVERVIEW

Clinically, we are interested in the properties of the pump that allow the generation of an adequate cardiac output with an adequate MAP. Cardiac output is a function of four interrelated factors: heart rate, intrinsic myocardial contractility, preload, and afterload. There are many ways of representing this ventricular pumping function. Each has its advantages and shortcomings. Since the heart is usually modeled as a hydraulic pump, the simplest method of describing ventricular pumping function is to relate the blood volume within the ventricle prior to ejection, or end-diastolic volume, to the resultant stroke volume delivered into the circulation. This analysis is referred to as the Frank-Starling relationship and is often used clinically to describe ventricular pump function. The ventricle pumps this stroke volume into the circulation under pressure. Thus, some consideration must be given to the pressure developed during ventricular contraction, systole, since it more accurately describes the work that the pump performs. The most direct way to evaluate the work performed by the pump is to relate preload to afterload. In a classical mechanical analysis these loads are both pressures. However, since the heart is really a volume-loaded pump, as we will discuss, it is better to think of the left ventricular (LV) preload as the volume in the LV at the end of diastole. Since volume is difficult to measure, the corresponding LV end-diastolic pressure is often used to infer preload. Similarly, afterload can be thought of as the pressure generated at the end of systole. This analysis is limited, however, because it does not take into account the time required for the ventricle to pump its stroke. Since myocardial work can be thought of as a function of pressure generated over time, it is clear that for the same preload and afterload, if ejection takes longer, the ventricle has had to work harder. This aspect is better accounted for when the relation between myocardial wall tension and time of ejection, the tension-time index, is used to assess ventricular pump function. In this chapter we will describe ventricular pump function as it relates first to the Frank-Starling relationship, then to the ventricular pressure-volume history of a cardiac cycle, and finally as it relates to wall tension, ejection velocity, and the time required for ejection to occur.

THE FRANK-STARLING RELATIONSHIP

The heart pumps the blood it receives into the arterial tree. In a steady state, it can eject no more blood out than it receives. For a given heart rate, as venous return increases, preload increases, and the force of ventricular ejection also increases. This allows the heart to empty to a nearly constant end-systolic volume. Similarly, as preload decreases, the force of ventricular ejection also decreases, again tending to maintain end-systolic volume. Since stroke volume is the difference between end-diastolic and end-systolic volume, it can be seen that changes in preload will induce proportionally similar changes in stroke volume. To the extent that heart rate is constant, then cardiac output will change as well. This preload-dependent effect on ventricular performance, referred to as Starling's law of the heart,[13, 20] is a central characteristic of cardiac myofibrils and separates them mechanically from skeletal and smooth muscle fibers, which do not increase their force of contraction as fiber length increases above resting length. The degree to which a ventricle ejects its preload into the circulation will be affected by the baseline level of contractility of the heart,[17] mechanical factors related to pump function,[4] and the afterload that the heart has to eject against.[16] Contractility can be directly affected by myocardial blood flow and oxygen delivery,[19] as well as by intracellular levels of Ca^{++}, K^+, and a wide variety of pharmacologic agents.

Figure 3–1 illustrates the relation between LV preload and stroke volume for two different conditions, labeled here A and B. This relation is usually referred to as the Starling curve, although a more correct term would be the Frank-Starling curve. Starling curves can be generated by either increasing or decreasing preload and observing the resulting change in stroke volume. In this figure, curve A has a steeper slope and is shifted to the left of curve B. Ventricular performance can be defined by the slope and position of the curve, while response to an intervention can be defined by the change in either the slope or the position

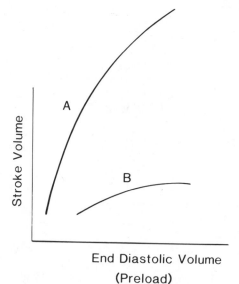

FIG 3–1.
The relation between left ventricular (LV) preload and LV stroke volume, the Frank-Starling curve. Increases in end-diastolic volume increase the force of contraction, increasing stroke volume. The slope and the position of this relation define the contractility of the ventricle. A shift of the Frank-Starling curve downward and to the right represents decreased ventricular performance, while a shift of the curve upward and to the left represents improved performance. The heart represented by curve A has a better performance than the heart represented by curve B.

of the curve. Using this analysis, curve A describes a heart with a better function than that described by curve B. For any given preload, the heart described by curve A will eject a greater stroke volume than the heart described by curve B. Similarly, for any given increase in preload, heart A will increase its stroke volume more than heart B will. In an operational sense, the relation between these two characteristics of heart A defines its performance as better than heart B's.

Many factors can alter the shape of the Starling curve.[17] Increased inotropy (contractile state), decreased afterload, and increased heart rate all improve ventricular pump function (systolic performance) and are associated with an improved ejection fraction. Changes in ejection fraction may therefore occur independently of changes in contractility. Decreased inotropy, increased afterload, and bradycardia all depress systolic performance. If the hearts described in Figure 3–1 represent the same heart at two different times, then the change in performance from a time corresponding to curve *A* to a time corresponding to curve *B* would represent a decreased systolic performance. If the shift were from *B* to *A*, the opposite would be true. If the only event that occurred between these two curves was an acute myocardial infarction, without any change in afterload, drug therapy, sympathetic tone, or blood chemistry, then the cause of the depressed ventricular performance could be rather confidently blamed on loss of myocardial muscle mass or change in LV compliance. Unfortunately, under most clinical conditions in which cardiac performance is altered, reflex mechanisms increase sympathetic tone, both increasing afterload and minimizing the infarction-induced decrease in inotropy. By our analysis of ventricular function, we are unable to ascertain the degree to which such depression in systolic performance is due to decreased cardiac contractility (inotropy) or to increased afterload. Since the management of these two processes is different, the use of stroke-volume-defined Starling curves to ascertain systolic performance is of limited value.

The pressure generated during systole can be measured relatively easily, using a pulmonary arterial catheter to measure pulmonary arterial wedge pressure and a sphygmomanometer or indwelling arterial cannula to measure MAP. This pressure difference defines the pressure generated by the LV during systole. LV stroke work, the product of pressure generated and stroke volume, can be substituted for stroke volume in the Frank-Starling relationship. When this is done, changes in afterload can be shown to have a minimal effect on systolic performance of the normal ventricle. If afterload increases in Figure 3–1 from the curve *A*, although the stroke volume will fall, creating a new curve *B*, it will not decrease the stroke work, since pressure generated will increase proportionally. When ventricular output is expressed as stroke work, depression of the Starling curve is usually due to decreases in contractility. These points are illustrated in Figure 3–2, which describes the Frank-Starling relationship in terms of stroke work instead of stroke volume. As in Figure 3–1, systolic performance can be described by the position and slope of the Starling curve generated for a ventricle. Again, the ventricle described by curve *B* has a depressed systolic performance compared with the ventricle described by curve *A*. In this analysis, because the calculation of stroke work takes into account

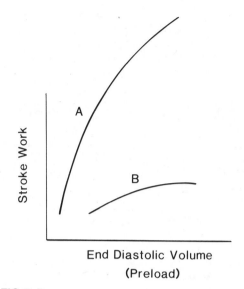

FIG 3–2.
The relation between left ventricular preload and its stroke work. This preload relation is also referred to as the Frank-Starling relation, as described in Figure 3–1. See text.

the variables that usually dominate afterload, it is unlikely that increases in afterload can account for the depression in curve *B* from curve *A*. Using stroke work to define systolic performance allows one to ascertain the performance of the ventricle relatively independent of changes in afterload. Unfortunately, this simplification does not hold true under some conditions. Afterload is a function not only of pressure generated during ejection, but also of systolic pressure generated during isometric contraction and of ventricular wall tension. In Figure 3–2, for a given stroke work, heart *B* is generating a greater wall tension than heart *A* because its volume is greater. Thus, even when stroke work is used, analyzing systolic performance using Starling curves is of limited value when changes in end-diastolic volume and afterload occur.

It is difficult to measure end-diastolic volume. As an approximation, end-diastolic pressure is often used. Clinically, wedge pressure is used as an estimate of end-diastolic pressure. Using wedge pressure as an estimate of preload in assessing ventricular pump function assumes that certain relations are constant, which may not be so. Conditions under which wedge pressure may not accurately reflect end-diastolic pressure or its change in response to therapy are described in chapter 15, "Technical Problems in Data Acquisition." Similarly, and of greater importance, end-diastolic pressure and its change may not reflect end-diastolic volume.[5] End-diastolic volume is a function of the diastolic compliance of the LV and its distending pressure. The diastolic compliance of the LV is not a straight-line relation between filling pressure and volume but is curvilinear; it becomes stiffer at higher volumes. Second, increases in pericardial pressure secondary to pericardial effusion or overdistention of the right ventricle (ventricular interdependence) or expansion of the lung will decrease the "perceived" diastolic compliance by decreasing the distending pressure. Diastolic compliance can be altered by ischemia,[14] heart rate,[15] and pharmacologic interventions.[3] For example, in the setting of an acute myocardial infarction, a greater wedge pressure is likely to be required to generate the same preload than was required prior to the ischemia. If Starling curves are generated for such a ventricle, with preload estimated as wedge pressure, then it would appear that a greater preload than was actually required is necessary to generate the given stroke volume. Since wedge pressure is commonly used to monitor LV preload, consideration of what is actually measured and how that might be affected independent of preload is important in the rational evaluation of Starling curves.

THE CARDIAC CYCLE: VENTRICULAR PRESSURE-VOLUME HISTORY

Ventricular pump function is often described as related to preload and afterload. By the Frank-Starling mechanism, as end-diastolic volume (preload) increases, the force of systolic contraction also increases, increasing stroke volume and tending to keep the resulting end-systolic volume constant. That this volume relation between preload and stroke volume is associated with corresponding intraventricular pressure changes allows us to describe this relation as the pressure-volume history of the ventricle as it travels through one cardiac cycle. In this analysis, preload is the volume in the ventricle at end-diastole. End-diastolic volume, in turn, is a function of the distending pressure of the ventricle and ventricular diastolic compliance. For any given level of cardiac contractility and afterload, the stroke volume is a

function of end-diastolic volume, not end-diastolic pressure.

The afterload can be considered as the average pressure that the heart must generate to pump blood into the systemic circulation. The afterload is therefore the difference between MAP and the pressure surrounding the heart. This afterload-preload analysis of LV function would be more precise if the forward flow of blood from the ventricle to the aorta always followed a positive pressure gradient between the LV and the aorta. This is not the case. Indeed, a positive-pressure gradient between the LV and the aorta is present for only about the first half of ventricular emptying.[12] The forward flow in a direction opposite from the pressure gradient is a result of the momentum of the blood, which requires an opposing force to decelerate. The greater the outflow impedance, the more quickly the column of blood decelerates. Although it is probably more precise to consider all the forces opposing ventricular emptying, consideration of the average pressure load can yield valuable insights.

The relation of afterload to preload, plotted on axes with LV volume on the abscissa and average pressure load of the ventricle on the ordinate, was first used by Frank in 1895.[6] An example of such an analysis is shown in Figure 3–3. With the heart relaxed in diastole, there is a relation of pressure to volume. There is an unstressed volume (V_0), that is, the volume that can be contained by the ventricle with no transmural pressure gradient, and a relation of stressed volume to transmural pressure. In the relaxed state this is the passive tension curve, or diastolic compliance curve (curve *A* in Fig 3–3). If the heart contracts from some stressed volume, the pressure in the chamber will rise. Within the physiologic range, the maximum pressure that can be generated by the contracting LV is a function of the end-diastolic volume: the greater the end-diastolic volume, the greater the developed pressure.[20] Experimentally this is determined by actually obstructing the aorta and observing the pressure generated (see Fig 3–3). If a series of contractions occurs at various end-diastolic volumes at each of several afterloads, a relation between the end-systolic volume and the developed pressure is described. This is the total tension curve, or end-systolic pressure-volume curve. The passive tension curve describes the maximal compliance, or minimal elastance, of the relaxed ventricle. The total tension curve is the end-sys-

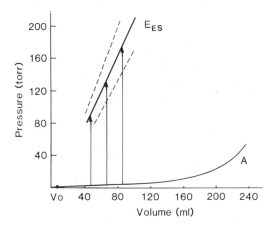

FIG 3–3.
Relation between ventricular pressure and volume during diastole and systole. Each vertical line represents contraction at the indicated diastolic volume while ejection is prevented by aortic clamping. The maximum pressures reached during systole at different volumes fall on a straight line. The maximum systolic pressure line will be higher or lower *(dashed lines)* with change in contractility. Note that left ventricular end-diastolic pressure (LVEDP) is not a straight-line function of volume.

tolic elastance, or E_{ES} (see · Fig 3–3). Cardiac contraction can then be thought of as an active change in cardiac elastance from the diastolic curve to a point on the E_{ES} curve. For a given passive tension curve, the better the cardiac contractility, the greater the end-systolic elastance. For a given passive tension curve and afterload, the lower the end-systolic volume, the better the cardiac contractility. Thus, the relation between end-systolic volume and MAP is an important indicator of ventricular contractility.

These points are illustrated in Figure 3–4. On the abscissa is plotted the volume of the left ventricle, and on the ordinate is plotted LV transmural pressure. Curve *A* is a passive tension curve. It shows the change in diastolic pressure with change in diastolic volume and therefore describes the diastolic elastance of the LV. Curve E_{ES} is the total tension curve, or end-systolic elastance, and relates end-systolic volume to afterload. Let us say that the afterload in the aorta is 90 torr. In order for the LV represented in this example to achieve this pressure, it must have a minimum volume of 50 ml. If the end-diastolic volume were less than 50 ml, the ventricle would be unable to attain a transmural pressure of 90

torr during systole. If the end-diastolic volume were exactly 50 ml, then the ventricle could attain the pressure but would eject no stroke volume. If the volume at end-diastole were greater than 50 ml, then all the volume above 50 ml would be ejected and the end-systolic volume would be 50 ml.

Figure 3–5 represents a normal contraction. The end-diastolic volume in this example is 140 ml (point *a*). The ventricle contracts until the aortic pressure is reached (line *a–b*). This contraction occurs isovolumetrically, because the pressure within the ventricle is still less than in the aorta. During isovolumetric contraction, potential energy is added to the blood within the ventricle. Once the afterload pressure is achieved, volume leaves the ventricle until the end-systolic elastance curve is reached (line *b–c*). When the systolic elastance is reached (point *c*), there can be no further emptying of the ventricle. In this example, this occurs at an afterload of 90 torr, when the ventricular volume is 50 ml, generating a stroke volume of 90 ml. The ventricle now relaxes (line *c–d*) and diastolic filling begins (point *d*).

The area under the curve within this boundary *(a, b, c, d)* represents the external mechanical work done by the ventricle. The triangle formed by *c*, *d*, and V_0, combined with the area de-

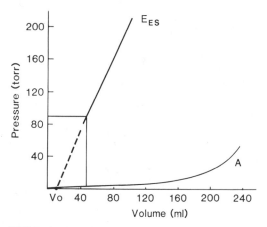

FIG 3–4.
The developed transmural pressure of the left ventricle is plotted as a function of LV volume. Curve *A* represents passive elastance and curve E_{ES} represents the end-systolic elastance that is developed by ventricular contraction. The ventricle represented must contain 50 ml to develop a transmural pressure of 90 torr.

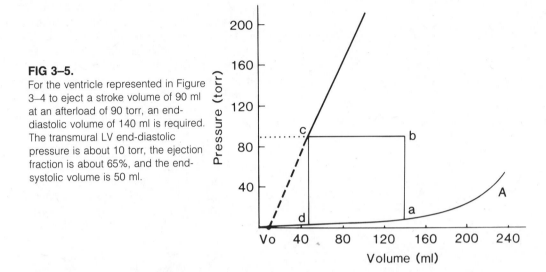

FIG 3–5.
For the ventricle represented in Figure 3–4 to eject a stroke volume of 90 ml at an afterload of 90 torr, an end-diastolic volume of 140 ml is required. The transmural LV end-diastolic pressure is about 10 torr, the ejection fraction is about 65%, and the end-systolic volume is 50 ml.

scribed by *a, b, c, d,* represents the entire energy expenditure of the contracting ventricle. This total described area correlates very highly with oxygen consumption.[8] Obviously, the more of this area that is related to the production of a stroke volume, which is the external mechanical work, the greater the efficiency of the pump.

If the afterload of the LV is increased, one can see from Figure 3–5 that the end-systolic volume will also increase. In order for the stroke volume to be maintained with this elevated afterload, the end-diastolic volume must increase, resulting in a decreased ejection fraction. The fall in ejection fraction under these conditions does not represent failure of the heart, because the heart is still operating on the normal systolic elastance curve. The reduction in the ejection fraction is the inevitable result of the increase in afterload and the Frank-Starling mechanism, whereby the heart increases volume to pump against a greater afterload. However, under these conditions the heart actually can improve its contractility in the face of a persistently increased afterload by mechanisms that are still poorly understood. This is observed in a heart that first increases in volume to meet the new afterload, then continues to pump an unchanged stroke volume but reduces its end-systolic and end-diastolic volume. This has been called homeometric autoregulation.[18] The phenomenon was first described by Knowlton and Starling in 1912.[9]

When myocardial contractility is reduced, as in congestive heart failure, there is a decrease in

the slope of the end-systolic pressure-volume curve, representing a decrease in the end-systolic elastance. This is demonstrated by curve *C* in Figure 3–6. Note that in this example the minimal LV volume necessary to develop the average afterload of 90 torr when contractility is reduced is much higher, about 100 ml. For the same stroke volume as before, 190 ml must be in the ventricle at end-diastole. Because the ventricle gets progressively stiffer at higher volumes, LV end-diastolic pressure has risen from about 8 torr to about 20 torr. The relation of the stroke volume area to the entire area encompassed by the E_{ES} curve and the stroke volume should be compared with the normal example in Figure 3–5. Note how inefficient the failing heart has become. If the stroke volume were not maintained, the heart rate would have to increase to keep cardiac output constant. This would further increase the heart's oxygen requirement, which is already increased and less efficiently utilized than normal. Notice also that the end-systolic volume is increased from 50 to 100 ml and the ejection fraction is reduced from about 65% to about 45%. Since in this example the afterload is maintained, these changes in ventricular volumes are due to decreased inotropic state of the heart. Thus, this analysis allows a simple graphic explanation for the events occurring in the cardiac cycle.

In the example discussed with the first model (see Figs 3–1 and 3–2), myocardial ischemia decreases cardiac contractility and will decrease

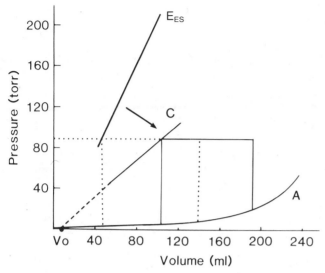

FIG 3–6.
Curves *A* and E_{ES} are as in Figure 3–4. Curve *C* represents a decrease in end-systolic elastance developed by the contracting ventricle. At the same afterload of 90 torr and the same stroke volume of 90 ml, the result of the change in contractility can be seen. The end-diastolic volume is now 190 ml, the transmural LV end-diastolic pressure is 19 torr, the ejection fraction is about 45%, and the end-systolic volume is 100 ml.

E_{ES}. In addition, myocardial ischemia decreases the diastolic compliance of the LV. Since the relevant preload is volume,[5] not pressure, as seen in Figure 3–7, the LV end-diastolic volume necessary to maintain stroke volume at the given afterload is associated with a substantially higher LV end-diastolic pressure, about 30 torr, compared with 19 torr. Yet for the given total tension curve the end-diastolic and end-systolic volumes are the same. This demonstrates that the heart is a volume load-dependent pump, not a pressure-dependent pump. As can be seen in Figure 3–5, the stroke volume is not a direct function of LV end-

diastolic pressure, but is a direct function of LV end-diastolic volume.

Figure 3–8 shows the result of an isolated improvement in contractility, such as might occur with administration of an inotrope. For the same stroke volume and afterload, the end-systolic volume is reduced. The end-diastolic volume is reduced, and oxygen utilization has become more efficient. Further improvement occurs when the afterload is reduced from 90 to 80 torr by an afterload-reducing agent, such as nitroprusside (Fig 3–9). If the afterload-reducing agent also improves LV compliance, as might occur with ni-

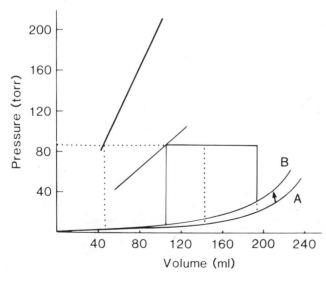

FIG 3–7.
The passive tension curve now shows a decrease in ventricular compliance (curve *B*). Compared to Figure 3–6, although ejection fraction and LV volumes are unchanged, the transmural LV end-diastolic pressure is now about 30 torr.

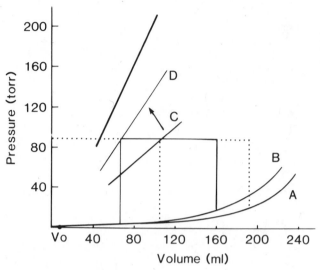

FIG 3–8.
At the same afterload and stroke volume, improvement in myocardial contractility (moving from curve *C* to curve *D*) is associated with a decrease in end-systolic volume, end-diastolic volume, and transmural LV end-diastolic pressure. Ejection fraction is increased to about 55%.

troprusside, then LV pressures are returned to a normal range despite the decreased contractility.

As diastolic pressures in the left side of the heart increase, pressures in the right side must increase to maintain the same flow from the right heart to the left heart. When this happens, further decreases in effective LV diastolic compliance may occur as a result of ventricular interdependence. With the pericardium as a limiting external membrane and the sharing of the interventricular septum, it is intuitively obvious that the pressure-volume relation of each ventricle depends to some extent on the pressure and volume of the other chamber, in that distention of one ventricle limits the filling of the other.

As pressure in the right side of the heart increases, the average pressure in the entire vascular bed must increase in order to maintain venous return and therefore cardiac output. Over time, fluid is retained by the kidneys, which increases intravascular volume. The constant increase in intravascular volume and pressure leads to peripheral signs of congestive heart failure. The increased pressures in the pulmonary circulation lead to increased extravascular fluid in the lung, with resulting dyspnea and orthopnea.

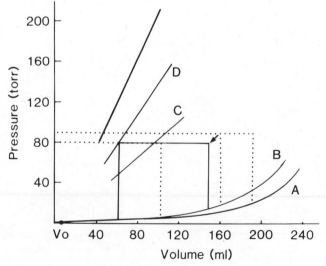

FIG 3–9.
When the afterload is reduced to 80 torr with the same stroke volume *(arrow)*, there is further improvement in all parameters. With relief of ischemia there may be an increase in ventricular compliance back to curve *A* and a reduction in LV transmural diastolic pressures back to within the normal range.

Many factors determine cardiac performance. Not all of these can be illustrated using the pressure-volume diagram. Ventricular pump efficiency is the external work performed by the heart relative to the amount of energy it uses to do that work. As illustrated above, in heart failure states, as the ventricle dilates to larger volumes, the area under the total work curve increases despite a constant stroke volume and pressure. This translates into a greater oxygen consumption by the failing heart to deliver the same cardiac output as a healthy heart. The cardiac output relative to myocardial oxygen consumption is used as an index of myocardial efficiency. Many factors determine oxygen consumption by the heart. Besides the total work performed by the heart, as described by the pressure-volume relation during the cardiac cycle, both heart rate[21] and the time required for ejection[11] also affect oxygen consumption and therefore ventricular pump efficiency. Since the LV pressure-volume axis has no units of time, it is unclear from this representation of ventricular pump function how long each segment of the cardiac cycle takes. Ventricular pump function can be described relative to the rate of ejection during systole. For the same stroke volume and pressure generated, a longer ejection time requires greater energy to maintain the wall tension. Therefore an analysis of ventricular pump function in the time domain is useful in order to evaluate systolic performance.

VENTRICULAR PUMP FUNCTION IN THE TIME DOMAIN

The LV develops active tension as it contracts from a point on its passive distention curve (diastolic compliance curve) to its end-systolic pressure-volume curve (E_{ES}). This contraction involves two separate but interrelated processes. First, before ejection, as contraction commences, wall tension within the ventricle increases without a change in myocardial muscle length. Once the pressure afterload is reached and the aortic valve opens, myocardial muscle fiber length decreases without a significant further increase in tension. Thus the tension developed by a muscle fiber can be studied separately from the velocity at which it contracts. If one were to take an isolated papillary muscle from the heart and connect

it to a fixed post at one end and a weight at the other, then one could define the relation between the weight lifted or tension generated and the velocity at which the weight was lifted. If no weight were hung from this muscle, then when it was activated to contract, it would decrease in length at a maximum velocity for that muscle (V_{max}). As the weight on the muscle was increased, the muscle would still continue to contract and shorten, but at a slower and slower velocity. At some point further increases in weight would exceed the muscle's ability to shorten. At this weight the muscle would have a velocity of zero (V_0), but would generate the greatest tension.[1] These points are illustrated in Figure 3-10, where tension developed is plotted on the x axis, and velocity is plotted on the y axis. Notice that the relation is not linear but hyperbolic, curving up from the axis to both V_{max} and V_0. This curve describes the relation between velocity and active tension for a papillary muscle of a given contractility. All the points along this curve represent the same contractility, but under different afterloading conditions. As the weight, which corresponds to the pressure load, increases, the velocity of contraction decreases. This inverse relation between load and velocity of fiber shortening holds true for the ventricle as a whole. Increases in afterload pressure decrease both the rate of ventricular ejection and the velocity of circumferential fiber shortening (V_{cf}).[20] If contractility improves, as would occur with the application of an inotrope, then the heart will not only increase the pressure it generates during systole, but it will increase the V_{cf} as well.

Clinically, the velocity of ventricular fiber shortening is assessed using echocardiography.[2] The technology allows visualization of the walls of the ventricle and, when recorded over time, documents the velocity of their shortening during ejection. Unfortunately, accurate estimation of V_{cf} requires two-dimensional echocardiography, which is not always available and is often difficult to perform. Analysis of the systolic time interval can bypass this problem.[10] This technique compares the external pressure pulse profile at the carotid artery as measured by a pressure sensor over the neck, phonocardiography, and electrocardiography. The time between the Q wave of the ECG and the A_2 sound, indicating closure of the aortic valve, represents the total systolic interval. The ejection interval represents the up-

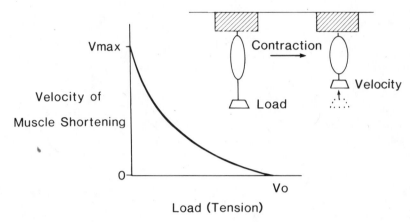

FIG 3–10.

The relation between velocity of shortening during systole and the load carried during that shortening for an isolated papillary muscle. The papillary muscle preparation is diagramed on the right. The velocity of muscle shortening (distance/time) decreases as the load (tension or weight) increases. For a given load, if the velocity of muscle shortening increases, then contractility of that muscle has also increased. The maximum velocity of fiber shortening occurs in the unloaded condition (V_{max}), while the maximum tension developed by the muscle occurs once the load is so great as to prevent any shortening (V_0).

stroke of the carotid pulse to its incisura or to the A_2. The pre-ejection period is calculated from the difference between these two intervals and represents the isovolumic contraction time. For a given afterload pressure, the pre-ejection period will vary in length inversely with preload and contractility. If preload increases, then the pre-ejection period decreases in length. Similarly, if cardiac contractility should decrease, as may occur with an acute myocardial infarction, then the pre-ejection period will increase. Measurement of systolic time intervals allows the noninvasive assessment of cardiac performance in man. This analysis, like all the analyses we have discussed, has its limitations. Since the pre-ejection period is affected by afterload, preload, and contractility, demonstration of a change in the pre-ejection period does not define the mechanism responsible.

In the assessment of ventricular pump function, discussed in chapter 15, "Technical Problems in Data Acquisition," modifications of most of these analyses will be discussed. That no one analysis defines all the characteristics of ventricular pump function illustrates the difficulties met in documenting the efficacy of a specific therapy or mechanism of a disease process or its progression. It is with the understanding of these limitations that one should approach the interpretation of hemodynamic data.

REFERENCES

1. Abbott BC, Wilkie DR: The relation between velocity of shortening and the tension-length curve of skeletal muscle. *J Physiol* 1953; 120:214–223.
2. Benzing G III, Stockert J, Nave E, et al: Evaluation of left ventricular performance: Circumferential fiber shortening and tension. *Circulation* 1974; 49:925–932.
3. Brodie BR, Grossman W, Mann T, et al: Effects of sodium nitroprusside on left ventricular diastolic pressure-volume relations. *J Clin Invest* 1977; 59:59–68.
4. Burton AC: Physical principles of circulatory phenomena: The physical equilibria of the heart and blood vessels, in *Handbook of Physiology*. Section 2: *Circulation,* vol 1, Hamilton WF, Dow P (eds). Washington, DC, American Physiological Society, 1962, pp 85–106.
5. Chatterjee MB, Parmley WW: Vasodilator therapy for acute myocardial infarction and chronic congestive heart failure. *J Am Coll Cardiol* 1983; 1:133–153.
6. Frank O: Zur Dynamik des Herzmuskels. Z. *Biol.* 1895; 32:370–447. [On the dynamics of cardiac muscle, Chapman CP, Wasserman E (trans). *Am Heart J* 1959; 58:282–317, 467–478.]
7. Karliner JS, Gault JH, Eckberg D, et al: Mean

velocity of fiber shortening: A simplified measure of left ventricular myocardial contractility. *Circulation* 1971; 44:323–333.

8. Khalafbeigui F, Suga H, Sagawa K: Left ventricular systolic pressure-volume area correlates with oxygen consumption. *Am J Physiol* 1972; 237:H566–H569.

9. Knowlton FP, Starling EH: The influence of variations in temperature and blood-pressure on the performance of the isolated mammalian heart. *J Physiol (Lond)* 1912; 44:206–219.

10. Martin CE, Shaver JA, Thompson ME, et al: Direct correlation of external systolic time intervals with internal indices of left ventricular function in man. *Circulation* 1971; 44:419–431.

11. Mommaerts WFHM: Energetics of muscular contraction. *Physiol Rev* 1969; 49:427–508.

12. Noble MIM: The contribution of blood momentum to left ventricular ejection in the dog. *Circ Res* 1968; 23:663–670.

13. Piper PH, Patterson SW, Starling EH: The regulation of the heart beat. *J Physiol* 1914; 48:465–513.

14. Rankin JS, Arentzen CE, McHale PA, et al: Viscoelastic properties of the diastolic left ventricle in the conscious dog. *Circ Res* 1977; 41(1):37–45.

15. Ricci DR, Orlick AE, Alderman EL, et al: Influence of heart rate on left ventricular ejection fraction in human beings. *Am J Cardiol* 1979; 44:447–451.

16. Ross J Jr: Afterload mismatch and preload reserve: A conceptual framework for the analysis of ventricular function. *Prog Cardiovasc Dis* 1976; 18(4):255–264.

17. Sarnoff S: Myocardial contractility as described by ventricular function curves: Observations on Starling's law of the heart. *Physiol Rev* 1955; 35:107.

18. Sarnoff SJ, Mitchell JH, Gilmore JP, et al: Homeometric autoregulation in the heart. *Circ Res* 1960; 8:1077–1091.

19. Scharf SM, Bromberger-Barnea B: Influence of coronary flow and pressure on cardiac function and coronary vascular volume. *Am J Physiol* 1973; 224(4):918–925.

20. Starling EH: *The Linacre Lecture on the Law of the Heart.* Delivered at St. John's College, Cambridge, England, 1915. London, Longmans, Green & Co., 1918.

21. Strobeck JE, Krueger J, Sonnenblick EH: Load and time considerations in the force-length relation of cardiac muscle. *Fed Proc* 1980; 39:175–182.

4 — Control of Cardiac Output by the Circuit

Howard S. Goldberg, M.D.

The circulation of blood in man requires a pump and a circuit. The pump adds sufficient energy to the column of blood so that circulation occurs. The properties of the circuit determine the distribution of the cardiac output, the arterial pressure for a given cardiac output, and the distribution of vascular volumes and pressures. Just as the systemic circuit depends on the output of volume from the heart, the heart depends on the return of volume from the circuit.

Most basically, the heart pumps at a given rate with a given stroke volume. This volume returns to the heart as the venous return, and is proportional to the difference between the average pressure in the combined venous and arterial circulation and the pressure in the right atrium. The venous return is inversely proportional to the resistance to return of blood to the heart.

The concept that the heart and the systemic circulation are linked and that cardiac output depends on the interaction of their mechanical properties is appealing because it is simple, accurate, and useful in understanding a wide variety of clinical problems. In this chapter we are concerned with the properties of the systemic circulation, and assume, unless we state otherwise, that the heart is functioning well. Under this circumstance the heart will pump all the blood returning to it, and cardiac output will be equal to venous return. A further simplifying assumption is that the volume of blood in the systemic circuit remains constant. When appropriate the limitations of these assumptions will be cast aside.

DISTRIBUTION OF STROKE VOLUME

The heart contracts and ejects a stroke volume. The volume enters the aorta, and the return of this bolus of blood to the heart has begun. The bolus is distributed to the various vascular beds of the body. Since the resistance of the arterial side of the circulation is about 20 times that of the venous side, it is the resistances on the arterial side that determine the distribution of the cardiac output. Therefore, the fractional distribution of the bolus is a function of the distribution of the resistances to arterial flow among the various vascular beds. A greater fraction of flow will go to a bed with less inflow resistance. If we consider the circulation as two parallel venous drainage systems, the superior vena cava (SVC) and the inferior vena cava (IVC), roughly one fourth of the cardiac output is distributed to the SVC system and three fourths to the IVC system.[3]

PRESSURE COST OF ARTERIAL FLOW

For a given cardiac output, the loss of pressure across the arterial bed is proportional to the total arterial resistance. The inflow or arterial resistance is an expression of the properties of the circuit that reduce energy in the flowing stream of blood. These properties are of two types: those that result in an energy loss because of flow itself, that is, the movement of blood from one place to another; and those that cause a potential energy loss, that is, the energy necessary to keep open a collapsible vessel with tone. These can be distinguished in a pressure-flow diagram (Fig 4–1). The loss in energy from flow is the incremental resistance and is represented as the change in pressure for a change in flow. For a vascular bed of fixed geometry perfused with blood, the change in driving pressure for a change in flow is the slope of a pressure-flow curve. The intercept of the extrapolation of this curve on the pressure

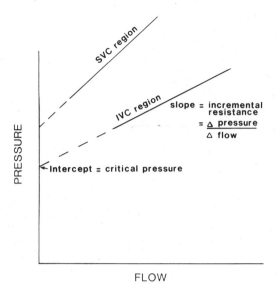

FIG 4–1.

The arterial pressure-flow resistance of the IVC and SVC drainage beds are diagramed. Notice the average critical pressure and incremental flow resistance of the SVC region are higher.

axis is the pressure that must be overcome before there can be any flow whatsoever and is the potential energy level that must be achieved before flow can commence. This pressure is called the critical pressure or sometimes the zero flow pressure.

These seemingly complicated relations can

be seen rather simply in an analogy. Suppose you have a cellophane tube. The least bit of pressure blown into one end of the tube causes it to distend to its full cross-sectional area. Further increases in pressure at one end of the tube change flow through the tube but not the cross-sectional area of the tube, nor of course its length. The pressure-flow relation of such a tube will be linear and will pass through the origin (Fig 4–2). Now imagine that a rubber band has been placed tightly around the middle of the tube. When one end is blown into, there will be no flow at all until sufficient pressure is generated to stretch the rubber band. At this point flow will begin, and as more and more pressure is applied to the inflow end of the cellophane tube the rubber band will stretch open farther and farther, allowing more and more flow, until the cellophane tube reaches its elastic limit. Now any given incremental increases in flow result in equal changes in inflow pressure (Fig 4–3). The slope of this relation will be the same as it was before the rubber band was placed around the tube. If a stronger rubber band were placed around the tube more pressure would be needed to fully open it, but the slope of the pressure-flow relation would be identical to that in the other two cases. If we plot the three pressure-flow curves on the same axes (Fig 4–4) we see that the third curve is displaced to the left of the second curve, which is displaced to the left of the first curve. The point at which the inflow pressure is sufficient to generate any flow is a

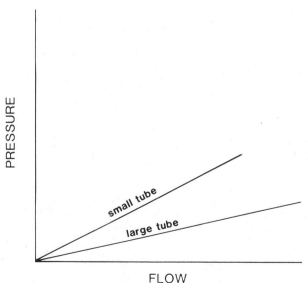

FIG 4–2.

The pressure-flow relations of two cellophane tubes are represented. One tube has a small and the other a large cross-sectional area. Flow is plotted on the abscissa and pressure on the ordinate. The slope of each pressure-flow curve is the resistance. The smaller tube has a greater resistance; that is, for any given change in flow there is a greater change in inflow pressure as compared to the large tube.

FIG 4–3.
The pressure-flow relation of the larger
cellophane tube is shown with and
without a constricting rubber band
around the tube. Once the constricted
tube is open to its full cross-sectional
area, the slope of the pressure-flow
relation of both tubes is the same. Thus
the incremental flow resistances are the
same. However, the constricted tube
will not allow any flow until the inflow
pressure is above that necessary to
open the constriction. The curvilinear
portion of the tube represents the
pressure-flow relation as the rubber
band stretches open until the elastic
limit of the cellophane tube *(E)* is
reached. The extrapolation of the
rectilinear portion of the curve
through the ordinate is the average
critical pressure and is the pertinent
backpressure to flow when flow is
sufficient to be on the rectilinear portion.

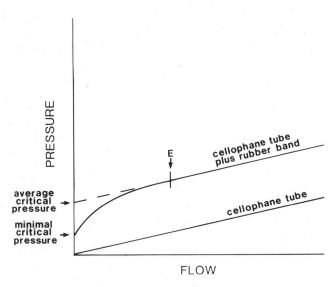

minimal critical pressure for any flow through the
system, and the extrapolation of the linear portion
of the curve through the pressure axis is an average critical pressure. The curvilinear portion of
the curve between the minimal pressure necessary
for flow to commence and the point at which the
curve becomes rectilinear is the result of the
stretching of the rubber band until the elastic
limit of the cellophane tube is reached.

The average critical pressure in an awake

standing dog is about 49 torr.[1] In the anesthetized
dog, the average critical pressure for the arterial
bed drained by the IVC is about 25 torr, and for
that drained by the SVC, about 35 torr.[3] For a
normal average pressure in the ascending aorta of
about 100 torr, the difference in critical pressures
would cause about 60% of the cardiac output to
be distributed to the IVC and about 40% to the
SVC. Yet at the same time 75% of the output is
drained by the IVC. This is accounted for by dif-

FIG 4–4.
The pressure-flow relation of the
cellophane tube with an even stiffer rubber
band is depicted and contrasted with the
previous two situations. *E* marks the elastic
limit of the tubes.

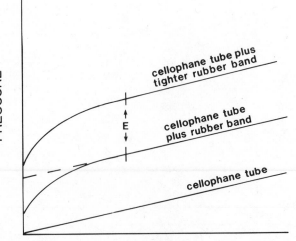

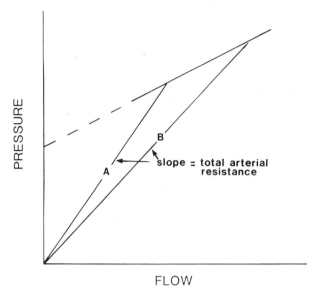

FIG 4–5.
An arterial pressure-flow curve is depicted as in Figure 4–1. The slope of the curve is the incremental flow resistance and the extrapolated intercept is the average critical pressure. With no change in the pressure-flow relation, the calculated total arterial resistance may change. For example, it will decrease as flow increases, as shown by the slopes of lines A and B.

ferences in the arterial incremental flow resistance, the change in pressure for a change in flow (see Fig 4–1).

ARTERIAL PRESSURE

At a given cardiac output, the total arterial resistance determines the mean arterial pressure (Fig 4–5). This is represented as the slope of a line drawn from the origin of the pressure-flow relation to the pertinent pressure-flow point. With no active change in the arterial bed, this resistance is lower the more the flow; but the incremental resistance, the slope of the pressure-flow curve, is unchanged. For the incremental resistance to change there must be a change in the vascular geometry, as might occur from active vasoconstriction. With no change in the vascular geometry but with greater arteriolar sphincteric tone, which increases the critical pressure, the slope of the pressure-flow curve is unchanged but the intercept is at a higher point on the pressure axis. This too will increase total arterial resistance. Therefore, changes in total arterial resistance can result from a simple change in flow with no active change in the arterial bed; or from an active change in vascular tone which might alter the vascular geometry and thus change the incremental resistance; or from an active change in vascular tone which might change the critical pressure;

or from any combination of these effects. For example, if a drug increases cardiac output but has no effect on the arterial pressure-flow relation, the calculated total arterial resistance will be lower. One might then erroneously conclude that the drug has vasoactive properties. On the other hand, an agent that does have vasoactive properties can change the incremental resistance, the critical pressure, or both. The only way to separate these effects is to determine the pressure-flow relation before and after administration of the drug.

Imagine the circulation with all blood flow completely stopped. Under this condition the arterial pressure in the two drainage beds will be the minimal critical pressure. At this time the heart ejects a stroke volume, and the pressure in each arterial bed rises and flow commences. However, not all of the stroke volume can empty before the next stroke volume is added to the circulation. The arterial pressure rises more, and more of this stroke volume can empty into the venous bed across the arterial resistance. This continues until the arterial pressure rises sufficiently to allow all of the preceding stroke volume to empty from the arterial bed before the next stroke volume is added. How high the arterial pressure must rise to completely empty the previous stroke volume is a function of the total arterial resistance. As described, the arterial pressure rises to this level by retaining ever-decreas-

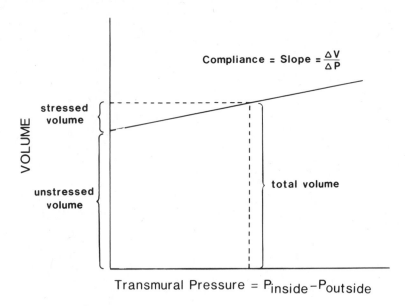

Compliance = Slope = $\frac{\Delta V}{\Delta P}$

VOLUME

stressed volume

unstressed volume

total volume

Transmural Pressure = $P_{inside} - P_{outside}$

FIG 4–6.
The pressure-volume relation of the systemic vascular bed.

ing portions of the stroke volume until, for a given heart rate and stroke volume, all the previous stroke volume empties before the next cardiac ejection.

STATIC MECHANICAL PROPERTIES

With four concepts—transmural pressure, unstressed volume, stressed volume, and compliance—the pertinent static mechanical properties of the vascular bed can be understood (Fig 4–6). The total blood volume in the arterial bed is the sum of the unstressed and stressed volumes. The stressed volume is a function of the compliance of the arterial bed and the transmural pressure of the bed when the steady state between emptying and filling is achieved. The unstressed volume is the maximum volume that the arteries can contain with no transmural pressure gradient. Transmural pressure is the pressure inside the vessel minus the pressure outside the vessel.

When considering the transmural arterial pressure, we usually assume that the pressure outside the vascular bed is atmospheric. In comparison, we relate cardiac chamber pressures either to atmospheric pressure, when we assess the pressure relation between the heart and the vas-

cular system, or to pleural pressure, when we assess the transmural pressure. For example, the right atrial pressure relative to atmospheric pressure is the pertinent downstream pressure for return of blood to the heart. On the other hand, left atrial pressure, or some reflection of it, is usually interpreted by taking into account the pressure surrounding it. If we are told a patient's left atrial pressure is 25 torr, we interpret the value much differently if we know that the patient is on 25 torr of positive end-expiratory pressure. For cardiac function we are more interested in transmural pressure.

Returning to the example of the bolus of stroke volume in a steady state, because of the distribution of arterial critical pressures and incremental flow resistances, 25% has gone to the SVC and 75% has gone to the IVC. The average arterial blood pressure of 100 torr has been determined by the flow and the total arterial resistance. The volume of blood in the arterial bed has been determined by the unstressed volume, which is a function of the arterial muscle tone, and the stressed volume, which is a function of the transmural arterial pressure and the arterial compliance. The bolus is now about to leave the high-pressure, high-resistance, low-compliance arterial bed and enter the venous bed where the pressure and resistance are an order of magnitude less and

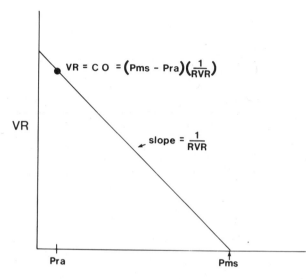

FIG 4–7.
A venous return curve as described in the text is shown. The mean systemic pressure *(Pms)* is equal to the vascular stressed volume divided by the systemic vascular compliance. The slope of the line is the reciprocal of the resistance to venous return *(RVR)*. The venous return *(VR)* in the steady state is equal to cardiac output *(CO)*. For any given right atrial pressure *(Pra)* above atmospheric pressure, VR is equal to the difference between Pms and Pra divided by RVR.

the compliance is an order of magnitude greater and where any critical pressure is an effect of the tissue pressure.

EFFECT OF VENOUS RESISTANCE AND COMPLIANCE

Since the downstream pressure draining the IVC and SVC venous beds is the right atrial pressure, the average pressure in each of these venous compartments will differ as a function of the resistance to outflow from each of the beds, the total flow through each of the beds, and the difference in tissue pressure for each bed. The average pressures in each of the venous compartments are important, since as we have seen they determine the amount of stressed volume in each of the venous beds. The IVC compliance is about four times that of the SVC for the same average pressure; and as the average venous pressure in a bed increases, for instance from increased flow, the compliance decreases. Even though the resistance to outflow in the IVC bed is about half that in the SVC bed, the average pressure in the IVC bed is greater than that in the SVC bed, primarily as a result of the greater flow. This tends to reduce the difference in compliance between the two beds. Nonetheless, the compliance in the IVC bed is greater. With the greater compliance and the higher average pressure, the IVC bed contains about four and a half times the stressed volume of the SVC bed.

Under the conditions of our example, the IVC bed has almost a four times greater compliance and half the venous resistance of the SVC bed. Therefore, the time constant (the product of the incremental flow resistance and the compliance) for drainage of the IVC bed is twice that of the SVC bed. The time constant is the time necessary for 63% of the stressed volume of an elastic container to empty across a resistance. With a heart rate of 60 beats/min and a stroke volume of 80 ml, the venous return required each second from the IVC bed would be about 60 ml, and from the SVC bed, about 20 ml. If the time constant of the IVC bed were 10 seconds and the SVC bed time constant were 5 seconds, then the stressed volume in the IVC bed would be about 575 ml and in the SVC bed about 125 ml in order for the steady state to be maintained. Because the time constant of each venous bed determines venous return from that bed, total venous return (and therefore cardiac output) can be regulated by distributing flow to beds with high or low time constant.

INFLUENCING CARDIAC OUTPUT

The cardiac output must equal the venous return in the steady state. As stated before, the venous return is proportional to the difference between the average pressure in the entire circulation, or the mean systemic pressure, and the right atrial pressure; it is inversely proportional to the resis-

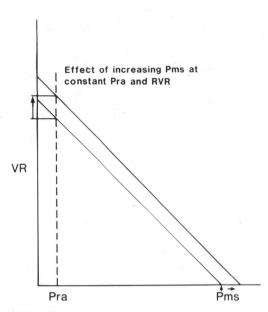

FIG 4–8.
The effect on venous return of a rise in mean systemic pressure *(Pms)*. Refer to Figure 4–7.

tance to venous return (Fig 4–7). The mean systemic pressure is a function of the stressed volume of the entire systemic circulation divided by the total systemic compliance. For a given right atrial pressure and resistance to venous return, cardiac output can be increased by increasing the mean systemic pressure (Fig 4–8).

The most familiar example of increasing the

cardiac output by increasing the mean systemic pressure is increasing the stressed volume by intravenous infusion of crystalloid or colloid solutions (Fig 4–9). Reflex or drug-related venoconstriction can also increase the stressed volume of the circulation. For the same total volume in the vascular bed, reducing the unstressed volume by venoconstriction results in a greater stressed volume, and thus an increase in the mean systemic pressure. Improvement of the inotropic state of the heart can also increase the systemic stressed volume. At a given cardiac afterload, improved contractility will reduce intracardiac and pulmonary blood volume. This volume is translocated to the systemic circuit and thereby increases the systemic vascular stressed volume.[5] Thus improvement in cardiac function increases cardiac output not only by reducing the right atrial pressure, but also by increasing the mean systemic pressure.

Cardiac output can also be increased by reducing the resistance to venous return (Fig 4–10). To understand the resistance to venous return we will consider the example of an arterial-to-venous (AV) fistula that is suddenly opened. In this case the stressed volume of the circulation is unchanged and, since the AV fistula has almost no compliance, the mean systemic pressure is unchanged. Right atrial pressure rises only slightly, yet cardiac output increases. The increase in cardiac output is the result of a decrease in the resistance to venous return.[2]

The AV fistula has a very low resistance and

FIG 4–9.
The pressure-volume relation of the circulation demonstrates the effect of venoconstriction or fluid infusion on the mean systemic pressure *(Pms)*. Both increase the stressed volume. Venoconstriction increases the stressed volume by decreasing the unstressed volume, and infusion increases the stressed volume by increasing the total blood volume.

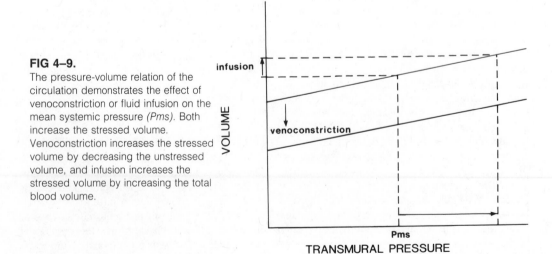

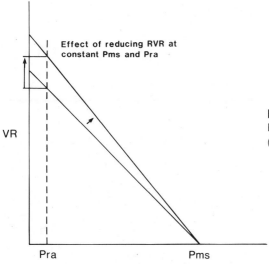

FIG 4–10.
Effect of a change in the resistance to venous return *(RVR)* on venous return *(VR).*

compliance, and therefore the time constant for drainage from the fistula is quite fast. One intuits that a red cell going through the fistula will return to the right atrium before a red cell leaving the heart simultaneously but going through the splanchnic circulation. So if the fraction of blood that goes through the fistula increases, more blood returns to the heart for any filling interval between beats, and cardiac output increases. More rigorously (Fig 4–11), it can be shown that the resistance to venous return is the sum of the fraction of cardiac output to each portion of the circulation, times the resistance to drainage from that portion of the circulation, times its fractional contribution to the total systemic vascular compliance. For any portion of the circulation this can be algebraically reduced to its fraction of the cardiac output times its time constant, divided by the total systemic compliance.[4] Such mathematical analyses become of greater interest as

therapeutic effort is directed toward pharmacologic manipulation of the distribution of perfusion.

Walking through the calculation for a 70-kg man with a systemic vascular compliance of about 140 ml/torr, an SVC time constant of 5 seconds with 25% of the cardiac output, an IVC time constant of 10 seconds with 75% of the cardiac output, and the whole arterial bed that gets 100% of the output with a time constant of about 3 seconds, the resistance to venous return is then 1.4 torr/L/min (Fig 4–12). With a mean systemic pressure of 7 torr and a right atrial pressure of zero, the cardiac output is 5 L/min. If we open an AV fistula (Fig 4–13) with a time constant of 0.05 second, which now receives 50% of the cardiac output at the expense of the IVC bed, which now receives 25% of the cardiac output, then with the right atrial pressure now 2 torr and all else being equal, the resistance to venous return

$$
\begin{aligned}
RVR &= R_{art}\left(\frac{C_{art}}{C_{tot}}\right)\left(\frac{F_{art}}{F_{tot}}\right) + R_{IVC}\left(\frac{C_{IVC}}{C_{tot}}\right)\left(\frac{F_{IVC}}{F_{tot}}\right) + R_{SVC}\left(\frac{C_{SVC}}{C_{tot}}\right)\left(\frac{F_{SVC}}{F_{tot}}\right) \\
&= \left(\frac{R_{art}\,C_{art}}{C_{tot}}\right)\left(\frac{F_{art}}{F_{tot}}\right) + \left(\frac{R_{IVC}\,C_{IVC}}{C_{tot}}\right)\left(\frac{F_{IVC}}{F_{tot}}\right) + \left(\frac{R_{SVC}\,C_{SVC}}{C_{tot}}\right)\left(\frac{F_{SVC}}{F_{tot}}\right) \\
&= \left(\frac{T_{art}}{C_{tot}}\right)\left(\frac{F_{art}}{F_{tot}}\right) + \left(\frac{T_{IVC}}{C_{tot}}\right)\left(\frac{F_{IVC}}{F_{tot}}\right) + \left(\frac{T_{SVC}}{C_{tot}}\right)\left(\frac{F_{SVC}}{F_{tot}}\right)
\end{aligned}
$$

FIG 4–11.
Equation for the resistance to venous return *(RVR).* *R*, resistance; *C*, compliance; *F*, flow; *T*, time constant (product of *R* and *C*) for the part of the circuit indicated by the subscript; *art,* arterial bed; SVC and IVC, venous bed drained by those veins; *tot,* the entire systemic circulation.

$$
\begin{aligned}
\text{RVR} &= \left(\frac{T_{art}}{C_{tot}}\right)\left(\frac{F_{art}}{F_{tot}}\right) + \left(\frac{T_{IVC}}{C_{tot}}\right)\left(\frac{F_{IVC}}{F_{tot}}\right) + \left(\frac{T_{SVC}}{C_{tot}}\right)\left(\frac{F_{SVC}}{F_{tot}}\right) \\
&= \left(\frac{3\text{ sec}}{140\text{ ml/torr}}\right)(1) + \left(\frac{10\text{ sec}}{140\text{ ml/torr}}\right)(.75) + \left(\frac{5\text{ sec}}{140\text{ ml/torr}}\right)(.25) \\
&= .021\,\frac{\text{torr}}{(\text{ml/sec})} + .054 + .009 \\
&= \frac{.084\text{ torr}}{\text{ml/sec}} \\
&= 1.4\text{ torr/(L/min)}
\end{aligned}
$$

$$
\begin{aligned}
\text{CO} = \text{VR} &= \frac{P_{ms} - P_{ra}}{\text{RVR}} \\
&= \frac{7\text{ torr} - 0\text{ torr}}{1.4\text{ torr/(L/min)}} \\
&= 5\text{ L/min}
\end{aligned}
$$

FIG 4–12.
Calculations of RVR and cardiac output *(CO).*

is now 0.8 torr/L/min, and the cardiac output is now 6.25 L/min.

Similarly, a redistribution of the cardiac output from the longer IVC bed to the SVC bed will also increase cardiac output. Considering the single bolus of stroke volume that left the heart at the beginning of our example, the fraction that went to the SVC bed will return to the heart before the fraction that went to the IVC bed. Intuitively, if a greater fraction of cardiac output went to the SVC bed, it would return faster to the right atrium and cardiac output would have to increase. In fact, the actual portion of the bolus that went to the IVC bed is additionally delayed in returning to the right atrium because of the larger volume of distribution that is present in the portion of the vascular bed drained by the IVC.

To this point we have considered the IVC

$$
\begin{aligned}
\text{RVR} &= \left(\frac{T_{art}}{C_{tot}}\right)\left(\frac{F_{art}}{F_{tot}}\right) + \left(\frac{T_{IVC}}{C_{tot}}\right)\left(\frac{F_{IVC}}{F_{tot}}\right) + \left(\frac{T_{SVC}}{C_{tot}}\right)\left(\frac{F_{SVC}}{F_{tot}}\right)\left(\frac{T_{av}}{C_{tot}}\right)\left(\frac{F_{av}}{F_{tot}}\right) \\
&= \left(\frac{3\text{ sec}}{140\text{ ml/torr}}\right) 1 + \left(\frac{10\text{ sec}}{140\text{ ml/torr}}\right)(.25) + \left(\frac{5\text{ sec}}{140\text{ ml/torr}}\right)(.25) + \left(\frac{.05\text{ sec}}{140\text{ ml/torr}}\right)(.5) \\
&= .021\text{ torr/(ml/sec)} + .018 + .009 + .0002 \\
&= \frac{.0482\text{ torr}}{(\text{ml/sec})} \\
&= 0.8\text{ torr/L/min}
\end{aligned}
$$

$$
\begin{aligned}
\text{CO} = \text{VR} &= \frac{P_{ms} - P_{ra}}{\text{RVR}} \\
&= \frac{7\text{ torr} - 2\text{ torr}}{0.8\text{ torr/(L/min)}} \\
&= 6.25\text{ L/min}
\end{aligned}
$$

FIG 4–13.
Effect of a short time constant bed [systemic arteriovenous (AV) fistula] on RVR and CO.

bed as a single drainage system. If the splanchnic and renal and adrenal circulations are considered separately, then the remainder of the IVC bed is muscle and skin. Since the time constant for drainage of the muscle and skin portion of the IVC is as fast as that of the SVC and if more of the cardiac output to the region drained by the IVC goes to muscle and skin, then the time constant for the whole IVC will be reduced. In this case the cardiac output will also be increased. This can partially explain the increase in cardiac output seen with exercise or hyperthermia, which is discussed in detail in the next chapter.

REFERENCES

1. Ehrlich W, Schrijen FU, Solomon TA, et al: Arterial pressure-flow relations in the awake standing dog. *Am J Physiol* 1975; 229:1261–1267.
2. Guyton AC, Sagawa K: Compensations of cardiac output and other circulatory functions in areflexic dogs with large a-v fistulae. *Am J Physiol* 1961; 200:1157–1165.
3. Malo J, Goldberg HS, Graham R, et al: Effect of hypoxic hypoxia on systemic vasculature. *J Appl Physiol* 1984; 56:1403–1410.
4. Mitzner W, Goldberg HS: Effects of epinephrine on the resistive and compliant properties of the canine vasculature. *J Appl Physiol* 1975; 39:272–280.
5. Mitzner W, Goldberg HS, Lichtenstein S: Effects of thoracic blood volume changes on steady state cardiac output. *Circ Res* 1976; 38:255–261.

Patterns of Hemodynamic Response

James V. Snyder, M.D.

NORMAL VASOREGULATION

Autoregulation

The circulation must supply enough blood flow to sustain the necessary metabolic functions of the tissues if the organism is to survive. Therefore, tissues with widely varying energy requirements must have the ability to influence delivery of flow to match their local needs, or sometimes must have blood flow much greater than those needs. The existence of this form of metabolic vasoregulation is supported by a large body of experimental data. Unless stated otherwise, the term autoregulation will refer to regulation of local flow by some response in the tissue. The pertinent physiology, as reviewed by Sparks[72] and Shepherd et al.,[66] includes the following features. (1) As metabolic activity increases in heart and skeletal muscle, increases in $\dot{V}O_2$ precede increases in blood flow. (2) Within a given skeletal muscle tissue bed, arteriolar diameter varies inversely with venular PO_2 at 30 torr. This relationship is attenuated at higher venous PO_2 values, being totally abolished at $PO_2 > 40$ torr. (3) Arterial wall hypoxia does not directly cause arterial dilation except possibly at precapillary sphincters. (4) Different tissue and arterial systems vary regarding their hypoxic sensitivity.

Besides local autoregulation of oxygen supply, regulation of oxygen supply to the entire body has also been demonstrated in dogs,[66] such that $\dot{V}O_2$ is maintained despite sudden changes in arterial pressure and PaO_2. The effectivity of this systemic response was mirrored by changes in $C(a - \bar{v})O_2$. $C(a - \bar{v})O_2$ and cardiac output alterations that occur during hypoxia and hypotension also suggest that $\dot{V}O_2$ determines oxygen transport, not vice versa. Overall, the gain of the tissue response correlated highest with the availability/need ratio (equivalent to $C\bar{v}O_2/\dot{V}O_2$). Although in tissues that are hypoxic, oxygen delivery determines oxygen consumption, adequately oxygenated tissues regulate oxygen delivery according to their own need.

Although hypoxia-induced autoregulation alone can define many of the responses associated with increased $\dot{V}O_2$, it cannot by itself account for the maintenance of normal resting cardiac output. In fact, at rest tissues are generally perfused in excess of their needs. That excess local blood flow is determined primarily by the *myogenic response of the arterioles;* that is, they dilate when luminal pressure falls and constrict when it rises, independent of metabolic demand. A metabolic feedback may underlie the myogenic response, although none has been found. The myogenic response maintains capillary pressure constant and is checked, and sometimes counteracted, by sympathetic and metabolic influences. The myogenic mechanism probably dominates the circulation in most beds by regulating hydrostatic pressure and fluid exchange to establish local flow in excess of metabolic needs. As the body adapts to changing internal and external demands on the circulation, the myogenic control of local flow is overridden.

Normal Distribution and Responsive Capacity

As reviewed by Folkow and Neil, basal (resting) vascular tone varies widely in different tissues: "Tissues that evince a wide range of metabolic activity, such as muscles, and salivary glands, manifest an especially high basal vascular tone which is correspondingly reduced when the tissue does work. In contrast, in the kidney, which works steadily, basal vascular tone is low."[29] The relationship between maximal blood flow and resting blood flow in a number of tissues is schematically illustrated in Figure 5–1.

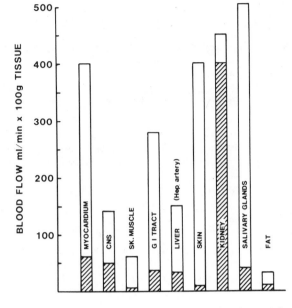

FIG 5–1.
Regional blood flows per 100 gm of tissue at "rest" *(shaded areas)* and at maximal dilation *(total areas)*. Figures below bars are approximate figures for a 70-kg man. The flow figures are given both for 100 gm of tissue and for the entire organs. (Modified from Mellander et al.,[45] by permission. Values for skin blood flow are from Rowell.[57])

Rest.blood flow (l/min):	0.21	0.75	0.75	0.7	0.5	0.2	1.2	0.02	0.8 ≈ 5.1
Max. blood flow (l/min):	1.2	2.1	18.0	5.5	3.0	7.5	1.4	0.25	3.0 ≈ 38
Organ weight (kg):	0.3	1.5	30	2.0	1.7	2.0	0.3	0.05	10 ≈ 48

This observation of normally high basal vascular tone, along with observed responses to various stresses in normal and compromised humans, creates a paradigm that can be applied to critically ill patients. Parallels to critical illness are suggested in some of the following sections in which experimental observations are described. Patterns of flow in which the dilation of specific beds is maximal occur during exercise and exogenous heat stress.

Exercise

The close matching of blood flow and oxygen consumption in exercise requires both augmentation and redistribution of cardiac output.[58] If pulmonary and cardiovascular systems are normal, exercise capacity depends on maximal cardiac output and $C(a - \bar{v})_{O_2}$.[47] As reviewed by Mitchell and Blomqvist, normally during submaximal work a nearly linear relation exists between cardiac output and $\dot{V}o_2$. From standing at rest to maximal exercise the consumption of oxygen increases 12 times. This is accomplished by increases of four times in cardiac output and almost three times in $C(a - \bar{v})_{O_2}$. The augmented cardiac output results from a doubling of both heart rate and stroke volume. The increase in heart rate and stroke volume is important in keeping right atrial pressure low and thus facilitating a maximal venous return. Because the $C(a - \bar{v})_{O_2}$ across the heart at rest is large, oxygenation of the myocardium is almost completely dependent on the increase in coronary blood flow to obtain its increased oxygen requirements.[47] Cerebral blood flow remains the same during maximal exercise as at rest. Renal and splanchnic blood flow is markedly diminished and partially compensated for by a wider $C(a - \bar{v})_{O_2}$ during heavy exercise. The common occurrence of abdominal pain during exercise after eating suggests that diversion of flow from abdominal viscera can be excessive. These regional responses are explored in more detail in chapter 7, "Control of Organ Blood Flow."

In the steady state, cardiac output can never be increased more than venous return. Venous return is increased during exercise by the constriction of inflow vessels to venous beds with high compliance (splanchnic vessels), thereby reducing their fraction of the cardiac output and allowing them to empty more completely. Similarly, blood flow is diverted into vascular beds with low compliance (muscle). Venous return is thus increased, reducing the unstressed volume (splanchnic circulation) and increasing the stressed volume (muscle circulation), which increases the mean systemic pressure (see chapter 4, "Control of Cardiac Output by the Circuit"). Vasoconstriction in other beds helps divert as much as 85% of total cardiac output to working skeletal muscles.[58] The range of response to exercise is exemplified by endurance athletes, normal sedentary subjects, and patients with "pure" mitral stenosis.[57, 58] In all of these subjects, cardiac output is distributed in the same way during exercise (Fig 5–2). In addition to the progressive reduction of visceral flow and the increased flow needed by the heart, note how the blood flow to the skin increases with exercise that is moderate (relative to the subject's capacity), then decreases again as muscle work (and heat generation) is increased maximally. This strongly suggests an element of competition for flow between maximally working muscle and the system for controlling heat loss. Similar competition is likely in critically ill patients.

Hyperthermia

Environmental heating in man causes redistribution of blood volume and flow that is different from that due to autoregulation (Fig 5–3).[57, 58] Environmental heat stress results in activation of a neurogenic vasodilator system in the skin, which permits a high rate of cutaneous perfusion. Skin blood flow increases by a remarkable 3 L/min per °C increase in core temperature.[57] The normally tight coupling between local $\dot{V}O_2$ and tissue blood flow persists except in the skin, where flow greatly exceeds that required for oxygenation. The response to heat stress is shown

in Figure 5–3, where right atrial pressure is lowered by 5 torr and renal and splanchnic blood flow is reduced 30%–40% while cardiac output doubles. In addition, the cutaneous venous network is capacious and highly distensible, in contrast to the vessels of working muscle, which act as conduits to return blood quickly to the heart. As a result, a considerable proportion of the blood volume is shifted to the larger capacitance skin vessels, and the higher cardiac output is maintained with a lower right atrial pressure. The cutaneous vasodilation system in man is activated by central thermoreceptors. Redistribution of blood flow away from visceral organs is probably initiated by the same central mechanism.[58]

Thermal stress in the ICU environment, although rarely so severe as used by Rowell, can vary widely. Cardiovascular adjustments to thermal stress are complex and can be dramatic.[57] As hypothalamic regulation of cutaneous circulation responds to endogenous pyrogens, antipyretics, and environmental cold stresses, the degree to which the patient's systemic vascular resistance, distribution of blood volume, and cardiac output are influenced is unknown but potentially significant when local or systemic oxygen transport is compromised. Although the response to environmental heat stress is different from the effect of fever, clinicians should still consider the shifts in distribution of cardiac output and changes in preload and afterload that patients might be undergoing during, for example, prolonged elevations of temperature or when fever "breaks."

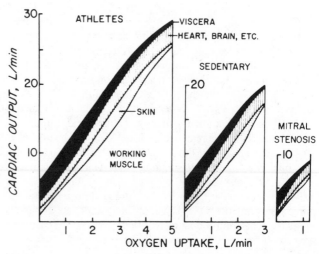

FIG 5–2.
Distribution of cardiac output during upright exercise in endurance athletes with high maximal $\dot{V}O_2$ (5 L/min), in sedentary men (maximal $\dot{V}O_2$, 3 L/min), and in patients with pure mitral stenosis (maximal $\dot{V}O_2$, 1.4 L/min). All subjects redistribute blood away from visceral organs to the same degree at any given percentage of their maximal $\dot{V}O_2$. (From Rowell LB: The distribution of blood flow and its regulation in humans, in Loeppky JA, Riedesel ML (eds): *Oxygen Transport in Human Tissues.* New York, Elsevier North-Holland, 1982, pp. 113–124. © 1982, reproduced by permission.)

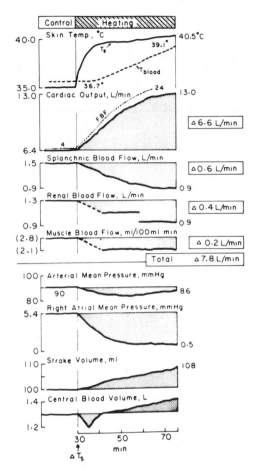

FIG 5–3.
Average circulatory changes in men directly heated by raising body skin temperature to 40°–41° C by means of water-perfused suits. Boxes on the right show average changes in flow to the specified regions; the sum of these changes (7.8 L/min) must go to skin. Note the decline in atrial pressure. (*FBF* = forearm blood flow.) (From Rowell.[59] Reproduced by permission.)

Heat and Exercise

The combination of heat and exercise presents humans with two severe regulatory problems,[58] because blood volume is shifted into cutaneous veins when skin vasodilates, and central blood volume and cardiac filling pressure are lower. Hence, cardiac output cannot be augmented to the same degree. In addition, there are two competing demands for the limited cardiac output. During moderate and heavy exercise, an increase in heart rate (which at a given venous return will

serve to keep right atrial pressure low) is necessary to achieve higher cardiac output. When venous return is limited, as when the unstressed blood volume is increased by filling cutaneous veins, heart rate approaches maximal values at submaximal levels of $\dot{V}O_2$. As expressed by Rowell, "During exercise, forearm [skin blood flow] is reduced below what it would be at the same core temperature during rest in hyperthermic subjects. Once [the core temperature] exceeds 38° C, the [skin blood flow] response tends to saturate at values that are only half of those attainable at rest. Thus a relative cutaneous vasoconstriction reduces or delays the peripheral displacement of blood volume and helps to compensate for the reduced ability to raise cardiac output so that blood pressure is maintained, but temperature regulation is impeded."[58] Therefore, when increased work load and need for heat loss are combined, both reduced work capacity and severe hyperthermia may be observed. These limitations in organ blood flow that result from competition for limited blood flow resemble the respiratory death seen in cardiogenic shock resulting from inadequate blood flow to respiratory muscles.[42, 62] The effect of superimposition of heat stress on the normal pattern of blood flow distribution during exercise is shown in Figure 5–4.

The Stress Response

As Cannon summarized his classic observations, "The adrenin secreted in times of stress . . . cooperates with sympathetic nerve impulses in calling for stored carbohydrate from the liver, thus flooding the blood with sugar; it helps in distributing the blood to the heart, lungs, central nervous system, and limbs, while taking it away from the inhibited organs of the abdomen; it quickly abolishes the effects of muscular fatigue; and it renders the blood more rapidly coagulable."[13] The acute response to stress includes an increase in oxygen transport relative to demand with lower $C(a-\bar{v})O_2$ and increased $P\bar{v}O_2$, as well as a redistribution of blood flow away from viscera. The response involves both neural and humoral elements and is almost instantaneous (Fig 5–5).

Stress is inherent in virtually all patients admitted to intensive care, and we sometimes see striking similarity between the stress response described by Cannon and the hyperdynamic states commonly seen in septic and other critically ill

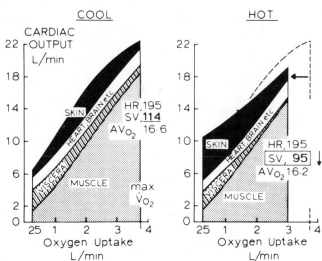

FIG 5–4.
Approximate distribution of cardiac output during upright exercise in 6 normal subjects in cool (25° C) and hot (43° C) environments. At 43° C, the reduction in stroke volume *(SV)* ultimately led to reduced cardiac output, and maximal heart rate *(HR)* and systemic arteriovenous oxygen difference *(AV$_{O_2}$)* were reached at submaximal levels of $\dot{V}_{O_2}$. Note the fall-off in blood flow to skin, which was observed by Brengelmann et al.[7] in the forearm. (From Rowell.[59] Reproduced by permission.)

patients.[1, 4, 36, 65] It is interesting to compare the experiences ICU patients encounter with a list of stressors used in animal studies, used typically because they are severely stressful (Table 5–1), and with stressors typically used in human research (Table 5–2).[20] It is obvious from these tables that responses to stress that are independent of or in addition to those related to the primary organic illness may be a major determinant of the hemodynamic response in any ICU patient. In addition, unpredictability adds significantly to the potency of a potential stress stimulus.[20] Unpredictability (for the patient) is characteristic of any intensive care experience and might be a major determinant of the stress of that experience. It is reasonable to expect that the unpredictability and related stress of admission to the ICU would be diminished by introducing preoperative patients to the ICU, establishing schedules for awake patients, and clearly stating plans in advance. Natural support systems can be effective in buffering stressful experiences.[21] Perhaps these observations should influence such practices as limiting visiting hours in ICUs.[78] External environmental factors also may strongly mediate stress. The effect of gardens and open space, light-colored rooms, or quiet surroundings in reducing the stressful effects of a high population density[26] can be used to advantage in ICUs.

The stress response, although almost uniformly experienced by all patients in an ICU, still has an ill-defined and variable cardiovascular effect. The Institute of Medicine has recently reviewed stress.[20] They suggest a conceptual framework of stresses *(x)*, reactions *(y)*, consequences *(z)*, and mediators. "Stressors are events or conditions that elicit physical or psychosocial reactions. To avoid the tautology inherent in such a definition, the committee recommended that events or conditions be identified as potential stressors based on the probability that they will be stressors in a particular individual under a given circumstance. *Reactions* are biologic and psychosocial responses of an individual to a stressor. *Consequences* are physical or psychosocial results of such reactions. And *mediators* are filters and modifiers that define the context in which the stressor-reaction-consequence *(x-y-z)* sequence occurs."[22]

Although stressors have often been associated with consequences *(x-z)*, the intervening steps have not been elucidated. Potential stressors may or may not elicit a definable response in an individual, depending on the strength, the repetition or chronicity, and the context of the stimulus, the individual's interpretation of the stimulus, and genetic and environmental predisposition.[22]

Stressors are not all noxious, and stress responses are not necessarily detrimental to the subject. Thus, "stressors, reactions, and mediators are neither 'good' nor 'bad'; only consequences can appropriately be qualified as being desirable or undesirable."[24]

If physical stressors are not viewed as noxious or alarming, they produce smaller or even

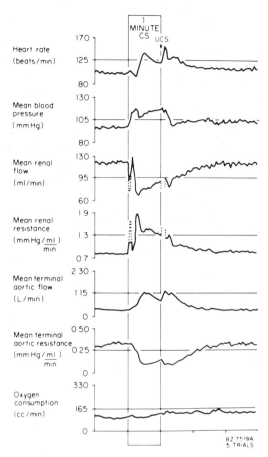

FIG 5–5.
Cardiovascular response to acute stress. Cardiovascular variables during a conditioned emotional response of a baboon to an auditory signal *(CS)* followed by an electrical shock *(UCS)* are plotted. The initial decrease in renal blood flow is due to neurally mediated constriction of renal vessels. The second renal blood flow decrease and the delayed increase in terminal aortic flow appear due to circulating epinephrine. The somatic vasodilation that causes increased terminal aortic flow and the increase in heart rate could be prevented by administration of a β-blocking agent (propranolol). The decreases in renal blood flow may be prevented by α-blockade (phentolamine). (From Smith et al.[69] Reproduced by permission.)

opposite physiologic responses. For example, monkeys exposed to a rapid rise in the environmental temperature show a brisk rise in adrenal corticosteroid secretion, a classic stress response; yet if the temperature is raised just as high but at a much slower rate to avoid the perception of it as novel, steroid secretion is suppressed. Determining whether an event is a stressor may depend on the subject's cognitive appraisal or on subcortical responses.

That these responses may have important sequelae and be modifiable in the setting of acute illness is suggested by recent observations in patients with coronary artery disease.[37] In these subjects, ST-segment depression was specifically associated with mental arithmetic. In this task, autonomic changes occurred that suggest β-sympathetic activation.

While the concept of a single response to stress is useful, it may be important to recognize a variation in the components and even direction of stress responses. In addition to catecholamines and corticosteroids, prolactin, insulin, growth hormone, testosterone, and luteinizing hormone have been found to be responsive to stress. The pattern of hormones released may vary with the emotion or activity involved[23, 31] or with personality traits.[25, 30, 35, 37, 44, 63, 75]

Stress has important interactions with the immune system, and the science of psychoneuroimmunology has developed a broad foundation.[17] This is the study of the interactions between the CNS and the immune system. It is founded on the concept that the immune system is integrated with other physiologic processes, and on considerable evidence that the CNS modulates the course of immunogenesis.[2, 34] Observations have advanced from those by Galen that melancholic women are more prone to cancer,[71] to the effect of psychological conditioning on antibody responses in mice.[32] Terman and colleagues have concluded that "the experience of 'helplessness' is important for the immunosuppressive and tumor-enhancing effects of stress, and that opioid peptides causing analgesia associated with 'helplessness' are also involved in mediating these immunologic and oncologic effects."[74] In some observations the response of immunologic reactivity varies with time, being first depressed and then increased.[2] While stress is clearly documented as a risk factor, the effects of stress are neither uniformly detrimental nor beneficial to the organism.[2]

In summary, a stress response almost invariably influences cardiovascular homeostasis, but the effect may vary from the extremes of hyperdynamic states resembling high output sepsis to more subtle patterns of myocardial dysfunction. Modification of the environment and of personal interaction can significantly lessen the severity of

TABLE 5–1.

Typical Stressors Used in Animal Research*

Cardiac catheterization	Immobilization
Cold exposure	Maternal deprivation
Competitive social interaction	Novel environments
Electric shock	Prolonged forced swimming
Food deprivation	Sensory deprivation
Handling	Sleep deprivation
Heat exposure	Social crowding
Immersion in ice water	Social isolation

*From Elliott and Eisdorfer,[20] p. 14. Reproduced by permission.

the stress response. However, stress can enhance as well as impair not only the hemodynamic responses but the psychological and immunologic defense systems as well. Hence, it is not always clear that the avoidance or relief of stress is bene-

TABLE 5–2.

Typical Stressors Used in Human Research*

EXPERIMENTAL STIMULI
   Acute stressors
      Threatening, unpleasant films
      Understimulation/demand underload
      Overstimulation/demand overload
      Noise, unexpected or uncontrollable
      Prestige or status loss
      Electric shock
      Approach-avoidance conflicts
      Uncontrollable situations
   Chronic stressors
      Sleep deprivation

NATURAL EVENTS
   Acute stressors
      Physical illness (including surgery,
         hospitalization)
      Threats to self-esteem
      Traumatic experiences
   Stress-event sequences
      Bereavement
      Losses of any type (physical, psychological, or
         social)
      Migration
      Retirement
      Status change (e.g., job change, salary change,
         marriage)
   Chronic and chronic intermittent stressors
      Daily "hassles"
      Demand overload or underload
      Role strains
      Social isolation

*From Elliott and Eisdorfer,[20] p. 16. Reproduced by permission.

ficial.[41] It is clear, however, that stress is an important factor to consider when interpreting hemodynamic patterns in patients.

Blood Loss

The cardiovascular response to simulated hemorrhage (lower body negative pressure) in humans is illustrated in Figure 5–6. First, right atrial pressure falls, resulting in a reflex vasoconstriction of cutaneous and skeletal muscle vascular beds followed by a 15% decrease in splanchnic blood flow. The subsequent decline in aortic pulse pressure (mean pressure constant) is closely paralleled by a rising heart rate, a falling splanchnic blood flow, and little additional change in forearm blood flow.[56] The arteriolar constriction allows passive drainage of downstream capacitance beds in mild hemorrhage. If hemorrhage continues, active venoconstriction also occurs.[33] Of the total compensatory decrease in vascular conductance in normal man, an estimated one third is contributed by vasoconstriction of the splanchnic bed, 39% by skin and muscle beds, and 28% by the kidneys.[58] Indirectly, these figures suggest that patients with compromised or no renal blood flow and/or diminished muscle mass may have a reduced ability to maintain blood pressure and flow after blood loss. Under normal conditions, decreasing arterial pressure induces a local vasodilation to maintain tissue blood flow. However, in hemorrhage, strong sympathetic discharge "overrides" this vasodilator response, presumably in an attempt to maintain central arterial pressure high enough for vital organ perfusion. The lower arterial pressure and the greater increase in the ratio of precapillary to postcapillary vascular resistance both reduce capillary pressure. This capillary pressure fall reverses the normal tendency for edema formation, promoting an influx of fluid from extracellular

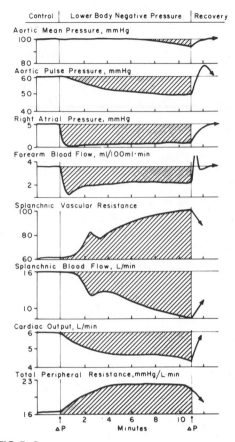

Control | Lower Body Negative Pressure | Recovery

Aortic Mean Pressure, mmHg
100
80

Aortic Pulse Pressure, mmHg
60
50
40

Right Atrial Pressure, mmHg
5
0

Forearm Blood Flow, ml/100ml·min
4
2

Splanchnic Vascular Resistance
100
80
60

Splanchnic Blood Flow, L/min
16
10

Cardiac Output, L/min
6
5
4

Total Peripheral Resistance, mmHg/L·min
23
16

ΔP 2 4 6 8 10 ΔP
Minutes

FIG 5–6.
Schematic illustration of cardiovascular responses when blood is sequestered in the lower extremities by application of −50 torr pressure below the iliac crests. (From Rowell.[60] Reproduced by permission.)

space.[33] Sympathetic stimulation also stimulates glucagon release, with resulting hyperglycemia. The oncotic pressure difference created by this hyperglycemia may further contribute to tissue fluid resorption.[33] Accordingly, the adaptive response to mild or moderate blood loss allows optimal regulation of flow according to local needs by sacrificing excess flow to nonvital tissue and by resorption of interstitial and intracellular fluid.

In hypovolemic patients, patients in cardiogenic shock, and exercising subjects, the algebraic concepts of the oxygen transport model are seen most clearly, and the implications of the model (for the interpretation of $P\bar{v}_{O_2}$, for example) are most reliable. The algebraic model is less reliable when the distribution of flow is influenced by factors other than current metabolic need. Thus, cutaneous vasodilation and the stress response each cause total oxygen transport to be greater than need. Local autoregulation remains intact, and local oxygenation usually remains adequate, but any factor that changes distribution of flow according to other than metabolic needs will inevitably compromise our ability to assess the adequacy of oxygen transport. More familiar than stress and thermal regulation as causes of confusion in assessment are the hemodynamic effects of sepsis and cirrhosis.

ABNORMAL PATTERNS OF RESPONSE

In the broad and complex range of insults and responses involved in the critically ill, there is often no clear line between physiology and pathology. Normal vasoregulation includes autoregulation, the maintenance of local flow according to local needs, and an increase in flow independent of metabolic need, such as during cutaneous vasodilation for heat loss and during the stress response. Vasodilation and perfusion in excess of oxygen need are also normal components of the inflammatory response. Inflammation, therefore, causes a blurring of the oxygen supply/demand relation similar to that caused by cutaneous vasodilation to control body temperature. Normally the demands for increased flow over that required for metabolism can be met, but when they are excessive or when the ability of the cardiovascular system to respond is compromised, a competition for flow like that seen during combined exercise and hyperthermia (see Fig 5–4) may occur, and the probability of ill consequences increases. Local ischemia is more likely and will occur at higher cardiac output than in normals when sepsis, cirrhosis, or other conditions cause widespread perturbation of normal adaptive vasoregulation. When vasoregulation is disturbed, loss of perfusion to a small vascular bed can easily be missed or discerned only through a secondary metabolic consequence or a loss of function. Within these disturbances, it is often difficult to discern when functional problems are primarily a result of a "steal" by overdilated vessels or when they are due primarily to vascular obstruction. A hyperdynamic state may be an ominous sign (of sepsis) but may also indicate simply the presence of stress and the capability of a vigorous response. A normal cardiac index, systemic vascular resistance, and $P\bar{v}_{O_2}$ may be an ominous conjunction in a septic or cirrhotic patient. A rising $P\bar{v}_{O_2}$ may indicate improvement in tissue oxygenation or may be the first sign of sepsis. The hyperdynamic responses associated with various conditions and the loss of metabolic regulation that commonly accompanies these states are discussed in the following section.

Sepsis

The hyperdynamic response in sepsis has both similarities to and differences from the stress response. The stress response is a highly sophisticated response in which high-capacitance reservoirs of blood are mobilized and flow is shifted from the slower splanchnic circuit to higher-flow somatic beds.[55] Flow to the viscera is markedly depressed, but normally a fine degree of control is maintained, and the viability of those tissues is not threatened acutely. Similarities in high output sepsis include the increase in cardiac index and the decrease in systemic vascular resistance, although the mechanisms of these changes are probably different. Because local vasoregulation is compromised and mobilization of blood from venous capacitance beds is much less effective in sepsis, aggressive intravascular volume loading may be required to maintain perfusion of all beds.

In our experience the hemodynamic and metabolic changes in sepsis usually remain logical when the following items are considered. (1) *Severe untreated sepsis in the absence of liver cirrhosis is associated characteristically with low cardiac output without major anomalies of distribution.* The low output is due largely to failure to mobilize blood from the venous capacitance system, and may not be seen if volume administration is sufficient. Bacteremia can produce hypotension (apparently by interfering with mobilization of capacitance blood, releasing of endogenous vasodilators, increasing capillary permeability, and simultaneously inhibiting the normal cardiac response) within seconds in experimental animals.[14] (2) The inflammatory process causes blood flow at the site of infection to increase in excess of apparent metabolic need. In systemic sepsis this occurs over wide areas. (3) As in any stressed state, after volume loading cardiac output can be supranormal. The nonspecific nature of the high output response in sepsis is suggested by the inability to distinguish gram-negative, gram-positive, and fungal sepsis hemodynami-

cally.[77] (4) The increase in cardiac output in experimental sepsis is associated with capillary hyperperfusion and not with the opening of larger arteriovenous anastomoses[14] (see chapter 28, "Pathology and Treatment of Septic Shock"). Thus, the hyperdynamic response associated with sepsis may be basically a normal stress response in a patient who is volume loaded sufficiently to compensate for a compliant vascular bed; inflammatory hyperfusion may contribute to this picture but is not essential. A similar distribution of cardiac output to vascular resistance ratios (Fig 5–7) indicates that the response is a systemic one and not related directly to features of the organism such as endotoxin. (5) The occluded pulmonary artery or wedge pressure (WP) in sepsis may exceed the left atrial pressure because of collateral pulmonary circulation and, therefore, mislead the clinician to think that fluid resuscitation is adequate when it is not.[70] (6) Microvascular perfusion can deteriorate quickly, and fluid resuscitation may reestablish perfusion only slowly or inadequately if blood in the microvasculature has become too viscid. Maximal fluid resuscitation may, therefore, resolve all ischemia or may diminish only the outward progression of ischemia from established islands. (7) The carotid baroceptors can reset in response to a change in pressure in as little as 2 hours. Therefore, resuscitation need be carried only to the point of restoring function, and a satisfactory arterial pressure may be considerably lower than normal for that patient. (8) Caution is appropriate when calculated systemic vascular resistance is used in defining hemodynamic responses because incorrect assumptions are made in the customary calculation (see chapter 15, "Technical Problems in Data Acquisition") and because there are other elements in vascular resistance besides tone. For example, blood viscosity is often reduced by fluid resuscitation, thereby reducing systemic vascular resistance.[73]

Thus, the expression of sepsis as a high output state appears to combine features of a stress response with an increase in venous capacitance but still adequate intravascular volume and compromise of local autoregulation.

The most viable paradigm in systemic sepsis is that some beds acquire flow well in excess of need and at the same time that flow is deficient in other beds. The underperfusion and overperfusion might occur within the same microvascular bed in capillaries with increased resistance to

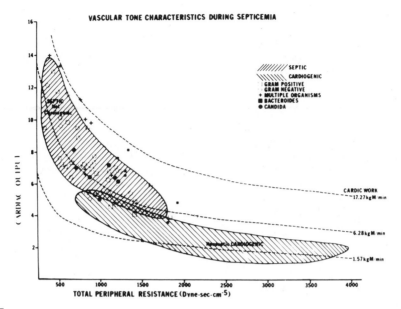

FIG 5–7.

Vascular tone characteristics during septicemia, illustrated with reference to nonseptic cardiogenic patients and septic noncardiogenic patients. The cardiac output/total peripheral resistance ratios are similarly distributed for all organisms, indicating that the septic physiologic response is a systemic one and is largely independent of the organism. (From Wiles et al.[77] Reproduced by permission.)

flow and via collateral bypass capillaries.[33] Thus, the high cardiac output state is still potentially associated with local hypoperfusion. The threat is not in the hyperdynamic state (unless heart function is compromised) but in the simultaneous local underperfusion. Local increase in microvascular resistance may be due to local viscous changes or to increased tissue edema, microemboli, or endothelial cell swelling, as postulated for trauma patients.[65] The high flow may be due to impaired vasoregulation or may in part show an appropriate local response to hypoxia in adjacent tissue to maximize oxygen delivery. Signs of tissue ischemia, such as organ dysfunction or lactic acidemia associated with high cardiac output or $P\bar{v}_{O_2}$, should not be presumed to be due to arteriovenous (AV) anastomoses or histotoxicity,[4] but may be due to focal hypoperfusion, which might respond to an increase in overall cardiac output or to specific vasoactive drugs. If this paradigm is correct, microcirculatory vasoderegulation would be characterized by a dependence of $\dot{V}_{O_2}$ on $\dot{D}_{O_2}$, such that both local circulation and the consumption of oxygen might be increased to normal or above normal as oxygen transport is improved. Indeed, this dependence of $\dot{V}_{O_2}$ on

$\dot{D}_{O_2}$ has been observed when $\dot{D}_{O_2}$ is increased in septic patients.[36, 38, 39]

We could also see increased $\dot{V}_{O_2}$ independent of changes in $\dot{D}_{O_2}$ if distribution of oxygen transport were altered beneficially. This would appear as an improvement in vasoregulation, in contrast to an increase in $\dot{V}_{O_2}$ related to increased perfusion of all vessels. Improving flow to all vascular beds may be a useful therapy but does not improve vasoregulation. Improved vasoregulation would not necessarily correlate with changes in measured individual hemodynamic indices such as cardiac output, $\dot{D}_{O_2}$, $C(a-\bar{v})_{O_2}$, or $P\bar{v}_{O_2}$. Indeed, these indices could improve without a change in vasoregulation. For example, the increase in limb and total $\dot{V}_{O_2}$ accompanying increased $\dot{D}_{O_2}$ with hypertonic mannitol in adult respiratory distress syndrome[54] may be due to reduction of endothelial cell swelling or interstitial edema or to microcirculatory viscosity changes.[65] The increased oxygen uptake that has been observed following phlebotomy and simultaneous fluid replacement in polycythemic patients also may be due to improved viscosity.[64] Unfortunately, neither obtaining very high cardiac output, nor lowering viscosity, nor instituting osmotherapy ensures perfusion of all tissues, because blood in the microcirculation may have become excessively viscid before adequate resuscitation.

When cardiac output is normal or high and arterial pressure is low, physicians often consider the use of vasoconstricting drugs to increase arterial pressure. When these agents constrict the excessively dilated beds, they may be useful in "normalizing" blood flow; however, if they act on hypoperfused beds, they are detrimental. Vasoconstricting drugs may also be beneficial by increasing venous tone and ventricular preload, or by raising arterial pressure to improve coronary perfusion. These distinctions cannot usually be made by analyzing changes in the hemodynamic profile. (They can only be suggested by related changes in derived values such as $\dot{V}O_2$.) Although there is little clinical evidence to support specific therapy now, it is likely that further investigation will identify the appropriately selective pharmacologic support for vasodilated septic patients. It is certain that restoration of a low systemic pressure by vasoconstricting agents is a salve to attending personnel; whether there is benefit to the septic patient is less clear. Until effective monitoring of local perfusion is available, improved status can only be told by changes in the secondary signs of tissue ischemia, such as acidemia, urine output, and changes in $\dot{V}O_2$.

In summary, sepsis causes hypoperfusion and a neuroendocrine stress response. Adequate volume loading then results in capillary hyperperfusion (where vascular obstruction has not occurred) at a lower than normal arterial pressure. Hyperperfusion of some beds and loss of perfusion in others may cause dissociation of clinical signs from all hemodynamic indices.[4] The following case illustrates the application of these thoughts with a successful outcome.

CASE 5–1.—An 88-year-old man was evaluated because of hypotension and dyspnea. Sepsis from an intra-abdominal source was apparent and bowel ischemia was considered likely. At laparotomy, large retroperitoneal collections of urine were found bilaterally. The infected left kidney was removed. The right kidney was hydronephrotic and studded with cysts, one of which had ruptured. A right ureterostomy was performed, wound drains were placed, and the abdomen was closed. In the ICU, the patient was hypothermic (95° F) and hypoperfused (arterial pressure 60/30 torr), with WP and central venous pressure (CVP) both 21 torr. Admin-

istration of 4 units of red cells, 250 ml of plasmanate, dopamine (8 μg/kg/min), and dobutamine (10 μg/kg/min) resulted in minimal improvement: blood pressure was 110/60 torr, but $P\bar{v}_{O_2}$ was 30 torr, and cardiac index was only 1.1 L/min/m² despite a WP of 25 torr. Despite increases in dopamine and dobutamine, the systemic arterial pressure drifted downward over the next 15 hours to a nadir on the third postoperative day. The cardiac index was then 2.0 L/min/m², and WP was still 25 torr. The patient was slightly edematous. Nevertheless, because of his refractoriness to current therapy and because of the possibility that WP was not accurately estimating the left ventricular end-diastolic volume, a brisk fluid challenge was begun with normal saline at 1 ml/kg/min. After 2 L of fluid had been given in this manner, the blood pressure was 100/50 torr, the cardiac index was 2.5 L/min/m², and the WP decreased to 18 torr. Urine output, which was 15 ml/hour before the fluid challenge, increased to 20 ml/hour, then gradually improved over the next 4 days, but the systemic systolic arterial pressure remained between 80 and 100 torr. Mechanical ventilation continued to be required, and positive end-expiratory pressure (PEEP) was raised to 20 cm H_2O because of extensive bilateral infiltrates with normal heart size on the fourth day. PEEP could not be reduced below 20 cm H_2O without a notable decrease in Pa_{O_2} until the ninth day. Systemic arterial pressure gradually returned to the patient's baseline value of 140/70 torr. The patient was extubated successfully on the 12th postoperative day. He continued his slow recovery and was discharged from the ICU on the 27th postoperative day.

Discussion: The response to fluid challenge despite an elevated WP suggests either dissociation of WP from left ventricular end-diastolic volume or reversible left ventricular failure from severe intravascular volume depletion sufficient to produce systemic hypotension and impaired myocardial perfusion. Increasing pulmonary edema and need for PEEP may have been the costs of providing sufficient volume to sustain a high cardiac output and to compensate for continuing losses into the interstitial space. Survival and recovery, despite depression of arterial pressure, suggests resetting of baroreceptors and reemphasizes the primary importance of flow rather than pressure.

Other Causes of Vasoderegulation

Cirrhosis

In patients with cirrhosis, the circulatory state is hyperkinetic.[43] Cardiac index is commonly about 5 L/min/m², and SVR is less than two-thirds normal. There is an increase in blood flow to the skin, muscles, lung, and spleen but a decrease to the kidney and, of course, to the liver.[43] It is clear that AV anastomoses contribute to the high output state, but capillary hyperperfusion might also be present. It is of interest to what degree vasoregulation remains intact. Because some patients with cirrhosis can undertake moderate exercise, some of those adaptive responses are still available; on the other hand, the degree to which oxygen supply exceeds need in stable cirrhosis indicates that vasoregulation is compromised. Similarly, the observation, in late stages of liver failure, of dysfunction of other organs due to ischemia despite high oxygen transport relative to need, shows that control is compromised. Recent observations in patients with fulminant hepatic failure suggest that severe loss of vasoregulation is a primary problem in acute as well as in chronic liver failure.[5, 6] Of 32 patients with grade IV hepatic encephalopathy, many had low SVR and an elevated cardiac index. Although there were no clinical differences between surviving and nonsurviving patients, patients who subsequently died had lower SVR and higher $\dot{D}O_2$ than did survivors; also, the $P\bar{v}O_2$ and blood levels of lactic acid were higher in the nonsurvivors, and they consumed a lower fraction of the $\dot{D}O_2$. The paradigm applied in sepsis is useful here. $\dot{D}O_2$ is more than adequate for current needs but is maldistributed; perfusion of some vascular beds is excessive but other vascular beds are underperfused, leaving tissues ischemic. As in septic shock, vasoconstrictors may be helpful in cirrhosis if only overperfused vessels respond, or they may be detrimental if low perfusion is made worse. Manipulations that increase $\dot{D}O_2$ may relieve ischemia, but the improvement may be detectable only by monitoring organ function or other secondary signs of adequate perfusion.

Pulmonary Diseases: ARDS and COPD

Several reports have shown venous oxygen values to be dissociated from $\dot{D}O_2$ in adult respiratory distress syndrome (ARDS).[18, 51, 54, 64] This could occur if vasoregulation were impaired or if local tissue oxygen needs varied widely. A significant degree of vasoderegulation has also been reported in a subgroup of patients with chronic obstructive pulmonary disease (COPD), as manifested by the failure of $P\bar{v}O_2$ to fall during exercise. Unlike in other COPD patients studied at the same time and earlier,[46] in whom $P\bar{v}O_2$

dropped to nearly 20 torr with exercise, the $P\bar{v}O_2$ stayed as high as 33 torr at maximal exercise in some patients at the same time that blood lactate levels were significantly elevated.[59] The observation of vasoderegulation in selected patients with ARDS and during exercising in patients with COPD suggests that the lung may have a more significant role in vasoderegulation than was previously thought. However, other patients with ARDS and COPD of equal severity do not show dependence of $\dot{V}O_2$ on $\dot{D}O_2$,[27, 28, 52] which suggests that depression of vasoregulation in ARDS and COPD may be a coincident rather than an inherent phenomenon of the lung disease. Contributing factors could include sepsis, stress, an elevated core temperature, and vasodilating drug therapy, because each of these may increase perfusion over current local tissue needs and dissociate venous oxygen from $\dot{D}O_2$. As discussed, any microvascular impairment would also diminish the correlation between venous oxygen and $\dot{D}O_2$ and tend to make $\dot{V}O_2$ dependent on higher $\dot{D}O_2$. Cain has nicely summarized the potential for activation of complement, arachidonic acid, and xanthine oxidase cascades to contribute both to acute respiratory failure and systemic microcirculatory failure with adjacent vasodilation.[12] This is an appealing explanation for much of the observed data. However, independence of $\dot{V}O_2$ from $\dot{D}O_2$ as seen by Fallat in patients with ARDS on extracorporeal membrane oxygenation must still be accounted for.[27, 28] It may be that the cascade phenomena have come under control in these end-stage patients, their respiratory failure now a result of established fibrosis rather than intravascular dynamics.

Drugs

Vasoactive agents with similar effects on gross hemodynamic indices may have different effects on local vessel tone and local perfusion. It would be valuable to identify drugs that constrict flow to overperfused but not to ischemic tissue (enhancement of metabolic autoregulation), and it may be detrimental to use drugs that depress that control. For example, blockade of α-receptors with phenoxybenzamine depressed vasoregulatory response to hypoxia in dogs, as a result of which oxygen uptake was lower at the same oxygen delivery rate.[10] In a seemingly parallel observation, administration of nitroprusside to patients with COPD resulted in a depression of $\dot{V}O_2$ when $P\bar{v}O_2$ was not as low (32 ± 3 torr) as is normally associated with $\dot{D}O_2$-dependent depression of $\dot{V}O_2$.[8] Because histotoxic depression of $\dot{V}O_2$ by nitroprusside is unlikely at the drug dosage administered in this study, some loss of vasoregulation is the most likely explanation. Hence, phenoxybenzamine and nitroprusside may adversely alter local oxygen metabolism and may be inappropriate agents to decrease afterload in patients with compromised cardiac output. But inappropriate relative to what? In the nitroprusside study, hydralazine, another afterload-reducing agent, did not cause a decrease in $\dot{V}O_2$—in fact, $\dot{V}O_2$ increased slightly—and thus, hydralazine appears preferable to nitroprusside. However, hydralazine was also associated with a significant increase in $\dot{D}O_2$, which might explain the improved $\dot{V}O_2$. Hydralazine might have impaired vasoregulation as seriously as nitroprusside, but in this study the impaired distribution of perfusion was compensated for by a simultaneous increase in total $\dot{D}O_2$. Further studies on the pharmacologic support of the failing cardiovascular system need to direct considerably more attention to the influence of these agents on the distribution of perfusion to ischemic versus normally and excessively perfused tissues. Following the effect of such interactions on the $\dot{V}O_2$-$\dot{D}O_2$ relationship (see Fig 5–10) and on the distribution of perfusion by xenon-enhanced CT scanning (see chapter 14, "Functional Imaging of the Critically Ill Patient") may be helpful in understanding this complex interaction.

Studies in the area of vasomotor control should include the effect of the drug on pulmonary as well as systemic vasculature. Drugs that increase flow to hypoxic tissues might also decrease adaptive hypoxic pulmonary vasoconstriction (HPV) and increase venous admixture. Similarly, almatrine increases HPV and might improve the distribution of ventilation/perfusion ratios in the lung, but might decrease flow to hypoxic tissue,[61] resulting in further tissue dysfunction.

Metabolic Vasoregulation and the Relation Between $\dot{V}O_2$ and $\dot{D}O_2$

When distribution of perfusion is tightly regulated according to the oxygen needs of the tissues and there is no excess $\dot{D}O_2$, then $\dot{V}O_2$ is maximal ($\dot{V}O_{2max}$). These points are illustrated in Figure 5–8, where $\dot{V}O_2$ is plotted relative to $\dot{D}O_2$ for man. $\dot{V}O_2$ can never be greater than $\dot{D}O_2$ in a stable situation. If $\dot{D}O_2$ is sufficient to meet oxygen

needs and vasoregulation remains intact, then changes in $\dot{D}O_2$ will cause no change in $\dot{V}O_2$. Resting $\dot{V}O_2$ is normally about 2 ml/kg/min, and $\dot{V}O_2$ is almost constant above a $\dot{D}O_2$ of about 7–9 ml/kg/min. Normally there is a reserve $\dot{D}O_2$ above what is needed to meet metabolic demand. Thus, the normal state (N in Fig 5–8) lies to the right of the line of $\dot{V}O_{2max}$ on a standard $\dot{D}O_2$–$\dot{V}O_2$ curve. Below that threshold (H in Fig 5–8), $\dot{V}O_2$ is $\dot{D}O_2$-dependent, decreasing as $\dot{D}O_2$ decreases and increasing as $\dot{D}O_2$ increases. Since autoregulation normally restricts local flow to only a limited excess over that needed, $\dot{D}O_2$ is relatively fixed under resting conditions. Therefore, testing the response of $\dot{V}O_2$ to higher $\dot{D}O_2$ usually entails control of $\dot{D}O_2$ by the observer, such as by cardiopulmonary bypass. Observations of the effects of $\dot{D}O_2$ higher than the normal reserve have therefore been limited to such artificial conditions. Figure 5–8 diagrams a reasonable paradigm of this relationship rather than a well-documented relation.

There are several perturbations of the normal relation to be considered. (1) During exercise, when the metabolic demand for oxygen is higher, the threshold of $\dot{D}O_2$ below which $\dot{V}O_2$ is $\dot{D}O_2$-dependent and above which it is not will naturally be higher. Exercise is represented in Figure 5–8 by the letter E. When oxygen needs increase, oxygen transport increases by a comparable amount, thereby maintaining a reserve oxygen transport (*arrow up* in Fig 5–8). If that level of $\dot{V}O_2$ is maintained but $\dot{D}O_2$ cannot be increased, as in cardiac failure, normal vasoregulation will adjust local vascular tone to be appropriate for local need, and systemic dysfunction due to ischemia or hypoxia should not become apparent until after the $\dot{V}O_{2max}$ is reached (*arrow left* in Fig 5–8). With exercise, as in the normal state, elevation of $\dot{D}O_2$ above the level at which oxygen needs are satisfied would result in no further increase in $\dot{V}O_2$. (2) Deviation from metabolic regulation of local flow will blur or splay the threshold and also raise the $\dot{D}O_2$ at which the threshold occurs, and this will occur in proportion to the severity of loss of vasoregulation. For example, increasing blood flow to the skin to increase heat loss detracts from the regulation of flow according to oxygen needs (line HS in Fig 5–9). Then, if $\dot{D}O_2$ is compromised by cardiac failure, the impairment of vasoregulation allows some tissues to be inadequately perfused before the $\dot{V}O_{2max}$ is reached. The threshold above which $\dot{V}O_2$ is con-

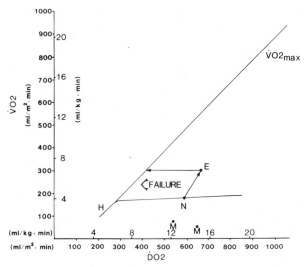

FIG 5–8.

Patterns of relation between $\dot{V}O_2$ and $\dot{D}O_2$. $\dot{V}O_2$ is established by the current metabolic needs of the tissues when $\dot{D}O_2$ is sufficient. The $\dot{D}O_2$ anaerobic threshold is the $\dot{D}O_2$ above which increasing $\dot{D}O_2$ does not cause a significant increase in $\dot{V}O_2$. Adequacy of $\dot{D}O_2$ to meet needs depends heavily on appropriate regulation of local flow. Normally there is an excess of flow relative to need; that is, the $\dot{D}O_2$ (point *N*) is well in excess of the $\dot{D}O_2$ threshold. Depression of oxygen transport from normal, as in progressive cardiac failure, is accompanied by increasingly tight regulation of the distribution of flow (movement from *N* to the left), so that $\dot{V}O_2$ is preserved until maximal regulation is achieved ($\dot{V}O_{2\,max}$). The increasingly tight vasoregulation (movement to the left) is manifest in, and effectively monitored by, changes in venous oxygen. Points on the curve below the normal threshold (hemorrhagic shock, *H*) represent as nearly perfect metabolic regulation of flow as the body is capable of, and make up the stages passed through in hemorrhagic shock of increasing severity, whereby perfusion of less vital tissue is sacrificed until vasoregulation fails. The $\dot{D}O_2$ varies with exercise according to the $\dot{V}O_2$ required *(E)*; $\dot{D}O_2$ is increased only by approximately the increase in $\dot{V}O_2$. Heart failure again moves the relation to $\dot{V}O_{2\,max}$.

stant occurs at a higher $\dot{D}O_2$ than when vasoregulation is normal (point *A* in Fig 5–9). In the hyperdynamic conditions seen in sepsis and cirrhosis, the threshold is similarly blurred and increased by vasoderegulation and may also be elevated because oxygen consumption is greater than normal. Microemboli (experimental or due to trauma or sepsis) can cause the same rightward

shift of the threshold (see Fig 5–9),[65] as can tissue edema (see chapter 10, "Oxygen Transport From Capillary to Cell"). (3) Cessation of flow to any tissue will lower both $\dot{V}O_2$ and the threshold $\dot{D}O_2$ (not diagramed). (4) Patients who have lost perfusion of extensive microvascular beds but still have a widely dilated central circulation may show severe depression of $\dot{V}O_2$ but less sig-

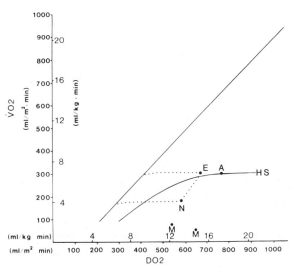

FIG 5–9.

Any compromise of local metabolic regulation of flow, by normal homeostatic changes in renal or skin blood flow as well as by pathologic processes, blurs the $\dot{D}O_2$ threshold and moves it to the right. This is represented by line *HS*, which represents hyperthermia and sepsis. Occasionally, late shock is characterized by marked depression of $\dot{V}O_2$ while $\dot{D}O_2$ remains normal or higher *(M)*. Apparently many beds are lost to the circulation, while vessels remaining open are overperfused. The graph is a conceptual construction based on the discussion in the text and on data in the literature.[1, 18, 27, 28, 38, 47, 49, 53, 58, 59, 67] *E*, exercise; *N*, normal; *HS*, hyperthermia and sepsis; *M*, moribund.

nificant or no depression of $\dot{D}O_2$ (*M* in Fig 5–9).[49, 68] This condition can sometimes be sustained for days, although the practice is not beneficial to the patient if no reversible process can be found. Note that increasingly severe loss of metabolic regulation increases the dependence of $\dot{V}O_2$ on high $\dot{D}O_2$ and therefore increases the $P\bar{v}O_2$ at which oxygen needs will be adequately met. This suggests that both high and low values of hemodynamic indices indicate severe illness and a poor prognosis. In contrast to arterial hypoxemia in cardiogenic and hypovolemic shock (vasoregulation intact), the hyperdynamic state is associated with loss of vasoregulation, and the patients with highest cardiac index, $\dot{D}O_2$, and $P\bar{v}O_2$ and lowest $C(a-\bar{v})O_2$ may be more likely to show signs of tissue hypoxia and die than septic patients with normal values.[5, 6, 40, 68] This statement presupposes adequate circulatory blood volume. A patient with severe loss of vasoregulation may have a normal or low $P\bar{v}O_2$ if preload is inadequate.

Changing relations between $\dot{D}O_2$, $\dot{V}O_2$, and $P\bar{v}O_2$ may provide clues regarding the distribution of blood flow to excessively or poorly perfused tissue. If only the flow in well-perfused tissue changes, $P\bar{v}O_2$ will follow $\dot{D}O_2$, but $\dot{V}O_2$ will not change. An increase in flow to both hyperperfused and ischemic tissue beds will be characterized by an increase in both $\dot{D}O_2$ and $\dot{V}O_2$. The change in $P\bar{v}O_2$ is not predictable; restored perfusion could bring a lower $P\bar{v}O_2$ from a bed that was not represented in venous blood before the change. A redistribution of flow to ischemic tissue with no change in cardiac output will increase $\dot{V}O_2$ and lower $P\bar{v}O_2$.

In the paradigm described, the finding of dependence of $\dot{V}O_2$ on $\dot{D}O_2$ suggests that oxygenation is threatened in some tissues, either because $\dot{D}O_2$ is low relative to $\dot{V}O_2$ or because metabolic vasoregulation is impaired, and that maintaining or increasing a high $\dot{D}O_2$ may be justified. Increasing local oxygen delivery may increase oxygen consumption at levels above the normal anaerobic threshold. These points will be addressed in the next section. Alternatively, the tissues may be unable to utilize the delivered oxygen appropriately because of derangement of intracellular metabolism, mitochondrial function, or membrane permeability. This pathologic process of abnormal oxygen metabolism, or dysoxia, is discussed in chapter 11, "Cellular Oxygen Utilization."

DEPENDENCE OF OXYGEN CONSUMPTION ON OXYGEN DELIVERY: CLASSIC PHYSIOLOGIC CONTROL VERSUS ABERRANT PHYSIOLOGIC STATES

The correlation between $\dot{D}O_2$ and $\dot{V}O_2$, even when $\dot{V}O_2$ is quite elevated, during many generalized disease states could be explained by a true dependence of $\dot{V}O_2$ on $\dot{D}O_2$. Nonshivering thermogenesis requires oxygen and would explain the findings for $\dot{D}O_2$-dependent $\dot{V}O_2$ in sepsis. Whalen et al.[76] demonstrated in isolated muscle groups from cats that normal autoregulation was lost and oxygen consumption was dependent on $\dot{D}O_2$. Decreases in skin temperature increased skin arteriolar resistance and, instead of decreasing cardiac output to meet the lower demand, diverted flow to underlying muscle. These muscle groups appeared to be capable of increased $\dot{V}O_2$ when flow was increased. The increase in $\dot{V}O_2$ was not coupled to muscle contraction or adenosine triphosphate generation but to heat generation. This phenomenon occurred at a tissue PO_2 much higher than that needed to effect hypoxic vasoregulation. If high-$\dot{D}O_2$-dependent increases in $\dot{V}O_2$ are due to increased perfusion of heat-generating tissues, the beneficial effect may be limited to temperature regulation. Preventing heat loss or providing radiant heat to the patient might achieve the same goals at less physiologic cost.

It is also possible that the observed $\dot{D}O_2$-dependent increases in $\dot{V}O_2$ are related to subtle variations in laboratory techniques. Duran et al.[19] made an interesting observation in their report of 35 dog muscle preparations. In 25, $\dot{V}O_2$ was constant at all blood flows above 2 ml/100 gm/min. In nine muscles, $\dot{V}O_2$ increased with blood flow up to at least 10 ml/100 gm/min. In one muscle the pattern changed spontaneously from one to the other. While the authors could not define a related change in technique, they noted that eight of the nine muscles showing $\dot{V}O_2$ dependence on flow belonged to the first 16 experiments. In the subsequent 19 experiments, only two muscle preparations showed $\dot{V}O_2$ dependence after 2–3 hours of perfusion.

Other mechanisms by which $\dot{V}O_2$ might be $\dot{D}O_2$-dependent are discussed in chapter 11, "Cellular Oxygen Utilization." If oxygen uptake is really related to $\dot{D}O_2$ and not to tissue needs, then monitoring of oxygen transport by any method using cardiopulmonary indices, including $\dot{V}O_2$, is of questionable value. Useful monitoring would then be reduced to observing for signs of inadequate perfusion, such as lactic acidemia or oliguria.

On the other hand, the supposition that in ARDS or any other condition $\dot{V}O_2$ will increase as long as cardiac output or $\dot{D}O_2$ increases may be in error. Experimentally, $\dot{V}O_2$ measured directly clearly plateaus above a threshold $\dot{D}O_2$ in dogs without pulmonary insult.[9, 11, 14, 15, 50] Likewise, when Carroll and Snyder[14] directly measured $\dot{V}O_2$ they did not find cardiac-output–dependent maximum $\dot{V}O_2$ in septic monkeys. For example, when intravenous fluid resuscitation was given to septic monkeys, $\dot{V}O_2$ increased by the greatest amount (160% of baseline) despite a persistently depressed cardiac output (44% of baseline). Furthermore, the one monkey in that study whose cardiac output improved most with fluid resuscitation (382% of baseline) had no increase in $\dot{V}O_2$ (92% of baseline). Overall, $\dot{V}O_2$ and cardiac output correlated significantly during the low cardiac output shock phase in that study, but once fluid resuscitation had restored cardiac output and mean arterial pressure, the $\dot{V}O_2$ no longer correlated with cardiac output. Subsequent increases in cardiac output above normal did not produce changes in $\dot{V}O_2$. These observations have since been duplicated by others.[16, 36] Specifically in ARDS, $\dot{V}O_2$ was found to be dependent on cardiac output only up to a threshold, albeit a higher threshold than normal.[49] Most decisively, when $\dot{D}O_2$ was varied from 7 to 27 ml/kg in patients with severe ARDS on extracorporeal membrane oxygenation, CO_2 production did not vary significantly, which suggests that tissue respiration remained constant.[27, 28]

When $\dot{V}O_2$ is not directly measured but rather calculated as the product of cardiac output and $C(a-\bar{v})O_2$, the expected coefficient of correlation between $\dot{V}O_2$ and $\dot{D}O_2$ is .71.[3] This is to be expected since both $\dot{V}O_2$ and $\dot{D}O_2$ terms have in common cardiac output and Ca_{O_2}. Therefore, the significance of the coefficients comparing $\dot{V}O_2$ with $\dot{D}O_2$ using this indirect method to measure $\dot{V}O_2$ should be determined as $>.71$ rather than as >0. One should be suspicious of any calculated $\dot{V}O_2$ that lacks clinical explanation, and one should suspect sustained increases in calculated $\dot{V}O_2$ above 200 ml/m^2/min to be artifactual unless they can be verified with a directly measured $\dot{V}O_2$.

Thus, the correlation of high $\dot{D}O_2$ and $\dot{V}O_2$ reported in ARDS patients appears to be due to wide variation in oxygen needs combined with vasoderegulation and a vigorous but sometimes inadequate response by the oxygen transport system. Some of the observed correlation may be due to the use of common terms (cardiac output and Ca_{O_2}), but it is not necessary to invoke this explanation. We have not seen reason to discard the concept of a $\dot{D}O_2$ threshold.

Thus, there is a widely variable but generally increased tissue need for oxygen in shock, sepsis, and other conditions associated with ARDS. The increased oxygen demand influences the location of the $\dot{D}O_2$ threshold below which $\dot{V}O_2$ is flow-dependent and above which it is flow-independent. The relation is complicated by stress states in which $\dot{D}O_2$ is more excessive than normal and $P\bar{v}O_2$ is subsequently increased, and by vasoderegulation in which the increased flow capacity of dilated beds must be satisfied before higher resistance beds will be perfused. Any disturbance of metabolic regulation of flow moves the $\dot{D}O_2$ threshold higher for any $\dot{V}O_2$ and blurs the presence of that threshold. $\dot{V}O_2$ may continue to increase with increases in $\dot{D}O_2$ in such cases, but only to levels compatible with the metabolic needs of stressed critically ill patients as classically described. These relations are diagramed in Figure 5–9. If the relation between $\dot{V}O_2$ and $\dot{D}O_2$ is sought when both values are calculated from measured cardiac output, the significance of the coefficient should be determined as $>.71$ rather than as >0. When calculated oxygen consumption is more than 200% of normal, error in measurement is the most likely cause. Significant errors doubtless occur at lower values of $\dot{V}O_2$. It also seems possible that there is an aberrant physiologic state wherein no threshold delimits the influence of cardiac output on $\dot{V}O_2$; however, we have not found such a state to be characteristic of any disease.

Interpretation of Changes in the $\dot{V}O_2$-$\dot{D}O_2$ Relation

Appropriate guidelines for treating patients who are or may be in shock are not precisely defined and treatment by prescription is not yet realistic. It is useful to assess repeatedly the patient's response over time and the patient's response to therapy, to test impressions regarding cause and course. Vasoderegulation complicates analysis in all cases, and no variable is completely satisfactory. While there remain significant technical problems, monitoring and plotting the $\dot{V}O_2$ and $\dot{D}O_2$ responses can be useful in treating such patients and in related models.

In the relationship between oxygen consumption and oxygen delivery, equal changes in each variable (movement up or down the line of identity) suggest that all change in flow has been in nutritional flow. Observations here are subject to statistical questioning when cardiac output measured by the same technique is used to calculate both $\dot{V}O_2$ and $\dot{D}O_2$, as described earlier. However, deviation from the line of identity is not subject to that error. Therefore, when changes in $\dot{V}O_2$ and $\dot{D}O_2$ are unequal (or opposite in direction) some useful observations can be made about the distribution of perfusion to nutritional or nonnutritional function. For our purposes here, any flow greater than that needed to prevent dysfunction is called nonnutritive. This term includes the reserve flow that is an impor-

tant safety feature of normal physiology. Nonnutritive flow, therefore, includes capillary flow that is in excess of the needs of the perfused tissues, in addition to flow that bypasses capillary beds, such as through AV anastomoses. Assuming no spontaneous change in oxygen need (primary change in metabolic rate), any increase in $\dot{V}O_2$ (upward movement on the $\dot{V}O_2$-$\dot{D}O_2$ plot, Fig 5–10) represents improvement in nutritional flow, and any movement downward represents loss of nutritional flow. Equally obvious, movement directly to the right or left indicates change in total oxygen transport and specifically a change in nonnutritive flow. Plotting changes in the $\dot{V}O_2$-$\dot{D}O_2$ relation, as in Figure 5–10, suggests whether vasoregulation is impaired or improved by a given therapy. Because $\dot{V}O_2$ varies spontaneously with stress, temperature, and activity, these measurements should be made at short intervals before and after changes in therapy. As illustrated in Figure 5–10, movement upward and to the left

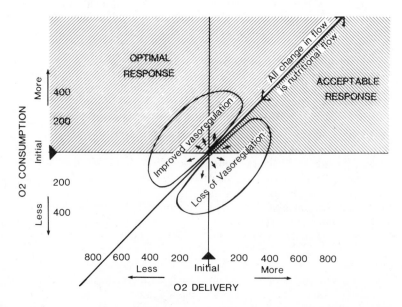

FIG 5–10.

Interpretation of changes in $\dot{V}O_2$–$\dot{D}O_2$ relation. When there has been no change in oxygen need the effect of a given treatment on both nutritional flow and on vasoregulation may be readily appreciated when a second set of data is plotted relative to the first set at the intersection of lines in the figure. When metabolic demand is unchanged, any movement upward in the figure indicates an increase in nutritional flow and improved oxygenation of hypoxic tissues. A move to the right is an increase in oxygen transport. A move up and to the left is always an improvement in vasore-

gulation. Administration of a drug that causes an increase in $\dot{V}O_2$ (other than can be related to increased myocardial oxygen consumption) greater than $\dot{D}O_2$, or even causes a decrease in $\dot{D}O_2$, has improved nutritional perfusion, and done so in part by improving vasoregulation. A drug that causes a greater increase in $\dot{D}O_2$ than $\dot{V}O_2$ can be recognized to have caused loss of vasoregulation, but can still be of potential benefit to the patient by increasing nutritional flow.

from a line of identical changes indicates tighter metabolic regulation of flow. Movement downward and to the right indicates a decrease or loss of metabolic regulation of flow. A vasodilator that affects vessels in both underperfused and adequately perfused tissue will appear in the right upper quadrant, but if it is influencing primarily underperfused vessels it will appear above the line of identity. A greater influence on vessels in overperfused tissue is indicated by less of an increase in $\dot{V}o_2$ than $\dot{D}o_2$ (above the horizontal line but below the line of identity). Movement into the right lower quadrant suggests a steal phenomenon. Movement upward is probably always beneficial when caused by a vasoactive agent unless there is a simultaneous increase in metabolic demand. An increase in metabolic demand might be due to a nonspecific increase in tissue metabolism caused by catecholamines, or to an increase in cardiac work. Upward movement due to administration of an inotropic agent also may indicate increased myocardial oxygen consumption rather than better perfusion of ischemic tissue.

Vasoconstrictors generally cause movement to the left. Rare exceptions are possible, as when improved coronary perfusion enhances contractility and oxygen transport. If arterial pressure is increased by constriction of overperfused vessels sufficient to compensate for any simultaneous constriction of underperfused vessels, perfusion of ischemic tissue may be improved (inverse steal) and the relationship between $\dot{V}o_2$ and $\dot{D}o_2$ will move into the left upper quadrant. Changes in the oxygen utilization coefficient have the same implications as movement of data relative to the line of identity in Figure 5–10; that is, an increase indicates better vasoregulation, and a decrease, less regulation.

REFERENCES

1. Abraham E, Bland RD, Cobo JC, et al: Sequential cardiorespiratory patterns associated with outcome in septic shock. *Chest* 1984; 85:75.
2. Ader R: Psychoneuroimmunology, in Ballieux RE (ed): *Breakdown in Human Adaptation to 'Stress'*. Boston, Martinus Nijhoff Publishers, 1984, vol II, part III, pp 653–670.
3. Archie JP: Mathematical coupling of data may produce invalid results and unjustified conclusions (abstract). *Crit Care Med* 1980; 8:252.
4. Bell H, Thal A: The peculiar hemodynamics of septic shock. *Postgrad Med* 1970; 48:106.
5. Bihari D, Gimson A, Waterson M, et al: Tissue hypoxia during fulminant hepatic failure: A major determinant of prognosis (abstract). *Crit Care Med* 1984; 12:233.
6. Bihari D, Gimson A, Lindridge J, et al: The pathogenesis of lactic acidosis in fulminant hepatic failure (abstract). *Crit Care Med* 1984; 12:255.
7. Brengelmann GL, Wyss C, Rowell LB: Control of forearm skin blood flow during periods of steadily increasing skin temperature. *J Appl Physiol* 1973; 35:77–84.
8. Brent BN, Matthay RA, Mahler DA, et al: Relationship between oxygen uptake and oxygen transport in stable patients with chronic obstructive pulmonary disease. *Am Rev Respir Dis* 1984; 129:682–686.
9. Cain SM: Oxygen delivery and uptake in dogs during anemic and hypoxic hypoxia. *J Appl Physiol* 1977; 42:228–234.
10. Cain SM: Effects of time and vasoconstrictor tone on O_2 extraction during hypoxic hypoxia. *J Appl Physiol* 1978; 45:219.
11. Cain SM, Adams RP: O_2 transport during two forms of stagnant hypoxia following acid and base infusions. *J Appl Physiol* 1983; 54:1518–1524.
12. Cain SM: Review: Supply dependency of oxygen uptake in ARDS—Myth or reality? *Am J Med Sci* 1984; 288:119.
13. Cannon WB (ed): *Bodily Changes in Pain, Hunger, Fear and Rage*. New York, Harper & Row, Publishers, 1953.
14. Carroll G, Snyder J: Hyperdynamic severe intravascular sepsis depends on fluid administration in cynomolgus monkeys. *Am J Physiol* 1982; 243:R131–R141.
15. Chapler CK, Cain SM: Effects of α-adrenergic blockade during acute anemia. *J Appl Physiol* 1982; 52:16–20.
16. Chappell TR, Rubin LJ, Markham RV Jr, et al: Independence of oxygen consumption and systemic oxygen transport in patients with either stable pulmonary hypertension or refractory left ventricular failure. *Am Rev Respir Dis* 1983; 128:30–33.
17. Cullen J, Siegrist J, Wegmann HM, et al (eds): *Breakdown in Human Adaptation to 'Stress'*. Boston, Martinus Nijhoff Publishers, 1984.
18. Danek SJ, Lynch JP, Weg JG et al: The dependence of oxygen uptake on oxygen delivery

in the adult respiratory distress syndrome. *Am Rev Respir Dis* 1980; 122:387.

19. Duran WN, Renkin EM: Oxygen consumption and blood flow in resting mammalian skeletal muscle. *Am J Physiol* 1974; 226:173.

20. Elliott GR, Eisdorfer C (eds): *Stress and Human Health: Analysis and Implications of Research*. New York, Springer, 1982.

21. Elliott GR, Eisdorfer C (eds): *Stress and Human Health: Analysis and Implications of Research*. New York, Springer, 1982, p XVIII.

22. Elliott GR, Eisdorfer C (eds): *Stress and Human Health: Analysis and Implications of Research*. New York, Springer, 1982, p 9.

23. Elliott GR, Eisdorfer C (eds): *Stress and Human Health: Analysis and Implications of Research*. New York, Springer, 1982, p 15.

24. Elliott GR, Eisdorfer C (eds): *Stress and Human Health: Analysis and Implications of Research*. New York, Springer, 1982, p 29.

25. Elliott GR, Eisdorfer C (eds): *Stress and Human Health: Analysis and Implications of Research*. New York, Springer, 1982, p 64.

26. Elliott GR, Eisdorfer C (eds): *Stress and Human Health: Analysis and Implications of Research*. New York, Springer, 1982, p 172.

27. Fallat RJ, Eberhart R: Independence of CO_2 production (V_{CO_2}) and systemic O_2 delivery (SOD) in severe adult respiratory distress syndrome (ARDS). *Am Rev Respir Dis* 1984; 129(suppl):A96.

28. Fallat RJ, Eberhart R: Unpublished data, 1984.

29. Folkow B, Neil E: The principles of vascular control, in Folkow B, Neil E (eds): *Circulation*. New York, Oxford University Press, 1971, p 289.

30. Friedman M, Thoresen CE, Gill JJ, et al: Alteration of type A behavior and reduction in cardiac recurrences in postmyocardial infarction patients. *Am Heart J* 1984; 108:237.

31. Funkenstein DH: The physiology of fear and anger. *Sci Am* 1955; 192:74.

32. Gorczynski RM, MacRae S, Kennedy M: Factors involved in the classical conditioning of antibody responses in mice, in Ballieux RE (ed): *Breakdown in Human Adaptation to 'Stress'*. Boston, Martinus Nijhoff Publishers, 1984, vol. II, part III, pp 704–712.

33. Gow BS: Circulatory correlates: Vascular impedance, resistance, and capacity, in Bohr DF, Somlyo AP, Sparks HV Jr (eds): *Handbook of Physiology: The Cardiovascular System*. Bethesda, American Physiological Society, 1980, vol II, pp 353–408.

34. Hall NR, McGillis JP, Spangelo BL, et al: Immune regulation of the hypothalamic-hypophyseal-adrenal axis. A role for thymosins and lymphokines, in Ballieux RE (ed): *Breakdown in Human Adaptation to 'Stress'*. Boston, Martinus Nijhoff Publishers, 1984, vol II, part III, pp 722–731.

35. Herd JA: Cardiovascular response to stress in man. *Annu Rev Physiol* 1984; 46:177–185.

36. Houtchens BA, Westenskow DR: Oxygen consumption in septic shock: Collective review. *Circ Shock* 1984; 13:361–384.

37. Jennings JR, Follansbee WP: Task-induced ST segment depression, ectopic beats, and autonomic responses in coronary heart disease patients. *Psychosom Med,* in press.

38. Kaufman BS, Rackow EC, Falk JL: The relationship between oxygen delivery and consumption during fluid resuscitation of hypovolemic and septic shock. *Chest* 1984; 85:336.

39. Kruse JA, Puri VK: The relationship of oxygen consumption to oxygen delivery in shock (abstract). *Chest* 1984; 86:283.

40. Kruse JA, Puri VK: Mixed venous oxygen tension is a poor predictor of lactic acidosis (abstract). *Chest* 1984; 86:288.

41. Longnecker DE: Stress free: To be or not to be? *Anesthesiology* 1984; 61:743.

42. Macklem PT: Respiratory muscles: The vital pump. *Chest* 1980; 78:753.

43. Martini GA, Baltzer G, Arndt H: Some aspects of circulatory disturbances in cirrhosis of the liver, in Popper H, Schaffner F (eds): *Progress in Liver Disease*. New York, Grune & Stratton, Inc, 1972, p 231.

44. Matthews KA, Jennings JR: Cardiovascular responses of boys exhibiting the type A behavior pattern. *Psychosom Med* 1984; 46:484–497.

45. Mellander S, Johansson B: Control of resistance, exchange, and capacitance functions in the peripheral circulation. *Pharmacol Rev* 1968; 20:117.

46. Minh VD, Lee HM, Dolan GF, et al: Hypoxemia during exercise in patients with chronic obstructive pulmonary disease. *Am Rev Respir Dis* 1979; 120:787.

47. Mitchell JH, Blomqvist G: Maximal oxygen uptake. *N Engl J Med* 1971; 284:1018.

48. Mithoefer JC: Indications for oxygen therapy

in chronic obstructive pulmonary disease. *Am Rev Respir Dis* 1974; 110:S35.

49. Mohsenifar Z, Goldbach P, Tashkin DP, et al: Relationship between O_2 delivery and O_2 consumption in the adult respiratory distress syndrome. *Chest* 1983; 84:267.

50. Pepe PE, Culver BH: Dependence of oxygen consumption on oxygen delivery during cardiac output reduction by positive end-expiratory pressure. *Am Rev Respir Dis* 1982; 125:84.

51. Powers SR Jr, Mannal R, Neclerio M, et al: Physiologic consequences of positive end-expiratory pressure (PEEP) ventilation. *Ann Surg* 1973; 178:265.

52. Raffestin B, Escourrou P, Legrand A, et al: Circulatory transport of oxygen in patients with chronic airflow obstruction exercising maximally. *Am Rev Respir Dis* 1982; 125:426–431.

53. Rashkin MC, Bosken C, Baughman RP: Oxygen delivery in critically ill patients: Relationship to blood lactate survival. *Chest* 1985; 87:580.

54. Rhodes GR, Newell JC, Shah D, et al: Increased oxygen consumption accompanying increased oxygen delivery with hypertonic mannitol in adult respiratory distress syndrome. *Surgery* 1978; 84:490.

55. Riley RL: Biophysics of gas and blood flow, in Loeppky JA, Riedesel ML (eds): *Oxygen Transport to Human Tissues*. New York, Elsevier North-Holland, Inc, 1982, pp 103–124.

56. Rowell LB: Regulation of splanchnic blood flow in man. *Physiologist* 1973; 16:127.

57. Rowell LB: Human cardiovascular adjustments to exercise and thermal stress. *Physiol Rev* 1974; 54:75.

58. Rowell LB: The distribution of blood flow and its regulation in humans, in Loeppky JA, Riedesel ML (eds): *Oxygen Transport to Human Tissues*. New York, Elsevier North-Holland, 1982, pp 113–124.

59. Rowell LB: Cardiovascular adjustments to thermal stress, in Shepherd JT, Abboud FM, Geiger ST (eds): *Handbook of Physiology*. Section 2: *The Cardiovascular System*. Bethesda, Maryland, American Physiological Society, 1983, vol 3, pp 967–1023.

60. Rowell LB: Reflex control of regional circulations in humans. *J Auton Nerv Syst* 1984; 11:101–114.

61. Romaldini H, Rodriguez-Roisin R, Wagner PD, et al: Enhancement of hypoxic pulmonary vasoconstriction by almitrine in the dog. *Am Rev Respir Dis* 1983; 128:288–293.

62. Roussos C, Macklem PT: The respiratory muscles. *N Engl J Med* 1982; 307:786–797.

63. Ruberman W, Weinblatt E, Goldberg JD, et al: Psychosocial influences on mortality after myocardial infarction. *N Engl J Med* 1984; 311:552.

64. Shah DM, Powers SR Jr, Bernard HR, et al: Increased oxygen uptake following phlebotomy and simultaneous fluid replacement in polycythemic patients. *Surgery* 1980; 88:686.

65. Shah DM, Newell JC, Saba TM: Defects in peripheral oxygen utilization following trauma and shock. *Arch Surg* 1981; 116:1277.

66. Shepherd AP, Granger HG, Smith EE, et al: Local control of tissue oxygen delivery and its contribution to the regulation of cardiac output. *Am J Physiol* 1973; 225:747–755.

67. Shibutani K, Komatsu T, Kubal K, et al: Critical level of oxygen delivery in anesthetized man. *Crit Care Med* 1983; 11:640.

68. Siegel JH, Greenspan M, Del Guercio LPM: Abnormal vascular tone, defective oxygen transport and myocardial failure in human septic shock. *Ann Surg* 1967; 165:504–517.

69. Smith OA, Hohimer AR, Astley CA, et al: Renal and hindlimb vascular control during acute emotion in the baboon. *Am J Physiol* 1979; 236:R198.

70. Snyder JV: Wedge higher than left atrial pressure in sepsis? (letter). *Ann Intern Med* 1984; 101:879.

71. Solomon G: Emotions, immunity and disease: An historical and philosophical perspective, in Ballieux RE (ed): *Breakdown in Human Adaptation To 'Stress'*. Boston, Martinus Nijhoff Publishers, 1984, vol II, part III, pp 671–680.

72. Sparks HV Jr: Effect of local metabolic factors on vascular smooth muscle, in Bohr DF, Somlyo AP, Sparks JV (eds): *Handbook of Physiology: The Cardiovascular System*. Washington, DC, American Physiological Society, 1980, vol 2, p 409.

73. Steingrub JS, Carroll GC: Viscosity and systemic vascular resistance index (SVRI) in sepsis (abstract). *Circ Shock* 1982; 9:192.

74. Terman GW, Shavit Y, Lewis JW, et al: Intrinsic mechanisms of pain inhibition: Activation by stress. *Science* 1984; 226:1270.

75. Verrier RL, Lown B: Behavioral stress and cardiac arrhythmia. *Annu Rev Physiol* 1984; 46:155–176.

76. Whalen WJ, Buerk D, Thuning CA: Blood flow-limited oxygen consumption in resting cat skeletal muscle. *Am J Physiol* 1973; 224:763–768.

77. Wiles J, Cerra F, Siegel J, et al: The systemic septic response: Does the organism matter? *Crit Care Med* 1980; 8:55.

78. Youngner SJ, Coulton C, Welton R, et al: ICU visiting policies. *Crit Care Med* 1984; 12:606–608.

6 — Neurohumoral Regulation of Cardiovascular Function

Robert R. Ruffolo, Jr., Ph. D.

J. Paul Hieble, Ph.D.

The cardiovascular system is under the control of or is modulated by a variety of neural and humoral factors. The neurotransmitters norepinephrine and acetylcholine influence cardiovascular function under normal circumstances and in a variety of pathophysiologic conditions. The actions of the neurotransmitters, circulating blood-borne hormones, and exogenously administered drugs are largely mediated through interaction with specific receptors in the major effector organs of the cardiovascular system, such as the heart, vasculature, and kidney. An understanding of these receptors in terms of their function, location, and distribution is of primary importance in treating the critically ill patient, inasmuch as the best available pharmacologic treatments for these patients involve the stimulation or blockade of drug, neurotransmitter, or hormone receptors in the cardiovascular system.

There have been many recent developments in our understanding of these receptors and the functions they subserve in the regulation of the cardiovascular system. This chapter addresses such recent developments with an emphasis on the clinical setting and on the use of drugs currently available or being developed that perturb the cardiovascular system through stimulation or antagonism of the critical drug, neurotransmitter, and hormone receptors.

CONTROL OF THE CARDIOVASCULAR SYSTEM

Organization of the Autonomic Nervous System

The cardiovascular system is under the control and regulation of the autonomic nervous system.

While effector organs of the cardiovascular system (heart, vasculature, kidneys) function in the absence of autonomic nerves, the sympathetic and parasympathetic divisions of the autonomic nervous system provide a delicate balance involving closed reflex loops to maintain these organs in their optimal functional state.

The autonomic nervous system is composed of the parasympathetic division, in which the neurotransmitter at the effector organ is acetylcholine, and the sympathetic division, in which the neurotransmitter is norepinephrine. The parasympathetic division exits the CNS from the brain stem (vagus) and the sacral region of the spinal cord. These nerves are characterized by long preganglionic neurons and short postganglionic neurons, the latter innervating the effector organs. The neurotransmitter in the parasympathetic ganglia is acetylcholine. The heart receives a dense cholinergic innervation from the vagus, and cholinergic ''tone'' in the heart predominates over adrenergic tone. In general, there is no significant parasympathetic innervation to the vasculature, although blood vessels nonetheless contain muscarinic cholinergic receptors that are stimulated by acetylcholine and mediate vasodilation through release of an endothelial-derived relaxant factor.[39]

The sympathetic division of the autonomic nervous system originates from the intermediolateral cell column of the thoracic and lumbar portions of the spinal cord. The relatively short preganglionic fibers characteristic of sympathetic nerves terminate in the sympathetic ganglia chain where again the neurotransmitter is acetylcholine. The postganglionic sympathetic neurons are long and liberate norepinephrine, which interacts postsynaptically with adrenoceptors in the heart, vasculature, and kidney. The innervation to the vasculature is almost exclusively sympathetic where the end-organ response is vasoconstriction.

Although the sympathetic and parasympathetic components of the autonomic nervous system originate in the spinal cord and are considered peripheral nerves, both divisions are under the control of nuclei located in the brain stem that in turn receive input from higher centers in the brain. Most of the cardiovascular reflex loops consist of afferent nerves from various peripheral chemoreceptors and baroreceptors in the periphery, which travel to these regulatory nuclei in the brain stem where the information is integrated. The efferent component of the reflex loop involves descending pathways originating from the brain stem nuclei, which ultimately recruit the sympathetic and parasympathetic divisions of the autonomic nervous system to make the necessary alterations in the functional state of the various effector organs of the cardiovascular system.

Cardiovascular Reflexes

Cardiovascular reflexes maintain cardiovascular function, in particular blood pressure, within a relatively narrow optimal range. A sensitive and highly efficient series of positive and negative feedback loops detect deviations from normal cardiovascular function and then "upregulate" or "downregulate" the function of peripheral organs of the cardiovascular system after integration in the CNS. Pressure receptors in the carotid sinus and aortic arch sense changes in peripheral arterial blood pressure and initiate the cardiovascular reflex. Afferents from the carotid sinus and aortic arch enter the CNS through cranial nerves IX (glossopharyngeal) and X (vagus), respectively, and form, in part, the solitary tract in the medulla. The first synapse in the cardiovascular reflex loop occurs in the nucleus tractus solitarii where the neurotransmitter appears to be L-glutamate.[89] Synapses are made within the nucleus tractus solitarii with inhibitory neurons that course to the ventrolateral medulla, which ultimately regulates sympathetic outflow, and with excitatory neurons that send connections to the dorsal motor nucleus of the vagus, which in turn regulates parasympathetic outflow.

Increases in systemic arterial blood pressure activate the afferent component of the cardiovascular reflex loop. As a result, the inhibitory neurons originating in the nucleus tractus solitarii and terminating in the ventrolateral medulla are activated, reducing sympathetic outflow to the heart, vasculature, and kidney. As a direct consequence, heart rate, stroke volume (and therefore cardiac output), and total peripheral vascular resistance are reduced, and blood pressure subsequently returns to within normal limits. In addition, the excitatory neurons that originate from the nucleus tractus solitarii and terminate in the dorsal motor nucleus of the vagus are activated and cholinergic outflow is increased, further decreasing heart rate and cardiac output[63] and thus augmenting the reduction of arterial blood pressure.

NEUROTRANSMITTER, DRUG, AND HORMONE RECEPTORS IN THE CARDIOVASCULAR SYSTEM

α-Adrenoceptors

Adrenoceptors may be subdivided into α and β types. β-Adrenoceptors are selectively activated by epinephrine, norepinephrine, and isoproterenol. α-Adrenoceptors are also stimulated by epinephrine and norepinephrine but are resistant to isoproterenol. β-Adrenoceptors may be subdivided further into the β_1 and β_2 subtypes; isoproterenol and epinephrine stimulate both subtypes, and norepinephrine stimulates only the β_1 subtype. Likewise, α-adrenoceptors have been subdivided into the α_1 and α_2 subtypes, and epinephrine and norepinephrine stimulate both subtypes. Although the naturally occurring catecholamines cannot distinguish between α_1- and α_2-adrenoceptors, many synthetic drugs do. Thus, phenylephrine and methoxamine are potent and highly selective α_1-adrenoceptor agonists, whereas clonidine and α-methylnorepinephrine (the active metabolite of α-methyldopa) are potent and selective α_2-adrenoceptor agonists.[93]

Central α-Adrenoceptors

Clonidine is an α_2-adrenoceptor agonist with antihypertensive activity resulting from an action within the CNS.[53] Clonidine is believed to interrupt the normal cardiovascular reflex loop. The primary site of action of clonidine is now believed to be the ventrolateral medulla, where α_2-adrenoceptors exist postsynaptically on dendrites of neurons that terminate in the intermediolateral cell column of the spinal cord.[89] When these postsynaptic α_2-adrenoceptors in the ventrolateral medulla are stimulated by clonidine, the neurons traversing to the intermediolateral cell column of the spinal cord are inhibited, resulting in inhibition of sympathetic outflow to the heart, vasculature, and kidneys. The net effect is vasodilation, which produces a decrease in total peripheral vascular resistance and a concurrent decrease in heart rate and cardiac output.[53, 63]

The antihypertensive activity of α-methyldopa likewise results from α_2-adrenoceptor stimulation in the brain, although the major site of action appears to differ from that of clonidine. α-Methyldopa is actively transported into the brain by an aromatic amino acid transport system. In the brain, α-methyldopa is subsequently decarboxylated and β-hydroxylated to form α-methyl-norepinephrine, a potent and selective α_2-adrenoceptor agonist[93] that interacts with α_2-adrenoceptors in the nucleus tractus solitarii[89] to produce a decrease in sympathetic outflow, in turn decreasing blood pressure and heart rate.

Peripheral α-Adrenoceptors

Presynaptic α-Adrenoceptors. The postsynaptic α-adrenoceptors that are located on effector organs and mediate their response have been known for many years. However, presynaptic α-adrenoceptors that, when activated, reduce neurotransmitter release by a negative feedback mechanism were identified more recently.[67, 104] The presynaptic α-adrenoceptor that inhibits neurotransmitter release is of the α_2 subtype.[67] The presynaptic α_2 adrenoceptor is stimulated by nor-

epinephrine released from the sympathetic nerve itself, which activates the negative feedback system to inhibit further release and thereby maintain synaptic levels of norepinephrine within a relatively narrow and optimal range (Fig 6–1).

The postganglionic nerve terminals innervating the vasculature, heart, and kidney all possess presynaptic α_2-adrenoceptors whose function is to inhibit neurotransmitter release. The presynaptic α_2-adrenoceptor appears to be similar at all neuroeffector junctions in the cardiovascular system, regardless of the receptor type (i.e., α_1, α_2, β_1, or β_2) located postsynaptically.

Postsynaptic Vascular α-Adrenoceptors. Defining the postsynaptic or postjunctional α-adrenoceptor that mediates vasoconstriction has been the target of many recent investigations. It is now widely accepted that α_1- and α_2-adrenoceptors coexist postsynaptically in the vasculature of most mammalian species, including humans, and that both α-adrenoceptor subtypes mediate vasoconstriction.[35, 38, 84, 99]

Although vasoconstriction may be mediated by a mixed population of postsynaptic vascular α_1- and α_2-adrenoceptors, the physiologic function and/or distribution of these receptors is just now beginning to be understood. It has recently been shown in most vascular beds in the *arterial* circulation that postsynaptic α-adrenoceptors located close to the neuroeffector junction (i.e., junctional receptors) are of the α_1 subtype,

Vascular Neuroeffector Junction

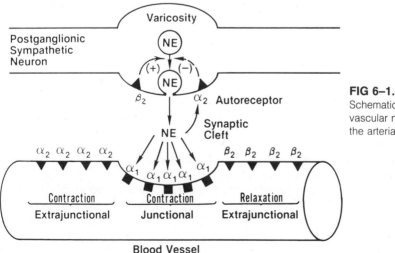

FIG 6–1.
Schematic representation of vascular neuroeffector junction in the arterial circulation.

whereas those postsynaptic vascular α-adrenoceptors located extrajunctionally are of the α_2 subtype (see Fig 6–1).[68] The physiologic role of the postsynaptic junctional α_1-adrenoceptors in the arterial circulation appears to be maintaining normal vascular tone. Presumably, these receptors, which are located in the vicinity of the synapse, would interact with norepinephrine liberated from sympathetic nerves. In contrast, the physiologic role of the extrajunctional α_2-adrenoceptors is not fully understood. It has been proposed that the extrajunctional α_2-adrenoceptors in the arterial circulation do not normally interact with norepinephrine liberated from sympathetic nerves since they are located at a distance from the adrenergic nerve terminal.[68] It has been suggested, therefore, that the extrajunctional α_2-adrenoceptors may respond to circulating epinephrine (and to a lesser extent, norepinephrine) released by the adrenal glands and acting as a blood-borne hormone.[68] On the *venous* side, in marked contrast to the arterial circulation, it appears that both α_1- and α_2-adrenoceptors may be postjunctional in the synaptic cleft, perhaps with even the α_2-adrenoceptor being selectively innervated.[37]

Postsynaptic Cardiac α-Adrenoceptors. The predominant postsynaptic adrenergic receptor in the heart is the β_1-adrenoceptor, which mediates a positive inotropic and chronotropic response.[18] However, there are postsynaptic α_1-adrenoceptors in the hearts of most mammalian species, including humans, that mediate a positive inotropic response without notably changing heart rate.[97] The mechanism by which cardiac α_1-adrenoceptors increase force of contraction has not been established, but it appears not to be associated with accumulation of cyclic adenosine monophosphate (cAMP) or stimulation of adenylate cyclase.[19] In this respect, α_1-adrenoceptors differ from β_1-adrenoceptors in the myocardium. Other differences between myocardial α_1- and β_1-adrenoceptors are the longer rate of onset and duration of action for α_1-adrenoceptor-mediated inotropic responses.[96] Differences among electrophysiologic actions mediated by α_1- and β_1-adrenoceptors have also been observed.[44] β_1-Adrenoceptor-mediated inotropic responses occur at all rates of contraction, but the effect mediated by α_1-adrenoceptors is most prominent at lower rates.[18]

Renal α-Adrenoceptors. α-Adrenoceptors in the kidney have been known for many years,

and α-adrenergic drugs produce a variety of renal effects. The functions and locations of the renal α-adrenoceptors are now only beginning to be understood.[108] Radioligand binding studies indicate that α_1- and α_2-adrenoceptors coexist in the kidneys of a variety of mammalian species; however, the number, proportion, and distribution of each α-adrenoceptor subtype may vary from one species to another.[108]

It is believed that α_1-adrenoceptors predominate in the human renal vasculature and mediate a vasoconstrictor response, thereby modulating renal blood flow.[51] α_2-Adrenoceptors have been identified in the juxtaglomerular apparatus and appear to inhibit renin release.[108] Recently it has been demonstrated that stimulation of renal α_2-adrenoceptors can inhibit the effects of vasopressin on water and sodium excretion.[101] This effect, mediated by α_2-adrenoceptors, appears to involve inhibition of adenylate cyclase and reductions in cellular cAMP, and may occur at the level of the cortical collecting tubule.[66] The α_2-adrenoceptor-mediated enhancement in sodium and water excretion occurs simultaneously with a decrease in potassium secretion. α-Adrenoceptors may also enhance sodium and water reabsorption in the proximal convoluted tubules.[108] In addition, gluconeogenesis in the proximal convoluted tubule has been shown to be under α_1-adrenergic control.[62]

The density of renal α_2-adrenoceptors is higher in spontaneously hypertensive and Dahl salt-sensitive hypertensive rats than in their normotensive controls, and high-sodium diets may increase α_2-adrenoceptor number even further.[45, 86] Thus, renal α_2-adrenoceptors may be involved in certain forms of genetic hypertension.

The nonuniform and differential distribution of α_1- and α_2-adrenoceptors in the kidney and the various functions these α-adrenoceptor subtypes subserve, such as regulation of renal blood flow, renin secretion, sodium and water excretion and reabsorption, and gluconeogenesis, indicate the complex nature of α-adrenergic effects in this organ.

Cardiovascular Effects of α-Adrenergic Drugs
Peripheral α-Adrenoceptor Blocking Agents as Antihypertensives. Since vascular tone is mediated predominantly by α-adrenoceptors, it is logical to assume that pharmacologic antagonists of α-adrenoceptors would abate hypertension. Indeed, the α-adrenoceptor antago-

nists, tolazoline (Priscoline) and phentolamine (Regitine), were introduced as clinical antihypertensive agents many years ago. These competitive α-adrenoceptor antagonists do in fact lower blood pressure, but their clinical efficacy has been unaccountably low. One explanation that has been proposed for the ineffectiveness of these agents in hypertension is their ability to potentiate neuronal norepinephrine release.[106] Both tolazoline and phentolamine are nonselective α-adrenoceptor antagonists and therefore have potent antagonist activity at prejunctional α₂-adrenoceptors in addition to their postjunctional α-adrenolytic effects. Their prejunctional α₂-adrenoceptor antagonist activity appears to interrupt the inhibitory negative feedback loop that regulates neurotransmitter release (see Fig 6–1), thereby increasing synaptic levels of norepinephrine. The elevated levels of norepinephrine in the synaptic cleft may partially overcome the postjunctional α₁-adrenoceptor antagonist effects and thus limit antihypertensive efficacy. This hypothesis has been widely accepted, primarily in light of the high antihypertensive efficacy observed with prazosin (Minipress), a highly selective α₁-adrenoceptor antagonist.[31] Since prazosin possesses only weak antagonist activity at presynaptic α₂-adrenoceptors, the neuronal negative feedback loop remains intact to prevent synaptic concentrations of norepinephrine from becoming elevated.[31]

In the human forearm, yohimbine, a selective α₂-adrenoceptor antagonist, produces arterial vasodilation and increases blood flow.[14] This finding suggests that at least in this vascular bed, the postsynaptic extrajunctional α₂-adrenoceptor may also play a significant role, along with the junctional α₁-adrenoceptor, in maintaining vascular tone. Vasoconstrictor activity mediated by postsynaptic extrajunctional α₂-adrenoceptors may play more of a role in the hypertensive state, as shown both in animal studies[78, 81] and in clinical studies in which increased vasodilatory activity of yohimbine and increased pressor potency to epinephrine have been observed in patients with essential hypertension.[15]

Circulating catecholamines are known to be elevated in a major subpopulation of patients with essential hypertension,[43] and these high plasma catecholamine levels have been proposed to contribute to the increased vascular resistance characteristic of essential hypertension.[3] The fact that circulating catecholamines appear to be the endogenous agonists for the extrajunctional vascular α₂-adrenoceptors suggests that in this subgroup of

patients, postjunctional α₂-adrenoceptors may in fact contribute to the elevated peripheral vascular resistance. As such, α₂-adrenoceptor blockade may prove to be beneficial in clinical antihypertensive therapy. To date, α₂-adrenoceptor-blocking drugs given orally have been poorly absorbed or are of only short duration of action. Phentolamine administered orally produces only very low plasma levels in humans[100] and short-lived antihypertensive activity in DOCA-salt hypertensive rats.[52] Improved α₂-adrenoceptor antagonists showing a superior profile to phentolamine in animal models have been identified[52, 90] and are currently being evaluated in humans to determine whether α₂-adrenoceptor blockade may also be a useful therapeutic approach in hypertension.

α-Adrenoceptor Antagonists in Congestive Heart Failure. Vasodilators have assumed a more prominent role in the treatment of congestive heart failure during the past decade, in part because technical advances have shown their desirable hemodynamic effects.[16] In most patients with congestive heart failure the optimal vasodilator is one that acts relatively equally on the arterial and venous beds. Sodium nitroprusside does so, but must be administered intravenously. Prazosin, an orally active selective α₁-adrenoceptor antagonist, has been shown to mimic the hemodynamic effects of nitroprusside in congestive heart failure, increasing cardiac output, decreasing left ventricular filling pressure and systemic and pulmonary vascular resistance, and maintaining heart rate.[8, 9] Although acute tolerance has been observed after multiple doses of prazosin over a period of 24–72 hours,[5] the beneficial effect often returns with continued therapy, and long-term clinical trials with prazosin show chronic efficacy in patients with congestive heart failure.[103] Prazosin improves symptoms most during exercise.[92]

Since there is evidence that the degree of sympathetic tone is proportional to the severity of heart failure,[85, 111] and since the level of plasma catecholamines has been implicated as a primary risk factor in patients with congestive heart failure,[28] the use of α-adrenoceptor antagonists in low output cardiac failure may have a rational advantage over other vasodilators. An additional benefit may be that anginal frequency decreases with reduced afterload, and cardiac oxygen needs may be diminished.[11]

The factor that correlates best with mortality in patients with heart failure is a high level of circulating catecholamines.[28] Since, as discussed earlier, circulating catecholamines may be the natural substrates for postsynaptic extrajunctional α_2-adrenoceptors in the arterial circulation, and since high plasma catecholamine levels may contribute to the increased total peripheral vascular resistance characteristic of congestive heart failure,[17, 85] the evaluation of an α_2-adrenoceptor antagonist in low output cardiac failure is indicated.

β-Adrenoceptors

Central β-Adrenoceptors

β-Adrenoceptors have been identified on many neurons of the CNS,[56] but their role in cardiovascular regulation is unclear. Activation of central β-adrenoceptors has been shown to elevate blood pressure and heart rate.[33] This observation is supported by the fact that injection of β-adrenoceptor antagonists into the CNS decreases blood pressure and heart rate.[33] In addition, systemic administration of β-adrenoceptor antagonists produces decreases in resting splanchnic sympathetic nerve discharge that correlate with reductions in arterial blood pressure.[70] Intravenously administered propranolol has been reported to interrupt the cardiovascular reflex loop in the CNS and inhibit sympathetic outflow.[34] Increases in blood pressure and heart rate evoked by sinoaortic denervation may be attenuated by injecting small doses of propranolol into the CNS.[83] These results are highly suggestive of a centrally mediated tonic β-adrenergic influence to increase blood pressure, and of a possible central mechanism for the antihypertensive effects of β-blockers.[65] However, those β-adrenoceptor antagonists that do not penetrate the blood-brain barrier, such as atenolol, are also highly effective antihypertensive agents, which suggests that the peripheral antihypertensive effects of β-adrenoceptor antagonists are also significant.

Peripheral β-Adrenoceptors

Presynaptic β-Adrenoceptors. The most intensely studied presynaptic adrenoceptor is the α_2-adrenoceptor, which inhibits neurotransmitter liberation. More recently, presynaptic β_2-adrenoceptors have been identified and shown to facilitate neurotransmitter release (see Fig 6–1). It has been shown that presynaptic β_2-adrenoceptors enhance stimulus-evoked norepinephrine release, which suggests that prejunctional β_2-adrenoceptors mediate a positive feedback on sympathetic

neurotransmission. The prejunctional β_2-adrenoceptor has been found in a variety of species, including humans.[22, 76, 77]

Most experiments characterizing the prejunctional β_2-adrenoceptor have used either epinephrine or isoproterenol as agonists. Norepinephrine is not a potent presynaptic β_2-adrenoceptor agonist,[78] acting instead on the presynaptic α_2-adrenoceptor to inhibit neurotransmitter release. It is therefore logical to assume that epinephrine is the physiologic ligand for the presynaptic β_2-adrenoceptor. This has led to the "epinephrine hypothesis" of essential hypertension, which suggests that activation of prejunctional β_2-adrenoceptors by neuronally released epinephrine may initiate the disease process.

Epinephrine Hypothesis of Essential Hypertension. Epinephrine, synthesized and released by the adrenal gland, has a short half-life in the systemic circulation. Although circulating epinephrine levels during stress are equivalent to the threshold concentration for in vitro activation of prejunctional β_2-adrenoceptors,[67] any β_2-adrenoceptor-mediated effect of circulating epinephrine on neuronal norepinephrine release should be transient. However, circulating epinephrine is readily accumulated by sympathetic nerve terminals via the neuronal uptake pump for sympathomimetic amines (uptake$_1$). In the sympathetic nerve terminal, epinephrine can be co-stored and co-released with norepinephrine.[78] Increases in the epinephrine content of tissues with dense sympathetic innervation are observed after stimulation-induced adrenal epinephrine secretion.[87] Since epinephrine, but not norepinephrine, will activate the prejunctional β_2-adrenoceptor, epinephrine co-released with norepinephrine will shift the balance toward increased β_2- relative to α_2-adrenoceptor-mediated prejunctional effects, thus increasing the net efficiency of sympathetic neurotransmission. Increased norepinephrine release in response to neuronally released epinephrine has been demonstrated both in vitro in guinea pig and rat atrial tissue[77] and in vivo in humans.[22]

Continuous infusion of low doses of epinephrine induces hypertension in rats.[77, 112] This effect is not mimicked by norepinephrine infusion and can be blocked by propranolol, suggesting an action on prejunctional β_2-adrenoceptors. Tachycardia is often an additional consequence of epinephrine infusion; this tachycardia is attenuated by neuronal uptake blockade and is much more persistent after epinephrine infusion than after isoproterenol administration, the latter not being a substrate for neuronal uptake.[21]

The results of a large-scale clinical study in Great Britain correlating blood pressure and plasma catecholamine levels in hypertensive and prehypertensive subjects support a role for epinephrine in the development of the hypertensive state.[20] While the mechanism(s) of the antihypertensive activity of β-adrenoceptor blocking agents has not been established, the blockade of presynaptic facilitory β-adrenoceptors and the resulting inhibition of neurotransmitter liberation must be considered.

Myocardial β-Adrenoceptors. The postsynaptic β-adrenoceptor of the heart that mediates an increase in both the rate and force of contraction is predominantly the β_1 subtype.[18] Biochemical studies indicate that the positive inotropic and chronotropic responses to catecholamines are mediated by β_1-adrenoceptor activation of adenylate cyclase, with the ultimate generation and accumulation of AMP.[18]

Recent studies have shown that there also may exist myocardial β_2-adrenoceptors in the sinoatrial node in some mammalian species. The functional significance of these β_2-adrenoceptors is not known and they appear not to be innervated.[18] It has been proposed that noninnervated extrajunctional β_2-adrenoceptors in the heart may represent "hormonal" adrenoceptors that are responsive to circulating blood-borne epinephrine.[4, 18]

Vascular β-Adrenoceptors. Postsynaptic vascular β_2-adrenoceptors mediate vasodilation. It appears that the vascular β_2-adrenoceptors, like the vascular α_2-adrenoceptors, are not innervated (i.e., are located extrajunctionally) (see Fig 6–1).[4] It has been proposed, therefore, that extrajunctional vascular β_2-adrenoceptors are "hormonal" receptors that mediate vasodilation in response to circulating epinephrine in certain vascular beds at times of stress, when plasma levels of epinephrine are elevated. It has recently been shown that the vasodilatory response mediated by vascular β_2-adrenoceptors after ganglionic stimulation is abolished by bilateral adrenalectomy, indicating that this response results from the action of circulating epinephrine liberated by the adrenal glands.[4]

Renal β-Adrenoceptors. The kidney is also heavily under adrenergic control. Probably the most important adrenergic effect in the kidney is the regulation of renin release from the juxtaglomerular apparatus.[61] Renin release from the juxtaglomerular cells is enhanced by β_1-adrenoceptor stimulation and/or stimulation of renal adrenergic nerves.[61] The increase in renin release evoked by the exogenous administration of β-adrenoceptor agonists or by adrenergic nerve stimulation is antagonized by β-adrenoceptor blocking agents such as propranolol. It appears that the juxtaglomerular cells are under a constant adrenergic tone since β-adrenoceptor blocking agents also inhibit basal renin release.[61] It has been suggested that the magnitude of the antihypertensive response to β-adrenoceptor antagonists depends on the initial plasma renin activity and the degree of its suppression by β-adrenoceptor blockade.[23] However, the relevance of the decrease in renin release mediated by β-adrenoceptor antagonists to the antihypertensive effects of these compounds has been questioned, since the reduction in blood pressure does not always parallel the reduction in renin release. In addition, some β-adrenoceptor blockers with intrinsic sympathomimetic activity may themselves promote renin release by their inherent β-adrenoceptor agonist properties,[61] yet these compounds nonetheless are effective antihypertensive agents in humans.

Renal β-adrenoceptors also appear to regulate renal blood flow at the vascular level. β-Adrenoceptors in the vasculature have been identified pharmacologically and mediate the expected vasodilatory response resulting in an increase in renal blood flow.

β-Adrenoceptors may also affect renal salt and water metabolism, but these effects are controversial and the results are often contradictory.[61]

Cardiovascular Effects of β-Adrenergic Drugs

β-Adrenoceptor Antagonists Used in the Management of Hypertension. β-Adrenoceptor blocking agents are commonly used to treat hypertension. Several β-adrenoceptor antagonists are available, and they are significantly different. Certain β-adrenoceptor antagonists, such as propranolol, are nonselective in that they antagonize both β_1- and β_2-adrenoceptors. Other β-adrenoceptor antagonists, such as atenolol, are termed "cardioselective" because they may preferentially antagonize myocardial β_1-adrenoceptors. Finally, a class of β-adrenoceptor antagonists with intrinsic sympathomimetic activity is now available, the prototype being pindolol. These different classes of β-adrenoceptor antagonists produce qualitatively and quantitatively distinct hemodynamic responses in humans and therefore should not be considered one homogeneous class of drugs possessing similar pharmacologic activities.

As indicated earlier, the mechanism of action of β-adrenoceptor antagonists in hypertension is still a matter of controversy. On the basis of the previously discussed effects that may be attributed to central β-adrenoceptors, and peripheral presynaptic and postsynaptic β-adrenoceptors in the heart, vasculature, and kidney, four logical mechanisms for the antihypertensive activity of β-blocking agents may be postulated: (1) an action within the CNS to antagonize the central β-adrenoceptor-mediated increases in blood pressure and heart rate; (2) presynaptic β-adrenoceptor blockade to inhibit the β-adrenoceptor-mediated positive feedback mechanism on neurotransmitter (norepinephrine) liberation in the heart and vasculature; (3) blockade of postsynaptic cardiac β_1-adrenoceptors to decrease the rate and force of myocardial contraction and thereby decrease cardiac output; and (4) inhibition of renin release, which is stimulated by β_1-adrenoceptor activation (in humans).

All classes of β-adrenoceptor antagonists lower blood pressure regardless of β-adrenoceptor subtype selectivity or the presence of intrinsic sympathomimetic activity. Furthermore, no one mechanism will adequately account for the antihypertensive activity of β-adrenoceptor antagonists in general. Thus, some β-adrenoceptor blockers do not penetrate the blood-brain barrier, whereas others with intrinsic sympathomimetic activity may enhance renin release. In addition, β-adrenoceptor antagonists decrease heart rate and cardiac output acutely, yet the antihypertensive effect of β-adrenoceptor blockers may take days to develop. It is likely, therefore, that several of these mechanisms may contribute to the antihypertensive activity of any one β-adrenoceptor blocker.

When β-adrenoceptor antagonists (without intrinsic sympathomimetic activity) are first administered, there is an acute decrease in heart rate and cardiac output and a reflex increase in total peripheral vascular resistance, such that no net change in blood pressure results. After a period of latency, total peripheral vascular resistance begins to decrease toward initial values in the face of continued reduced cardiac output, and the net effect is a decrease in blood pressure.[64] At times, total peripheral resistance may only return to normal levels, but cardiac output remains low and the net effect is still a reduction in blood pressure.[82]

In spite of the initial elevation in total peripheral vascular resistance, it has been shown that the antihypertensive effect of propranolol follows closely the secondary fall in peripheral resistance that occurs with time, even when there is some restoration in cardiac output.

β-Adrenoceptor Blocking Agents in Angina. The β-adrenoceptor blocking agents are useful in angina pectoris because they decrease myocardial oxygen demand. There are three determinants of myocardial oxygen demand: (1) myocardial wall tension, which is a function of ventricular pressure and the radius of the ventricle, (2) heart rate, and (3) contractility. β-Adrenoceptor antagonists produce a decrease in heart rate and contractile force, resulting simply from β-adrenoceptor blockade. The chronic antihypertensive effect of β-adrenoceptor blockers also serves to reduce myocardial wall tension by decreasing ventricular systolic developed pressure and by decreasing the size of the hypertrophied left ventricle. Therefore, the utility of β-adrenoceptor antagonists in treating angina pectoris results from the ability of these compounds to decrease the demand made by the myocardium for oxygen by each of the three factors known to create an oxygen demand.[48]

β-Adrenoceptor Agonists in Congestive Heart Failure. In heart failure, the goal of therapy is usually to increase cardiac output, and this is often done by increasing the contractile state of the myocardium. One mechanism that may be used to augment cardiac function is activation of myocardial β_1-adrenoceptors, which increases heart rate and contractility and therefore increases cardiac output. The increase in heart rate that occurs with isoproterenol may be undesirable since it increases myocardial work and oxygen demand. With certain inotropic agents, it is possible to selectively increase myocardial contractility while producing little or no increase in heart rate.

Intravenous infusion of dobutamine generally increases cardiac output by augmenting stroke volume,[1] the latter occurring directly from enhanced left ventricular contractility (dp/dt max).[57] Total peripheral vascular resistance (afterload) is reduced in part by reflex withdrawal of sympathetic tone[71] and in part by direct arterial vasodilation.[94] The reduction in afterload produced by dobutamine further increases left ventricular stroke volume by reducing the impedance to left ventricular ejection. Furthermore, the decrease in total peripheral vascular resistance offsets the contribution made by cardiac output to blood pressure such that mean arterial pressure is only minimally affected while cardiac output is significantly increased.[69]

Dobutamine infusion is generally associated with decreases in central venous pressure, right and left atrial pressures, pulmonary artery pressure and resistance, and pulmonary capillary wedge pressure.[69] Consequently, left ventricular end-diastolic volume (preload, represented by left ventricular end-diastolic pressure) is lowered, allowing the hypertrophied myocardium characteristic of congestive heart failure to reduce to a more efficient size.[102] The decrease in left ventricular end-systolic volume also decreases myocardial wall tension, an important determinant of myocardial oxygen consumption.[48]

With doses of isoproterenol and dobutamine that produce comparable increases in cardiac output, larger decreases in total peripheral vascular resistance, and hence greater reductions in blood pressure, are observed with isoproterenol.[102] In addition, tachycardia is more pronounced with isoproterenol,[57] resulting from a greater direct positive chronotropic effect of isoproterenol as well as from an additional reflex increase in cardiac rate secondary to the greater reduction in vascular tone. The more profound increase in cardiac rate observed with isoproterenol relative to dobutamine at doses that produce equivalent increases in cardiac output indicates that a smaller contribution to cardiac output is derived from augmentation of stroke volume with isoproterenol relative to dobutamine.

When dopamine and dobutamine are infused at doses that produce equivalent increases in cardiac output, dobutamine is generally associated with greater reductions in left ventricular filling pressure and pulmonary capillary wedge pressure.[69] Quite commonly, dopamine is associated with no change or even an increase in pulmonary artery pressure, pulmonary capillary wedge pressure, and left ventricular end-diastolic pressure. Whereas dobutamine tends to have minimal effects on blood pressure, dopamine is more likely to produce an increase in total peripheral vascular resistance and mean arterial blood pressure.[69] At low doses, dopamine has been shown to produce a selective increase in renal blood flow, secondary to a decrease in renal vascular resistance.[41] This action of dopamine, which is lacking with dobutamine, has been ascribed to selective renal vasodilation resulting from activation of renal DA_1-dopamine receptors. In contrast, the improvement in renal function observed with dobutamine appears to be secondary to an increase in cardiac output and a reflex decrease in total peripheral vascular resistance.[69]

At doses that produce comparable increases in cardiac output, epinephrine and norepinephrine tend to cause more tachycardia and greater increases in total peripheral vascular resistance than dobutamine. Consequently, dobutamine tends to increase stroke volume while not greatly affecting blood pressure or heart rate, whereas epinephrine and norepinephrine may cause a smaller increase in stroke volume due to the increased impedance to left ventricular ejection resulting from elevation of afterload, the latter serving to limit increases in stroke volume elicited by improved myocardial contractility.

Dopamine Receptors

Central Dopamine Receptors

Administration of dopamine or other dopamine receptor agonists into various brain regions may elicit a hypotensive and bradycardic response that is antagonized by dopamine receptor antagonists.[10] It has also been reported that dopamine administered directly into the brain produces an increase in blood pressure and heart rate.[32] However, in the latter studies, only dopamine was used, and it is established that dopamine will exert effects on α- and β-adrenoceptors[94] as well as on dopamine receptors, making the results of such studies difficult to interpret. In spite of the complexities in studying the central cardiovascular regulatory effects of dopamine, the use of selective and relatively specific dopamine receptor agonists suggests a minor inhibitory effect mediated by dopamine receptors on blood pressure and heart rate, although a much less significant effect than the one elicited by norepinephrine and α_2-adrenoceptors.

Peripheral Dopamine Receptors
Subclassification of Dopamine Receptors. As observed with α- and β-adrenoceptors, dopamine receptors have been identified both on sympathetic nerve terminals (presynaptic, or DA_2) and on smooth muscle cells of certain vascular beds (postsynaptic, or DA_1). The presynaptic DA_2 dopamine receptors mediate an inhibition of neurotransmitter release, whereas the postsynaptic DA_1 dopamine receptors on vascular smooth muscle mediate a vasodilatory response. Although the presence of specific receptors for dopamine has been conclusively established, the presence of dopamine-releasing neurons in the periphery is still controversial, except for the interneurons in sympathetic ganglia.

Presynaptic Dopamine (DA_2) Receptors. Neurotransmission at the vascular and cardiac sympathetic neuroeffector junctions can be modulated via presynaptic DA_2 receptors, which exert an inhibitory influence on stimulus-evoked neurotransmitter release from sympathetic nerve terminals.[26, 73] In the vasculature, which is under a dominant adrenergic control, stimulation of presynaptic DA_2 receptors on sympathetic neurons leads to inhibition of norepinephrine release, thereby producing passive vasodilation. This passive vasodilation results in a decrease in total peripheral resistance and a concomitant reduction in blood pressure.

In the heart, a similar response to presynaptic dopamine receptor activation occurs; however, the heart, unlike the vasculature, is under both cholinergic inhibitory and adrenergic facilitory neurogenic tone, and the cholinergic input dominates. Stimulation of presynaptic DA_2 receptors on postganglionic sympathetic nerve terminals produces the expected inhibition of norepinephrine release and subsequent decrease in adrenergic tone to the heart, with bradycardia resulting from an even further dominance of cholinergic tone. This effect has been demonstrated in vivo as inhibition of the chronotropic response to electrical stimulation of the cardioaccelerator nerve[12, 49] or as inhibition of reflex tachycardia resulting from nitroglycerin-induced hypotension.[13]

Stimulation of DA_2 receptors on sympathetic nerve terminals removes the input that these nerves provide to their effector organs by inhibiting norepinephrine release. The consequent loss of vascular and cardiac sympathetic tone results in an antihypertensive response and bradycardia.

Postsynaptic Vascular Dopamine (DA_1) Receptors. Postsynaptic vascular dopamine receptors mediate an active vasodilatory response in renal, mesenteric, hepatic, coronary, and cerebral vascular beds in a variety of species, including humans.[40, 42, 116] The use of selective dopamine agonists and antagonists has shown this receptor to be of the DA_1 subtype. The presence of vascular DA_1 receptors mediating an active postsynaptic (versus passive presynaptic) vasodilatory response in some, but not all, vascular beds offers a potentially important opportunity for selective drug action, especially since the vascular beds containing these DA_1 receptors include those most involved in cardiovascular disorders.

Dopamine Receptors in Sympathetic Ganglia. Dopamine-containing neurons have been identified in sympathetic ganglia.[72] These dopaminergic neurons are postulated to be short interneurons between preganglionic and postganglionic sympathetic nerves.[46] When activated by preganglionic sympathetic neurons, these interneurons release dopamine, which produces a long-lasting inhibitory postsynaptic potential of the postganglionic sympathetic neuron to inhibit efferent sympathetic outflow.[119] This neuroinhibitory action is thought to be mediated via a dopamine-sensitive adenylate cyclase.[60]

Recent evidence suggests that DA_1 receptors may be involved in the ganglia to inhibit sympathetic outflow, since the selective DA_1 agonist, fenoldopam, inhibits ganglionic neurotransmission.[2, 74, 95] Further evidence for DA_1-mediated inhibition in sympathetic ganglia has been provided by the observation that the neuroinhibitory effect of fenoldopam could not be blocked by the S-enantiomer of sulpiride, which has high DA_2 receptor selectivity, but was attenuated by R,S-sulpiride, an antagonist of both DA_1 and DA_2 receptors.[74] The ability of fenoldopam to produce cutaneous and skeletal vasodilation in the canine forelimb has been ascribed to DA_1 receptor–mediated inhibition of neurotransmission in the sympathetic ganglia.[47]

The possible therapeutic significance of the ganglionic dopamine receptor is unclear. Since activation of the ganglionic dopamine receptor inhibits neuronal activity of postganglionic sympathetic nerve fibers to the vasculature and heart,[54] a DA_1 agonist such as fenoldopam could produce a sympathoinhibitory effect similar to that seen on activation of presynaptic DA_2 receptors on postganglionic nerve terminals. Hence, DA_1 receptor activation may have both direct (postsynaptic) and indirect (ganglionic) vasodilator effects, and such drugs may prove to be effective antihypertensive agents in humans.

Dopaminergic Drugs Used in the Treatment of Cardiovascular Disorders

Dopamine in the Treatment of Shock. Dopamine is an agonist at presynaptic and postsynaptic dopamine receptors, DA_2 and DA_1, respectively, in the cardiovascular system. In addition, dopamine is also a potent indirectly acting sympathomimetic amine that is capable of entering the sympathetic nerve terminal and releasing endogenous stores of norepinephrine into the synapse. As such, some of the effects of the liberated norepinephrine (e.g., α_1-, α_2-, and β_1-adrenoceptor activation) also are observed following dopamine administration. In addition, dopamine itself will stimulate α- and β-adrenoceptors directly. It is now clear that this multitude of activities of dopamine contributes to the mostly beneficial effects of the compound in shock of multiple etiologies.[80] Thus, the dopaminergic effects of dopamine result in increases in renal, cerebral and coronary perfusion by an action on postsynaptic vascular DA_1-dopamine receptors to produce vasodilation in these critical vascular beds. The presynaptic DA_2 receptor effects of dopamine also inhibit norepinephrine release from nerves innervating the vasculature, and may further contribute to vasodilation in the renal, cerebral, and coronary beds. Vasoconstriction produced by dopamine in the less vital skeletal muscle and skin vascular beds, which is mediated by stimulation of α_1- and α_2-adrenoceptors, as well as the positive inotropic effect of dopamine mediated by myocardial β_1-adrenoceptors, all contribute to the redistribution of blood to the kidney, brain, and heart. These multiple effects of dopamine tend to sustain cardiac function while enhancing distribution of blood flow to vital organs.

Presynaptic (DA_2) Dopamine Receptor Agonists in the Management of Hypertension and Congestive Heart Failure. Presynaptic DA_2-dopamine receptors that inhibit norepinephrine release from adrenergic nerve terminals innervating the vasculature and heart are logical targets for drug action. Activation of these presynaptic dopamine receptors will decrease sympathetic tone to the vasculature and heart, leading to a decrease in blood pressure and heart rate.[73] In a preliminary clinical trial, N-n-propyl,N-n-butyldopamine (PBDA), a selective dopamine agonist, has been shown to be effective in lowering blood pressure in patients with essential hypertension at doses that were well tolerated.[110] The reduction in blood pressure was proposed to be mediated by stimulation of presynaptic DA_2 receptors. The observed increase in renal blood flow most likely results from stimulation of renal vascular DA_1 receptors.

Presynaptic dopamine DA_2 receptor agonists may also be useful in managing severe congestive heart failure as a direct consequence of their ability to reduce afterload by inhibiting norepinephrine release and thereby reducing total peripheral vascular resistance. In a recent study of risk factors in patients with congestive heart failure, plasma catecholamine level was the only variable to correlate significantly with mortality; higher plasma catecholamine levels were associated with a poorer prognosis.[28] The sympatholytic effect of a prejunctional DA_2 agonist may be especially beneficial in low output cardiac failure by producing peripheral arterial vasodilation and reduction in afterload without lowering inotropic state. Although the clinical efficacy of a DA_2 agonist in heart failure has not been established conclusively, PBDA has been shown to have a beneficial effect on the hemodynamic profiles of patients with low output cardiac failure, producing dose-dependent reductions in mean arterial pressure, left ventricular filling pressure, pulmonary vascular resistance, and systemic vascular resistance, accompanied by an increase in stroke volume and cardiac index.[36] Heart rate and stroke work index were unchanged.[36] Furthermore, it has recently been shown that the administration of levodopa, a precursor to dopamine in the periphery, increases cardiac index and stroke volume and decreases total peripheral vascular resistance with no change in blood pressure or heart rate in patients with congestive heart failure.[88]

Postsynaptic (DA_1) Dopamine Receptor Agonists Used in the Treatment of Hypertension and Renal Insufficiency. Agonists of postsynaptic DA_1 receptors produce active vasodilation of certain vascular beds, among the most important of which is the renal vasculature. Such compounds produce an antihypertensive response in humans, which may be secondary to diuresis resulting from enhanced renal blood flow, as well as from a possible tubular action of DA_1 receptors to inhibit sodium and water reabsorption. Currently, no selective postsynaptic DA_1-dopamine receptor agonists are clinically available. However, fenoldopam, a potent and selective DA_1 receptor agonist, has been shown to be effective in reducing blood pressure in patients with essential hypertension[24, 50, 117] and increasing renal plasma flow in normal volunteers,[24, 107] and is currently under clinical evaluation as an antihypertensive drug.

Serotonin (5-HT) Receptors

Central 5-HT Receptors

Low doses of serotonin injected into the brains of rats produce an increase in blood pressure and heart rate.[65] Centrally administered 5-HT also increases the firing rate of peripheral preganglionic sympathetic nerves, an effect that is presumably responsible for the observed hypertension and tachycardia.[65] Centrally administered 5,6-dihydroxytryptamine, which destroys serotonin-containing nerves and thereby releases 5-HT, produces tachycardia and hypertension.[65] Some data indicate that the tachycardia observed following stimulation of 5-HT receptors in the brain results from inhibition of cholinergic outflow, whereas the increase in blood pressure appears to coincide with an increase in sympathetic outflow to the vasculature.[65]

Peripheral Postsynaptic 5-HT Receptors

The peripheral effects of serotonin are complex, sometimes increasing and at other times decreasing blood pressure. It appears that the occasional decrease in blood pressure elicited by serotonin is not a direct effect of serotonin on the vasculature, but rather is due to stimulation by serotonin of a nonadrenergic, noncholinergic vasodilatory pathway, possibly involving a peptide neurotransmitter,[114] or to stimulation of presynaptic 5-HT receptors on adrenergic neurons that inhibit norepinephrine release. The more commonly observed vasoconstrictor effect of serotonin results from direct activation of postsynaptic vascular 5-HT receptors. On the basis of studies with selective serotonin agonists and antagonists, the postsynaptic vascular 5-HT recep-

tor mediating vasoconstriction has been classified as the $5-HT_2$ subtype,[29, 115] whereas the presynaptic serotonin receptor that inhibits norepinephrine release is of the $5-HT_1$ subtype.

Serotonin also potentiates the vasoconstrictor effect of α-adrenoceptor agonists and angiotensin II. This potentiation can be observed with concentrations of serotonin that have no vasoconstrictor activity.[114, 115] This effect, like the direct vasoconstrictor activity of serotonin, is mediated by $5-HT_2$ receptors.

Recent studies have shown that serotonin can also interact with receptors on vascular endothelium. Serotonin can dilate dog and pig coronary arteries contracted with a thromboxane agonist.[27] This dilation is seen only in vessels with intact endothelium and is not sensitive to $5-HT_2$ blockade with ketanserin, suggesting that endothelial $5-HT_1$ receptors are involved. Endogenous serotonin can also interact with endothelial receptors, since the vasoconstrictor response of dog coronary rings induced by aggregating platelets (which release serotonin) is significantly potentiated by removal of vascular endothelium.[30]

In a perfused coronary artery preparation with intact endothelium, serotonin can have opposite effects when administered extraluminally or intraluminally. Extraluminal administration of serotonin, which exposes predominantly vascular smooth muscle to serotonin, produces a contractile response, whereas with intraluminal administration of serotonin, in which the endothelium is preferentially exposed to serotonin, relaxation commonly occurs. In fact, intraluminal administration of serotonin can relax contractions induced by extraluminal serotonin. Relaxation can also be produced in this preparation by endogenous serotonin released from aggregating platelets.[30]

It is likely that at least some of these vasodilatory effects of serotonin may result from 5-HT_1 receptor activation. The relaxation induced by serotonin in isolated vascular tissues with intact endothelium can be blocked by methiotepin, a moderately selective $5-HT_1$ receptor antagonist, but not by ketanserin, a potent and selective $5-HT_2$ antagonist. In anesthetized rats treated with ketanserin (to block $5-HT_2$-mediated pressor activity), the hypotensive activity of a series of serotonin agonists correlated well ($r = 0.92$) with their affinity for $5-HT_1$ receptors.[58] This hypotensive effect suggests that $5-HT_1$ agonists may offer a unique approach to the treatment of hypertension.

Serotonergic Drugs Used in Cardiovascular Disorders

Serotonin Antagonists in Hypertension. The significance of peripheral serotonin receptors in hypertension is not clear. It has been proposed that peripheral 5-HT$_2$ receptors, by virtue of their ability to produce vasoconstriction, may be involved in the regulation of blood pressure. Ketanserin is a relatively selective 5-HT$_2$ receptor antagonist now being clinically evaluated as an antihypertensive drug. In humans, ketanserin is an effective antihypertensive agent,[113, 118] suggesting that peripheral vascular 5-HT$_2$ receptors may in fact play a role in hypertension in at least some patients. This observation is somewhat surprising since the vasculature receives no serotonergic innervation. Peripheral serotonin is formed in the enterochromaffin cells of the gastrointestinal tract; it escapes, is actively accumulated by platelets, and then is released upon aggregation.[114] It has been proposed that higher levels of serotonin could reach vascular 5-HT$_2$ receptors to mediate vasoconstriction in patients with hypertension if platelet uptake of serotonin were reduced and/or platelet aggregation accelerated.[114] Both of these phenomena have been observed in hypertensive patients, which raises the possibility, in theory, of a nonneuronal serotonergic tone to the vasculature in certain hypertensive states. This explanation has recently been proposed to account for the antihypertensive activity of ketanserin.[114]

However, this explanation for the antihypertensive activity of ketanserin has recently been challenged.[59] The basis for the argument against an antiserotonergic mechanism for the antihypertensive effects of ketanserin is twofold: (1) other 5-HT$_2$ antagonists fail to lower blood pressure,[55] and (2) ketanserin is also an α_1-adrenoceptor antagonist,[59] and it is well documented that α_1-adrenoceptor antagonists (e.g., prazosin) are effective antihypertensive agents because vascular tone is maintained largely by postsynaptic junctional α_1-adrenoceptors that respond to neuronally liberated norepinephrine (see Fig 6–1). It has been shown that the antihypertensive activity of ketanserin in spontaneously hypertensive rats may be completely accounted for by the α_1-adrenoceptor blocking activity of the compound.[59] Whether the same is true for the antihypertensive effects of ketanserin in humans is still not known and awaits further clinical evaluation.

Cholinergic Receptors

Muscarinic Cholinergic Receptors

Presynaptic Muscarinic Receptors. Presynaptic muscarinic cholinergic receptors have been identified on adrenergic nerve terminals that innervate the heart and blood vessels.[105] When stimulated, these presynaptic muscarinic receptors inhibit norepinephrine release and thereby decrease sympathetic tone to the various cardiovascular effector organs. The effects of presynaptic muscarinic receptor stimulation are usually not observed since they are relatively small in comparison to the response mediated by postsynaptic muscarinic receptors in the effector organs.

Postsynaptic Muscarinic Receptors. Although the heart is under a dual adrenergic and cholinergic innervation, it is clear that vagal cholinergic tone dominates.[98] The postjunctional cholinergic receptor in the heart is of the muscarinic type and mediates a decrease in both the rate and force of myocardial contraction. Intravenous administration of acetylcholine or other muscarinic cholinergic agonists will inhibit the spontaneous discharge of the sinoatrial node and thereby slow or abruptly stop spontaneous rhythm.

With only a few exceptions, such as in the genitals, the vasculature does not receive cholinergic innervation. Nevertheless, postsynaptic muscarinic receptors exist in the endothelium of the vasculature, and when activated by acetylcholine or exogenously administered muscarinic receptor agonists, these receptors mediate a pronounced vasodilatory response and hypotension through the release of a vascular smooth muscle relaxing factor of endothelial origin.[39]

Nicotinic Cholinergic Receptors

Presynaptic Nicotinic Receptors. Presynaptic nicotinic receptors have been identified on adrenergic nerve terminals. Their function is to facilitate norepinephrine release, in contrast to presynaptic muscarinic receptors, which inhibit neurotransmitter release.

Postsynaptic Nicotinic Receptors. Postsynaptic nicotinic receptors on cardiovascular effector organs play little if any role in the end-organ response. However, nicotinic cholinergic receptors mediate neurotransmission in autonomic ganglia and are located postsynaptically on the cell body and/or dendrites of the postganglionic sympathetic and postganglionic parasympathetic neurons. Hence, stimulation of ganglionic nicotinic receptors will activate the respective cholinergic or adrenergic outflows. The effect seen at the cardiovascular effector organ will depend on which component of the autonomic nervous system predominates. For example, since the adrenergic innervation dominates in the vasculature, stimulation of nicotinic ganglionic receptors will result in a selective stimulation of adrenergic nerves to the vasculature, which produces vasoconstriction and a subsequent increase in blood pressure. As expected, ganglionic blocking agents, which antagonize the nicotinic cholinergic receptor in the autonomic ganglia, will produce a dramatic decrease in blood pressure, and these agents have been used as antihypertensives. In the heart, where cholinergic tone dominates, ganglionic stimulation produces an effect that is predominantly cholinergic, and heart rate and force of contraction will decrease.

Use of Nicotinic (Ganglionic) Receptor Antagonists in Hypertension

One of the first classes of antihypertensives developed was the ganglionic blockers that antagonize the postjunctional nicotinic receptor in the autonomic ganglia. Since the innervation to the vasculature is predominantly sympathetic, interruption of ganglionic neurotransmission will decrease sympathetic tone to the vasculature and consequently decrease blood pressure.[98] Ganglionic blockers such as hexamethonium and mecamylamine are infrequently used because of their debilitating side effects, including orthostasis, syncope, and inhibition of gastric and bladder function. They may still be given, however, in severe hypertension in patients resistant to other forms of therapy. Their use is commonly associated with tachycardia resulting not from reflex but rather from removal, by ganglionic blockade, of the dominant inhibitory cholinergic tone to the heart.

Renin-Angiotensin System

Renal-Adrenal Axis

In the kidney and adrenal gland there is a closed loop feedback system that regulates electrolyte balance and is critical to the regulation of blood pressure. It is currently undergoing intensive study as a target of antihypertensive drug action.

The enzyme renin is released into the blood from the juxtaglomerular apparatus in the kidney. Renin in plasma enzymatically converts angiotensinogen into angiotensin I, which is relatively inert. However, angiotensin I is a substrate for angiotensin-converting enzyme, which generates angiotensin II. Angiotensin II is a potent vasoconstrictor that acts by stimulating postsynaptic vascular angiotensin II receptors to elevate blood pressure by producing systemic arterial vasoconstriction. Another mechanism was recently discovered that may contribute to the elevation in blood pressure elicited by angiotensin II and involves an effect of angiotensin II on presynaptic angiotensin II receptors associated with sympathetic neurons to facilitate norepinephrine release. The elevated synaptic levels of norepinephrine resulting from the presynaptic facilitory effect of angiotensin II will stimulate postsynaptic α_1-adrenoceptors to cause systemic vasoconstriction. In addition, angiotensin II will stimulate aldosterone release from the adrenal cortex which, in turn, causes tubular sodium and water retention, further elevating blood pressure. Elevated blood pressure and increased sodium normally inhibit further renin release to complete the closed loop (long loop) system. In addition, angiotensin II has been shown to directly inhibit renin release (short loop reflex). Clearly, the inability of the kidney to regulate renin release because of damage or an imbalance in the delicate reflex mechanism can result in the elevation of blood pressure with a concomitant electrolyte imbalance that may produce additional kidney damage, exacerbating the condition and leading to an even greater elevation in blood pressure and further electrolyte imbalance.

Angiotensin-Converting Enzyme Inhibitors in the Treatment of Hypertension

Angiotensin-converting enzyme converts angiotensin I to angiotensin II, and the latter is responsible directly for vasoconstriction and indirectly, through aldosterone release, for sodium and water retention. It is now known that angiotensin-converting enzyme is not restricted to plasma or lung, but may be found in many organs of the body, including the vasculature.[91] It has recently been established that inhibiting angiotensin-converting enzyme and subsequently decreasing angiotensin II formation is an effective method of lowering blood pressure in animals and humans. Captopril (Capoten) is a potent competitive inhibitor of angiotensin-converting enzyme and has recently been introduced clinically as an antihypertensive agent.

While originally thought to be useful only in those hypertensive patients with high plasma renin activities, captopril has been shown to be effective in most forms of hypertension (except primary aldosteronism) characterized by either high or low renin activities. However, greater reductions in blood pressure by captopril have been reported in patients with high plasma renin activity.[7] Administration of captopril to humans increases plasma renin activity by abolishing the negative feedback effect elicited by angiotensin II.[25] As a direct consequence of inhibiting angiotensin-converting enzyme, captopril increases circulating angiotensin I and decreases angiotensin II. Since angiotensin II levels are lowered after captopril administration, aldosterone levels likewise fall.[6]

The effectiveness of captopril in patients with normal or low plasma renin activities has led to the proposal that the renin-angiotensin system may be a contributing factor to most forms of hypertension.[91] For this reason, it is clear that measurements of plasma renin activity are not necessary to predict the likelihood of a response to captopril. Still, the effectiveness of captopril in patients with low renin activities has been an enigma. It is now known that the arterial wall of animals and humans contains all of the factors necessary to generate angiotensin II locally.[109] As indicated earlier, the vasculature also contains angiotensin-converting enzyme, which is capable of converting angiotensin I into angiotensin II, the latter possibly responsible for local vasoconstriction leading to elevated blood pressure. It is possible that the antihypertensive efficacy of captopril in patients and animals with low plasma renin activity may result from inhibition of angiotensin-converting enzyme, and subsequent blockade of angiotensin II formation, in the vasculature.[91]

Angiotensin-Converting Enzyme Inhibitors in Congestive Heart Failure

Although originally developed for hypertension, the angiotensin-converting enzyme inhibitor captopril has proved to be a highly effective agent in the management of congestive heart failure. The primary effect of angiotensin-converting enzyme inhibitors in low output cardiac failure is derived principally from a decrease in total peripheral vascular resistance (afterload). Secondary to the reduction in afterload is a marked increase in cardiac output due primarily to an augmentation in stroke volume, since heart rate is not markedly affected. As expected, the stroke work index increases.

Angiotensin-converting enzyme inhibitors also produce vasodilation on the venous side, and this, combined with improved left ventricular ejection, causes a profound reduction in left ventricular filling pressure (preload). Thus, in patients with congestive heart failure, angiotensin-converting enzyme inhibitors produce a significant reduction in right atrial pressure, pulmonary artery pressure, and left ventricular end-diastolic pressure.

Acknowledgment

The authors are indebted to Ms. Stephany Ruffolo for her assistance in the preparation of this manuscript.

REFERENCES

1. Akhtar N, Mikulik E, Cohn JN, et al: Hemodynamic effect of dobutamine in patients with severe heart failure. *Am J Cardiol* 1975; 36:202.
2. Alkhadhi KA, Sabouni MH, Lokhandwala MF: Characterization of dopamine receptors in a mammalian sympathetic ganglion. *Fed Proc* 1984; 43:1094.
3. Amann FW, Bolli P, Kiowski W, et al: Enhanced α-adrenoceptor-mediated vasoconstriction in essential hypertension. *Hypertension* 1981; 3(suppl 1):I–119.
4. Ariens EJ: The classification of β-adrenoceptors: 2. *Trends Pharmacol Sci* 1981; 2:170.
5. Arnold SB, Williams RL, Ports TA, et al: Attenuation of prazosin effect on cardiac output in chronic heart failure. *Ann Intern Med* 1979; 91:345.
6. Atlas SA, Case DB, Sealey JE, et al: Interruption of the renin-angiotensin system in hypertensive patients by captopril induces sustained reduction in aldosterone secretion, potassium retention and natriuresis. *Hypertension* 1979; 1:274.
7. Atlas SA, Case DB, Sealey JE, et al: Involvement of the renin-angiotensin-aldosterone axis in the antihypertensive action of captopril (SQ 14,225). *Circulation* 1978; 57/78(suppl II):II–143.

8. Awan NA, Miller RR, Maxwell KS, et al: Effects of prazosin on forearm resistance and capacitance vessels. *Clin Pharmacol Ther* 1977; 22:79.

9. Awan NA, Miller RR, Miller MP, et al: Clinical pharmacology and therapeutic application of prazosin in acute and chronic refractory congestive heart failure. *Am J Med* 1978; 65:146.

10. Barrett RJ, Lokhandwala MF: Central dopaminergic mechanisms on the cardiovascular actions of intracisternally-administered pergolide. *Fed Proc* 1982; vol 41, abstract 30064.

11. Bertel O, Burkart R, Buhler FR: Sustained effectiveness of chronic prazosin therapy in severe chronic congestive heart failure. *Am Heart J* 1981; 5:529.

12. Bhatnagar RK, Arneric SP, Cannon JG, et al: Structure activity relationships of presynaptic dopamine receptor agonists. *Pharmacol Biochem Behav* 1982; 17(suppl):11.

13. Blumberg AL, Wilson JW, Hieble JP: Neuroinhibitory effects of SK&F 85174, a novel dopamine receptor agonist. *J Cardiovasc Pharmacol* 1985; 7:723.

14. Bolli P, Erne P, Kiowski W, et al: Important contribution of post-junctional α_2-adrenoceptor-mediated vasoconstriction to arteriolar tone in man. *J Hypertension* 1983; 1(suppl 2):257.

15. Bolli P, Erne P, Block LH, et al: Adrenaline induces vasoconstriction through postjunctional α_2-adrenoceptor stimulation which is enhanced in essential hypertension. *J Hypertension* 1984; 2(suppl 3):115.

16. Breckenridge A: Vasodilators in heart failure. *Br Med J* 1982; 284:765.

17. Bristow MR: The adrenergic nervous system in heart failure. *N Engl J Med* 1984; 311:850.

18. Broadley KJ: Cardiac adrenoceptors. *J Auton Pharmacol* 1982; 2:119.

19. Brodde O-E, Motomura S, Endoh M, et al: Lack of correlation between the positive inotropic effect evoked by α-adrenoceptor stimulation and the levels of cyclic AMP and/or cyclic GMP in the isolated ventricle strip of the rabbit. *J Molec Cell Cardiol* 1978; 10:207.

20. Brown MJ: Adrenalin and essential hypertension in man, in Bevan JA, Godfraind T, Maxwell RA, et al (eds): *Vascular Neuroeffector Mechanisms*. Amsterdam, Elsevier Press, 1985, pp 251–256.

21. Brown MJ, Brown DC, Murphy MB: Hypokalemia from β_2-receptor stimulation by circulating epinephrine. *N Engl J Med* 1983; 309:1414.

22. Brown MJ, Macquin I: Is adrenaline the cause of essential hypertension? *Lancet* 1981; 2:1079.

23. Buhler FR, Laragh JH, Baer JH, et al: Propranolol inhibition of renin secretion: A specific approach to the diagnosis and treatment of renin-dependent hypertensive disease. *N Engl J Med* 1972; 287:1209.

24. Carey RM, Townsend LH, Rose CE, et al: The specific dopamine agonist, SK&F 82526-J, increases renal blood flow and lowers blood pressure in essential hypertension. *Clin Res* 1983; 31:487A.

25. Case DB, Atlas SA, Laragh JH, et al: Clinical experience with blockade of the renin-angiotensin-aldosterone system by an oral converting-enzyme inhibitor (SQ 14,225, captopril) in hypertensive patients. *Prog Cardiovasc Dis* 1978; 21:195.

26. Cavero I, Massingham R, Lefevre-Borg F: Peripheral dopamine receptors; potential targets for a new class of antihypertensive agents. Part II. Sites and mechanisms of action of dopamine receptor agonists. *Life Sci* 1982; 31:1059.

27. Cocks JM, Angus JA: Endothelium-dependent relaxation of coronary arteries by noradrenaline and serotonin. *Nature* 1983; 305:627.

28. Cohn JN, Levine TB, Olivari MM, et al: Plasma norepinephrine as a guide to prognosis in patients with chronic congestive heart failure. *N Engl J Med* 1984; 311:819.

29. Cohen ML, Fuller RW, Wiley KS: Evidence for 5-HT$_2$ receptors mediating contraction in vascular smooth muscle. *J Pharmacol Exp Ther* 1981; 218:421.

30. Cohen RA, Shepherd JJ, Vanhoutte PM: Inhibitory role of the endothelium in the response of isolated coronary arteries to platelets. *Science* 1983; 221:273.

31. Davey MJ: Relevant features of the pharmacology of prazosin. *J Cardiovasc Pharmacol* 1980; 2(suppl 3):S287.

32. Day MD, Roach AG: Cardiovascular effects of dopamine after central administration into conscious cats. *Br J Pharmacol* 1976; 58:505.

33. Day MD, Roach AG: Central α- and β-adrenoceptors modifying arterial blood pressure

and heart rate in conscious cats. *Br J Pharmacol* 51:325, 1974.

34. Dorward PK, Korner PI: Effect of *dl*-propranolol on renal sympathetic baroreflex properties and aortic baroreceptor activity. *Eur J Pharmacol* 1978; 52:61.

35. Elliott HL, Reid JL: Evidence for postjunctional vascular α_2-adrenoceptors in peripheral vascular regulation in man. *Clin Sci* 1983; 65:237.

36. Fennell WH, Taylor AA, Young JB, et al: Propylbutyldopamine: Hemodynamic effects in conscious dogs, normal human volunteers and patients with heart failure. *Circulation* 1983; 67:829.

37. Flavahan NA, Rimele TJ, Cooke JP: Characterization of postjunctional α_1- and α_2-adrenoceptors activated by exogenous or nerve-released norepinephrine in canine saphenous vein. *J Pharmacol Exp Ther* 1984; 230: 699.

38. Fowler PJ, Grous M, Price W, et al: Pharmacological differentiation of postsynaptic α-adrenoceptors in the dog saphenous vein. *J Pharmacol Exp Ther* 1984; 229:712.

39. Furchgott RF, Zawadzki JV: The obligatory role of endothelial cells in the relaxation of arterial smooth muscle by acetylcholine. *Nature* 1980; 288:373.

40. Furster C, Whalley ET: Dopamine receptors mediating relaxation of the human basilar artery in vitro. *Br J Pharmacol* 1981; 74:944P.

41. Goldberg LI, Hsieh YY, Resnekov L: Newer catecholamines for treatment of heart failure and shock: An update on dopamine and a first look at dobutamine. *Prog Cardiovasc Dis* 1977; 19:327.

42. Goldberg LI, Sonneville PF, McNay JL: An investigation of the structural requirements for dopamine-like renal vasodilation: Phenylethylamines and apomorphine. *J Pharmacol Exp Ther* 1968; 163:188.

43. Goldstein DS: Plasma catecholamines and essential hypertension: An analytical review. *Hypertension* 1983; 5:86.

44. Govier WC: Prolongation of the myocardial functional refractory period by phenylephrine. *Life Sci* 1967; 6:1367.

45. Graham RM, Pettinger WA, Sagalowsky A, et al: Renal α-adrenergic receptor abnormality in the spontaneously hypertensive rat. *Hypertension* 1982; 4:881.

46. Greengard P, Kebabian JW: Role of cyclic AMP in synaptic transmission in the mammalian peripheral nervous system. *Fed Proc* 1974; 33:1059.

47. Grega GJ, Barrett RJ, Adamski SW, et al: Effects of dopamine and SK&F 82526, a selective DA_1-receptor agonist, on vascular resistances in the canine in forelimb. *J Pharmacol Exp Ther* 1984; 229:756.

48. Gross GJ, Urquilla PR: Antianginal drugs, in Craig CR, Stitzel RE (eds): *Modern Pharmacology*. Boston, Little, Brown & Co, 1982, pp 283–294.

49. Hamed AT, Jandhyala BS, Ginos JZ, et al: Presynaptic dopamine receptors and α-adrenoceptors as mediators of the bradycardic action of N-n-propyl-N-n-butyldopamine. *Eur J Pharmacol* 1981; 74:83.

50. Harvey JN, Worth DP, Gregeen R, et al: Fenoldopam (SK&F 82526), a dopaminergic vasodilator: Studies in essential hypertension. *Br J Pharmacol* (in press).

51. Hepburn ER, Bentley GA: The effects of α-agonists on various vascular beds, in Bevan JA, Godfraind T, Maxwell RA, et al (eds): *Vascular Neuroeffector Mechanisms*. New York, Raven Press, 1980, pp 249–251.

52. Hieble JP, Roesler JM, Fowler PJ, et al: A new approach to antihypertensive therapy via blockade of the postjunctional α_2-adrenoceptor, in Bevan JA, Godfraind T, Maxwell RA, et al (eds): *Vascular Neuroeffector Mechanisms*. Amsterdam, Elsevier Press, 1985, pp 159–164.

53. Hoefke W, Kobinger W, Walland A: Relationship between activity and structure in derivatives of clonidine. *Arzneimittelforsch* 1975; 25:786.

54. Horn PT, Kohli JD, Goldberg LI: Facilitation of sympathetic ganglionic transmission by R-sulpiride. *Fed Proc* 1981; vol 40, abstract 320.

55. Humphrey PPA, Feniuk W, Watts AD: Ketanserin: A novel antihypertensive drug. *J Pharmacol* 1982; 34:541.

56. Iversen LL: Catecholamine-sensitive adenylate cyclases in nervous tissue. *J Neurochem* 1977; 29:5.

57. Jewitt D, Mitchell A, Birkhead J, et al: Clinical cardiovascular pharmacology of dobutamine. *Lancet* 1974; 2:363.

58. Kalkman HO, Boddeke WGM, Doods HN, et al: Hypotensive activity of serotonin receptor agonists in rats related to their affinity for 5-HT_1 receptors. *Eur J Pharmacol* 1983; 91:155.

59. Kalkman HO, Timmermans PBMWM, van Zwieten PA: Characterization of the antihypertensive properties of ketanserin (R 41 468) in rats. *J Pharmacol Exp Ther* 1982; 222:227.

60. Kebabian JW, Greengard P: Dopamine-sensitive adenyl cyclase: Possible role in synaptic transmission. *Science* 1971; 174:1346.

61. Keeton TK, Campbell WB: The pharmacologic alteration of renin release. *Pharmacol Rev* 1980; 32:81.

62. Kessar P, Saggerson ED: Evidence that catecholamines stimulate renal gluconeogenesis through an α_1-type of adrenoceptor. *Biochem J* 1980; 190:119.

63. Kobinger W: Central α-adrenergic system as targets for hypotensive drugs. *Rev Physiol Biochem Pharmacol* 1978; 81:39.

64. Korner PI: Discussion, in: Systemic hemodynamic effects of centrally acting antihypertensive agents, in Onesti G, Fernandes M, Kim KE (eds): *Regulation of Blood Pressure by the Central Nervous System*. New York, Grune & Stratton, Inc, 1976, p 412.

65. Korner PI, Angus JA: Central nervous control of blood pressure in relation to antihypertensive drug treatment. *Pharmacol Ther* 1981; 13:321.

66. Krothapalli RK, Suki W: Functional characterization of the α-adrenergic receptor modulating the hydroosmotic effect of vasopressin on the rabbit cortical collecting tubule. *J Clin Invest* 1984; 73:740.

67. Langer SZ: Presynaptic receptors and their role in the regulation of transmitter release. *Br J Pharmacol* 1977; 60:481.

68. Langer SZ, Massingham R, Shepperson N: Presence of postsynaptic α_2-adrenoreceptors of predominantly extrasynaptic location in the vascular smooth muscle of the dog hind limb. *Clin Sci* 59:225s, 1980.

69. Leier CV, Unverferth DV: Dobutamine. *Ann Intern Med* 1983; 99:490.

70. Lewis PJ, Haeusler G: Reduction in sympathetic nervous activity as a mechanism for hypotensive effect of propranolol. *Nature* 1975; 256:440.

71. Liang CS, Hood WB: Dobutamine infusion in conscious dogs with and without autonomic nervous system inhibition: Effects of systemic hemodynamics, regional blood flows and cardiac metabolism. *J Pharmacol Exp Ther* 1979; 211:698.

72. Libet B, Tosaka T: Dopamine as a synaptic transmitter and modulator in sympathetic ganglia: A different mode of synaptic action. *Proc Natl Acad Sci* 1970; 67:667.

73. Lokhandwala MF, Barrett RJ: Cardiovascular dopamine receptors: Physiological pharmacological and therapeutic implications. *J Auton Pharmacol* 1982; 3:189.

74. Lokhandwala MF, Watkins H, Alkhadhi KA: Involvement of DA_1-receptors in the neurogenic vasodilation produced by SK&F 82526 in the canine hindlimb. *Fed Proc* 1984; 43:1094.

75. Majewski H, Rand MJ, Tung LH: Activation of prejunctional β-adrenoceptors in rat atria by adrenaline applied exogenously or released as a co-transmitter. *Br J Pharmacol* 1981; 73:669.

76. Majewski H, Hedler L, Starke K: The noradrenaline release rate in the anesthetized rabbit: Facilitation by adrenaline. *Naunyn Schmiedebergs Arch Pharmacol* 1982; 321:20.

77. Majewski H, Tung LH, Rand MJ: Adrenaline activation of prejunctional β-adrenoceptors and hypertension. *J Cardiovasc Pharmacol* 1982; 4:99.

78. Majewski H, Tung LH, Rand MJ: Adrenaline-induced hypertension in rats. *J Cardiovasc Pharmacol* 1981; 3:179.

79. McCafferty JP, Hieble JP, Roesler JM, et al: Activation of both vascular α-adrenoceptor subtypes is required for maintenance of blood pressure in DOCA-salt hypertensive rats. *Fed Proc* 1982; 41:1668.

80. McCannel KL, McNay JL, Meyer MD, et al: Dopamine in the treatment of hypotension. *N Engl J Med* 1966; 275:1389.

81. Medgett IC, Hicks PE, Langer SZ: Smooth muscle α_2-adrenoceptors mediate vasoconstrictor responses to exogenous norepinephrine and to sympathetic stimulation to a greater extent in spontaneously hypertensive than in Wistar Kyoto rat tail arteries. *J Pharmacol Exp Ther* 1984; 231:159.

82. Meier M, Orwin J, Rogg H, et al: β-Adrenoceptor antagonists in hypertension, in Scriabine A (ed): *Pharmacology of Antihypertensive Drugs*. New York, Raven Press, 1980, pp 179–194.

83. Montastruc J-L, Montastruc P: Effect of intracisternal application of 6-hydroxydopamine on the antihypertensive action of propranolol

in the dog. *Eur J Pharmacol* 1980; 63: 103.

84. Muller-Schweinitzer E: α-Adrenoceptors, 5-hydroxytryptamine receptors and the action of dihydroergotamine in human venous preparations obtained during saphenectomy procedures for varicose veins. *Naunyn Schmiedebergs Arch Pharmacol* 1984; 327:299.

85. Ogasawara B, Ogawa K, Hayashi H, et al: Plasma renin activity and plasma concentration of norepinephrine and cyclic nucleotides in heart failure after prazosin. *Clin Pharmacol Ther* 1981; 29:464.

86. Pettinger WA, Gandler T, Sanchez A, et al: Dietary sodium and renal α₂-adrenoceptors in Dahl hypertensive rats. *Clin Exp Hypertension* 1982; A4(4&5):819.

87. Raab W, Gigee W: Die Katecholamine des Herzens. *Naunyn Schmiedebergs Arch Pharmacol* 1953; 219:248.

88. Rajfer SI, Anton AH, Rossen JD, et al: Beneficial hemodynamic effects of oral levodopa in heart failure. *N Engl J Med* 1984; 310:1357.

89. Reis DJ: The brain and hypertension: Reflections on 35 years of inquiry into the neurobiology of the circulation. *Circulation* 1984; 70:III-31.

90. Roesler JM, McCafferty JP, DeMarinis RM, et al: Characterization of the antihypertensive activity of SK&F 86466, a selective alpha-2 antagonist, in the rat. *J Pharmacol Exp Ther* 1986; 236:1.

91. Rubin B, Antonaccio MJ: Captopril, in Scriabine A (ed): *The Pharmacology of Antihypertensive Drugs*. New York, Raven Press, 1980, pp 21–42.

92. Rubin SA, Chatterjee K, Gelberg HJ, et al: Paradox of improved exercise but not resting hemodynamics with short term prazosin in chronic heart failure. *Am J Cardiol* 1979; 43:810.

93. Ruffolo RR Jr: Structure-activity relationships of α-adrenoceptor agonists, in Kunos G (ed): *Adrenoceptors and Catecholamine Action—Part B*. New York, John Wiley & Sons, Inc, 1983, pp 1–50.

94. Ruffolo RR Jr, Morgan EL: Interaction of novel inotropic agent, ASL-7022, with α- and β-adrenoceptors in the cardiovascular system of the pithed rat: Comparison with dobutamine and dopamine. *J Pharmacol Exp Ther* 1984; 229:364.

95. Sabouni MH, Lokhandwala MF: Effects of selective DA₁- and DA₂-receptor agonists on responses to pre- and postganglionic cardiac sympathetic nerve stimulation. *Fed Proc* 1984; 43:1094.

96. Schumann HJ, Endoh M, Brodde O-E: The time course of the effects of β- and α-adrenoceptor stimulation by isoprenaline and methoxamine on the contractile force and cAMP level of the isolated rabbit papillary muscle. *Naunyn Schmiedebergs Arch Pharmacol* 1975; 289:291.

97. Schumann HJ, Wagner J, Knoor A, et al: Demonstration in human atrial preparations of α-adrenoceptors mediating positive inotropic effects. *Naunyn Schmiedebergs Arch Pharmacol* 1978; 302:333.

98. Scriabine A: Ganglionic blocking drugs, in Scriabine A (ed): *The Pharmacology of Antihypertensive Drugs*. New York, Raven Press, 1980, pp 113–118.

99. Shoji T, Tsuru T, Shigei T: A regional difference in the distribution of postsynaptic α-adrenoceptor subtypes in canine veins. *Naunyn Schmiedebergs Arch Pharmacol* 1983; 324:246.

100. Sioufi A, Pommier F, Mangoni P, et al: Gas chromatographic determination of phentolamine (Regitine) in human plasma and urine. *J Chromatogr* 1981; 222:429.

101. Smyth DD, Umemura S, Pettinger WA: α₂-Adrenoceptors and sodium reabsorption in the isolated perfused rat kidney. *Am J Physiol* (in press).

102. Sonnenblick EH, Frishman WH, LeJemtel TH: Dobutamine: A new synthetic cardioactive sympathetic amine. *N Engl J Med* 1979; 300:17.

103. Stanaszek WF, Kellerman D, Brogden RN, et al: Prazosin update: A review of its pharmacological properties and therapeutic use in hypertension and congestive heart failure. *Drugs* 1983; 25:339.

104. Starke K: Regulation of noradrenaline release by presynaptic receptor systems. *Rev Physiol Biochem Pharmacol* 1977; 77:1.

105. Starke K, Taube H, Borowski E: Presynaptic receptor system in catecholaminergic transmission. *Biochem Pharmacol* 1977; 26:259.

106. Stokes GS, Marwood JF: Review of the use of α-adrenoceptor antagonists in Hypertension. *Meth Find Exp Clin Pharmacol* 1984; 6:197.

107. Stote RM, Dubb JW, Familiar RG, et al: A new oral renal vasodilator, fenoldopam. *Clin Pharmacol Ther* 1983; 34:309.

108. Summers RJ, McPherson GA: Radioligand studies of α-adrenoceptors in the kidney. *Trends Pharmacol Sci* 1982; 3:291.

109. Swales JD: Arterial wall or plasma renin in hypertension. *Clin Sci* 1979; 56:293.

110. Taylor AA, Fennell WA, Ruud CO, et al: Propylbutyldopamine: Mechanism of blood pressure lowering in hypertensive patients. *Hypertension* 1984; 6(suppl 1):I–40.

111. Thomas JA, Marks BH: Plasma norepinephrine in congestive heart failure. *Am J Cardiol* 1978; 41:233.

112. Tung LH, Rand MJ, Majewski H: Adrenaline-induced hypertension in rats. *Clin Sci* 1981; 61:191s.

113. van der Starre PJA, Scheijgrond HW, Reneman RS, et al: The use of ketanserin, a 5-hydroxytryptamine antagonist for treatment of postoperative hypertension following coronary artery bypass surgery. *Anesth Analg* 1983; 62:63.

114. Vanhoutte PM: Does 5-hydroxytryptamine play a role in hypertension? *Trends Pharmacol Sci* 1982; 3:370.

115. van Neuten JM, Janssen PAJ, van Beek J, et al: Vascular effects of ketanserin (R41468), a novel antagonist of 5-HT$_2$ serotonergic receptors. *J Pharmacol Exp Ther* 1981; 218:217.

116. Veda S, Yuno S, Sakanashi M: In vitro evidence for dopaminergic receptors in human renal artery. *J Cardiovasc Pharmacol* 1982; 4:76.

117. Ventura HO, Messerli FH, Oigmun W, et al: Immediate hemodynamic effects of SK&F 82526—dopamine agonist—in hypertension. *Circulation* 1983; 68(2)(suppl III):46.

118. Wenting GJ, Man in't Veld AJ, Woittiez AJ, et al: Treatment of hypertension with ketanserin, a new selective 5-HT$_2$ receptor antagonist. *Br Med J* 1982; 284:537.

119. Willems JL: Dopamine-induced inhibition of synaptic transmission in lumbar paravertebral ganglia of the dog. *Naunyn Schmiedebergs Arch Pharmacol* 1973; 279:115.

7 _____ Control of Organ Blood Flow

Frank J. Bruns, M.D.

Donald S. Fraley, M.D.

John Haigh, M.D.

Jose M. Marquez, M.D.

Douglas J. Martin, M.D.

George M. Matuschak, M.D.

James V. Snyder, M.D.

The flow of blood to any tissue depends primarily on perfusion pressure and the caliber of the resistance vessels. The major site of vascular resistance is the arterioles, as can be inferred from the large pressure drop that occurs in these vessels (Fig 7–1). Arteriolar resistance is controlled by inherent tone, autonomic nervous stimulation, humoral stimulation, local vasodilators, and tissue pressure. The inherent tone in each major vascular bed is shown by the change in flow between resting and maximally dilated states (see Fig 5–2).[155b] The principles of neural and humoral control were summarized in chapter 6, "Neurohumoral Regulation of Cardiovascular Function." A fundamental mechanism underlying control of local blood flow is the maintenance of a high arterial tone, which is estimated as calculated systemic vascular resistance (SVR). High SVR allows wide variation in local resistance to direct flow to metabolically active tissue without significantly affecting other vascular beds. *The precapillary microcirculation must compensate not only for changes in metabolic rate, but also for changes in perfusion pressure (whether this be a drop in systemic pressure or an increase in venous or tissue pressure), pathologic obstructions, viscosity, and concentration of nutrients.* Such local regulation must also compete with

systemic neural and humoral control mechanisms. Changes in caliber are dictated by chemical and physical changes that originate within and immediately surrounding the resistance vessels (Fig 7–2), by alterations in activity of the nerves to the vessels, and by circulating vasoactive agents (Fig 7–3). The regulation of local blood flow is complex, and no simple paradigm can integrate the diverse observations that have been made. In this chapter we review the mechanisms of local blood flow control: the general aspects of resistance and mediators and their action in specific vascular beds.

CRITICAL CLOSURE AND THE COMPARTMENT SYNDROME

The concept of critical closure arose because of the observation that flow ceases at pressures greater than zero; that is, the pressure-flow intercept does not pass through the origin (Fig 7–4). There are two important implications in the concept of critical closure. The first is that using the slope of the pressure-flow relation as a measure of arterial tone can be misleading. Resistance is the change in flow caused by a change in pressure. Using the difference between mean arterial

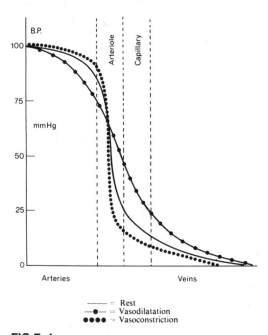

FIG 7–1.
Profile of decreases in pressure through the systemic circulation, demonstrating the major site of vascular resistance in precapillary vessels and showing increases and decreases in capillary pressure that occur during precapillary vasodilation and vasoconstriction, respectively. (From Keele and Neil.[122] Reproduced by permission.)

pressure (MAP) and central venous pressure (CVP) to determine tone leads to inaccurate estimates of tone and may lead one to believe arterial tone has changed when it has not (see discussion of SVR in chapter 15, "Technical Problems in Data Acquisition").

The second implication of the critical closure concept is the importance of vessel transmural pressure as the limiting factor in tissue perfusion. This phenomenon presents itself in pathology as the various compartment syndromes. Just as we commonly neglect pleural pressure when considering intrathoracic vascular pressures, so we ignore interstitial pressure when considering systemic perfusion. This lapse is inconsequential when pleural and interstitial pressure are both low and constant, but leads to confusion when those pressures vary. When the influence of increased interstitial pressure on critical closure is considered, it is obvious that perfusion can depend on tissue pressure as much as on arterial pressure.

We can then appreciate that the pathophysiologic concepts related to compartment syndrome apply in more than just muscle compartments in extremities. Intracranial hypertension and herniation are also forms of compartment syndrome, and related dynamics participate in the compromise of myocardial perfusion in cardiac tamponade, of splanchnic perfusion from increased intraperitoneal pressure, and perhaps of liver and kidney perfusion when those organs swell within their capsules. An argument could be made that, except for the intracranial space, pressures in these examples rarely reach 40 torr, and in the compartment syndrome deleterious sequelae are not usually seen until pressures of 45–60 torr are reached.[153] However, these observations have been made primarily in otherwise healthy subjects, and the lower arterial pressure often seen in critically ill patients reduces the threshold at which interstitial pressure becomes significant. Thus, any elevation of interstitial pressure, such as that due to an increase in interstitial fluid, can threaten local flow, especially when viscosity is increased or arterial pressure is low.

LOCAL MECHANISMS AND MEDIATORS

Normally, we think of local blood flow regulation as tied to the need of the tissue for oxygen, but in fact the mechanism by which flow is regulated varies widely in various physiologic circumstances. Dissociation of flow from oxygen need may represent only a change in the primary regulating system and is not necessarily an inappropriate flow. Renal blood flow is an example of flow grossly in excess of oxygen need, as are skin blood flow in individuals in warm environments, and local blood flow in response to any inflammation. Some tissues exhibit a postischemic hyperperfusion, which is again in excess of current oxygen need; examples are cerebral hyperperfusion following anoxia or ischemia or trauma, and flushed skin after the release of pressure dressings. Flows to most tissues are normally regulated to deliver oxygen in excess of current need, yet vascular tone usually changes quickly to maintain that level of oxygen delivery. Mechanical forces also cause prompt change in tone, yet chemical mediators seem certain to play a role. Several mediators will be mentioned as

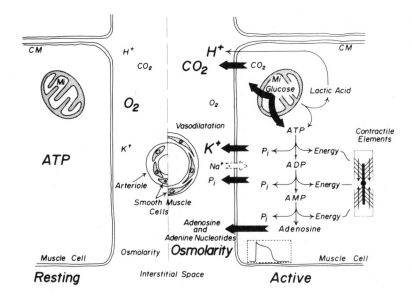

FIG 7–2.
Possible mediators of local vasoregulation in muscle causing major changes in composition of interstitial fluid during contraction of muscle cells. When muscles are inactive *(left)*, (1) arterioles are constricted, (2) concentration of metabolites and CO_2 in interstitial fluid is low, and (3) little O_2 is used. When muscles become active *(right)*, (1) depolarization of the cell membrane (CM) increases $[K^+]$ in the extracellular space; (2) regeneration of adenosine triphosphate *(ATP)* by mitochondria *(Mi)* augments CO_2 production, which diffuses to the extracellular space; (3) anaerobic production of ATP in the cytoplasm results in formation of lactic acid, which slowly diffuses out of the cell; (4) increases in amounts of lactic acid and CO_2 cause an increase in $[H^+]$ of the extracellular fluid and thus a decrease in pH; (5) breakdown of ATP to adenosine diphosphate *(ADP)* and monophosphate *(AMP)* and to adenosine, with liberation of inorganic phosphate (P_i), augments concentration of adenosine and adenine nucleotides in the extracellular space; and (6) osmolarity of the extracellular fluid increases. Each change can relax contracted smooth muscle cells. (From Shepherd and Vanhoutte.[232] Reproduced by permission.)

candidates for physiologically significant roles. It seems likely that all of them serve in some circumstances.*

Autoregulation[233]

The vasculature exhibits pressure autoregulation, which protects the capillary beds from high pressures and ensures a relatively constant flow over a range of perfusion pressures. A passive vasculature behaves in the manner depicted in Figure 7–5. At low flow the resistance is high, but it decreases rapidly because of an increase in radius of the vessel caused by passive distention of the elastic elements of the vessel wall. Connective tissue components with low compliance limit di-

*An invaluable resource, from which much of this introductory material has been extracted, is the *Handbook of Physiology*.[78a, 233]

lation, and at higher pressures the fall in resistance begins to level off. The flow curve of such a system reflects an increasing flow/pressure ratio in the low-pressure range, but becomes more linear at higher pressures.

A system that actively autoregulates is shown in Figure 7–6. At low pressures the system behaves as a passive system. Within the autoregulatory range, however, active constriction (when perfusion pressure increases) or dilation (when perfusion pressure falls) matches resistance to pressure, such that the flow remains relatively constant. When the upper limits of the autoregulatory range are reached the pressure exceeds the tension capabilities of the vascular muscle. The resistance can no longer compensate and may begin to fall because of forced dilation. Flow therefore increases. Resistance falls until the connective tissue limits distention. Autoregu-

FIG 7–3.
Regulation of resistance vessels in skeletal muscle by local, nervous, and humoral factors. Metabolites produced in muscles enter interstitial space and cause relaxation of adjacent resistance vessels, thus adjusting blood flow to meet local metabolic needs. An increase in transmural pressure can cause vessels to constrict and vice versa, partly because of a local myogenic mechanism, which results in autoregulation of blood flow. Prostaglandins synthesized in vessel wall can contribute to vasodilation. Vessel caliber adjusts in response to changes in sympathetic noradrenergic activity governed by arterial and cardiopulmonary mechanoreceptors, arterial chemoreceptors, and afferents from contracting muscles. Histamine release from cells near arterioles can cause vasodilation; this release is governed by sympathetic nerve activity. Emotional stress dilates muscle vessels by activating cholinergic nerves and by increasing epinephrine output from the adrenal medulla. *ACh,* acetylcholine; α, α-adrenergic receptor; β$_2$, β-adrenergic receptor; *Ne,* norepinephrine. (From Shepherd.[233] Reproduced by permission.)

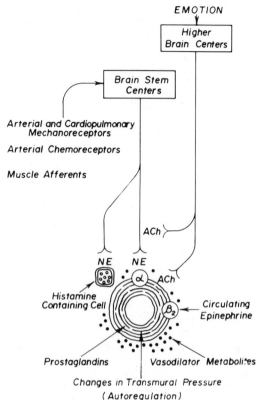

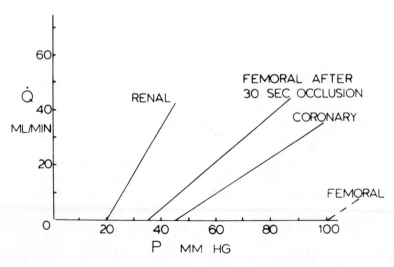

FIG 7–4.
Arterial pressure-flow curves from several vascular beds. Femoral artery before 30 sec occlusion *(extreme right)* could not be studied accurately. (From Riley[207] and Ehrlich.[61] Reproduced by permission.)

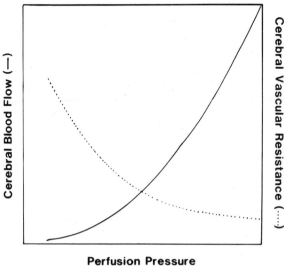

Perfusion Pressure

FIG 7–5.
Relation between cerebral blood flow and cerebral vascular resistance to perfusion pressure when vascular bed responds passively. (From Heistad and Kontos.[101] Reproduced by permission.)

lation occurs in arteries devoid of nerves and is therefore a local phenomenon, but whether it is blood flow or wall tension that is being regulated is not clear. The mechanisms involved depend on the pressure range studied and the means used to change the pressure. The myogenic and metabolic hypotheses are diagramed in Figure 7–7.

Local Mediators

Metabolically active tissues produce chemical substances that regulate the resistance vessels to match oxygen supply to demand. As Shepherd has summarized for muscle blood flow, a muscle contraction lasting 0.3 sec causes an increase in blood flow within 1 sec, resulting in venous ox-

ygen content well above the control value. The increased flow is apparently not used for metabolic purposes. The dilation could be caused by a metabolite(s), which may be removed by diffusion, local degradation, or cell uptake. Thus the duration of effect may not be dependent on the induced change in flow, the substance may not appear in the blood emerging from the muscle, and the concentration of a substance in muscle does not necessarily reflect the time course of its action.[233]

Oxygen Lack

Hypoxia may influence resistance vessels directly or indirectly. Although severe reductions in

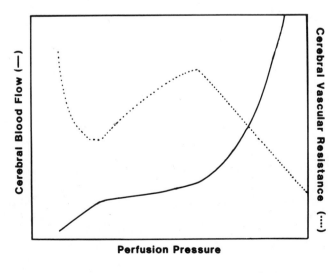

Perfusion Pressure

FIG 7–6.
Relation between cerebral blood flow and cerebral vascular resistance to perfusion pressure when vascular bed displays autoregulation. (From Heistad and Kontos.[101] Reproduced by permission.)

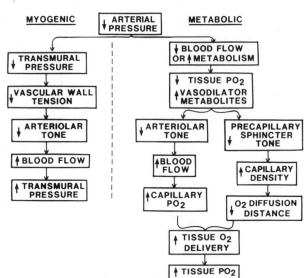

FIG 7–7.
Autoregulation of blood flow and oxygen delivery to the small intestine. The myogenic and metabolic hypotheses both explain the tendency of the small intestine to maintain blood flow and oxygen delivery when the arterial pressure falls. (From Granger et al.[80] Reproduced by permission.)

oxygen pressure (Po_2) can contribute to sustained vasodilation, a direct depressant action of Po_2 on vascular smooth muscle is not the primary cause of vasodilation in muscle during exercise. The contractile activity of vascular smooth muscle cells is not affected by oxygen lack until the Po_2 falls below about 8 torr. Therefore the vascular adjustments that follow imbalance in oxygen supply and demand are probably due indirectly to change in Po_2 by way of some chemical mediator produced by the parenchymal cells. Only under abnormal circumstances, such as restricted flow or perfusion with hypoxic blood, is it likely that the vessel wall Po_2 would be low enough to cause vasodilation. There is evidence that in reactive hyperemia, vascular dilation in the first 10–30 sec is due to loss of myogenic tone, whereas dilation after 60-120 sec might be caused by accumulation of vasodilator metabolites.

Lactic Acid, pH, and CO₂

Moderate to severe exercise increases $[H^+]$ in the venous blood of muscle, and elevation of $[H^+]$ in arterial blood perfusing resting skeletal muscle decreases vascular resistance, but the changes in $[H^+]$ that occur physiologically are too small to account for the increase in blood flow through active tissues. Thus the role of change in pH in exercise hyperemia must at best be only contributory in muscle and probably in most tissues. The response of cerebral vessels to increased $[H^+]$ is more pronounced.

Local exposure of perfusing blood to increased carbon dioxide tension (Pco_2) decreases vascular resistance in limb muscles of animals and humans. In the human the available evidence suggests that carbon dioxide produces vasodilation by direct action on vascular smooth muscle, probably by decreasing intracellular pH.

Potassium

The potassium ion (K^+) is also thought to be a transient mediator of vasomotor tone and of local blood flow. A small increase in extracellular K^+ concentration secondary to hypoxia will alter resting membrane potential directly. It can also diminish sodium ion (Na^+) permeability and decrease inward Na^+ current during electrical excitation. Finally, increases in extracellular K^+ can alter intracellular Na^+, which in turn will influence Ca^{++} transport. Increases in extracellular K^+ ion concentration can also decrease release of norepinephrine from nerve endings within the vessel wall and thereby modulate resting arteriolar tone.

The calculated time course of interstitial K^+ accompanying a 1-sec tetanic stimulation indicates that interstitial $[K^+]$ changes rapidly enough to precede and therefore partially cause the vascular response. These changes in interstitial $[K^+]$ could transiently cause as much as a fivefold to sixfold decrease in vascular resistance.[233] Although K^+ is an important factor in regulation of muscle blood flow during exercise, the effect is generally transient, and it is unlikely that K^+ release is essential in long-continued exercise hyperemia.

Osmolarity

Tissue osmolarity changes during exercise because osmotically active particles form during increased muscle metabolism. Also, the infusion of hypertonic solution into the arterial blood supply to resting muscle causes vasodilation that is not related to prostaglandins or histamine,[194] and the external application of hyperosmolar solutions can dilate terminal arterioles. Hyperosmolarity acts on resistance vessels by shrinking tissue, inhibiting spontaneous electrical and mechanical activity, inhibiting sympathetic nerve activation, inhibiting the response to α-adrenergic stimulation, depressing spontaneous myogenic activity, and increasing microvascular permeability. Hyperosmolarity may also have a direct contractile effect on smooth muscle cells. The rapid onset of hyperemia in exercising muscles is unlikely to be caused by an increase in tissue hyperosmolarity, and although hyperosmolarity might contribute to the dilation after a few minutes, its effect becomes less important as the exercise continues.

Prostaglandins

The lack of influence of prostaglandin inhibitors on local perfusion in many studies suggests that these ubiquitous chemicals have little role in basal regulation of flow. It is apparent, however, that arachidonic acid derivatives can have significant effects on vascular tone and on blood pressure in stress and pathologic states. In general PGI_2, PGE_1, and PGE_2 are vasodilators, whereas thromboxane A_2, PGF_2, and leukotrienes C_4 and D_4 are vasoconstrictors, but the results vary from one vascular bed to another. (See chapter 9, "Role of Prostacyclin, Thromboxane A_2, and Leukotrienes in Cardiovascular Function and Disease," for a partial review.)

Adenosine and Adenine Nucleotides

The potency of adenine and adenosine triphosphate (ATP) in dilating the resistance blood vessels of skeletal muscle, heart, and cerebral vessels, together with the rapidity of local inactivation and the absence of sensation accompanying the vasodilation when they are infused in humans, suggest that these agents play a key role in exercise and reactive hyperemia. Adenosine may act by decreasing K^+ and Na^+ permeability and interfering with the inward movement of Ca^{++}.

Conjugates of adenosine with high molecular weight are as effective as adenosine as dilators of coronary resistance vessels, suggesting that adenosine acts at a receptor site on the cell membrane. There is evidence for two types of receptors on vascular smooth muscle, one of which is more sensitive to ATP and the other to adenosine. Either chemical might be a principal mediator of local coronary blood flow, whereas adenosine seems likely to be the principal mediator of blood flow to skeletal muscle. When infused into the human brachial artery, ATP can increase muscle blood flow as much as maximal exercise of the forearm muscles does. However, the dilator effect of ATP may be a result of its rapid conversion to adenosine.

Summary

In summary, microvascular control by local mediators is complex. In muscle, the initial vasodilation during exercise is probably due to K^+ release and hyperosmolarity; adenosine becomes increasingly important after 10–15 minutes. After exercise during which flow is restricted, vasodilation is prolonged far beyond the time required for oxygen consumption to return to the resting value; this dilation is not caused by the release of K^+, lactic acid, hyperosmolarity, or decreased vessel wall Po_2. Prostaglandin release also appears to contribute, because it increases late in the postexercise period, and histamine may also contribute, because the dilation is reduced by tripelennamine.

CORONARY BLOOD FLOW

The heart is a tissue that cannot sustain an oxygen debt and is more important than any other to the survival of the organism. In addition, the heart provides the force necessary for its own blood supply, and the process of contraction affects myocardial flow by compressing the coronary vessels.[85]

Relative to skeletal muscle, the myocardium has an extremely dense capillary network and large capillary surface area. Because of the thin myofibrils and the density of capillaries, the myocardium has 2,500–4,000 capillaries/mm^3, compared with 300–400/mm^3 in skeletal muscle. Despite this extensive capillary arborization there is poor artery-to-artery connection in more proximal parts of the circuit such that after an acute arterial obstruction, these collaterals can supply less than 10% of the normal flow.

Regulation of Coronary Blood Flow

Under basal conditions the level of oxygen in the coronary sinus is very low, about 5–6 ml O_2/100 ml of blood (Table 7–1).[224] Consequently, greater oxygen needs can be met only by an increase in coronary blood flow. Normal myocardial oxygen consumption ($\dot{M}v_{O_2}$) in awake sedated humans is 8–10 ml/100 gm/min.[213] Assuming a 300-gm heart, the total oxygen consumption of the heart is therefore 24–30 ml/min, or approximately 10% of the total body oxygen consumption. Even when asystolic the heart shows a considerably greater oxygen consumption (1.0–2.0 ml/100 gm/min) than does resting skeletal muscle (0.1–0.2 ml/100 gm/min).

Coronary blood flow at rest is 75–80 ml/100 gm/min or 225–240 ml/min, comprising 4%–5% of resting total cardiac output. During maximal dilation, coronary blood flow can increase as much as fivefold.

Metabolic Factors

The major factor regulating coronary blood flow is myocardial oxygen consumption ($\dot{M}v_{O_2}$). In the healthy heart coronary blood flow changes parallel changes in $\dot{M}v_{O_2}$. $\dot{M}v_{O_2}$ is closely related to myocardial work. A clinical approximation of myocardial work is the arterial pressure times the cardiac output. However, work done primarily by generating pressure consumes more oxygen than flow work. When the transmural systolic pressure increases, the oxygen consumption increases proportionately to the increase in pressure. In contrast, an increase in cardiac output without an increase in pressure results in only a minimal increase in oxygen consumption.

Pressure Effects

Coronary blood flow depends on the perfusion pressure and the coronary vascular resistance. The effective perfusion pressure is the coronary arterial pressure minus the pressure in the wall of the ventricle.[86] The effective perfusion pressure, therefore, is not constant throughout the cardiac cycle or throughout the thickness of the ventricular wall. Since the left ventricular (LV) myocardial wall develops more tension than the right ventricle (RV), coronary blood flow to the LV is much more restricted during contraction than is flow to the RV. Flow to the LV during systole ranges from 7% to 45% of diastolic flow and may represent primarily outer wall flow.[87] In contrast, RV systolic flow is greater than RV diastolic flow because the high systolic aortic pressure vastly exceeds the relatively moderate rise in intramural tension.

Because ventricular systole exerts such a profound effect on blood flow to the LV, it is clear that flow to the LV will be reduced by conditions that increase the total systolic ejection time relative to the cardiac cycle, such as tachycardia, decreased LV contractility, and increased aortic outflow resistance.

Endocardial to Epicardial Pressure Differences

Studies using small pressure-sensitive probes inserted into the myocardium show that LV myocardial pressure is greatest in the subendocardium and falls off linearly to zero in the subepicardium.[125] Under normal conditions coronary blood flow is distributed equally to the epicardium and endocardium as a consequence of preferential dilation of subendocardial vessels.[6] However, endocardial blood flow selectively decreases when diastolic coronary blood flow is severely compro-

TABLE 7–1.

Myocardial Oxygenation in Awake Sedated Man at Rest

INDEX	VALUE
Myocardial oxygen consumption	8–10 ml O_2/kg/min[213]
Coronary blood flow	75–80 ml blood/kg/min[213]
$D(a-cs)_{O_2}$	11–13 ml O_2/100 ml blood[237]
Ccs_{O_2}	5–6 ml O_2/100 ml blood[224]
Scs_{O_2}	26%–32%[204]

$D(a-cs)_{O_2}$ = difference in oxygen content between arterial and coronary sinus blood.
Ccs_{O_2} = oxygen content of coronary sinus blood.
Scs_{O_2} = saturation of hemoglobin of coronary sinus blood.

mised by increased extravascular compression, tachycardia, or reduced diastolic perfusion pressure.[54, 127, 165] Since the peak wall pressure can be higher than peak systolic blood pressure, flow to the subendocardial layers may occur only during diastole, whereas subepicardial muscle is perfused throughout the cardiac cycle. Therefore the effective coronary perfusion pressure for the endocardium is the gradient between the diastolic coronary pressure and the LV diastolic pressure. When either diastolic pressure rises, as in heart failure, or coronary artery pressure falls, as in atherosclerotic coronary disease, subendocardial ischemia and infarction may occur.[176] Following occlusion of a major coronary artery the ratio of blood flow to the endocardium versus the epicardium also becomes significantly less than 1.[5]

Autoregulation

There is an approximately linear relation between coronary blood flow and perfusion pressure. It could be concluded that perfusion pressure is the primary determinant of coronary blood flow. This conclusion, however, falsely assumes a constant oxygen consumption at different perfusion pressures; instead, $\dot{M}v_{O_2}$ increases with increases in arterial pressure. When a coronary artery is cannulated and perfused with blood from an external reservoir, the heart is able to maintain a constant flow over a broad range of perfusion pressures (pressure autoregulation). Following an increase in coronary arterial pressure, coronary blood flow increases temporarily, but then returns to control levels as vascular resistance increases to the new perfusion pressure. Subsequent restoration of the perfusion pressure to normal levels results in a transient reduction in coronary blood flow that slowly returns to normal. This capacity for regulation of flow according to metabolic need is most prominent with perfusion pressures from 40 to 160 torr.[57]

Neurohumoral Factors

The sympathetic nervous system can affect coronary blood flow indirectly, by increasing $\dot{M}v_{O_2}$, and directly, by changing coronary vascular resistance. Both α- and β$_2$-adrenergic receptors have been demonstrated on the coronary vessels, and β$_1$ receptors appear to be the site of action of sympathetic activity on the myocardium. The effect of neurohumoral stimulation is to increase $\dot{M}v_{O_2}$. Coronary blood flow changes are secondary to the increase in $\dot{M}v_{O_2}$ rather than direct responses to neural or humoral stimulation of the vessels (see chapter 6, "Neurohumoral Regulation of Cardiovascular Function). The distribution of parasympathetic innervation to the ventricular coronary system is so slight that parasympathetic stimulation has almost no direct effect on coronary flow.

Clinical Problems

Tachycardia

Under resting conditions extravascular compression of the coronary arteries accounts for about 25% of the total resistance to coronary blood flow. During tachycardia the proportion of coronary resistance due to compression increases to about 55% because the percentage of time during the cycle length the heart spends in systole increases.[143] Because most of LV flow occurs during diastole, decreasing the percent time spent in diastole reduces coronary blood flow, especially to "vulnerable" regions of the heart such as the endocardium. Paradoxically, tachycardia causes an increase in demand for coronary blood flow secondary to the increase in $\dot{M}v_{O_2}$. Vatner et al.[252] have estimated that tachycardia alone accounts for approximately one third of the increase in coronary blood flow during heavy exercise.

Hypotension

When coronary perfusion pressure falls to below 60–70 torr, coronary vasodilation is maximal and further autoregulation of coronary blood flow cannot occur. Flow becomes pressure-dependent.[171] Reduced coronary blood flow during periods of decreased aortic pressure is due to a combination of decreased perfusion pressure and decreased $\dot{M}v_{O_2}$ since the pressure load on the ventricle is also reduced. In hypovolemic shock the changes in coronary blood flow are more complex than simply decreased perfusion pressure. Initially the coronary vascular resistance increases owing to neurohumoral stimulation as a part of the generalized sympathetic response.[79] Increased interstitial pressure from the higher force of contraction and heart rate may also contribute to increasing resistance.[63] This is followed by a decrease in coronary vascular resistance, locally mediated in response to the oxygen supply/demand imbalance, that is, in response to the greatly reduced perfusion pressure and the increased myocardial oxygen debt.

Hypertension

If SVR is acutely increased, coronary blood flow initially increases in response to a rise in coronary perfusion pressure and remains elevated because of the elevated $\dot{M}v_{O_2}$. In chronic hypertension, total coronary blood flow is increased in proportion to $\dot{M}v_{O_2}$, but flow per unit of weight of LV myocardium is unchanged.[209, 262]

Progressive Coronary Artery Stenosis

In coronary artery disease, the coronary arterial pressure distal to a narrowed section is reduced such that coronary perfusion is decreased. This is especially true during diastole. With slowly progressive stenosis, coronary blood flow is initially well maintained by progressive dilation of the resistance vessels.[123] The coronary vascular reserve or ability to further dilate if necessary is diminished, as evidenced by a reduction in the degree of reactive hyperemia. With further progression of the stenosis, coronary blood flow diminishes as this coronary artery dilator reserve is exhausted. At this time the resistance vessels are maximally dilated and reactive hyperemia disappears. If the stenotic process is slow enough, by the time of complete occlusion collateral arterial vessels have appeared, and an infarct usually does not occur.

Collaterals

The most potent stimulus for the development of collateral circulation is the gradual occlusion of a coronary artery. Although the stimulus to collateral formation is poorly defined, most investigators favor either the effects of hypoxia or a decreased pressure gradient. Schaper[219] has provided evidence that collaterals develop from microscopic vascular communications between branches of major coronary arteries. These thin-walled vessels become damaged by distention in response to myocardial ischemia, and in the reparative process, larger, thicker-walled vessels develop.

Acute Occlusion

Acute occlusion of either the left anterior descending or the circumflex coronary artery increases coronary blood flow in the nonoccluded vessel,[58, 103] primarily by increasing the work of the nonischemic myocardium. When the occlusion is abrupt and collateral vessels have not developed, myocardial edema and infarction occur.

The extent of restoration of myocardial function is determined by the duration of occlusion before reperfusion.[23]

Aortic Stenosis

Patients with aortic stenosis may have symptoms of angina secondary to the increased $\dot{M}v_{O_2}$ caused by chronic increased LV pressure work. Long-standing elevations in pressure work provide a potent stimulus for myofibril protein synthesis and ultimately muscle hypertrophy. The enlarged muscle mass has a greatly increased oxygen demand, which frequently results in symptoms of coronary insufficiency in the presence of normal coronary arteries. In valvular and subvalvular stenosis, LV pressure rises but aortic pressure and cardiac output do not change.[25] Despite an increase in extravascular compression, coronary blood flow increases in response to a greater $\dot{M}v_{O_2}$.[88] The compromise is a progressive exhaustion of the coronary vasodilator reserve.

Aortic Insufficiency

In aortic insufficiency, increases in LV diastolic volume and stroke volume impose an increased work load on the LV. Thus oxygen needs are increased at a time when perfusion pressure is reduced. Diastolic coronary blood flow decreases, but frequently systolic pressure and flow both increase, while the total coronary flow does not change.[225] Nevertheless, with severe reductions in diastolic pressure, subendocardial regions manifest evidence of ischemia. Indeed, more than one third of patients with severe aortic insufficiency have symptomatic angina pectoris in the absence of coronary artery disease.[225]

Summary

Coronary blood flow is the product of metabolic, mechanical, and neurohumoral stimuli. The most important regulatory mechanism determining this blood flow is the metabolic demand of the myocardium for oxygen.

SPLANCHNIC BLOOD FLOW

Overview

The distinct vascular beds that together comprise blood flow to the gut, spleen, and liver are the largest regional circulation in the body, receiving up to 25% of the cardiac output.[55, 71] For a 70-kg man, this amounts to 1,500 ml/min. Moreover, the vascular volume contained within this circulation (splanchnic blood volume, SBV) represents 20%–25% of the total blood volume, a third of which is contained within the liver.[55] Because of the magnitude of inflow to this regional circuit and its large capacitance, changes in the pressure-flow and pressure-volume relations of the splanchnic circulation can have significant effects on cardiovascular homeostasis.[211] Because of the relative inaccessibility of the splanchnic circulation to direct study in humans, and the insensitivity of commonly measured biochemical variables to splanchnic ischemia, the functional significance of changes in splanchnic blood flow in the critically ill is not well understood. Yet, because of the central role of the liver in metabolic and immunologic regulation and the importance of adequate nutrition in systemic host defense, compromise of splanchnic and hepatic cellular performance may contribute to the development of irreversible multisystem organ failure in this patient population.[74, 216]

General Anatomical and Functional Considerations

A general anatomical characteristic of the splanchnic circulation is the presence of discrete tissue compartments in the gastrointestinal (GI) wall.[71, 80] Current experimental methods permit separation of these into an inner mucosal-submucosal layer specialized for absorptive and secretory functions and an outer muscularis-serosal layer that facilitates propulsion of intestinal contents. The fractional transmural blood flow distribution between these two layers may be significantly altered during normal and pathologic GI circulatory changes.

Another major physiologic determinant of splanchnic blood flow regulation is the complex series of changes associated with digestion. Because of the large capacitance of the splanchnic blood reservoir, if the observed regional postprandial hyperemic responses were all to occur simultaneously, flow to the splanchnic circulation would approximate 4 L/min.[71] Although large increases in flow occur, they are regional and occur sequentially, so that the total increment in postprandial splanchnic blood flow is about 50% of control.[71] After the increases in oxygen demand imposed by intraluminal solutes, both metabolic and myogenic mechanisms participate in the local control of GI blood flow, and the relative contribution of these two mechanisms appears to be

governed by the baseline level of oxygen extraction.[81, 231] Postprandial increases in gut flow are reflected by increments in portal flow, and thus total hepatic blood flow is also increased during digestion.

A third anatomic characteristic of the splanchnic circulation is the series-coupled arrangement of the GI tract (including the spleen) with the liver. As a result, a significant fraction of total hepatic inflow is determined by influences acting outside of the liver. This circulatory "linkage" of the gut-liver axis results in multiple potential points of control of splanchnic blood flow regulation. For example, the entire extrahepatic splanchnic outflow comprises portal venous inflow, and the entirety of this portion of systemic venous return must pass through the extensive low-pressure sinusoidal network of the liver before returning to the systemic circulation. Consequently, changes in prehepatic vascular pressure-flow and pressure-volume relations in both the preintestinal and postintestinal vascular bed can significantly modulate SBV and portal flow. Up to 75% of hepatic blood flow derives from the portal vein, and flow in the portal vein does not exhibit autoregulation; rather, constancy of portal venous pressure appears to be the regulated variable.[28, 82, 206] However, decrements in portal flow are buffered to a variable extent by large compensatory increases in hepatic arterial flow. Also, large decreases in portal venous pressure can be offset by reflex increases in hepatic venous resistance, which results in a return of portal pressure toward normal. As a result of this mechanism, however, significant increases in transsinusoidal plasma movement may cause large losses of fluid into the peritoneal cavity.[140]

Respiration is an important determinant of hepatic blood flow and capacitance. Variations in hepatic outflow normally occur during spontaneous breathing. Moreno et al. have shown in a canine model that inspiration is associated with a decrease in hepatic outflow relative to expiration and that this respiratory cycle–related flow variation is 180 degrees out of phase with concurrent changes in systemic venous return.[167] These changes are depicted in Figure 7–8. Despite decreases in downstream hepatic venous and right atrial pressure,[28] hepatic compression by the descending, contracting diaphragm has been postulated to increase intrahepatic resistance to flow out of the liver. This causes hepatic engorgement during inspiration.[1] This thesis is supported by

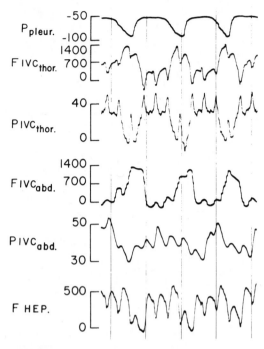

FIG 7–8.
Respiratory alternation of systemic and splanchnic venous return. The hepatic (splanchnic) venous contribution is derived from the differences in flows in the thoracic vena cava and the infrahepatic abdominal vena cava. Corresponding changes in pressures are also indicated. Increased thoracic caval flow during inspiration primarily reflects the splanchnic component of venous return. Tracings from top to bottom: P_{pleur}, intrapleural pressure; $FIVC_{thor}$, thoracic (suprahepatic) inferior vena cava flow; $PIVC_{thor}$, thoracic (suprahepatic) inferior vena cava pressure; $FIVC_{abd}$, abdominal (infrahepatic) inferior vena cava flow; $PIVC_{abd}$, abdominal (infrahepatic) inferior vena cava pressure; FHEP, hepatic (splanchnic) outflow. Flows are in ml/min; pressures are in cm H_2O. (Gain for hepatic outflow is 3 × the caval flows.) Time lines indicate 1-sec intervals. (From Moreno et al.[167] Reproduced by permission.)

the findings that phrenicotomy or isolation of the liver from diaphragmatic impact reverses the alternation between splanchnic and systemic venous return.[167] The normal liver contains little intrahepatic connective tissue support and thus is compressible by relatively low pressures acting at the liver surface and at the hepatic veins. Variations in flow that occur with respiration may be decreased or reversed when cirrhosis is present.[168]

Regulation of Gastric Blood Flow

Autoregulation in most tissues permits compensatory changes in vascular resistance to prevent decreases in blood flow and oxygen uptake during circulatory stresses. However, autoregulation of blood flow to the gastric vascular bed does not occur to any appreciable degree.[107] The dependence of oxygen uptake on arterial pressure before and after loss of sympathetic tone is shown in Figure 7–9. It is apparent in the figure that gastric autoregulation of oxygen uptake is impaired during normal sympathetic innervation of the stomach.

Changes in the intramural distribution of gastric blood flow may be more significant than total flow in determining the adequacy of gastric oxygenation. Therefore, conceptualization of flow "compartments" is valuable to understanding more clearly the functional significance of changes in GI blood flow regulation. Under rest-

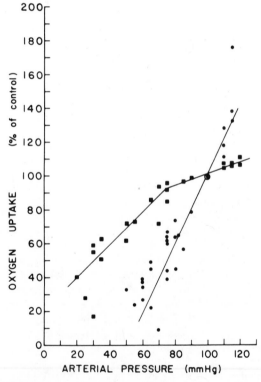

FIG 7–9.
Dependence of gastric oxygen uptake on arterial pressure in sympathetically innervated *(circles)* and denervated *(squares)* preparations. (From Holm-Rutili et al.[107] Reproduced by permission.)

ing conditions, gastric wall blood flow is 20–40 ml/kg/min and accounts for 12%–15% of total portal flow.[71] A greater portion of flow goes to the mucosal-submucosal compartment (50–80 ml/kg/min) than to the smooth muscle compartment (10–15 ml/kg/min). During postprandial hyperemia, however, total flow may increase to as much as 150 ml/kg/min, with mucosal-submucosal perfusion increasing maximally to 300–400 ml/kg/min.[71] These changes may be modulated by the ability of the gastric vascular bed to autoregulate its flow better in the postprandial state; autoregulatory ability may also differ between the two flow compartments. As in the intestine, autoregulation of flow by the mucosal-submucosal compartment occurs to preferentially preserve flow to this metabolically active region when nutrients are present in the lumen.[71, 80] Preferential redistribution of total gastric flow to the active mucosal-submucosal compartment can occur such that significant regional changes may be present without differences in total flow values. Parasympathetic stimulation also induces greater proportional hyperemia of the mucosal-submucosal compartment as part of the interrelated local mechanisms leading to acid secretion during digestion.[71]

Focal mucosal-submucosal ischemia during changes in perfusion pressure consequent on direct or reflex-mediated systemic hemodynamic changes may contribute to the clinical syndrome of stress-mediated gastric ulceration. Focal ischemia of this flow compartment represents a final common pathway for ulceration.[157] Because under these conditions mucosal integrity is further compromised by the presence of excessive gastric acid and bile, cytoprotective therapies designed to reduce gastric acidity and to redistribute flow to areas prone to stress ulceration have been studied. Prostaglandins are produced by the gastric mucosa and appear to be cytoprotective against stress-mediated ulceration; exogenous prostacyclin has been evaluated experimentally and has been found to result in significant gastric mucosal flow redistribution.[75] Prostaglandin inhibitors such as aspirin may inhibit this protection.

Intestinal Blood Flow and Oxygen Uptake

In the critically ill, acute mesenteric ischemia remains a serious problem because of its high mortality rate.[190] Even though differential autoregulatory ability appears to exist within the layers of the intestinal wall, and the mucosal-submucosal

compartment may be better able to preserve flow, the most constant pathologic response to ischemia in the intestine is mucosal edema, followed by hemorrhage and sloughing.[190] Since mesenteric ischemia is a continuum, various expressions of ischemia may occur, ranging from absorption, secretion, and motility impairments through compromise of mucosal integrity to frank infarction. Independent of the clinical problems of nutritional failure and stress-induced GI bleeding, significant impairment of mucosal integrity may lead to increased enteric absorption of bacteria and their products, which may overwhelm hepatic clearance mechanisms. Spillover of these vasoactive and vasotoxic substances into the systemic circulation may result.[26, 113, 201] In addition to reductions in cardiac output and systemic arterial perfusion pressure, increases in intrathoracic pressure during positive pressure ventilation, particularly during use of high levels of positive end-expiratory pressure (PEEP), may increase portal venous pressure owing to backtransmission of hepatic venous pressure through the liver.[116] Since progressive reductions in blood flow to the mucosal-submucosal layer and reductions in capillary density occur experimentally as venous pressure is increased from 0 to 20 torr,[80] such supportive therapy in the critically ill has the potential to compromise GI homeostasis even as it improves arterial oxygenation.

General Anatomical and Functional Considerations for Intestinal Blood Flow

There are three primary determinants of blood flow to the intestine: (1) intrinsic factors, including local metabolic and myogenic responses of the resistance vessels; (2) extrinsic factors, such as sympathetic nervous system activity, which can alter both transmural intestinal flow distribution and SBV; and (3) circulating substances of endogenous (humoral) or exogenous (vasoactive drugs) origin.[80] Total resting blood flow values for the small intestine in humans range approximately from 29 to 70 ml/kg/min, with most (50–90 ml/kg/min) of this perfusion supplying the mucosal-submucosal layer.[80] The high metabolic oxygen demands generated by intestinal absorption and secretion are reflected in the large distribution of flow to the villi and intestinal crypts in the submucosa, each of which receives about 25% of total intestinal blood flow. However, localization of the functional hyperemic response appears to vary with the type of nutrient placed within the lumen. Hyperemia is limited to involved segments after instillation of glucose, amino acids, or fatty acids in the duodenum, but hyperemia is more widespread in response to high-fat feedings.[65]

The ability of the intestine to autoregulate its blood flow and the corresponding changes in tissue oxygenation have been characterized during the presence of four hemodynamic and metabolic stresses: (1) reductions in arterial perfusion pressure, (2) increases in the oxygen metabolic rate, (3) increases in venous outflow pressure, and (4) arterial hypoxia.[81, 91, 138, 139, 230] Under resting, fasted conditions, reductions in intestinal perfusion pressure elicit weak and inconstant pressure-flow autoregulation, and flow usually falls accordingly.[138, 186, 231] If control arteriovenous oxygen values are low, reflecting a low metabolic rate, then modulation of intestinal oxygen uptake during changes in oxygen delivery occurs by compensatory increases in oxygen extraction.[81] However, the presence of intraluminal food or absorbable solutes significantly enhances autoregulation of blood flow during reductions in perfusion pressure,[186, 231] which in some studies has led to the observation of superregulation (increased flow above control values when perfusion pressure is reduced) in the fed condition.[81] Metabolic and myogenic mechanisms interact under stress conditions, as evidenced by the response to venous pressure elevation during control and hypermetabolic states. Evidence for a myogenic mechanism exists when venous pressure elevation in fasted states increases vascular resistance and reduces capillary perfusion owing to precapillary sphincter vasoconstriction. Metabolic control is more obvious in the presence of intraluminal solutes; elevation of venous pressure then causes a vasodilatory response.

The effects of arterial hypoxia and combined hypoxia-ischemia on intestinal blood vessels and oxygen uptake have been studied to further define the limits of autoregulation.[212, 230] Using an acute canine model, Grum et al. found a high correlation between changes in intramural pH and intestinal oxygen consumption during reductions in oxygen delivery and showed that these variables were initially maintained during progressive reductions in oxygen delivery.[91] However, a critical threshold, below which they decreased, developed at about 60% of control oxygen delivery in the ischemic group and at about 50% of control during hypoxia-ischemia. Similar reductions

in intramural pH and oxygen consumption did not appear during hypoxia alone despite significant reductions in oxygen delivery (36% of control). These data support the concept that blood flow, not arterial oxygenation alone, is the major limiting factor of oxygen consumption in the splanchnic response to these hemodynamic stresses. Rowell et al. studied the splanchnic vasomotor and metabolic adjustments to hypoxia and exercise in humans and found that splanchnic $\dot{V}o_2$ was maintained at control levels during the breathing of 11% oxygen, by increased oxygen extraction.[212]

Extrinsic regulation of intestinal flow is primarily limited to the sympathetic nervous system. Splanchnic sympathetic nerve stimulation reduces intestinal flow by directly acting on resistance vessels by increasing their vascular resistance.[55, 147] Although progressive increases in resistance occur with increasing frequency of nerve stimulation, flow recovery eventually occurs despite continuation of stimulation. This phenomenon is termed autoregulatory escape. As described by Granger et al.,[80] three distinct phases occur during splanchnic nerve stimulation: initial flow reduction, autoregulatory escape, and the hyperemic phase. The mechanism of autoregulatory escape remains unclear but may involve mucosal flow autoregulation. No direct parasympathetic innervation of intestinal vessels has been described, and changes in motility due to increased activity do not seem to be associated with increases in intestinal oxygen consumption.[71]

Hepatic Blood Flow and Oxygen Uptake

The liver plays a central role in systemic homeostasis. Although the liver accounts for only 2%–3% of total body weight, optimal hepatic performance is critical in systemic host defense and in the support of the extensive metabolic functions of the liver. Similarly, the significance of changes in hepatic vascular capacitance on total body circulatory control[211] derives from the fact that hepatic blood volume is about 25 ml/kg/min, large in comparison to the intestine (8 ml/kg/min) or skeletal muscle (3 ml/kg/min).[75] Hepatic oxygen uptake varies with systemic and intestinal circulatory conditions, but averages from 2 to 7 ml O_2/kg/min.[82] Most studies of total hepatic blood flow have been performed in anesthetized animals, particularly dogs. In such preparations, total flow is partitioned between the hepatic artery, supplying 15%–30% of the total (approximately

50 ml/100 gm/min), and the portal vein, supplying the rest.[206] In humans, total hepatic flow is 800–1,200 ml/min, with similar flow partitioning.[206]

The unique sinusoidal network of the liver permits the enormous amount of blood from its dual vascular inputs to mix completely. Because of the large hepatic capacitance, sinusoidal vascular pressures range from about 4 to 10 torr.[28, 46, 82] At the microcirculatory level, well-defined topographical areas of metabolic function within the liver correspond to the Po_2 gradient of sinusoidal blood. Rappaport has defined three circulatory zones relative to their major metabolic functions (Fig 7–10).[200] For example, the main area of protein synthesis and metabolism is in circulatory zone 1, whereas reductase activity and

glycogen storage are predominant in zone 3, following the Po_2 and concentration gradient of materials. Lower sinusoidal Po_2 levels near the terminal hepatic venules appear to explain the susceptibility of the centrilobular area to hypoxic liver injury.

Central to an analysis of the effects of changes in hepatic flow and vascular pressures on hepatic parenchymal performance is consideration of the anatomical properties of the hepatic microvasculature. The sinusoidal endothelium is perforated by fenestrae of various sizes such that dissolved substances freely enter the extracellular space of the liver (space of Disse). Goresky has defined the processes of cellular uptake and exchange in the liver using multiple indicator dilution techniques.[77] The sinusoidal wall permits un-

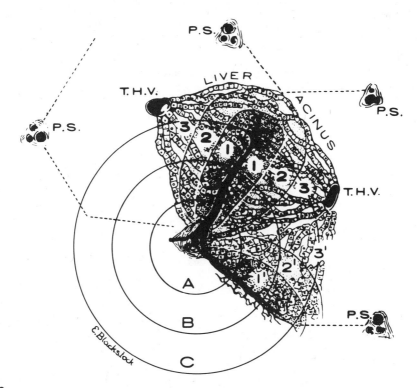

FIG 7–10.
Blood supply of the simple liver acinus and the zonal arrangement of cells. The acinus occupies adjacent sectors of neighboring hexagonal fields. Zones 1, 2, and 3, respectively, represent areas supplied with blood of first, second, and third quality with regard to oxygen and nutrients. These zones center about the terminal afferent vascular branches, terminal bile ductules, lymph vessels, and nerves, and extend into the triangular portal field from which these branches crop out. Zones 1′, 2′, and 3′ designate corresponding areas in a portion of an adjacent acinar unit. In zones 1 and 1′, the afferent vascular twigs empty into the sinusoids. Circles *B* and *C* indicate peripheral circulatory areas as commonly described around a "periportal" area *A*. *PS,* portal space; *THV,* terminal hepatic venules ("central veins"). (From Rappaport.[200] Reproduced by permission.)

restricted entry of all vascular labels, including labeled water, into their respective intrahepatic "spaces" via delayed wave flow–limited distribution. This barrier demonstrates an exclusion phenomenon with increasing molecular size of the label. These data suggest that significant increases in the sinusoidal filtration of plasma containing dissolved substances will occur with increases in backpressure to hepatic outflow (venous hypertension). The extent of transsinusoidal passage of these substances will be governed by their molecular size. Such changes in transsinusoidal flow have been demonstrated by Laine et al.: 90% of the increase in inferior vena caval pressure was transmitted back to the sinusoids, resulting in increases in transsinusoidal fluid filtration manifested by increases in hepatic lymph flow and surface exudation.[140] In other studies by Bennett and Rothe, elevations in hepatic venous pressure in dogs resulted in sustained increases in fluid movement across the sinusoidal walls that persisted as long as the pressure remained elevated.[15] These findings may be relevant to the critically ill patient in whom persisting elevations in backpressure to hepatic venous outflow due to right heart dysfunction or secondary to positive pressure ventilation with PEEP may lead to enhanced transsinusoidal fluid movement into the space of Disse, changes in hepatic performance,[27] and augmented rates of ascitic fluid formation.

Because of the homeostatic significance of the magnitude and intrahepatic distribution of hepatic blood flow, it is important to understand the determinants of changes in liver perfusion. The main determinants of hepatic blood flow are (1) intestinal vascular resistance, which defines the magnitude of mesenteric inflow and thus portal inflow, (2) hepatic arterial resistance, and (3) intrahepatic portal venous resistance.[28, 82, 206] Hepatic arterial pressure-flow autoregulation appears to be relatively weak and in many studies has been absent, such that there is an approximately linear relationship between pressure and flow. The hepatic portal vascular circuit exhibits no autoregulation and thus behaves "passively," with corresponding linear reductions in flow as perfusion pressure falls. However, interpretation of changes in total hepatic flow during systemic hemodynamic alterations is complicated by hepatic arterial-portal venous interactions, by which an increase in flow through one circuit leads to partial reductions in flow in the other by increasing its respective inflow resistance. Conversely, occlusion of one inflow circuit leads to an approximately 20% reduction in vascular resistance in the other, resulting in a partial restoration of flow toward control. The hepatic vascular response to experimental venous pressure elevation is an increase in hepatic arterial resistance, while the hepatic portal vascular resistance may fall,[206] suggesting that portal pressure and not portal venous flow per se is the regulated variable. Moderate levels of arterial hypoxia (arterial Po_2 approximately 45 torr) do not appear to be accompanied by significant hepatic hemodynamic changes in experimental preparations.[141] Flow remains constant and the hypoxemia is compensated for by an increase in hepatic oxygen extraction to levels approaching 100%. The concomitant effects on liver parenchymal function [plasma clearance, extraction ratio, and biliary recovery of indocyanine green (ICG) dye] were not apparent until the hepatic venous Po_2 fell below 5–10 torr. However, when arterial hypoxia was induced in humans by breathing of a gas mixture of 11% oxygen (arterial Po_2 approximately 32 torr), Rowell et al. found significant increases in splanchnic blood flow concomitant with elevations in heart rate and plasma catecholamine concentrations, which were accompanied by increases in hepatic glucose release and lactate uptake.[212] Similar to the situation in experimental animals, oxygen uptake was maintained by increased oxygen extraction. However, hypoxia selectively reduced ICG extraction by 28%, despite preservation of other hepatic metabolic functions. Other studies have shown that hepatic lactate uptake is more closely related to hepatic venous oxygen tension than to either blood flow or oxygen delivery; that hypoxemia of the perfusing blood causes greater changes in hepatic lactate metabolism than do comparable reductions in oxygen delivery, owing to increased extraction; and that a critical hepatic venous oxygen threshold exists, after which hepatic lactate uptake is reduced (Po_2 approximately 24 torr).[240] That variations in the oxygen content of portal blood can affect hepatic circulatory autoregulation was shown by Gelman and Ernst in anesthetized dogs, in which increases in portal oxygen content caused a decrease in portal venular resistance, an increase in portal flow, and a reduction in hepatic arterial flow.[76] Additionally, changes in systemic and portal Pco_2 levels can influence the hepatic circulation and hepatic $\dot{V}o_2$. Sustained decreases in portal pH and increases in Pco_2 can increase portal venous pressure and portal venous resistance, leading to reductions in portal venous flow.[76] Hughes et al. found in anesthetized dogs that graded arterial hypocapnia (Pco_2 values of 30, 22, and 17 torr) led to progressive decreases in hepatic arterial blood flow, although such reductions in flow diminished over time, presumably because of autoregulatory escape.[108] Reversal of hypocapnia during continuation of raised AWP in these studies led to normalization of hepatic blood flow and oxygen consumption.

Two additional major influences on hepatic blood flow are digestion and respiration. Portal flow increases in the postprandial state, owing to intestinal hyperemia; there is suggestive evidence that hepatic arterial flow similarly increases.[206] The effect of respiration on hepatic blood flow during spontaneous breathing has been alluded to; however, the effects of positive pressure ventilation with PEEP merit further description. Because of the importance of the diaphragm in regulating hepatic outflow during spontaneous breathing and because up to 77% of patients in intensive care units ventilated with PEEP show evidence of hepatic dysfunction,[95] it would be important to know if this ventilatory mode compromises hepatic performance. This is especially the case because it has been well documented that

PEEP may have significant extrathoracic effects.[151, 248] During PEEP, cardiac output usually decreases as right atrial pressure (RAP) increases. PEEP of 10 cm H_2O affects total hepatic blood flow only to the degree to which cardiac output is also affected.[154] Restoration of cardiac output to pre-PEEP levels by intravascular volume infusions during continuation of PEEP also returns hepatic blood flow to control values (Fig 7–11). However, knowledge of the relationship between changes in portal venous and hepatic arterial flows and hepatic cellular performance under conditions in which hepatic blood flow is varied by PEEP is incomplete. Johnson et al. found that 10 cm H_2O PEEP decreased sulfobromophthalein sodium (BSP) excretion by the liver in dogs, although no estimates of hepatic blood flow or cardiac output were obtained.[118] PEEP also appears to increase choledochoduodenal biliary flow resistance.[117]

Relationships Among Hepatic Blood Flow, Phagocytosis, and Multiple Organ Function

Nearly 90% of the body's reticuloendothelial system (RES) mass is located in the liver, where the phagocytic Kupffer cells line the hepatic sinusoids. Foremost among the functions of these macrophages and associated phagocytic sinusoi-

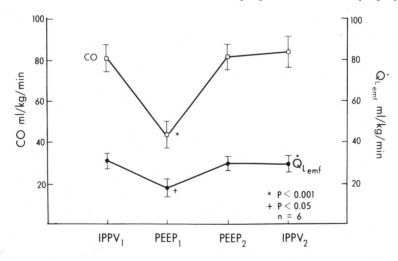

FIG 7–11.
Variation in cardiac output *(CO) (open squares)* and in steady-state mean hepatic outflow *(Q_{Lemf}) (closed circles)* as measured by electromagnetic flow probes around the suprahepatic and infrahepatic segments of the inferior vena cava in closed-chest dogs.[154] *IPPV$_1$*, intermittent positive pressure ventilation (Vt = 12 ml/kg); *PEEP$_1$*, addition of 10 cm H_2O to IPPV$_1$; *PEEP$_2$*, continuation of PEEP with restoration of CO to IPPV$_1$ by intravascular volume infusions; *IPPV$_2$*, removal of PEEP and excess volume to return CO to IPPV$_1$ levels. (Modified from data reported in Matuschak et al.[155a])

dal lining cells is phagocytosis of blood-borne particulate matter, foreign substances, and several classes of vasoactive materials that have been implicated in the development of acute lung injury and multisystem organ failure during critical illness.[2, 3, 208, 214] As a corollary, the concept of the protective role of the liver in ameliorating extrahepatic organ dysfunction has been emphasized by several investigators.[72, 92, 214] In a canine model of intestinal ischemic shock, Selkurt found that diversion of blood past the liver reduced survival time, and postulated that compromise of normal liver function permitted the entry of vasotoxic substances into the systemic circulation, with consequent impairment of cardiovascular function.[227] We have found a markedly increased incidence of lethal acute respiratory failure (ARF) associated with multisystem organ failure in patients with end-stage liver failure awaiting hepatic transplantation, which was irreversible despite vigorous cardiopulmonary support including PEEP.[154] The complex interactions among hepatic blood flow, hepatic RES function, and multisystem organ failure therefore necessitate an understanding of the determinants of hepatic RES phagocytic function under normal conditions.

Phagocytic clearance by the hepatic RES is influenced by both the volume and velocity of hepatic blood flow and the status of cellular and humoral (opsonic) components of the clearance mechanism.[2, 24, 92, 185, 214, 215, 217] Changes in the volume or velocity of flow can significantly affect phagocytic uptake by affecting transport to the sinusoidal vascular space, while changes in intrahepatic blood volume due to variations in hepatic venous outflow resistance may represent an additional factor determining the efficiency of blood:cell exchange processes.[27] These relationships may be markedly influenced by significant hepatic ischemia or by sustained changes in hepatic blood flow distribution during critical illness. In addition, hepatic RES depression during several types of experimental shock has been shown to be due to humoral factor depletion (plasma fibronectin), which can modulate RES function independent of change in hepatic blood flow.[121, 145]

In contrast to the hepatic handling of substances dissolved in plasma, uptake of RES-specific substances by Kupffer cells is governed by the Fick principle (conservation of mass) when their size restricts them to the sinusoidal vascular space. Thus, changes in blood flow rates and

blood flow distribution through the liver may have important effects on not only hepatocellular[263] but also phagocytic uptake.[27, 214] Application of these principles has been used to measure hepatic blood flow and to explain the effects of changes in the clearance velocity on phagocytic uptake. The mathematical relationships underlying the removal of IV injected particulate matter from the bloodstream have been well defined.[185] It has been shown that the rate equations for phagocytosis show similarity to enzyme kinetics, where the order of the reaction depends on substrate concentration. Thus: (1) as particle concentration increases, clearance velocity approaches a maximum phagocytic velocity, (2) the order of the reaction varies with the particle concentration, and (3) a particle-membrane rate constant (Kp) exists corresponding to the Michaelis-Menton constant (Km). The latter constant describes the affinity of particle binding to the phagocyte surface. Since larger doses of particles are not usually given, an approximation of clearance velocity is conventionally made assuming first-order kinetics. The initial clearance velocity is then estimated as the product of Kp and the particle dose injected: initial clearance velocity = Kp (dose). Since the vascular clearance of RES-specific substances conforms to surface saturation kinetics and obeys rate equations consistent with the formation of a particle-membrane intermediate, the clearance of test substances has been modeled using double-reciprocal plots of clearance velocity versus the particle concentration (Lineweaver-Burk plot).[184]

A variety of test substances have been used to quantify RES function,[185] although particulate colloid uptake by the liver may not be specific to RES cells.[198] Furthermore, as indicated above, hepatic clearance of particulates depends on both hepatic blood flow and circulating plasma fibronectin. Hepatic extraction at constant flow will vary with the dose and nature of the RES-specific particles administered. Similarly, at constant dose but with varying flows, changes in the extraction ratio and therefore in the clearance velocity of substances may be, within limits, directly related to hepatic blood flow. Thus, reductions in portal venous and hepatic arterial flows consequent to reductions in cardiac output may result in decreased clearance rates for RES-specific substances. The observation that hepatic artery flow and portal vein flow normally subserve different physiologic functions extends to considerations regarding hepatic RES performance. That differences in hepatic uptake occur with selective portal venous or hepatic arterial input has been shown by Wolter et al.: the hepatic clearance of endotoxin in pigs was higher with portal vein injections.[269] This was presumably due to the observed slower portal venous perfusion velocity.

In summary, splanchnic hemodynamic changes may impair hepatic RES phagocytic function and compromise systemic host defense, and thereby have the potential to contribute to extrahepatic organ dysfunction and resulting multisystem organ failure. These pathophysiologic interactions are schematically depicted in Figure 7–12. For example, lung function in particular may be compromised by reductions in hepatic RES function. Schumacker et al. have shown in dogs that low-grade intravascular coagulation in the presence of RES blockade can lead to significant pulmonary hemodynamic and gas exchange abnormalities.[223] Although the lung can act as a passive secondary filter for substances escaping hepatic phagocytic uptake, the consequent release of bioactive materials within the lung and impairment of pulmonary metabolic function may lead to further release of vasoactive agents into the systemic circulation. Thus, alteration in the liver-lung axis of cardiopulmonary homeostasis secondary to reductions in cardiac output affecting splanchnic blood flow may significantly impair systemic homeostasis in the critically ill.

BRAIN BLOOD FLOW

The cerebral circulation, like other vascular beds, regulates its blood flow in an attempt to maintain nutrient flow and also to protect its microcirculation from high intravascular pressures. Total cerebral blood flow (CBF) is approximately 0.75 L/

min and may increase roughly threefold to 2.1 L/min. The average blood flow is about 55 ml/100 gm/min, depending on the method of measurement.[246] This represents 14% of the total cardiac output and 18% of the total body oxygen consumption for an organ that constitutes roughly 2% of total body mass.[73] The flow is not homogenous, flow to gray matter being three to four times higher than flow to white matter (75–80 ml/100 gm/min in gray matter, 20–25 ml/100 gm/min in white matter). Unlike total CBF, which remains relatively constant over a wide range of mental activities, regional flow increases markedly in areas anatomically linked to the function being performed.[111, 150, 235]

Similarly, the blood flow required for function and viability is not uniform throughout the brain.[97] The EEG begins to change when cortical flow is reduced to 20 ml/100 gm/min and becomes isoelectric around 15 ml/100 gm/min. This is also the level at which synaptic transmission fails, as indicated by the loss of the postsynaptic component of the evoked potential. The presynaptic component of the evoked potential remains until the flow decreases to about 12 ml/100 gm/min. Individual cells vary in their sensitivity, spontaneous activity ceasing at flows ranging from 22–6.4 ml/100 gm/min.[97]

Cell death is also variable and is associated with levels of ischemia that result in massive potassium efflux. This phenomenon is a function of both flow and time, that is, 5 ml/100 gm/min for 20 minutes is as damaging as 15 ml/100 gm/min for 80 minutes. Above 18 ml/100 gm/min the time threshold for ischemic necrosis approaches infinity.[97]

The cerebral vascular bed responds to a variety of metabolic and neural influences, as do other vascular beds. Both qualitative and quantitative differences, however, make the response of

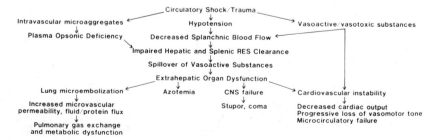

FIG 7–12.
Potential pathophysiologic sequences after circulatory shock/trauma that contribute to multisystem organ failure. (Adapted from Saba et al.[216] with permission.)

the cerebral circulation unique. This section describes these distinguishing aspects as well as the fundamental regulation of blood flow in the brain. For a more detailed discussion the reader is referred to an excellent review by Heistad and Kontos.[101]

Anatomy

In humans, blood is supplied to the brain via the internal carotid and basilar arteries. Although these vessels and the major vessels of the brain anastomose at the circle of Willis, there is little mixing of blood unless one of the major vessels supplying blood to the circle is obstructed.[101] The anterior, posterior, and middle cerebral arteries behave as endarteries, and the boundary zones of the cortex they supply are extremely susceptible to ischemic injury.[32] However, collateral arterial channels do exist and may become significant. These include subarachnoid collaterals between the major cerebral vessels, collaterals between the internal and external carotid arteries around the orbit, and collaterals from the cervical arteries to the vertebral and external carotid arteries.[67]

The blood-brain barrier is maintained primarily by the endothelial cells. It has structural and enzymatic components[192] and isolates the vascular smooth muscle from many circulating vasoactive substances. Less than 5% of circulating norepinephrine, serotonin, and epinephrine leaves the bloodstream, and this amount is readily metabolized before it reaches neural parenchyma. However, the barrier may be disrupted by a variety of conditions such as hypertension, administration of intraarterial hyperosmolar solutions, hypoxia/ischemia, infection, and radiation.[195] If the blood-brain barrier is disrupted, catechols and related compounds exert both primary and secondary vascular effects, the latter in response to changes in neuronal metabolic activity. Norepinephrine is a primary arteriolar vasoconstrictor, but increases CBF by increasing metabolism via a β-mediated effect. Serotonin, on the other hand, markedly reduces CBF by direct constriction and perhaps by a reduction in metabolism.[192] Such effects may be clinically significant when these agents are administered systemically in patients who have a damaged blood-brain barrier.

Metabolic Regulation

Changes in cerebral function result in demonstrable changes in metabolism and flow. EEG frequency correlates with the metabolic rate of the brain, and total CBF correlates with oxygen consumption.[112] Activation of specific areas of the brain associated with sensory, motor, and mental functions has been shown to cause concomitant increases in flow and metabolism.[111, 236] The mechanism by which flow is coupled to metabolism is still not clear, but the most widely accepted hypothesis is that neural activity results in the release of vasoactive compounds.[101] The local resistance of the blood vessels and, therefore, local flow would be proportional to the local concentration of metabolites. There are a number of proposed metabolites.

Adenosine

The following observations suggest that adenosine may be the mediator responsible for the local coupling of blood flow and metabolism. Adenosine dilates pial arteries in a dose-dependent manner, and smaller vessels respond more vigorously than do larger vessels.[254] Adenosine concentration in the brain increases during arterial hypoxemia (6-fold within 30 sec), during profound ischemia (2.5-fold within 5 sec of a decrease in blood pressure to zero), with decreases in blood pressure within the autoregulatory range, and during drug-induced seizures (especially with concomitant hypoxia or reduction in blood pressure).[265, 267] Adenosine may be produced by the breakdown of adenosine triphosphate (ATP) released with neural transmitters or by dephosphorylation of 5'-AMP by 5'-nucleotidase located on the membrane of astrocytic footplates enveloping intracerebral vessels.[267]

Carbon Dioxide and pH

These relations merit more detailed discussion because of their importance in therapy. The CBF response is curvilinear, but for Pa_{CO_2} values between 20 and 80 torr the response is almost linear, increasing 1.8 ml/100 gm/min/torr Pa_{CO_2}.[89, 203] The response is greater in gray than in white matter, probably because gray matter has greater vascular density. Consequently, the response to carbon dioxide varies in different regions of the brain according to their gray matter content.[189] The lower limit of the vasoconstrictor response to respiratory alkalosis represents either vasodilation resulting from ischemia[77a] or the effects of extreme alkalosis.[268] The upper limit represents maximal vasodilation. The response to carbon dioxide therefore depends on the resting caliber of the vessel and on other competing metabolic influences. Hypercapnia has a greater effect on vessels less than 100 μ in diameter than on larger vessels. However, if the increase in sympathetic tone caused by the hypercapnia is blocked, the response in all vessels is similar. The response of large and small pial vessels to hypocarbia is comparable because these vessels lack resting sympathetic tone.[259]

The mechanism of carbon dioxide vasoactivity appears to be a direct action of H^+ on the vascular smooth muscle that is situated on the brain side of the blood-brain barrier. The response to arterial carbon dioxide depends on diffusion of carbon dioxide across the blood-brain barrier and the exclusion of HCO_3^-. This results in a decrease in the pH of the periarteriolar CSF and subsequent dilation. The response of cerebral blood vessels to changes in arterial Pa_{CO_2} occurs within 20–30 sec.[129] Changing arteriolar carbon dioxide or pH does not change flow if CSF pH is kept constant,[19] and changing CSF carbon dioxide and HCO_3^- changes pial arteriolar caliber only if pH is allowed to change.[130] Thus, carbon dioxide and HCO_3^- have no intrinsic vascular effects. The pH response is not unique to the cerebral vasculature, but the high solubility of carbon dioxide and the exclusion of H^+ and HCO_3^- by the blood-brain barrier make the brain vasculature very sensitive to Pa_{CO_2}. With time, the normalization of CSF pH by active changes in HCO_3^- negates the effects of carbon dioxide on CBF. This adaptation has a half-life of about 6 hours and is complete by 30 hours.[43] This limits the long-term use of sustained hyperventilation in the treatment of elevated intracranial pressure (ICP).

The change in flow associated with increased metabolism is not dependent on a change in pH.[104, 182] Therefore, it appears that $[H^+]$ is not the primary factor coupling metabolism with blood flow.

A number of pathologic states negate or obtund the response to carbon dioxide. After 12 minutes of global ischemia the response to carbon dioxide is almost totally abolished for 24 hours.[129] Impairment has also been reported after transient focal ischemia and seems related to the severity of the ischemia.[226] Loss of response to carbon dioxide after head injury is common and is associated with severe brain injury. With clinical recovery the response gradually returns.[62] Also, any process that disrupts the blood-brain barrier markedly reduces the response to Pa_{CO_2} by

allowing HCO_3^- to enter the CSF and minimize the change in pH.[193]

Cerebral blood volume increases by approximately 0.04 ml/100 gm/torr CO_2.[89] The reduction in vascular resistance that causes flow to increase is a result of an increase in the diameter, and therefore volume, of the arteries. Venous volume also increases as flow increases. Cerebral blood volume does not increase linearly with CBF, but as the cube root of CBF.[89] This has important clinical implications for intracranial pressure when carbon dioxide and blood flow are manipulated.

Oxygen

Hypoxemia causes pial arteriolar dilation and increases CBF.[101] The response to arterial hypoxemia is a function of a decrease in arterial oxygen content. Because of the sigmoid nature of the hemoglobin dissociation curve, the increase in flow with decreasing Pa_{O_2} is semilogarithmic and begins to increase dramatically at a Pa_{O_2} of about 60 torr.[120] The maximum dilation achieved by hypoxia is equivalent to that observed with hypercarbia. At submaximal levels of dilation, hypoxic dilation is additive with that of hypercarbia.[229] The vasodilation induced by ischemic hypoxia is unresponsive to hypocarbia.[132]

The response to hypoxia appears to depend on the level of neural tissue oxygenation rather than arterial Pa_{O_2}.[132] However, the way in which neural hypoxia induces vasodilation in blood flow is not firmly established. It does not seem to involve prostaglandins[258] or potassium,[104] and at least the initial increase in blood flow that occurs with induction of hypoxia is not caused by CSF acidosis.[182] Adenosine may be the mediator.[266]

Potassium

Elevation of perivascular potassium dilates pial arterioles,[136] and the time course and concentrations achieved during stimulation of the brain are compatible with potassium being a primary regulator of CBF.[250] Potassium may be the major vasodilator during seizures.[267]

Calcium

Calcium concentration exerts major effects on pial vessels, elevation causing vasoconstriction and depression causing vasodilation.[20] Calcium levels in the brain have been shown to decrease during electrical stimulation and seizures,[96] and changes in calcium flux may be the final pathway of many vasodilators.[267]

Prostaglandins

Pial vessels react to a large variety of prostaglandins, the majority of which dilate small cerebral vessels.[101] Although their effects on the normal control of CBF and their involvement in the carbon dioxide response are not clear, prostaglandins appear to have major effects in certain pathologic conditions. During energy failure caused by ischemia, enhanced lipolysis liberates free fatty acids that are synthesized into prostaglandins on recirculation and delivery of oxygen.[234] The most damaging aspect of such synthesis is the formation of free oxygen radicals. Postischemic vascular abnormalities have been inhibited by the use of indomethacin and blunted by the addition of free radical scavengers.[133] Similarly, vascular abnormalities following concussive brain injury and hypertensive brain injury have been inhibited by the use of free radical scavengers.[134, 260]

Neural Regulation of Blood Flow

Sympathetic innervation has little influence on resting CBF[69, 98, 173] but appears to attenuate flow increases caused by fluctuations in blood pressure in both physiologic[39] and hypertensive pressure ranges.[60, 99] Sympathetic stimulation constricts large arteries but has minimal effect on small arteries.[137, 257] However, both large and small pial vessels may be under dual sympathetic and metabolic control, the latter predominating as pial vessel size decreases.[249]

Sympathetic tone may be important in pathologic states. CBF is decreased by sympathetic stimulation in situations where smaller downstream vessels are maximally dilated, and the vasodilation of larger cerebral vessels is partially inhibited by reflex increases in sympathetic action, such as in hemorrhagic shock,[69, 152] hypercarbia,[93] and hypoxia.[40] Sympathetic tone may be protective in chronic hypertension. In stroke-prone spontaneously hypertensive rats, denervation attenuates the development of vascular hypertrophy[94] and is associated with a higher incidence of both ischemic and hemorrhagic infarction.[218] The hemorrhagic infarction is thought to occur because the autoregulatory response to high blood pressure is impaired, and the ischemic infarction may occur because blood vessels are exposed to vasoconstrictive substances that are able to penetrate the blood-brain barrier made permeable by high vascular pressure.[100]

Pressure Autoregulation

Perfusion pressure for the brain is defined as the MAP of the major arteries at the entrance to the skull minus the venous pressure at the outflow of the skull (or minus ICP if ICP is greater than venous pressure). Pressure autoregulation in the brain is probably not absolute. In human studies, flow changes within the autoregulatory range have varied from 0 to 7%/10 torr.[101] The autoregulatory response is rapid, however. It begins in 3–7 sec and is complete in approximately 1 minute.[131]

The mechanism of pressure autoregulation in the brain is not firmly established. The mechanisms involved depend very much on the pressure range studied and the means used to change the pressure. The evidence suggests that metabolic, flow-dependent mechanisms predominate over myogenic, pressure-dependent mechanisms,[253, 261] and that the cerebral vascular response depends on the interplay of metabolic and neural influences on large and small vessels.[131, 148, 152, 249] Neither H^+ nor K^+ seems to be involved in the autoregulatory response,[255] but adenosine levels in the brain have been observed to increase during blood pressure reductions within the autoregulatory range.[264]

The role of neural influences in autoregulation seems to be in the high pressure range and involves constriction of large cerebral vessels. Though the major site of cerebrovascular resistance is at the arterioles, the larger pial arteries that respond to sympathetic stimulation contribute an unusually large percentage of the total resistance.[101] When pressure increases are within the normal range the major change in resistance is in the smaller vessels, but when increases are in the hypertensive range the increase in resistance occurs predominantly in large extracerebral arteries.[99, 131] In fact, the major function of the sympathetic innervation may be to protect the brain from transient increases in blood pressure associated with generalized sympathetic discharge.[9] Such increases in resistance may be detrimental. Hemorrhage results in increased sympathetic tone and increases the lower limit of autoregulation at a time when perfusion pressure is reduced.[69]

Both large and small vessels may be controlled by a combination of neutral and metabolic mechanisms. As the vessels become smaller, metabolic factors become increasingly important. With reduction in perfusion pressure and flow, metabolic factors gradually override the neural influences until the circulation is maximally dilated and pressure passive. This may explain why the slope of the pressure/flow relation is not constant but increases gradually below the autoregulatory plateau, and why the cerebral circulation becomes truly pressure passive only at pressures well below the lower limit of autoregulation.[152, 249]

These statements indicate the autoregulatory curve will be different in both its slope and its range depending on the method of pressure reduction.[101] Hypotension caused by hemorrhage, which induces sympathetic reflexes, will shift the curve to the right. Substances that cause vasodilation will tend to diminish the autoregulatory plateau, both increasing its slope and narrowing its range (Fig 7–13).

Autoregulation is abolished in many clinical conditions. After transient severe increases in pressure, the pial vessels remain dilated for several hours.[134] Loss of autoregulation is a common phenomenon after head injury, although "false autoregulation" may be observed. In the latter situation increased CBF causes a concomitant increase in intracranial or local tissue pressure, which limits perfusion pressure and flow.[62, 191] Vasodilators such as hypoxia,[146] carbon dioxide,[142] hydralazine,[210] nitroprusside,[102] and halothane[169] depress or ablate the response to autoregulation. Postischemic luxury perfusion is also a form of disrupted autoregulation that appears to be caused by small vessel dilation. CBF in this situation is not related to the metabolic needs of the tissue or to the correction of an oxygen debt.[78]

Interrelation of ICP, CBF, and CBV

Because the skull and meninges are structures with low compliance, the brain readily develops a compartmental syndrome in which the gradient of arterial to intracranial pressure rather than of arterial to central venous pressure determines cerebral perfusion.[199] ICP usually has little effect on the arterial circulation because intraluminal pressure is high. However, veins are more susceptible to compression, most likely at the region 1–2 mm proximal to the junction of the lateral lacunae and the sagittal sinus.[177] Elevation of ICP thereby restricts venous outflow, and increases cerebral venous blood volume and pressure. The decrease in perfusion pressure is overcome by autoregulation, which allows flow to continue until a perfusion pressure of around 30 torr is reached. Below this perfusion pressure blood flow decreases.[90]

The relation of ICP to CBF will vary according to the mechanism primarily responsible for the elevation in ICP. If it is loss of autoregulation, CBF becomes very high, causing vascular engorgement of the brain. Because the loss of resistance involves an increase in vessel radius, there is an increase in blood volume, which results in an increase in ICP. If, on the other hand, the elevation of ICP is caused by an increase in the volume of tissue or of CSF within the cranial

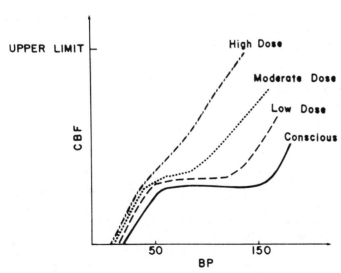

FIG 7–13.
Schematic representation of the effect of a progressively increased dose of a typical volatile anesthetic agent on CBF autoregulation. Both upper and lower thresholds are shifted to the left. (From Shapiro H.M.[227a] Reproduced by permission.)

vault, the pressure will be transmitted to the lacunar and arterial vessels, reducing flow by a Starling resistor effect. Flow will be maintained if autoregulation is still intact or if there is blood in the venous capacitance beds that can be expelled without markedly changing venous resistance. If the venous vascular compartment has already been maximally reduced, there will be false autoregulation, in which any increase in flow results in an increase in ICP, which keeps the flow constant.[42] These differences in the etiology of increased ICP may account for the observation that all possible CBF to ICP relations have been observed clinically: high CBF/high ICP, high CBF/low ICP, and low CBF/high ICP.[245]

Within the skull, increases in pressure can be balanced only by changes in the volume of tissue, CSF, or blood. The tissue structures, meninges, and dura are not very compliant and the response to a rapid addition of nonvascular volume results in a pressure increase. With chronic changes in ICP, changes in tissue volume or in CSF volume are possible, but with acute changes only shifts in blood volume can account for the rapid equilibration.[228] The apparent compliance of the brain is therefore dependent on the blood volume within the brain.[42] The compliance of the intracranial contents is not constant but decreases rapidly as intracranial volume is increased; that is, ICP increases exponentially with increases in volume. The underlying physical mechanism of intracranial compliance has been debated but the observed ICP response to the infusion of volume into the cranial vault is most likely a result of the compression of venous capacitance vessels and reflects resistance to the expulsion of the venous blood volume, rather than the stretching of elastic structures.[42, 228] When autoregulation is exhausted the observed compliance reflects a reduction in blood volume caused by a reduction in CBF. The true compliance of the rigid meninges and skull is assessed when ICP exceeds the arterial pressure.[42]

In summary, CBF is controlled predominantly by metabolic regulation. Adenosine may be the primary metabolic mediator. Carbon dioxide, pH, potassium, and prostaglandins also affect cerebral vascular tone and may be important in certain pathologic states. Many of the responses of the circulation require an intact blood-brain barrier, which is easily disrupted. Pressure autoregulation involves a balance between metabolic and neural influences, the former being more important to the regulation of small vessels and the latter to the regulation of larger vessels. Intrinsic myogenic regulation may also play a role. The cerebral circulation includes a variable, ICP-dependent resistance just proximal to the lacunar/sagittal sinus junction. The "compliance" of the intracranial contents is not constant. The response at lower pressures is a function of the venous volume and its resistance to drainage. When autoregulation is exceeded it is a function of reduction in blood volume secondary to reduction in blood flow. Finally, when ICP exceeds the arterial pressure, the compliance of the meninges and skull determines the pressure response.

RENAL CIRCULATION

The regulation of blood flow to the kidney is different from that of flow to other organs. In most tissues blood flow is only a fraction of the maximum, and flow may vary widely in response to changing oxygen needs. In contrast, renal blood flow (RBF) is usually near maximum and oxygen delivery greatly exceeds oxygen requirements. Changes in RBF are usually secondary to neurohumoral reflexes rather than to local metabolism. The prime determinant of oxygen consumption in the kidney is sodium reabsorption, which varies only a few percent in all but the most extreme circumstances. Therefore, changes in oxygen consumption do not significantly alter RBF.

While oxygen metabolism is not intimately tied to RBF, renal function is highly dependent on the distribution of blood flow to either deep or superficial cortex, and afferent and efferent glomerular vessel tone. Therefore, the control of RBF must include examination of factors that alter distribution of flow within the cortex, regulation of glomerulation filtration rate (GFR), and the determinants of Starling forces within the peritubular vessels.

Autoregulation

RBF is relatively independent of perfusion pressure over a wide range. This autoregulation appears to be an intrinsic property of the renal vasculature, and independent of humoral or neurogenic mechanisms.

Water and sodium excretion is regulated by the kidney to balance intake and can vary independent of GFR. However, variation in the amount of delivered sodium can dictate change in

GFR. This "tubuloglomerular feedback" phenomenon has been well described but the various explanations of the sensing system remain controversial. When increased filtered sodium is delivered to the distal tubule, absorption is increased, leading to activation of a feedback system increasing afferent glomerular arteriolar resistance, decreasing GFR, and ultimately decreasing distal sodium delivery. One favored theory concludes that the increased sodium results in increased release of renin from macula densa cells.[178, 222] By contrast, a decrease in GFR and sodium delivered to the macula densa cells will lead to diminished afferent arteriolar tone, which restores the GFR. This state of autoregulation is maintained until MAP reaches 70–80 torr.

Regulation of Cortical Blood Flow

The renal vasculature can be divided into three circulatory groups: glomerular, peritubular, and medullary.[13]

The glomerulus consists of a capillary tuft within the proximal tubule. Flow to and within the glomerulus is controlled by a variety of neurogenic and humoral factors. Investigators have shown that flow to the deep juxtamedullary nephrons of animals is the same, relative to glomerular volume and filtration, as flow to the more superficial nephrons.[181, 270] However, various stimuli can alter this pattern and increase flow to either deep or superficial nephrons. Fractional cortical flow to the outermost glomeruli is decreased while juxtamedullary flow is increased during renal arterial perfusion with acetylcholine and bradykinin as well as during saline diuresis,[34, 114] ureteral obstruction,[10] aortic constriction, and hemorrhagic hypotension.[238] Total renal resistance is decreased in these conditions. Prostaglandin inhibitors also decrease overall renal vascular resistance, leading to an increase in total blood flow, but the increase is to the superficial cortex, and deep cortical flow is inhibited.[11] Overall renal resistance is increased by infusion of norepinephrine or angiotensin,[202] renal nerve stimulation,[188] and hypoxia.[37] In general, conditions that increase total RBF increase the proportion of flow to deep glomeruli, but conditions associated with a decrease in total RBF are usually associated with a proportional decrease in flow to all glomeruli. Since sodium excretion is determined largely by changes in filtration fraction, alteration in regional single nephron filtration fractions is more closely associated with

changes in sodium reabsorption than might be estimated from change in regional plasma flow alone.[8, 31, 238]

Glomerular Filtration

The capillaries of the glomerulus are situated between two arterioles that work in consort to regulate the intraglomerular capillary pressure. Since the glomerular ultrafiltrate is nearly protein free, effective filtration pressure is the difference between the hydrostatic pressure and the colloid oncotic pressure. In rats, the hydrostatic pressure gradient between the capillary lumen and Bowman's space is 30–40 torr. As water ultrafilters, the protein concentration increases in the glomerular capillary lumen and raises the colloid oncotic pressure to approximately 30–40 torr, at which point filtration ceases.[49, 50] Single nephron glomerular filtration rate (SNGFR) is dependent on renal plasma flow (RPF) and can be altered by changes in the capillary hydrostatic pressure, oncotic pressure, or hydraulic permeability of the capillary wall. These relations are defined in the following formula:

$$\text{SNGFR} - K_f \times S \times (\overline{\Delta P} - \overline{\Delta \pi}) \qquad \text{(Eq. 7–1)}$$

where K_f denotes the effective hydraulic permeability of the capillary wall, S denotes the surface area for filtration, $\overline{\Delta P}$ is the capillary minus Bowman's space hydrostatic pressure, and $\overline{\Delta \pi}$ is the capillary minus Bowman's space oncotic pressure.[22]

Alterations in these factors determine the fraction of the plasma flow that is ultimately filtered. Increasing the intraglomerular hydrostatic pressure ($\overline{\Delta P}$) by volume expansion augments SNGFR, while reducing RPF by decreasing systemic blood pressure or cardiac output may decrease SNGFR. The effective surface area (S) is decreased with any form of renal parenchymal injury. In addition, many hormones can decrease the effective hydraulic permeability (K_f).[11, 109] Parathyroid hormone and angiotensin as well as some prostaglandin inhibitors decrease SNGFR by reducing K_f. Although PGE_1 and histamine decrease K_f, total GFR is not altered since there are compensatory changes in other factors, especially an increase in effective glomerular hydrostatic pressure ($\overline{\Delta P}$).

The hydrostatic pressure in the renal circulation drops as blood passes through the glomerulus into the peritubular plexus.[149] The hydrostatic pressure gradient across the glomerulus is higher than the oncotic gradient that works in the opposite direction, so that ultrafiltration is promoted.[30] In addition, the effective hydraulic permeability of the glomerular vessels is significantly higher than that of capillaries from other beds.[51] Beyond the glomerulus, vascular resistance falls sharply so that the oncotic pressure gradient exceeds the hydrostatic pressure gradient and the peritubular vessels are less permeable, all of which promote reabsorption of filtrate from the surrounding renal tubules.[128] These changes in intravascular oncotic and hydrostatic pressures can account for the bulk of proximal tubular reabsorption,[50, 64] and can therefore greatly influence the eventual delivery of water and sodium to more distal sites.

Extraction of tubular water to concentrate urine is carried out in the medulla. In primates, the medullary circulation has a very low hydraulic permeability, more outflow than inflow vessels, and a high ratio of capillary to tubule volume. The microanatomy, therefore, facilitates reabsorption of large volumes and promotes urine concentration.[244]

Renal Circulation During Hypoxia

Patients with pulmonary disease and hypoxia often have diminished RPF, GFR, sodium excretion,[68, 124] and water excretion.[53] Oxygen therapy has been shown to reverse these effects but it remains unclear whether the beneficial effect directly alters the renal circulation or augments some other mechanism such as the cardiac output.

Although human studies have demonstrated that acute hypoxia decreases urine output, a finding associated with increased antidiuretic hormone production, only a few studies directed at explaining the mechanisms that alter renal circulation have been reported. In patients with chronic lung disease studied acutely, a fall in arterial PO_2 to 30 torr is associated with sodium retention and a decrease in RBF and GFR.[124] Glomerular volume in patients with chronic bronchitis is larger than glomerular volume in nonbronchitic controls, but the distribution of RBF in these patients is undocumented.[41] From this paucity of data, no conclusion concerning therapy for renal circulatory abnormalities in hypoxic humans can be made. Studies during acute hypoxia in animals, however, suggest that adequate hydration and vascular volume expansion are important factors in maintaining normal renal circulatory function. In cases where sodium and water retention are of clinical concern, agents might be utilized that augment cardiac output, increase RBF directly, or promote renal vasodilation.

In hypervolemic dogs, hypoxia to 30 torr does not cause reduced renal function. Hypervolemic dogs respond to hypoxia with either no change or even a slight increase in glomerular filtration and sodium excretion.[4, 35] However, urine volume decreases and urine concentration increases, apparently as a result of an increase in arginine vasopressin production related to carotid chemoreceptor stimulation.[4, 44] If carotid chemoreceptors are denervated in dogs, vasopressin levels do not increase, nor does urine volume decrease. Baroreceptor denervation does not affect the vasopressin response to hypoxia. Renal denervation in a volume-expanded animal does not alter GFR, RPF, urine volume, or sodium excretion.[4]

Acute studies in hydropenic dogs have been performed in which the PO_2 was lowered without lowering cardiac output or changing arterial pH. Lowering the systemic arterial PO_2 to 30–40 torr decreased RPF, GFR, and sodium excretion approximately 30%.[37] The effect was reversed when the PO_2 was restored to normal. Furthermore, when one kidney was perfused with the vasodilator acetylcholine, there was no change in the renal circulation of that kidney during hypoxia, suggesting that the hypoxic decrease in RPF is a neurohumoral response to a decrease in metabolic rate rather than toxic injury to the vessel.

Studies in hydropenic dogs have attempted to explain the mechanisms of increased renal vascular resistance that occurs with hypoxemia. Both α-adrenergic blockade with dibenzylene and renal denervation prevent the fall in RPF, GFR, and sodium excretion,[36] demonstrating that the increase in vascular resistance is an α-adrenergic-mediated response rather than humoral. It is possible that in addition to the augmented α-adrenergic stimuli, there is a decrease in intrarenal vasodilation stimuli. Renal prostaglandin production is known to decrease in response to hypoxia in tissue preparations,[271] and prostaglandins are known α-adrenergic inhibitors. Unilateral renal infusion of PGE_1 prevents the hypoxia-induced decrease in RPF and GFR but fails to prevent the decrease in sodium excretion.[38] Thus, factors in addition to depressed prostaglandin production are needed to produce sodium retention during hypoxia. Results of studies in the conscious dog are different from those in anesthetized animals. In the conscious state, hypoxia is associated with an increase in urine volume and sodium excretion.[256] These findings may be secondary to an increase in cardiac output and an arterial pressure of more than 30%, since when the pressure increase is blunted with propranolol, urine volume does not increase significantly.

Renal Blood Flow During Acid-Base Disorders

Renal blood vessels appear to be exquisitely sensitive to changes in blood pH. Most studies[239] indicate that, in contrast to that in other vascular beds, renal vascular resistance increases in acidosis, and particularly in respiratory acidosis, resulting in a decrease in RBF. However, adaption occurs over time so that RBF may be normal in chronic acidosis. Alkalosis decreases renal vascular resistance and causes a sodium diuresis.[37] The effect of rapid correction of acidosis by administration of bicarbonate is less clear.

Renal Blood Flow and Acute Renal Failure

Acute renal failure (ARF) is characterized by an acute reversible depression of renal function found in association with hypotension or renal toxins.[106] Patients in ARF have oliguria, a high fractional sodium excretion, and a low urine to plasma creatinine ratio. Although RPF is diminished early in the disorder, flow rapidly returns to nearly normal levels while GFR remains depressed.[166, 205] Autopsy studies usually show tubular damage.[188]

The pathophysiology of ARF has been examined in detail by numerous investigators using models such as nephrotoxic injury and renal ischemia. Several mechanisms may explain the depressed GFR and urine output that occur despite a return to normal RPF. Tubular obstruction with or without backleak of filtered fluid has been demonstrated.[56] The extent of the backleak is dependent on the severity of the ischemic insult. Obstruction has not been demonstrated, however, in all models.[128] Intraglomerular shunting by reduction of ΔP as a result of efferent arteriolar dilation has been postulated.[7] A decrease in K_f produces a similar finding.[21] Marked fusion of glomerular foot process structure adds support to evidence that decreased K_f is a key alteration.[47]

In a given model, a combination of several mechanisms may be operative.

In animals, volume expansion by a high-salt diet prior to renal injury blunts the reduction in GFR and urine flow but does not alter histologic tubular damage.[52] This protection of GFR may be a result of depressed renin production with maintenance of RPF or of high urine flow rates, which may enhance the excretion of nephrotoxins. The role of renin and angiotensin in the genesis of ARF remains unclear since immunization against angiotensin II or treatment with converting enzyme inhibitor fails to protect the GFR in some models.[110] Intrarenal vasodilation with prostaglandins or kinins may be an important factor in resistance to ARF since inhibition of prostaglandin synthesis by indomethacin augments the severity of ARF induced by some nephrotoxins.[247] Since a decrease in prostaglandin synthesis decreases RPF, the alteration of function is probably a result of increased vascular resistance prior to the toxic insult rather than a direct effect of prostaglandin.

The protection against ARF provided by volume expansion has led to the investigation of various protective agents. Pretreatment with diuretics has been shown to protect against nephrotoxic injury.[243] This may be related to an increase in solute flow since furosemide does not change GFR when GFR and RBF are decreased with an aortic clamp.[119] Furosemide does not reverse ARF when the drug is given after the toxic injury.[175] Mannitol protects against ARF when administered before an ischemic injury.[48] In hypotensive rats, mannitol restored RBF and GFR.[119] The increased GFR and urine flow may prevent tubular obstruction by flushing debris or by decreasing ischemic tubular swelling. Increased RBF by volume expansion may also play a role. The beneficial effects of mannitol have prompted its use in open heart, complicated biliary, and major vascular surgery, although the effectiveness of this prophylactic use has not been proved in humans.[16]

There are few experimental data to dictate any specific therapy for ARF patients following renal injury. The recently increased incidence of nonoliguric renal failure remains unexplained,[156] but is associated with more aggressive treatment of critically ill patients with volume replacement, vasodilator therapy, and the use of inotropic agents. Preservation of RBF may prevent the development of severe oliguria and depressed GFR.

Since maintenance of RBF with volume expansion, vasodilation, cardiotonic agents, and certain diuretics may be protective, it seems prudent to use such measures to prevent ARF in critically ill and preoperative patients.

REFERENCES

1. Alexander RS: Influence of the diaphragm upon portal blood flow and venous return. *Am J Physiol* 1951; 167:738–748.

2. Altura BM: Reticuloendothelial cells and host defense. *Adv Microcirc* 1980; 9:252–294.

3. Altura BM: Endothelium, reticuloendothelial cells, and microvascular integrity: Roles in heart disease, in Altura BM, et al (eds): *Handbook of Shock and Trauma*. Vol 1: *Basic Science*. New York, Raven Press, 1983, pp 51–95.

4. Anderson RJ, Pluss RG, Berns PS, et al: Mechanism of effect of hypoxia in renal water excretion. *J Clin Invest* 1978; 62:768.

5. Bache RJ, Dymek DJ: Local and regional regulation of coronary vascular tone. *Prog Cardiovasc Dis* 1981; 24:191.

6. Baggar H: Distribution of coronary blood flow in the left ventricular wall of dogs evaluated by the uptake of Xe-133. *Acta Physiol Scand* 1977; 99:431.

7. Balint P, Scocs E: Intrarenal hemodynamics following temporary occlusion of the renal artery in the dog. *Kidney Int* 1976; 10:5128.

8. Bartoli E, Earley LE: The relative contribution of reabsorptive rate and redistributed nephron filtrate rate to changes in proximal tubular fractional reabsorption during acute saline infusion and aortic constriction in the rat. *J Clin Invest* 1973; 50:2191.

9. Baumbach GL, Heistad DD: Effects of sympathetic stimulation and changes in arterial pressure on segmental resistance of cerebral vessels in rabbits and cats. *Circ Res* 1983; 52:527–533.

10. Bay WH, Stein JH, Rector JB, et al: Redistribution of renal cortical blood flow during elevated ureteral pressure in the dog. *Am J Physiol* 1972; 222:33.

11. Bayliss C, Deen WM, Meyers BD, et al: Effects of some vasodilator drugs on transcapillary fluid exchange in the renal cortex. *Am J Physiol* 1976; 230:1148.

12. Becker LC, Fortuin JJ, Pitt B: Effect of ischemia and antianginal drugs on the distribution of radioactive microspheres in the canine left ventricle. *Circ Res* 1971; 28:263–269.

13. Beeuwkes R III, Ichikawa I, Brenner BM: The renal circulation, in Brenner BM, Rector KC Jr (eds): *The Kidney*. Philadelphia, WB Saunders Co, 1982, pp 215–250.

14. Belleau L, Earley LE: Autoregulation of renal blood flow in the presence of angiotensin infusion. *Am J Physiol* 1967; 213:1590.

15. Bennett TD, Rothe C: Hepatic capacitance responses to changes in flow and hepatic venous pressure in dogs. *Am J Physiol* 1981; 240:H18–H28.

16. Berman LB, Smith LL, Chisolm GD, et al: Mannitol and renal function in cardiovascular surgery. *Arch Surg* 1964; 88:239.

17. Berne RM, Blackmon JR, Gardner TH: Hypoxemia and coronary blood flow. *J Clin Invest* 1957; 36:1101–1106.

18. Berne RM, Levy MN: *Cardiovascular Physiology,* ed 3. St Louis, CV Mosby Co, 1977, p 225.

19. Betz E, Heuser D: Cerebral cortical blood flow during changes of acid-base equilibrium of the brain. *J Appl Physiol* 1967; 23:726–733.

20. Betz E, Csornai M: Action and interaction of perivascular H^+, K^+ and Ca^{++} on pial arteries. *Pflugers Arch* 1978; 374:67–72.

21. Blantz RC: Mechanism of acute renal failure after uranyl nitrate. *J Clin Invest* 1975; 55:621.

22. Blantz RC: Glomerular filtration, in Massry SG, Glassock RJ (eds): *Textbook of Nephrology*. Baltimore, Williams & Wilkins Co, 1983, pp 1.34–1.39.

23. Bloor CM, White FC: Coronary artery reperfusion: Effects of occlusion duration on reactive hyperemia response. *Basic Res Cardiol* 1975; 70:148–158.

24. Blumenstock F, Weber P, Saba TM, et al: Electroimmunoassay of alpha-2-opsonic protein during reticuloendothelial blockade. *Am J Physiol* 1977; 232:R80–R87.

25. Blumenthal MR, Wang HH, Wang SC: Effect of acute experimental aortic stenosis on coronary circulation. *Circ Res* 1962; 11:727–735.

26. Bradfield JWB: Control of spillover: The importance of Kupffer cell function in clinical medicine. *Lancet* 1974; 2:883–886.

27. Brauer RW, Holloway RJ, Leony GF: Changes in liver function and structure due to experimental passive congestion under controlled hepatic vein pressures. *Am J Physiol* 1959; 197:681–692.

28. Brauer RW: Liver circulation and function. *Physiol Rev* 1963; 43:115–193.

29. Bredenberg CE, Paskanik A, Fromm D: Portal hemodynamics in dogs during mechanical ventilation with positive end-expiratory pressure. *Surgery* 1981; 90:817–822.

30. Brenner BM, Troy JL, Daugherty TM: The dynamics of glomerular ultrafiltration to the rat. *J Clin Invest* 1971; 50:1776.

31. Brenner BM, Troy JL, Daugherty TM, et al: Dynamics of glomerular ultrafiltration in the rat: II. Plasma flow dependence of GFR. *Am J Physiol* 1972; 223:1184.

32. Brierley JB, Brown AW, Excell BJ, et al: Brain damage in the rhesus monkey resulting from profound arterial hypotension: 1. Its nature, distribution, and general physiological correlates. *Brain Res* 1969; 13:68–100.

33. Brown BG, Gundel WD, Gott VL, et al: Coronary collateral flow following acute coronary occlusion: A diastolic phenomenon. *Cardiovasc Res* 1974; 8:621–631.

34. Bruns FJ, Alexander ED, Riley AL, et al: Superficial and juxtamedullary nephron function during saline loading in the dog. *J Clin Invest* 1974; 53:971.

35. Bruns F, Todroff R: Prevention of hypoxia-induced decreases in GFR by volume expansion. *Clin Res* 1974; 22:518.

36. Bruns F, Losos K: The role of alpha adrenergic and renal nerve stimulation of GFR and sodium excretion during hypoxia. *Kidney Int* 1976; 10:579.

37. Bruns F: Decrease in renal perfusion, glomerular filtration and sodium excretion by hypoxia in the dog. *Proc Soc Exp Biol Med* 1978; 159:468.

38. Bruns F, Soroka K: The role of prostaglandin E₁ on glomerular filtration, renal plasma flow and sodium excretion during hypoxia. *Kidney Int* 1979; 16:849.

39. Busija DW, Heistad DD, Marcus ML: Effects of sympathetic nerves on cerebral vessels during acute, moderate increases in arterial pressure in dogs and cats. *Circ Res* 1980; 46:696–702.

40. Busija DW: Sympathetic nerves reduce cerebral blood flow during hypoxia in awake rabbits. *Am J Physiol* 1984; 247:H446–H451.

41. Campbell JL, Callerly PM, Lamb D, et al: The renal glomerulus in hypoxic cor pulmonale. *Thorax* 1982; 37:607–611.

42. Chopp M, Portnoy HD, Branch C: Hydraulic model of the cerebrovascular bed: An aid to understanding the volume-pressure test. *Neurosurgery* 1983; 13:5–11.

43. Christensen MS, Brodersen P, Olesen J, et al: Cerebral apoplexy (stroke) treated with or without prolonged artificial hyperventilation: 2. Cerebrospinal fluid acid-base balance and intracranial pressure. *Stroke* 1973; 4:620–631.

44. Claybaugh JR, Wade CE, Sato AK, et al: Antidiuretic hormone responses to encapric and hypoxcapric hypoxia in humans. *J Appl Physiol* 1982; 53:R815–R823.

45. Coffman JD, Gregg DE: Reactive hyperemia characteristics of the myocardium. *Am J Physiol* 1960; 199:1143–1149.

46. Cohn JN, Pinkerson AL: Intrahepatic distribution of hepatic arterial and portal venous flows in the dog. *Am J Physiol* 1969; 216:285–289.

47. Cox JW, Baehler RW, Sharma H, et al: Studies on the mechanisms of oliguria in a model of unilateral acute renal failure. *J Clin Invest* 1974; 53:1546.

48. Cronin RF, DeTorrente A, Miller PD, et al: Pathogenic mechanisms in early norepinephrine-induced renal failure: Functional and histological correlates of proteinuria. *Kidney Int* 1978; 14:115.

49. Deen WM, Robertson CR, Brenner BB: A model of glomerular ultrafiltration in the rat. *Am J Physiol* 1972; 223:1178.

50. Deen WM, Robertson CR, Brenner BB: A model of peritubular capillary control of isotonic fluid reabsorption by the renal proximal tubule. *Biophys J* 1973; 13:340.

51. Deen WM, Troy JL, Robertson CR, et al: Dynamics of glomerular ultrafiltration in the rat: IV. Determination of the ultrafiltration coefficient. *J Clin Invest* 1973; 52:1500.

52. DiBona GF, McDonald DF, Flamenbaum W, et al: Maintenance of renal function in salt loaded rats despite severe tubular renins induced by HgLI₂. *Nephron* 1971; 8:105.

53. Doberneck RC, Schwartz FD, Barry KG: A comparison of the prophylactic value of

20% mannitol, 4% urea, and 5% dextrose on the effect of renal ischemia. *J Urol* 1963; 89:300.

54. Domenech RJ, Hoffman JIE, Noble MIM, et al: Total and regional coronary blood flow measured by radioactive microspheres in conscious and anesthetized dogs. *Circ Res* 1969; 25:581–596.

55. Donald DE: Splanchnic circulation, in Shepherd JT, Abboud FM (eds): *Handbook of Physiology: The Cardiovascular System,* section 2, vol III, part 1. Bethesda, Md, American Physiological Society, 1983, pp 219–240.

56. Donohoe JF, Jenkatachalan MA, Bernard DB, et al: Tubular leakage and obstruction in acute ischemic renal failure. *Kidney Int* 1978; 13:208.

57. Driscol TE, Moir TW, Eckstein RW: Autoregulation and coronary blood flow: Effect of interarterial pressure gradients. *Circ Res* 1964; 15:103–111.

58. Driscol TE, Eckstein RW: Coronary inflow and outflow responses to coronary artery occlusion. *Circ Res.* 1967; 20:485–495.

59. Earley LE, Schrier RW: Intrarenal control of sodium excretion by hemodynamic and physical factors, in Orloff J, Berliner RW (eds): *Handbook of Physiology: Renal Physiology.* Washington, DC, American Physiologic Society, 1973, section 2, pp 721–762.

60. Edvinsson L, Owman C, Siesjö B: Physiologic role of cerebrovascular sympathetic nerves in the autoregulation of cerebral blood flow. *Brain Res* 1976; 117:519–523.

61. Ehrlich W: Unpublished data.

62. Enevoldsen EM, Jensen FT: Autoregulation and CO_2 responses of cerebral blood flow in patients with acute severe head injury. *J Neurosurg* 1978; 48:689–703.

63. Entman ML, Martin AM Jr, Mikat E, et al: Phasic myocardial blood flow in hemorrhagic hypotension: Effect of beta sympathetic blockade. *Am J Cardiol* 1968; 21:881–885.

64. Falchuk KH, Brenner BM, Tadokoro M, et al: Oncotic and hydrostatic pressures in peritubular capillaries and fluid reabsorption by proximal tubules. *Am J Physiol* 1971; 220:1427.

65. Fara JW, Rubinstein EH, Sonnenshein RR: Intestinal hormones in mesenteric vasodilation after intraduodenal agents. *Am J Physiol* 1972; 223:1058–1067.

66. Farber MD, Bright TP, Strawbridge RA, et al: Impaired water handling in chronic obstructive lung disease. *J Lab Clin Med* 1975; 85:41.

67. Fisher CM, Mohr JP, Adams RD: Cerebrovascular diseases, in Wintrobe MM, Thorn GW, Adams RD, et al (eds): *Harrison's Principles of Internal Medicine,* ed 7. New York, McGraw-Hill Book Co, 1974, pp 1752–1753.

68. Fishman TP, Maxwell MH, Crouder CH: Kidney function in cor pulmonale. *Circulation* 1951; 3:703.

69. Fitch W, Mackenzie ET, Harper AM: Effects of decreasing arterial blood pressure on cerebral blood flow in the baboon. *Circ Res* 1975; 37:550–557.

70. Flores J, DiBonna DR, Beck CH, et al: The role of cell swelling in ischemic renal damage and the protective effect of hypertonic solute. *J Clin Invest* 1972; 51:118.

71. Folkow B, Neil E: Gastrointestinal and liver circulations, in *The Circulation.* New York, Oxford University Press, 1971, pp 466–493.

72. Frank HA, Seligman AM, Finie J: Traumatic shock: XIII. The prevention of irreversibility in hemorrhagic shock by viviperfusion of the liver. *J Clin Invest* 1946; 25:22–29.

73. Ganong WF (ed): *Review of Medical Physiology.* Los Altos, Lange Medical Publications, 1971, p 439.

74. Gans H, Mori K, Lindsey E, et al: Septicemia as a manifestation of acute liver failure. *Surg Gynecol Obstet* 1971; 133:783–790.

75. Gaskill HV, Sirinek KR, Levine BA: Prostacyclin selectively enhances blood flow in areas of the GI tract prone to stress ulceration. *J Trauma* 1984; 24:397–402.

76. Gelman S, Ernst EA: Role of pH, pCO_2, and O_2 content of portal blood in hepatic circulatory autoregulation. *Am J Physiol* 1977; 233:E256–E262.

77. Goresky CA: The processes of cellular uptake and exchange in the liver. *Fed Proc* 1982; 41:3033–3039.

77a. Gotoh F, Meyer JS, Takagi Y: Cerebral effects of hyperventilation in man. *Arch Neurol* 1965; 12:410–423.

78. Gourley JK, Heistad DD: Characteristics of reactive hyperemia in the cerebral circulation. *Am J Physiol* 1984; 246:H52–H58.

78a. Gow BS: Circulatory correlates: Vascular

impedance, resistance, and capacity, in Bohr DF, Somlyo AP, Sparks HV Jr (eds): *Handbook of Physiology*. Vol 2: *The Cardiovascular System*. Bethesda, American Physiological Society, 1980, pp 353–408.

79. Granata L, Huvos A, Pasque A, et al: Left coronary hemodynamics during hemorrhagic hypotension and shock. *Am J Physiol* 1972; 216:1583–1589.

80. Granger DN, Richardson PDI, Kvietys PR, et al: Intestinal blood flow. *Gastroenterology* 1980; 78:837–863.

81. Granger HN, Norris CP: Intrinsic regulation of intestinal oxygenation in the anesthetized dog. *Am J Physiol* 1980; 238:H836–H843.

82. Greenway CV, Stark RD: Hepatic vascular bed. *Physiol Rev* 1971; 51:23–65.

83. Greenway CV: Role of splanchnic venous system in overall cardiovascular homeostasis. *Fed Proc* 1983; 42:1678–1684.

84. Gregg DE, Thornton JJ, Mautz FR: The magnitude, adequacy and source of the collateral blood flow and pressure in chronically occluded coronary arteries. *Am J Physiol* 1939; 127:161–175.

85. Gregg DE: Physiology of the coronary circulation: The George E. Brown Memorial Lecture. *Circulation* 1963; 28:1128–1137.

86. Gregg DE, Fisher LC: Blood supply to the heart, in Hamilton WF (ed): *Handbook of Physiology: Circulation*. Washington, DC, American Physiological Society, 1963, pp 1517–1584.

87. Gregg DE, Khouri EM, Rayford CR: Systemic and coronary energetics in the resting unanesthetized dog. *Circ Res* 1965; 16:102–113.

88. Griggs DM Jr, Chen CC: Coronary hemodynamics and regional myocardial metabolism in experimental aortic insufficiency. *J Clin Invest* 1974; 553:1599.

89. Grubb RL, Raichle ME, Eichling JO, et al: The effects of changes in $PaCO_2$ on cerebral blood volume, blood flow, and vascular mean transit time. *Stroke* 1974; 5:630–639.

90. Grubb RL, Raichle ME, Phelps ME, et al: Effects of increased intracranial pressure on cerebral blood volume, blood flow, and oxygen utilization in monkeys. *J Neurosurg* 1975; 43:385–398.

91. Grum CM, Fiddian-Green RG, Pittenger GL, et al: Adequacy of tissue oxygenation in intact dog intestine. *J Appl Physiol* 1984; 56:R1065–R1069.

92. Grun M, Brolsch CE, Wolter J: Influence of portal hepatic blood flow on RES function, in Liehr H, Grun M (eds): *Reticuloendothelial System and the Pathogenesis of Liver Disease*. New York, Elsevier/North Holland Biomedical Press, 1980, pp 149–158.

93. Harper AM, Deshmukh VD, Rowan JO, et al: The influence of sympathetic nervous activity on cerebral blood flow. *Arch Neurol* 1972; 27:1–6.

94. Hart MN, Heistad DD, Brody MJ: Effect of chronic hypertension and sympathetic denervation on wall/lumen ratio of cerebral arteries. *Hypertension* 1980; 2:419–423.

95. Hedley-Whyte J: Effect of pattern of ventilation on hepatic, renal, and splanchnic function, in Hedley-White J (ed): *Applied Physiology of Respiratory Care*. Boston, Little, Brown & Co, 1976, pp 27–30.

96. Heinemann U, Lux HD, Gutnick MJ: Extracellular free calcium and potassium during paroxysmal activity in the cerebral cortex of the cat. *Exp Brain Res* 1977; 27:237

97. Heiss WD: Flow thresholds of functional and morphological damage of brain tissue. *Stroke* 1983; 14:329.

98. Heistad DD, Marcus ML, Gross PM: Effects of sympathetic nerves on cerebral vessels in dog, cat, and monkey. *Am J Physiol* 1978; 235:H544–H552.

99. Heistad DD, Marcus ML: Effect of sympathetic stimulation on permeability of the blood-brain barrier to albumin during acute hypertension in cats. *Circ Res* 1979; 45:331–338.

100. Heistad DD, Marcus ML, Busija D, et al: Protective effects of sympathetic nerves in the cerebral circulation, in Heistad DD, Marcus ML (eds): *Cerebral Blood Flow: Effects of Nerves and Neurotransmitters*. New York, Elsevier-North Holland, Inc, 1982.

101. Heistad DD, Kontos HA: Cerebral circulation, in Shepherd JT, Abboud FM, Geiger SR (eds): *Handbook of Physiology*. Vol 3: *The Cardiovascular System*. Bethesda, Md, American Physiological Society, 1983, section 2, part 1, pp 137–182.

102. Henriksen L, Thorshauge C, Harmsen A, et al: Controlled hypotension with sodium nitroprusside: Effects on cerebral blood flow and cerebral venous blood gases in patients operated for cerebral aneurysms. *Acta Anaesthesiol Scand* 1983; 27:62–67.

103. Herzberg RM, Rubio R, Berne RM: Coro-

nary occlusion and embolization: Effect on blood flow in adjacent arteries. *Am J Physiol* 1979; 210:169–175.

104. Heuser JAD, Lassen NA, Nilsson B, et al: Evidence against H^+ and K^+ as the main factors in the regulation of cerebral blood flow during epileptic discharges, acute hypoxemia, amphetamine intoxication, and hypoglycemia: A microelectrode study, in Betz E (ed): *Ionic Actions on Vascular Smooth Muscle*. Berlin, Springer-Verlag, 1976, pp 110–116.

105. Hinshaw LB, Day SB, Carlson CH: Tissue pressure as a casual factor in the autoregulation of blood flow in the isolated perfused kidney. *Am J Physiol* 1959; 197:309.

106. Hollenberg N, Epstein M, Rosen R, et al: Evidence for preferential renal cortical ischemia. *Medicine* 1968; 47:435.

107. Holm-Rutili L, Perry MA, Granger DN: Autoregulation of gastric blood flow and oxygen uptake. *Am J Physiol* 1981; 241: G143–G149.

108. Hughes RL, Mathie RT, Fitch W, et al: Liver blood flow and oxygen consumption during hypocapnia and IPPV in the greyhound. *J Appl Physiol* 1979; 47:R290–R295.

109. Humes HD, Ichikawa J, Troy JL, et al: Evidence for a parathyroid hormone-dependent influence of calcium on the glomerular ultrafiltration coefficient. *J Clin Invest* 1978; 61:32.

110. Ichikawa J, Hollenberg N: Pharmacologic interruption of the renin-angiotensive system in myohemoglobinuric acute renal failure. *Kidney Int* 1976; 10:5183.

111. Ingvar DH: Functional landscapes of the dominant hemisphere. *Brain Res* 1976; 107:181.

112. Ingvar DH, Sjölund B, Ardö A: Correlation between dominant EEG frequency, cerebral oxygen uptake and blood flow. *Electroencephalogr. Clin Neurophysiol* 1976; 41:268–276.

113. Jacob AI, Goldberg PK, Bloom N, et al: Endotoxin and bacteria in portal blood. *Gastroenterology* 1977; 72:1268–1270.

114. Jamison RL, Lacey FB: Effect of saline infusion on superficial and juxtamedullary nephrons in the rat. *Am J Physiol* 1971; 221:69.

115. Johansson B, Linder E, Seeman T: Effects of heart rate and arterial blood pressures on coronary collateral blood flow in dogs. *Acta Physiol Scand Suppl* 1966; 272:33–46.

116. Johnson EE, Hedley-Whyte J: Continuous positive-pressure ventilation and portal flow in dogs with pulmonary edema. *J Appl Physiol* 1972; 33:385–389.

117. Johnson EE, Hedley-Whyte J: Continuous positive pressure ventilation and choledochodenal flow resistance. *J Appl Physiol* 1975; 39:937–942.

118. Johnson EE, Hedley-Whyte J, Hall SV: End-expiratory pressure ventilation and sulfobromophthalein sodium excretion in dogs. *J Appl Physiol* 1977; 43:714–720.

119. Johnstin P, Bernard DB, Donohoe JF, et al: Effect of volume expansion on hemodynamics of the hypoperfused rat kidney. *J Clin Invest* 1979; 64:550.

120. Jones MD Jr, Traystman RJ, Simmons MA, et al: Effects of changes in arterial O_2 content on cerebral blood flow in the lamb. *Am J Physiol* 1981; 240:H209–H215.

121. Kaplan JE, Saba TM: Humoral deficiency and reticuloendothelial depression after traumatic shock. *Am J Physiol* 1976; 230:7–14.

122. Keele CA, Neil E (eds): *Samson Wright's Applied Physiology*. London, Oxford University Press, 1971.

123. Khouri EM, Gregg DE, Lowensohn HS: Flow in the major branches of the left coronary artery during experimental coronary insufficiency in the unanesthetized dog. *Circ Res* 1968; 23:99–109.

124. Kilburn KH, Dowell AR: Renal function in respiratory failure: Effects of hypoxia, hyperoxia, and hypercarbia. *Ann Intern Med* 1971; 127:754.

125. Kirk ES, Honig CR: Non-uniform distribution of blood-flow and gradients of oxygen tension within the heart. *Am J Physiol* 1964; 207:661–668.

126. Kjekshus J, Aukland K, Kiil F: Oxygen cost of sodium reabsorption in proximal and distal parts of the nephron. *Scand J Clin Lab Invest* 1971; 23:307.

127. Kjekshus JK: Mechanism for flow distribution in normal and ischemic myocardium during increased ventricular preload in the dog. *Circ Res* 1973; 33:489–499.

128. Knox FG, Willis LR, Strandhoy JW, et al: Hydrostatic pressures in proximal tubules and peritubular capillaries in the dog. *Kidney Int* 1972; 2:11.

129. Koch KA, Jackson DL, Schmiedl M, et al:

Total cerebral ischemia: Effect of alterations in arterial PCO_2 on cerebral microcirculation. *J Cereb Blood Flow Metab* 1984; 4:343–349.

130. Kontos HA, Raper AJ, Patterson JL Jr: Analysis of vasoactivity of local pH, PCO_2, and bicarbonate on pial vessels. *Stroke* 1977; 8:358–360.

131. Kontos HA, Wei EP, Navari RM, et al: Responses of cerebral arteries and arterioles to acute hypotension and hypertension. *Am J Physiol* 1978; 234:H371–H383.

132. Kontos HA, Wei EP, Raper AJ, et al: Role of tissue hypoxia in local regulation of cerebral microcirculation. *Am J Physiol* 1978; 3:H582–H591.

133. Kontos HA, Wei EP, Povlishock JT, et al: Cerebral arteriolar damage by arachidonic acid and prostaglandin G_2. *Science* 1980; 209:1242–1245.

134. Kontos HA, Wei EP, Dietrich WD, et al: Mechanism of cerebral arteriolar abnormalities after acute hypertension. *Am J Physiol* 1981; 240:H511–H527.

135. Kramer K, Deetjen P: Beziehungen des O_2 Verbrauchs der Niere zu Durchblutung und Glomerulusfiltrat bei Änderung des arteriellen Druckes. *Arch Ges Physiol* 1960; 271:782.

136. Kuschinsky W, Wahl M, Bosse O, et al: Perivascular potassium and pH as determinants of local pial arterial diameter in cats. *Circ Res* 1972; 31:240–247.

137. Kuschinsky W, Wahl M: Alpha-receptor stimulation by endogenous and exogenous norepinephrine and blockade by phentolamine in pial arteries of cats. *Circ Res* 1975; 37:168–174.

138. Kvietys P, Miller T, Granger DN: Intrinsic control of colonic blood flow and oxygenation. *Am J Physiol* 1980; 238:G478–G484.

139. Kvietys PR, Granger DN: Relation between intestinal blood flow and oxygen uptake. *Am J Physiol* 1982; 242:G202–G208.

140. Laine GA, Hall JT, Laine SH, et al: Trans-sinusoidal fluid dynamics in canine liver during venous hypertension. *Circ Res* 1979; 45:317–373.

141. Larsen JA, Krarup N, Minck A: Liver hemodynamics and liver function in cats during graded hypoxic hypoxemia. *Acta Physiol Scand* 1976; 98:257–262.

142. Lassen NA: Autoregulation of cerebral blood flow. *Circ Res* 1964; 14(suppl 1): 201–204.

143. Lewis FB, Coffman JD, Gregg DE: Effect of heart rate and intracoronary isoproterenol, levarterenol, and epinephrine on coronary flow and resistance. *Circ Res* 1961; 9:89–95.

144. Lie M, Johannesen J, Kiil F: Glomerular tubular balance and renal metabolic rate. *Am J Physiol* 1973; 225:1181.

145. Loegering DJ: Humoral factor depletion and reticuloendothelial depression during hemorrhagic shock. *Am J Physiol* 1977; 232:H283–H287.

146. Lou HC, Lassen NA, Tweed WA, et al: Pressure passive cerebral blood flow and breakdown of the blood-brain barrier in experimental fetal asphyxia. *Acta Paediatr Scand* 1979; 68:57–63.

147. Lundgren O: Role of splanchnic resistance vessels in overall cardiovascular homeostasis. *Fed Proc* 1983; 42:1673–1677.

148. MacKenzie DT, Farrar JK, Fitch W, et al: Effects of hemorrhagic hypotension on the cerebral circulation: I. Cerebral blood flow and pial arteriolar caliber. *Stroke* 1979; 10:711–718.

149. Maddox DA, Deen WM, Brenner BM: Dynamics of glomerular ultrafiltration: VI. Studies in the primate. *Kidney Int* 1974; 5:271.

150. Mangold R, Sokoloff L, Conner E, et al: The effects of sleep and lack of sleep on the cerebral circulation and metabolism of normal young men. *J Clin Invest* 1955; 34:1092–1099.

151. Manny J, Justice R, Hechtman HB: Abnormalities in organ blood flow and its distribution during positive end-expiratory pressure. *Surgery* 1979; 85:425–432.

152. Marcus ML, Heistad DD: Effects of sympathetic nerves on cerebral blood flow in awake dogs. *Am J Physiol* 1979; 236:H549–H553.

153. Matsen FA III: *Compartmental Syndromes.* New York, Grune & Stratton, 1980.

154. Matuschak GM, Pinsky MR, Rogers RM: Respiratory variations in hepatic blood flow during positive pressure ventilation (abstract). *Fed Proc* 1984; 43:311.

155. Matuschak GM, Rinaldo JE, VanThiel DH, et al: Acute respiratory failure with pre-existing end-stage hepatic insufficiency is irreversible. *Am Rev Respir Dis* 1985; 1311:A135.

155a. Matuschak GM, Pinsky MR, Rogers RM, et al: Effect of positive pressure ventilation on hepatic blood flow and function (abstract). *Am Rev Respir Dis* 1984; 129:A99.

155b. Mellander S, Johansson B: Control of resistance, exchange, and capacitance functions in the peripheral circulation. *Pharmacol Rev* 1968; 20:117.

156. Meyers BD, Carrie BJ, Yee RR, et al: Pathophysiology of hemodynamically mediated acute renal failure in man. *Kidney Int* 1980; 18:495.

157. Mittermayer J, Riede UN: Human pathology of the gastrointestinal tract in shock, ischemia, and hypoxemia, in Cowley RA, Trump BE (eds): *Pathophysiology of Shock, Anoxia, and Ischemia.* Baltimore, Williams & Wilkins Co, 1982, pp 301–308.

158. Moffitt EA, Sethna DH, Busse U, et al: Haemodynamic responses to halothane or morphine anaesthesia for coronary artery surgery. *Anesth Analg* 1982; 61:979–985.

159. Moffitt EA, Sethna DH, Gary RJ, et al: Nitrous oxide added to halothane reduces coronary flow and myocardial oxygen consumption in patients with coronary oxygen consumption in patients with coronary disease. *Can Anaesth Soc J* 1983; 30:5–9.

160. Moffitt EA, Imrie D, Scouil JE, et al: Myocardial metabolism and haemodynamic responses with enflurane anaesthesia for coronary artery surgery. *Can Anaesth Soc J* 1984; 31:604.

161. Moffitt EA, Barker RA, Glenn JJ, et al: Myocardial metabolism and haemodynamic responses with isoflurane anesthesia for coronary artery surgery (abstract). *Anesth Analg* 1984; 63:252.

162. Moffitt EA, Scouil JE, Barker RA, et al: Myocardial metabolism and haemodynamic responses during high-dose fentanyl anaesthesia for coronary patients. *Can Anaesth Soc J* 1984; 31:611–618.

163. Moffitt EA, Scouil JE, Barker RA, et al: The effects of nitrous oxide on myocardial metabolism and hemodynamics during fentanyl or enflurane anesthesia in patients with coronary disease. *Anesth Analg* 1984; 63:1071–1075.

164. Moir TW, Eckstein RW, Discrol TE: Thebesian drainage of the septal artery. *Circ Res* 1963; 12:212–219.

165. Moir TW, DeBra DW: Effect of left ventricular hypertension, ischemia and vasoactive drugs on the myocardial distribution of coronary flow. *Circ Res* 1967; 21:65–74.

166. Montoreano R, Cunarro J, Mouzet MT, et al: Prevention of the initial oliguria of acute renal failure by the administration of furosemide. *Postgrad Med J* 1971; 47(suppl):7.

167. Moreno AH, Burchell AR, van der Woude R, et al: Respiratory regulation of splanchnic and systemic venous return. *Am J Physiol* 1967; 213:455–465.

168. Moreno AH, Burchell AR: Respiratory regulation of splanchnic and systemic venous return in normal subjects and in patients with hepatic cirrhosis. *Surg Gynecol Obstet* 1982; 154:257–267.

169. Morita H, Nemoto EM, Bleyaert AL, et al: Brain blood flow autoregulation and metabolism during halothane anesthesia in monkeys. *Am J Physiol* 1977; 233:H670–H676.

170. Morris CR, Alexander EA, Bruns FJ, et al: Restoration and maintenance of glomerular filtration by mannitol. *J Clin Invest* 1972; 51:1555.

171. Mosher P, Ross J Jr, McFate A: Control of coronary blood flow by an autoregulatory mechanism. *Circ Res* 1964; 14:250.

172. Mubarak SJ, Hargens AR: *Compartment Syndromes and Volkmann's Contracture.* Philadelphia, WB Saunders Co, 1981, vol 3.

173. Mueller SM, Heistad DD, Marcus ML: Total and regional cerebral blood flow during hypotension, hypertension, and hypocapnia: Effect of sympathetic denervation in dogs. *Circ Res* 1977; 41:350–356.

174. Munck O (ed): *Renal Circulation in Acute Renal Failure.* Oxford, England, Blackwell Scientific Publications, 1958, p 1.

175. Muth RG: Furosemide in acute renal failure, in Friedman EA, Eliahu HE (eds): *Proceedings of the Conference on Acute Renal Failure.* HEW (NIH) publication No. 75-608. Washington, DC, 1973, p 245.

176. Myers WW, Honig CR: Number and distribution of capillaries as determinants of myocardial oxygen tension. *Am J Physiol* 1964; 207:653–660.

177. Nakagawa Y, Tsuru M, Yada K: Site and mechanism for compression of the venous system during experimental intracranial hypertension. *J Neurosurg* 1974; 41:427–434.

178. Navar SG, Bruke TJ, Robinson RR, et al:

Distal tubular feedback and autoregulation of nephron filtration. *J Clin Invest* 1974; 53:516.

179. Nelimarkka O: Renal oxygen and lactate metabolism in hemorrhagic shock: An experimental study. *Acta Chir Scand* 51(suppl):1, 1984.

180. Neutz JM, Wyler F, Rudolph AM: Use of radioactive microspheres to assess distribution of cardiac output of microspheres. *Am J Physiol* 1968; 215:486.

181. Nissen OJ: Changes in the filtration fractions in the superficial and deep venous drainage area of the kidney due to fluid loading. *Acta Physiol Scand* 1968; 73:320.

182. Nolan WF, Davies DG: Brain extracellular fluid pH and blood flow during isocapnic and hypocapnic hypoxia. *J Appl Physiol* 1982; 53:R247–R252.

183. Norman JN, Shearer JR, Kapper AJ, et al: Action of oxygen on the renal circulation. *Am J Physiol* 1974; 227:740.

184. Normann SJ: Kinetics of phagocytosis: II. Analysis of in vivo clearance with demonstration of competitive inhibition between similar and dissimilar foreign particles. *Lab Invest* 1974; 31:161–169.

185. Normann SJ: Kinetics of vascular clearance of particles by phagocytes, in Reichard SM, Filkins JP (eds): *The Reticuloendothelial System: A Comprehensive Treatise*. 7A: *Physiology*. New York, Plenum Press, 1984, pp 73–101.

186. Norris CP, Barnes GE, Smith EE, et al: Autoregulation of superior mesenteric flow in fasted and fed dogs. *Am J Physiol* 1979; 237:H174–H177.

187. Nuutinen LS, Tuononen S: The effect of furosemide on renal blood flow and renal tissue oxygen tension in dogs. *Ann Chir Gynaecol* 1976; 65:272.

188. Oliver J, McDowell M, Tracy A: Pathogenesis of acute renal failure associated with traumatic and toxic injury. *J Clin Invest* 1951; 30:1305.

189. Orr JA, DeSoignie RC, Wagerle LC, et al: Regional cerebral blood flow during hypercapnia in the anesthetized rabbit. *Stroke* 1983; 14:802–807.

190. Ottinger LW: Acute mesenteric ischemia. *N Engl J Med* 1982; 307:535–537.

191. Overgaard J, Tweed WA: Cerebral circulation after head injury: Part 1. Cerebral blood flow and its regulation after closed head injury with emphasis on clinical correlations. *J Neurosurg* 1974; 41:531–541.

192. Owman C, Hardebo JE: Functional aspects of the blood brain barrier, with particular regard to effects of circulating vasoactive neurotransmitters, in Heistad DD, Marcus ML (eds): *Cerebral Blood Flow: Effects of Nerves and Neurotransmitters*. New York, Elsevier North-Holland, Inc, 1982.

193. Pannier JL, Leusen I: Cerebral blood flow in cats after an acute hypertensive insult with damage to the blood-brain barrier. *Stroke* 1975; 6:188–198.

194. Pinsky MR, Smith PL, Bleecker ER, et al: Effects of antihistamines and indomethacin on hyperosmolar-induced vasodilation. *Am J Physiol* 1982; 242:H450.

195. Pollay M, Roberts PA: Blood-brain barrier: A definition of normal and altered function. *Neurosurgery* 1980; 6:675–685.

196. Pomeranz BH, Birtch AG, Barger AL: Neural control of intrarenal blood flow. *Am J Physiol* 1968; 215:1067.

197. Portnoy HD, Chopp M, Branch C: Hydraulic model of myogenic autoregulation of the cerebrovascular bed: The effects of altering systemic arterial pressure. *Neurosurgery* 1983; 13:482–498.

198. Praaining van Oslen P, Braumer A, Knouk DL: Clearance capacity of rat liver endothelial and parenchymal cells. *Gastroenterology* 1981; 81:1036–1044.

199. Portnoy HD, Chopp M, Branch C, et al: Cerebrospinal fluid pulse waveform as an indicator of cerebral autoregulation. *J Neurosurg* 1982; 56:666–678.

200. Rappaport AM: Physioanatomic considerations, in Schiff L, Schiff ER (eds): *Disease of the Liver,* ed 5. Philadelphia, JB Lippincott Co, 1982, pp 1–57.

201. Ravin HA, Rowley D, Jenkins C, et al: On the absorption of bacterial endotoxin from the gastrointestinal tract of the normal and shocked animal. *J Exp Med* 1960; 112:783–792.

202. Rector JB, Steven OH, Bay WH, et al: Effect of hemorrhagic and vasopressor agents on distribution of renal blood flow. *Am J Physiol* 1972; 222:1125.

203. Reivich M: Arterial PCO$_2$ and cerebral hemodynamics. *Am J Physiol* 1964; 206:25–35.

204. Reiz S, Balfors E, Sorensen MB, et al: Iso-flurane: A powerful coronary vasodilator in patients with coronary artery disease. *Anesthesiology* 1983; 59:91–97.

205. Reubi FL, Vorburger C: Renal hemody-namics in acute renal failure after shock in man. *Kidney Int* 1976; 10:5137.

206. Richardson PDI, Withrington PG: Liver blood flow: I. Intrinsic and nervous control of liver blood flow. *Gastroenterology* 1981; 81:159–173.

207. Riley RL: Biophysics of gas and blood flow, in Loeppky JA, Riedesel ML (eds): *Oxygen Transport to Human Tissues*. New York, Elsevier North-Holland, Inc, 1982.

208. Rogers DE: Host mechanisms which act to remove bacteria from the blood stream. *Bacteriol Rev* 1960; 24:50–66.

209. Rowe GG, Castillo CA, Maxwell GM, et al: A hemodynamic study of hypertension in-cluding observations on coronary blood flow. *Ann Intern Med* 1961; 54:405–412.

210. Rowe GG, Maxwell GM, Crumpton CW: The cerebral hemodynamic response to ad-ministration of hydralazine. *Circulation* 1962; 25:970–972.

211. Rowell LB, Johnson JM: Role of the splanchnic circulation in reflex control of the cardiovascular system, in Shepherd AP, Granger DN (eds): *Physiology of the Intes-tinal Circulation*. New York, Raven Press, 1984, pp 153–163.

212. Rowell LB, Blackmon JR, Kenny MA, et al: Splanchnic vasomotor and metabolic ad-justments to hypoxia and exercise in hu-mans. *Am J Physiol* 1984; 247:H251–H258.

213. Rubio R, Berne RM: Regulation of coronary blood flow. *Prog Cardiovasc Dis* 1975; 18:105.

214. Saba TM: Physiology and physiopathology of the reticuloendothelial system. *Arch In-tern Med* 1970; 126:1031–1052.

215. Saba TM, Jaffe E: Plasma fibronectin (op-sonic glycoprotein): Its synthesis by vascular endothelial cells and role in cardiopulmo-nary integrity after trauma as related to reti-culoendothelial function. *Am J Med* 1980; 68:577–593.

216. Saba TM, Niehaus GD, Dillon BC: Reticu-loendothelial response to shock and trauma: Its relationship to disturbances in fibronectin and cardiopulmonary function, in Alterua BM, Saba TM (eds): *Pathophysiology of the Reticuloendothelial System*. New York, Raven Press, 1981, pp 131–157.

217. Saba TM: Plasma fibronectin and hepatic Kupffer cell function, in Popper H, Schaff-ner F (eds): *Prog Liver Dis* 1982; 7:109–131.

218. Sadoshima S, Busija D, Brody M, et al: Sympathetic nerves protect against stroke in stroke-prone hypertensive rats. *Hypertension* 1981; 3(suppl 1):I124–1127.

219. Schaper W: *The Collateral Circulation of the Heart*. Amsterdam, North Holland, 1971.

220. Scheel KW, Banet M, Ott C, et al: A quan-titative approach to collateral and antegrade flows after coronary occlusion. *Am J Physiol* 1972; 222:687–694.

221. Schlesinger MJ: Relation of anatomic pat-tern to pathologic conditions of the coronary arteries. *Arch Pathol* 1940; 30:403–415.

222. Schnermann J, Persson AEG, Agerup B: Tubuloglomerular feedback. *J Clin Invest* 1973; 57:862.

223. Schumacker PR, Saba TM: Pulmonary gas exchange abnormalities following intravas-cular coagulation: Reticuloendothelial in-volvement. *Ann Surg* 1980; 192:95–102.

224. Scott JC: Myocardial coefficient of oxygen utilization. *Circ Res* 1961; 9:906.

225. Segal J, Harvey WP, Hugnagel C: A clini-cal study of one hundred cases of severe aortic insufficiency. *Am J Med* 1956; 21:200.

226. Seki HT, Yoshimoto T, Ogawa A, et al: The CO_2 response in focal cerebral isch-emia-sequential changes following recircula-tion. *Stroke* 1984; 15:699–704.

227. Selkurt EE: Intestinal ischemic shock and the protective role of the liver. *Am J Physiol* 1959; 197:281–285.

227a. Shapiro HM: Anesthesia effects upon cere-bral blood flow, cerebral metabolism, and the electroencephalogram, in Miller RD (ed): *Anesthesia*, vol 2. New York, Church-ill Livingstone, 1981, p. 808.

228. Shapiro K, Marmarou A, Shulman K: Char-acterization of clinical CSF dynamics and neural axis compliance using the pressure-volume index: 1. The normal pressure-volume index. *Ann Neurol* 1980; 7:508–514.

229. Shapiro W, Wasserman AJ, Patterson JL Jr: Human cerebrovascular response to com-

bined hypoxia and hypercapnia. *Circ Res* 1966; 19:903–910.

230. Shepherd AP: Intestinal O_2 consumption and ^{86}Rb extraction during arterial hypoxia. *Am J Physiol* 1978; 3:E248–E251.

231. Shepherd AP: Intestinal blood flow autoregulation during foodstuff absorption. *Am J Physiol* 1980; 239:H156–H162.

232. Shepherd JT, Vanhoutte PM (eds): *The Human Cardiovascular System*. New York, Raven Press, 1979.

233. Shepherd JT: Circulation to skeletal muscle, in Shepherd JT, Abboud FM, Geiger SR (eds): *Handbook of Physiology*. Vol 3: *The Cardiovascular System*. Bethesda, Md, American Physiological Society, 1983, pp 319–370.

234. Siesjö BK: Cerebral circulation and metabolism. *J Neurosurg* 1984; 60:883–903.

235. Sokoloff L, Mangold R, Wechsler RL, et al: The effect of mental arithmetic on cerebral circulation and metabolism. *J Clin Invest* 1955; 34:1101–1108.

236. Sokoloff L: Relation between physiological function and energy metabolism in the central nervous system. *J Neurochem* 1977; 29:13–26.

237. Sonntag H, Larsen R, Hilfiker O: Myocardial blood flow and oxygen consumption during high-dose fentanyl anaesthesia for coronary patients. *Can Anaesth Soc J* 1984; 31:611–618.

238. Stein JH, Boohjaren S, Mark RC: Mechanism of the redistribution of renal cortical blood flow during hemorrhagic hypotension in the dog. *J Clin Invest* 1973; 52:39.

239. Stone JE, Wells J, Draper WB, et al: Changes in renal blood flow in dogs during inhalation of 30% CO_2. *Am J Physiol* 1958; 194:115.

240. Tashkin DP, Goldstein PJ, Simmons DH: Hepatic lactate uptake during decreased liver perfusion and hypoxemia. *Am J Physiol* 1972; 223:968–974.

241. Teschan PE, Lawson NL: Prevention by osmotic diuresis, and observations on the effect of plasma and extracellular volume expansion. *Nephron* 1966; 3:1.

242. Thaysen JH, Lassen WA, Munck O: Sodium transport and oxygen consumption in the mammalian kidney. *Nature* 1961; 190:919.

243. Thiel GF, Brenner F, Wunderlich M, et al:

Protection of rat kidneys against $HgLI_2$ induced acute renal failure by induction of high urine flow without serious suppression. *Kidney Int* 1976; 10:S191.

244. Tisher CC: Relationship between renal structure and concentrating ability in the Rhesus monkey. *Am J Physiol* 1971; 220:1100.

245. Todd MM, Shapiro HM, Obrist WD: Cerebral blood flow measurements in the critically ill patient, in Grenvik A, Safar P (eds): *Brain Failure and Resuscitation*. New York, Churchill Livingstone, 1981, pp 125–154.

246. Todd MM, Shapiro HM, Obrist WD: Cerebral blood flow measurements in the critically ill patient, in Grenvik A, Safar P (eds): *Brain Failure and Resuscitation*. New York, Churchill Livingstone, 1981, p 125.

247. Torres VW, Strong CG, Romero JC, et al: Indomethacin enhancement of glycerol-induced acute renal failure in rabbits. *Kidney Int* 1975; 7:170.

248. Tucker HJ, Murray JF: Effects of end-expiratory pressure on organ blood flow in normal and diseased dogs. *J Appl Physiol* 1973; 34:573–577.

249. Tuor UI, Farrar JK: Pial vessel caliber and cerebral blood flow during hemorrhage and hypercapnia in the rabbit. *Am J Physiol* 1984; 247:H40–H51.

250. Urbanics R, Leniger-Follert E, Lübbers DW: Time course of changes of extracellular H^+ and K^+ activities during and after direct electrical stimulation of the brain cortex. *Pflugers Arch* 1978; 378:47–53.

251. Vasko JS, Gutelius J, Sabiston DC: A study of predominance of human coronary arteries determined by arteriographic and perfusion techniques. *Am J Cardiol* 1961; 8:379–384.

252. Vatner SF, Higgins CB, Franklin D, et al: Role of tachycardia in mediating the coronary hemodynamic response to severe exercise. *J Appl Physiol* 1972; 32:380–385.

253. Wagner EM, Traystman RJ: Cerebral venous outflow and arterial microsphere flow with elevated venous pressure. *Am J Physiol* 1983; 244:H505–H512.

254. Wahl M, Kuschinsky W: The dilatory action of adenosine in pial arteries of cats and its inhibition by theophylline. *Pflugers Arch* 1976; 362:55–59.

255. Wahl M, Kuschinsky W: Unimportance of

perivascular H^+ and K^+ activities for the adjustment of pial arterial diameter during changes of arterial blood pressure in cats. *Pflugers Arch* 1979; 382:203–208.

256. Walker BR: Diuretic response to acute hypoxia in the conscious dog. *Am J Physiol* 1982; 243:F440.

257. Wei EP, Raper AJ, Kontos HA, et al: Determinants of response of pial arteries to norepinephrine and sympathetic nerve stimulation. *Stroke* 1975; 6:654–658.

258. Wei E, Ellis EF, Kontos HA: Role of prostaglandins in pial arteriolar response to CO_2 and hypoxia. *Am J Physiol* 1980; 238:H226–H230.

259. Wei EP, Kontos HA, Patterson JL Jr: Dependence of pial arteriolar response to hypercapnia on vessel size. *Am J Physiol* 1980; 238:H697–H703.

260. Wei EP, Kontos HA, Dietrich WD, et al: Inhibition by free radical scavengers and by cyclooxygenase inhibitors of pial arteriolar abnormalities from concussive brain injury in cats. *Circ Res* 1981; 48:95–103.

261. Wei EP, Kontos HA: Responses of cerebral arterioles to increased venous pressure. *Am J Physiol* 1982; 243:H442–H447.

262. West JW, Mercker H, Wendel H, et al: Effects of renal hypertension on coronary blood flow, cardiac oxygen consumption and related circulatory dynamics of the dog. *Circ Res* 1959; 7:476–485.

263. Wilkinson GR, Shand DG: A physiologic approach to hepatic drug clearance. *Clin Pharmacol Ther* 1975; 18:377–390.

264. Winn HR, Welsh JE, Rubio R, et al: Brain adenosine production in rat during sustained alteration in systemic blood pressure. *Am J Physiol* 1980; 239:H636–H641.

265. Winn HR, Welsh JE, Rubio R, et al: Changes in brain adenosine during bicuculline-induced seizures in rats. *Circ Res* 1980; 47:568–577.

266. Winn HR, Rubio R, Berne RM: Brain adenosine concentration during hypoxia in rat. *Am J Physiol* 1981; 241:H235–H242.

267. Winn HR, Rubio GR, Berne RM: The role of adenosine in the regulation of cerebral blood flow (editorial). *J Cereb Blood Flow Metab* 1981; 1:239–244.

268. Wollman H, Smith TC, Stephen GW, et al: Effects of extremes of respiratory and metabolic alkalosis on cerebral blood flow in man. *J Appl Physiol* 1968; 24:60–65.

269. Wolter J, Liehr M, Gran M: Hepatic clearance of endotoxins: Differences in arterial and portal venous infusion. *J Reticuloendothel Soc* 1978; 23:145–152.

270. Yarger WE, Boyd MA, Schroder NW: Evaluation of methods of measuring glomerular and nutrient blood flow in rat kidneys. *Am J Physiol* 1978; 235:H592.

271. Zenser TV, Levitt MJ, Davis BB: Possible modulation of rat renal prostaglandin production by oxygen. *Am J Physiol* 1977; 233:F539.

8 _____ Prostaglandins and Related Lipids

Jon Gerrard, M.D.

Prostaglandins, thromboxanes, leukotrienes, and related lipids are important intracellular and intercellular messengers. They currently have an aura of mystique, perhaps because of their newness and the complexity of their structure and function. The goal of this chapter is not to define the role of specific compounds in specific human disorders, but rather to provide a perspective on our current understanding to help the reader interpret the rapidly accumulating information on these agents.

WHERE DO THESE CHEMICALS COME FROM?

Critical to an understanding of prostaglandins and related chemicals is an understanding of their origin. *These compounds result from the breakdown of phospholipids in cellular membranes, either in response to a specific stimulus or as a side effect of membrane breakdown.* Figure 8–1 shows how a lipase can act to break down a phospholipid within a membrane to release arachidonic acid, which can then subsequently be converted to prostaglandin E_2 (PGE$_2$). Production of prostaglandins and related chemicals results largely from the effect of specific agonists that act on cellular receptors to activate phospholipases to release arachidonic acid. Examples of specific agonists acting to cause release of arachidonic acid that is then converted to prostaglandins and/or related lipids include thrombin and collagen in platelets, activated complement in neutrophils, immune complexes in monocytes, IgE-antigen complexes in mast cells, bradykinin in endothelial cells and fibroblasts, angiotensin II in the kidney, and oxytocin in the uterus.

However, it is clear from many studies that nonspecific breakdown of membranes is also associated with arachidonic acid release and for-

mation of prostaglandins and related chemicals.[58] The latter circumstance appears particularly important for situations of cell injury, as may occur during mechanical trauma or during tissue ischemia. *This means that prostaglandins and related messengers are important both as cellular responses to hormones and as side effects of nonspecific cell injury.* Elsewhere I have suggested that cellular responses to specific agonists that result in prostaglandin production may have evolved from a condition in more primitive cells where the cell needed to identify and respond to membrane injury or damaging stimuli.[27] Whether or not this occurred, an important first step in understanding these chemicals is to appreciate that they are produced as a result of the breakdown of the membrane bilayer.

THE CHEMICALS OF INTEREST AND THEIR STRUCTURE

We shall deal first in general terms with lipids produced by the breakdown of membrane phospholipids. A full catalogue of all the potential prostaglandins and related compounds is beyond the scope of this review, and the reader is referred elsewhere.[26, 45] In general, there are two groups of lipid mediators, those derived from arachidonic acid or a related fatty acid, and those that are not (Fig 8–2). Compounds that are not derived from arachidonic acid but that may be important intracellular or intercellular messengers include inositol trisphosphate, diglyceride, certain lysophospholipids, and platelet-activating factor. These chemicals are important in that they may help to explain processes in which phospholipids are involved but inhibitors of arachidonic acid metabolism are not effective. Note also that in certain circumstances, platelet-activating factor stimulates thromboxane synthesis in the respond-

FIG 8–1.

Arachidonic acid, the precursor of prostaglandins and other substances, as shown in Figure 8–2, is released from phospholipids present in the cellular bilayer membrane. Arachidonic acid may be released either by specific agonist-stimulated pathways, or as a result of nonspecific membrane damage. In the case of specific agonists, the agonist interacts with a specific receptor *(R)* which is coupled directly or indirectly to the action of a lipase *(L)*. The lipases produce both arachidonic acid and other chemicals shown in Figure 8–2. The initial conversion of arachidonic acid to prostaglandins is to the prostaglandin/ endoperoxide PGH_2 and then to other prostaglandins, such as PGE_2, as shown here.

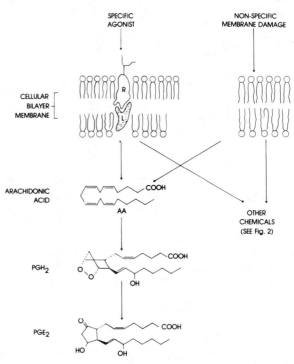

ing cell and can be inhibited by cyclo-oxygenase or thromboxane synthetase inhibitors. However, phospholipase inhibitors such as steroids and experimental compounds (Table 8–1) may inhibit the production of these chemicals as well as the production of chemicals derived from arachidonic acid.

A considerable array of products, including various prostaglandins, thromboxanes, leuko-

trienes, and hydroxy fatty acids, are derived from arachidonic acid by the action of specific intracellular enzymes. Arachidonic acid is pivotal because it is a major polyunsaturated fatty acid in most cells. Its four double bonds on a 20-carbon fatty acid chain allow many variations on a basic theme in which oxygen is added at the site of one of the double bonds, followed by further derivation of the initial oxygen, which becomes an

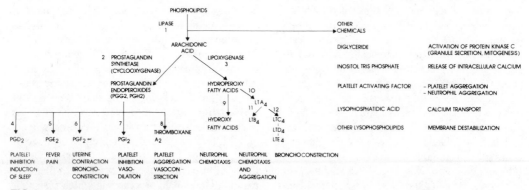

FIG 8–2.

The various products of arachidonic acid and other chemicals that can be produced as a result of the initial lipase action. Enzymes shown in this diagram are numbered, and reference is made to these in the text and in Table 8–1. *PG*, prostaglandin; *LT*, leukotriene. Examples of the actions of these compounds are given beside individual compounds. These are not meant to represent exclusive lists.

TABLE 8–1.

Enzyme Inhibitors and Receptor Antagonists*

ENZYME NO. SHOWN IN FIG 8–2	NAME OF ENZYME	INHIBITORS OF ENZYME
	Enzyme Inhibitors	
1	Lipases:	Steroids (e.g., dexamethasone)
	Phospholipase A_2	Quinacrine
		Calmodulin antagonists (e.g., trifluoperazine)
		U10029A
		Indomethacin (very high concentrations)
		Bromophenacyl bromide
	Phospholipase C	Spermine
	Diglyceride lipase	Octyl-glyceryl ether
		RHC 80267
		Indomethacin (very high concentrations)
2	Prostaglandin endoperoxide synthetase or fatty acid cyclo-oxygenase	Acetylsalicylate (aspirin)
		Indomethacin
		Phenylbutazone
		Ibuprofen
		Meclofenamic acid
		Naproxen
		Benoxaprofen
		Acetaminophen (for cells with low peroxide tone)
3	Lipoxygenases: 5-lipoxygenase, 12-lipoxygenase, and 15-lipoxygenase	Retinoids
		Phenidone
		Nordihydroguiaretic acid
		Sulfasalazine (specific for 5-lipoxygenase)
		Esculetin
		BW755C
		Benoxaprofen
4	PGD_2 synthetase	
5	PGE_2 isomerase	
6	PGF-reductase	
7	Prostacyclin synthetase	Alkyl hydroperoxides
		Tranylcypromine
8	Thromboxane synthetase	Imidazole
		OKY-1581
		UK-38,485
		Sulfasalazine
		9,11-azo-13-oxa-15-hydroxy-prostanoic acid
9	Leukotriene A synthetase	Diethylcarbamazine
10	Hydrolase	
11	Glutathione-s-transferase	
	Receptor Antagonists	
1	Thromboxane A_2	13-azaprostanoic acid
		9,11-azo-13-oxa-hydroxy-prostanoic acid
2	LTD_4	FPL 55712

*Consult references 8, 21 and 26 for more details.

epoxide, a hydroxy, a ketone, or even an oxygen-glutathione conjugate. The variety of possible mediators allows specific messages to go inside a cell or from cell to cell. Linoleic acid, the other major polyunsaturated fatty acid in most cells, has only two double bonds and is much more limited in its oxidation products; thus it has not developed as nearly so important a messenger. In certain cells and in organisms on specific diets, polyunsaturated fatty acids such as eicosapentaenoic acid (with 20 carbons and 5 double bonds), and dihomogammalinolenic acid (with 20 carbons and 3 double bonds), may to some extent replace the arachidonic acid. For most cells, dihomogammalinolenic acid is not of much significance, partly because of its rapid conversion to arachidonic acid. However, it is an important constituent of evening primrose oil, which is used in the treatment of eczema and certain inflammatory disorders. The effectiveness of this oil has been suggested to result from the formation of 1-series prostaglandins such as PGE_1 rather than the 2-series prostaglandins and thromboxanes, derived from arachidonic acid.

Eskimos in Greenland and other individuals with a diet that is rich in eicosapentaenoic acid, found in fish or fish-eating mammals, form TXA_3 instead of TXA_2 and PGI_3 instead of PGI_2.[19] The net effect clinically is a relatively larger vasodilator response and inhibition of platelet activity. A mild bleeding tendency and a lower incidence of atherosclerosis in Greenland Eskimos appear to result from these changes.

A considerable variety of metabolites of arachidonic acid are produced by cells. Figure 8–2 shows the pathways involved, Figure 8–3 gives details of some of the particular structures, and Table 8–1 lists major inhibitors.

The conversion of arachidonic acid to prostaglandins proceeds initially through the formation of two endoperoxides, PGG_2 and PGH_2. These endoperoxides are subsequently converted by various enzymes to the prostaglandin or thromboxane products. PGI_2, also called prostacyclin, has a bicyclic structure. It is unstable in acidic solutions but relatively stable in basic solutions. TXA_2 is a highly unstable derivative.

Hydroxy fatty acids formed through the lipoxygenase pathway have hydroxyl groups added on to the basic arachidonic acid structure. Other products of the lipoxygenase pathway include the leukotrienes, so named because they were first

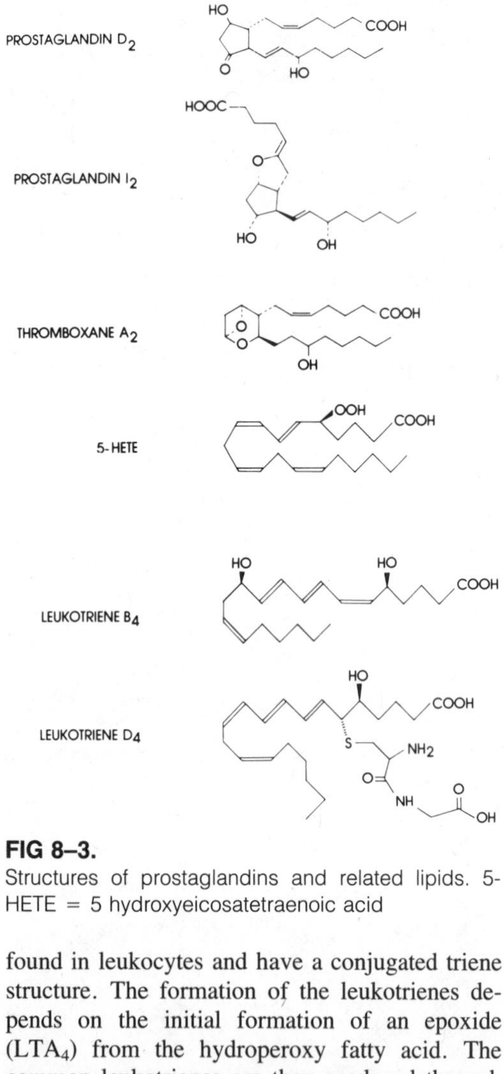

FIG 8–3.
Structures of prostaglandins and related lipids. 5-HETE = 5 hydroxyeicosatetraenoic acid

found in leukocytes and have a conjugated triene structure. The formation of the leukotrienes depends on the initial formation of an epoxide (LTA_4) from the hydroperoxy fatty acid. The common leukotrienes are then produced through the 5-lipoxygenase pathway (see Fig 8–2). Leukotrienes may also be produced through the 15-lipoxygenase pathway, but the functional importance of such leukotrienes is uncertain at present. LTB_4 contains two hydroxy groups. It is a highly potent chemotactic substance for neutrophils and facilitates the invasion of these cells during inflammation. Leukotrienes C_4, D_4, and E_4 are formed from LTA_4: the addition of glutathione forms LTC_4, the subsequent loss of one amino acid forms LTD_4, and the loss of two amino acids forms LTE_4. A few specific blocking agents are available (see Table 8–1), but many more are under development and should become widely available in the near future.

THE REACTIONS INVOLVED IN PRODUCTION OF THESE ACTIVE CHEMICALS

Phospholipases

Arachidonic acid can be released from cells either by a phospholipase A_2 or a phospholipase C coupled to a diglyceride lipase (*1* in Fig 8–2; see also Table 8–1).[6, 61] The involvement of a phospholipase A_2 specific for phosphatidic acid is possible under some circumstances.[5] Steroids such as prednisone, at pharmacologic levels, stimulate synthesis of a protein that inhibits all these lipases (see Fig 8–2). This protein, or proteins, has been termed lipomodulin and macrocortin.[8] Other enzymes, including triglyceride lipases, could be important in certain cells. Other products, notably inositol triphosphate, diglyceride, and lysophospholipids, may be produced by these same lipases (see Fig 8–2).

Enzymes Involved in the Oxidation of Arachidonic Acid

There are two major pathways for the metabolism of arachidonic acid. The first is through an enzyme called prostaglandin endoperoxide synthetase or fatty acid cyclo-oxygenase (*2* in Fig 8–2), which initially produces prostaglandin endoperoxides. The endoperoxides are then converted to other prostaglandins, including PGE_2, PGD_2, and $PGF_{2\alpha}$; to TXA_2; or to prostacyclin (PGI_2). The cyclo-oxygenase enzyme can be inhibited by many known nonsteroidal anti-inflammatory drugs, including aspirin (which acetylates a serine residue at the active site of the enzyme to irreversibly inactivate it), and indomethacin, phenylbutazone, ibuprofen, and mefenamic acid, which cause reversible inactivation.[64] The enzyme is activated by peroxides, including the product endoperoxides. Acetaminophen appears to inhibit prostaglandin synthesis in some cells with low resting levels of peroxides by decreasing the peroxide content of the cell.[44] A number of drugs that are specific thromboxane synthetase inhibitors (*8* in Fig 8–2), including imidazole, OKY-1581, and UK-38,485, are currently being tested. Certain drugs, including tranylcypromine and certain alkylhydroperoxides, will inhibit prostacyclin synthetase (*7* in Fig 8–2).

The second major pathway for arachidonic acid metabolism is through a lipoxygenase enzyme (*3* in Fig 8–2). This is the initial step in the production of hydroxy fatty acids and leukotrienes. As with cyclo-oxygenase, there is an initial peroxide activation.[70] A variety of lipoxygenase inhibitors have been described (see Table 8–1); however, many of these compounds have other actions in addition to inhibiting lipoxygenase enzymes, such as nonspecifically inhibiting neutrophil chemotaxis or granule secretion.[7, 23, 41, 66, 71]

THE CELLULAR BASIS FOR PROSTAGLANDIN ACTION

It is useful to consider the actions of prostaglandins and related substances as either stimulatory (for example, TXA_2 and LTB_4 stimulate platelet and neutrophil aggregation, respectively) or inhibitory (PGI_2 inhibits platelet and neutrophil function; PGE_2 inhibits lymphocyte function). This concept also applies to vascular smooth muscle cells, where TXA_2 and $PGF_{2\alpha}$ generally promote vasoconstriction, while PGI_2 and PGE_2 generally promote vasodilation. Since, for a given cell type, certain arachidonic acid derivatives are stimulatory whereas others are inhibitory, the balance of production of these metabolites is rather important, and agents that modify this balance can have considerable effect. While this generalization is useful, in some cells certain prostaglandins (e.g., PGE_2 in monocytes/macrophages) can be either stimulatory or inhibitory, depending on the circumstance.[26] The mechanism of stimulatory and inhibitory effects will be considered separately.

Stimulatory Effects: Calcium and Protein Kinase C

In platelets and other blood cells, prostaglandins and thromboxanes appear to generate intracellular messages, activated through two separate pathways. The situation has been most clearly demonstrated in platelets, where effects of prostaglandin endoperoxides and TXA_2 cause both calcium flux and activation of protein kinase C.[28, 65] The raised cytosol calcium, as a major effect, interacts with calmodulin to activate a protein kinase that phosphorylates myosin light chain.[16] This triggers actin-myosin contraction and produces a centralized movement of the granules, one component of the secretory and shape change response in platelets.[26, 30] TXA_2 also causes phosphorylation of an intracellular platelet protein

(47P) which results from activation of another protein kinase, protein kinase C.[26] It has recently become clear that activation of protein kinase C can occur independently of calcium flux.[42] This suggests that TXA_2 may deliver a second message to the platelet cytosol to activate this protein kinase. Activation of protein kinase C is associated, in platelets, with labilization and fusion of granules, a second component important for granule secretion.[31, 42] Evidence from other cells suggests it may be critical to granule secretion and/or cell division in many different cell types.

TXA_2, through these two effects (Fig 8–4), can promote granule secretion and also directly promote platelet aggregation.[26] It is likely that many of the other activating prostaglandins, thromboxanes, and leukotrienes work either by promoting calcium flux or by activating protein kinase C.

Inhibitory Effects and Cyclic AMP

PGI_2, PGE_1, and PGD_2 can inhibit platelet aggregation through a receptor-coupled mechanism to stimulate adenylate cyclase, resulting in the production of cyclic AMP (Fig 8–5).[38] Cyclic AMP inhibits platelet function by stimulating cyclic AMP-dependent protein kinases. One effect of this cyclic AMP action in platelets is to facilitate the removal of calcium from the cytoplasm, but there appear to be other inhibitory effects as well. In some cells cyclic AMP synthesis is stimulatory (e.g., epinephrine stimulates liver cells by producing an increase in cyclic AMP, which acti-

vates glycogen phosphorylase to stimulate glycogen breakdown, and thyroid-stimulating hormone stimulates thyroid cells in part by increasing cellular cyclic AMP).

PROSTAGLANDINS IN PHYSIOLOGIC PROCESSES

As a preliminary to evaluating the effects of prostaglandins and related chemicals in specific disease states, it is helpful to discuss individually a number of pathophysiologic processes in which these agents are involved.

Fever

Although prostaglandins are produced at the site of most infections, it is usually not these prostaglandins that are important in producing fever. Rather, since prostaglandins usually act only locally because of their rapid destruction, it appears that pyrogens produced in association with the bacterial infection reach the hypothalamus and stimulate hypothalamic prostaglandin production.[77] Acetaminophen and aspirin appear to control fever through their ability to inhibit prostaglandin synthesis in the hypothalamus.

Pain

Pain frequently develops at the site of a bacterial infection. This appears to result partly from the production of prostaglandins and related chemicals since many prostaglandin synthetase inhibi-

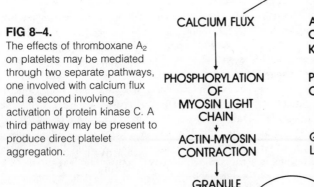
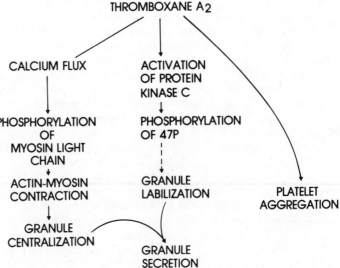

FIG 8–4.
The effects of thromboxane A_2 on platelets may be mediated through two separate pathways, one involved with calcium flux and a second involving activation of protein kinase C. A third pathway may be present to produce direct platelet aggregation.

THROMBOXANE A_2

CALCIUM FLUX

ACTIVATION OF PROTEIN KINASE C

PHOSPHORYLATION OF MYOSIN LIGHT CHAIN

ACTIN-MYOSIN CONTRACTION

GRANULE CENTRALIZATION

PHOSPHORYLATION OF 47P

GRANULE LABILIZATION

GRANULE SECRETION

PLATELET AGGREGATION

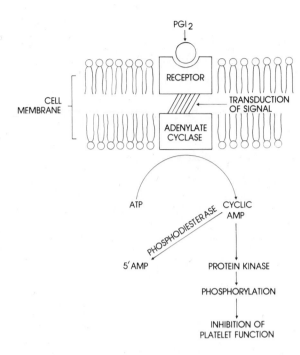

FIG 8–5.
PGI_2 and other inhibitory prostaglandins frequently produce their effects by acting on receptors coupled to adenylate cyclase, which produces cyclic AMP from ATP.

tors, such as aspirin, are effective in reducing pain. For the most part, prostaglandins alone do not produce pain, although prostaglandins will strongly potentiate the pain response to histamine and bradykinin. This suggests that inhibitors of prostaglandin synthesis are analgesic because they inhibit prostaglandin sensitization of pain receptors to other agonists.[21, 22, 40]

Inflammation

Studies with inhibitors suggest that prostaglandins enhance vasodilation, which contributes to the edema of inflammation, whereas the lipoxygenase products facilitate the infiltration of cells such as neutrophils.[9, 48, 83]

Bronchoconstriction and Bronchodilation

A variety of prostaglandins and related compounds, including PGD_2, $PGF_{2\alpha}$, TXA_2, leukotrienes C_4, D_4, and E_4, and platelet-activating factor, are generally bronchoconstrictive.[47, 76] PGI_2 is a bronchodilator and PGE_2 is usually a bronchodilator but can be a bronchoconstrictor in some individuals. The overall effect of prostaglandins and leukotrienes in a given circumstance (for example, asthma) will depend on the products generated and on the sensitivity of the airways to these specific products. However, administration of inhibitors of the enzymes shown in Figure 8–2 to most normal individuals causes no discernible change in airway resistance.

Vasoconstriction and Vasodilation

In general PGI_2, PGE_1, and PGE_2 are vasodilators, whereas TXA_2, $PGF_{2\alpha}$, and leukotrienes C_4 and D_4 are vasoconstrictors. However, the effects vary from one vascular bed to another and the reader is referred to chapter 9, "Role of Prostacyclin, Thromboxane A_2, and Leukotrienes in Cardiovascular Function and Disease," and to reviews elsewhere for more details.[26, 34, 46a] The remarkable lack of hemodynamic effect of blockade in most individuals is only evidence that these compounds do not regulate basal vascular tone. Their effects in stressed states can be marked, and the effect of blockade can then also be prominent.

Urine Flow

The regulation of urine flow is complex and depends on the blood flow as well as on more direct natriuretic, diuretic, and antidiuretic factors. However, under normal conditions, there is no significant effect of inhibition of prostaglandin production on urine volume or quality. However, under conditions of reduced plasma volume, hypotension, or shock, it appears that endogenous renal PGE_2 and PGI_2 are important in promoting renal perfusion and urinary flow.[24, 50] The use of inhibitors of prostaglandin synthesis in subjects with volume depletion, congestive heart failure, nephrotic syndromes, or cirrhosis of the liver with ascites decreases renal blood flow and urine output.[2, 10, 54, 78]

Hemostasis and Thrombosis

TXA_2, produced by platelets, is a potent platelet aggregating agent as well as a vasoconstrictor. PGI_2, or prostacyclin, produced largely by endothelial cells in the blood vessel wall, is a potent inhibitor of platelet aggregation as well as a vasodilator. The balance of PGI_2 and TXA_2 influences the overall extent of platelet aggregation and clot formation[32, 52] and affects the relative predisposition of an individual to bleed or to form a clot or thrombus. Inhibitors of thromboxane synthesis and effect appear likely to have a role in the prevention and treatment of thrombotic disorders. In this regard, one 300-mg tablet of aspirin causes greater than 90% inhibition of both platelet thromboxane and vascular prostacyclin production. Endothelial cell PGI_2 production will recover more quickly than platelet thromboxane production since endothelial cells can synthesize new protein. Marked inhibition of platelet thromboxane production is present for 12–16 hours after a single 40-mg dose, while endothelial cell prostacyclin production is normal.[81] The optimal dosage of aspirin has been suggested to be 40 mg every second day, but more research is needed to confirm this.

Gastrointestinal Protection and Motility

One of the major side effects of the prostaglandin synthetase inhibitors is gastric irritation and the propensity for development of gastritis and ulcers. This appears to result partly from the acidity of many synthetase inhibitors, but primarily because PGI_2 produced in the stomach has two effects: reduction of acid secretion, and nonspecific (and not well understood) protection of the membranes in the gastrointestinal (GI) tract.[46, 62, 82] Inhibition of the synthesis of the protective PGI_2 can therefore explain the increased incidence of gastritis associated with prostaglandin synthetase inhibitors. The lack of such an effect by acetaminophen is due to its different mechanism. Prostaglandins in the lower GI tract can cause diarrhea. Diarrhea is an important symptom in systemic mastocytosis, which appears to be due partly to PGD_2 production by the mast cells. This diarrhea can be reduced by prostaglandin synthetase inhibitors. However, most common forms of diarrhea do not appear to result from prostaglandin production, and synthetase inhibitors are not effective treatment.

PROSTAGLANDINS AND DISEASE STATES

Anaphylactic Shock

Platelet-activating factor is a structurally unusual phospholipid that has been implicated in pulmonary and cardiovascular symptoms of anaphylactic shock.[59] Other products, in particular arachidonic acid metabolites such as TXA_2 and LTD_4, may also contribute.

Septic Shock and Acute Respiratory Failure

A variety of animal studies suggest a prominent role for arachidonic acid metabolites, in particular TXA_2, in the genesis of septic shock. Beneficial effects of prostaglandin and thromboxane synthetase inhibitors in some animal models of shock are consistent with this concept.[84, 85] Recent studies suggest that pulmonary vasoconstriction produced by activated complement, endotoxin, and oxidants may be mediated by TXA_2, whereas leukotrienes may mediate hypoxia-induced pulmonary vasoconstriction.[15, 36, 53, 84] When complement-activated plasma, endotoxin, or live gram-negative organisms are infused into sheep or goats there is thromboxane synthesis and accompanying pulmonary vasoconstriction with increased pulmonary artery and pulmonary wedge pressure and an increase in pulmonary vascular permeability.[37, 53, 55, 72, 79, 85] Associated with these changes in the lung is a significant fall in cardiac output. Production of TXA_2 may be secondary in some circumstances to an initial synthesis of LTC_4 and LTD_4 or platelet-activating factor. Treatment with cyclo-oxygenase or thromboxane synthetase inhibitors largely prevents the acute pulmonary vasoconstriction and fall in cardiac output but has a lesser effect on the change in pulmonary vascular permeability and the development of pulmonary edema. There is some evidence to suggest that lipoxygenase products, derived from arachidonic acid, may play a part in the vascular permeability changes in the mild, late-appearing pulmonary hypertensive response to endotoxin seen in sheep. Production of TXA_2

may be secondary in some circumstances to an initial synthesis of LTC_4 and LTD_4 or platelet-activating factor.

Asthma

Accumulating evidence suggests that LTD_4 may have a role in the origin of asthma in humans.[17, 35] Approximately 10% of asthmatics have increased bronchoconstriction when they take aspirin or other prostaglandin synthetase inhibitors.[68] This effect may be due either to inhibition of bronchodilator prostaglandin production or to a shunting of arachidonic acid that increases synthesis of bronchoconstrictor leukotrienes. Bronchodilation occurs in rare patients given prostaglandin synthetase inhibitors.[74] The mediators causing bronchoconstriction in these patients are probably different from those in most patients.

Inflammatory Disorders

The efficacy of drugs that modify the production of arachidonic acid derivatives in a variety of inflammatory disorders suggests that prostaglandins and related chemicals are mediators of inflammation.[75] It is not possible here to detail all conditions, but the reader is referred elsewhere.[26, 33, 80] Four clinical conditions will be mentioned briefly. The effectiveness of colchicine in gout may be partly due to its inhibition of LTB_4 synthesis.[67] Lipoxygenase inhibitors may have promise in the treatment of psoriasis.[1] Sulfasalazine, used for the treatment of inflammatory bowel disease, has been found to inhibit the 5-lipoxygenase and thromboxane synthetase.[73] Some patients with rheumatoid arthritis have been found to have interferon-producing T lymphocytes that are exquisitely sensitive to PGE_2 so that in the presence of minute amounts of this prostaglandin they fail to generate the γ-interferon necessary to turn off the β-lymphocyte response.[39] It is also of note that high concentrations of prostaglandin synthetase inhibitors have now been shown to increase mortality in mice from bacterial infections,[20] whereas treatment with steroids increases mortality under some circumstances.[63] However, recent studies in animals suggest that mechanisms of host defense should be studied more carefully in humans on high therapeutic doses of aspirin, and the relationship between low aspirin doses and particular conditions such as Reye's syndrome needs to be further evaluated.[20]

Oxygen Toxicity

Oxygen is associated with toxic effects on the eyes and the lungs, especially in premature infants. High levels of oxygen may be associated with increased nonspecific fatty acid oxidation. This may produce increased amounts of hydroxy and hydroperoxy fatty acids. Both of these may have direct biologic effects such as promoting neutrophil chemotaxis; the fatty acid hydroperoxides are also potent inhibitors of prostacyclin synthetase, the enzyme that converts PGH_2 to PGI_2.[12] Some of the toxic effects of oxygen may therefore be due to perturbations in the synthesis of prostaglandins and related chemicals.

Ischemia and Reperfusion

Ischemic injury increases the release of free fatty acids as a result of hypoxia and cell damage.[3, 14] It is possible that during tissue ischemia, the level of tissue oxygen may sometimes fall below that needed for the synthesis of prostaglandins and related chemicals. If so, reperfusion would be expected to be associated with a rapid burst of these chemicals. Whether this occurs, and whether some of the injurious changes occurring during reperfusion may relate to effects of prostaglandins and related chemicals, is presently uncertain.

PROSTAGLANDINS AND THE TREATMENT OF DISEASES

Prostaglandins are currently used to treat some specific diseases, and research is being conducted to evaluate their potential in others. PGE_1 is known to dilate the ductus arteriosus, and this effect is clinically important in infants with congenital heart disease when it is desirable to maintain the patency of this vessel.[39] PGE_1 and PGI_2, both of which inhibit platelet aggregation and are generally vasodilators, have been used in certain circumstances when thrombosis is likely. These include cardiopulmonary bypass, hemodialysis, peripheral vascular disease, stroke, and thrombotic thrombocytopenic purpura.[13, 56, 60] However, to date, the benefit of these compounds has not been proved in any of these disorders in humans. The side effects of PGI_2, notably hypotension, limit its use. A compound that has antiplatelet effects without hypotensive actions is needed. Considerable potential exists for the use of prostaglandin derivatives with protective action on the GI tract in ulcer prophylaxis and therapy. Studies in mice suggest that a stable analogue of PGE_1 may be useful for the treatment of autoimmune disorders.[86]

SUMMARY

A review of the origins and actions of prostaglandins and related chemicals suggests that they probably have importance in a variety of disease states. Fundamental to understanding these agents is the realization that they arise from the breakdown of biologic membranes and that this breakdown may occur specifically in response to hormone action, or may occur nonspecifically whenever there is tissue damage or trauma. Thus when there is inflammation or when there are burns or trauma, these chemicals are likely to be produced and likely to be important in the production of effects, including shock, fever, and pain. Prostaglandin synthesis inhibitors have been used to treat pain and fever for many years. The potential use of drugs that modify the production and effects of prostaglandins and related chemicals and the uses of prostaglandins themselves in a variety of other conditions is being intensively studied. Laboratory observations should be cautiously extended to clinical conditions, since the effects of these agents vary in different species, in response to different stressors, and from one tissue to another. In some circumstances nonspecific side effects may occur when specific blocking agents are used.

REFERENCES

1. Allen BR, Littlewood SM: Benoxaprofen: Effect on cutaneous lesions in psoriasis. *Br Med J* 1982; 285:1241.
2. Arisz L, Donker AJ, Brentjens JR, et al: The effect of indomethacin on proteinuria and kidney function in the nephrotic syndrome. *Acta Med Scand* 1976; 199:121.
3. Aveldano MI, Bazan NG: Differential lipid deacylation during brain ischemia in a homeotherm and poikilotherm: Content and composition of free fatty acids and triacylglycerols. *Brain Res* 1975; 100:99.
4. Bell RL, Kennerly DA, Stanford N, et al: Diglyceride lipase: A pathway for arachidonate release from human platelets. *Proc Natl Acad Sci USA* 1979; 76:3238.
5. Billah MM, Lapetina EG: Formation of lysophosphatidylinositol in platelets stimulated with thrombin and ionophore A23187. *J Biol Chem* 1982; 257:5196.
6. Bills TK, Smith JB, Silver MJ: Selective release of arachidonic acid from the phospholipids of human platelets in response to thrombin. *Biochim Biophys Acta* 1976; 424:303.
7. Blackwell GJ, Flower RJ: 1-phenyl-3-pyrazolidone: An inhibitor of cyclo-oxygenase and lipoxygenase pathways in lung and platelets. *Prostaglandins* 1978; 16:417.
8. Blackwell GJ, Flower RJ: Inhibition of phospholipase. *Br Med Bull* 1983; 39:260.
9. Black AK, Greaves MW, Hensby CN, et al: The effects of indomethacin on arachidonic acid and prostaglandins E_2 and F_2 levels in human skin 24 h after u.v.B. and u.v.C irradiation. *Br J Clin Pharmacol* 1978; 6:261.
10. Boyer TD, Zia P, Reynolds TB: Effect of indomethacin and prostaglandin A_1 on renal function and plasma renin activity in alcoholic liver disease. *Gastroenterology* 1979; 77:215.
11. Brigham KL, Ogletree M, Snapper J, et al: Prostaglandins and lung injury. *Chest* 1983; 83(suppl):705.
12. Bunting S, Gryglewski R, Moncada S, et al: Arterial walls generate from prostaglandin endoperoxides a substance (prostaglandin X) which relaxes strips of mesenteric and coeliac arteries and inhibits platelet aggregation. *Prostaglandins* 1976; 12:897.
13. Carlson LA, Eriksson I: Femoral artery infusion of prostaglandin E_1 in severe peripheral vascular disease. *Lancet* 1973; 1:155.
14. Cenedella RJ, Galli C, Paoletti R: Brain free fatty acid levels in rats sacrificed by decapitation versus focused microwave irradiation. *Lipids* 1975; 10:290.
15. Cooper JD, McDonald JW, Ali M, et al: Prostaglandin production associated with the pulmonary vascular response to complement activation. *Surgery* 1980; 88:215.
16. Dabrowska R, Hartshorne DJ: Ca^{2+} and modulator-dependent myosin light chain kinase from non-muscle cells. *Biochem Biophys Res Commun* 1978; 85:1352.
17. Dahlen SE, Hansson G, Hedquist P, et al: Allergen challenge of lung tissue from asthmatics elicits bronchial contraction that correlates with the release of leukotrienes C_4, D_4

and E$_4$. *Proc Natl Acad Sci USA* 1983; 80:1712.

18. Drazen JM, Austen KF, Lewis RA, et al: Comparative airway and vascular activities of leukotrienes C and D in vivo and in vitro. *Proc Natl Acad Sci USA* 1980; 77:4354.

19. Dyerberg J, Bang DO: Haemostatic function and platelet polyunsaturated fatty acids in Eskimos. *Lancet* 1979; 2:433.

20. Esposito AL: Aspirin impairs anti-bacterial mechanisms in experimental pneumonia. *Am Rev Respir Dis* 1984; 130:857.

21. Ferreira SH: Prostaglandins, aspirin-like drugs and analgesia. *Nature* 1972; 240:200.

22. Ferreira SH, Nakamura M, de A Castro MS: The hyperalgesic effects of prostacyclin and prostaglandin E$_2$. *Prostaglandins Med* 1978; 16:32.

23. Fielder-Nagy C, Hamilton JG, Batula-Bernardo C, et al: Inhibition of 5-lipoxygenase, 12-lipoxygenase and prostaglandin endoperoxide synthetase by selected retinoids (vitamin A derivatives). *Fed Proc* 1982; 42:919.

24. Flamenbaum W, Kleinman JG: Prostaglandins and renal function, or "a trip down the rabbit hole," in Ramwell PW (ed): *Prostaglandins*. New York, Plenum Press, 1977.

25. Fletcher JR, Ramwell PW: Indomethacin improves survival after endotoxin in baboons. *Adv Prostaglandin Thromboxane Res* 1980; 7:821.

26. Gerrard JM: *Prostaglandins and Leukotrienes: Role in Blood and Vascular Cell Function*. New York, Marcel Dekker, Inc, 1985.

27. Gerrard JM: Phospholipid metabolism and cell stimulus activation coupling in platelets and other blood cells. *Surv Synth Pathol Res* 1984; 3:457.

28. Gerrard JM, Butler AM, Graff G, et al: Prostaglandin endoperoxides promote calcium release from a platelet membrane fraction in vitro. *Prostaglandins Med* 1978; 1:373.

29. Gerrard JM, Carroll RC: Stimulation of platelet protein phosphorylation by arachidonic acid and endoperoxide analogs. *Prostaglandins* 1981; 22:81.

30. Gerrard JM, Friesen LL, McCrae JM, et al: Platelet protein phosphorylation, in Westwick J, et al (eds): *Mechanisms of Stimulus Response Coupling in Platelets,* New York, Plenum Press (in press).

31. Gerrard JM, Schollmeyer JV, White JG: The role of contractile proteins in the function of the platelet surface membrane. *Cell Surface Rev* 1981; 7:217.

32. Gerrard JM, White JG: Prostaglandins and thromboxanes: 'Middlemen' modulating platelet function in hemostasis and thrombosis. *Prog Hemostas Thromb* 1978; 4:87.

33. Goldstein IM, Malmsten CL, Samuelsson B, et al: Prostaglandins, thromboxanes and polymorphonuclear leukocytes: Mediation and modulation of inflammation. *Inflammation* 1977; 2:309.

34. Greenberg S, Kadowitz PJ, Burks TF (eds): *Prostaglandins: Organ and Tissue-Specific Actions*. New York, Marcel Dekker, Inc, 1982.

35. Griffin M, Weiss JW, Leitch AG, et al: Effects of leukotriene D on the airways in asthma. *N Engl J Med* 1983; 308:436.

36. Gurtner GH, Knoblauch A, Smith PL, et al: Oxidant and lipid-induced pulmonary vasoconstriction mediated by arachidonic acid metabolites. *J Appl Physiol* 1983; 55:949.

37. Harlan J, Winn R, Weaver J, et al: Selective blockade of thromboxane A$_2$ synthesis during experimental *E. coli* bacteremia in the goat: Effects on hemodynamics and lung water. *Chest* 1983; 83(suppl):755.

38. Haslam RJ, Davidson MML, Davies T, et al: Regulation of blood platelet function by cyclic nucleotides. *Adv Cyclic Nucleotide Res* 1978; 9:533.

39. Hasler F, Bluestein HG, Zvaifler NJ, et al: Analysis of the defects responsible for the impaired regulation of EBV-induced B cell proliferation by rheumatoid arthritis lymphocytes. *J Immunol* 1983; 131:768.

40. Higgs EA, Moncada S, Vane JR: Inflammatory effects of prostacyclin (PGI$_2$) and 6-oxo-PGF$_{1\alpha}$ in the rat paw. *Prostaglandins Med* 1978; 16:153.

41. Higgs GA, Flower RJ, Vane JR: A new approach to anti-inflammatory drugs. *Biochem Pharmacol* 1979; 28:1959.

42. Kaibuchi K, Takai Y, Sawamura M, et al: Synergistic function of protein phosphorylation and calcium mobilization in platelet activation. *J Biol Chem* 1983; 258:6701.

43. Karim SMM, Adaikan PG, Kottegoda SR: Prostaglandins and human respiratory tract smooth muscle: Structure activity relationship. *Adv Prostaglandin Thromboxane Res* 1980; 7:969.

44. Lands WEM, Cook HW, Rome LH: Prostaglandin biosynthesis: Consequence of oxygenase mechanism upon in vitro assays of drug effectiveness. *Adv Prostaglandin Thromboxane Res* 1976; 1:7.

45. Lee JB (ed): *Prostaglandins*. New York, Elsevier-North Holland, 1982.

46. Main IH, Whittle BJ: Investigation of the vasodilator and antisecretory role of prostaglandins in the rat gastric mucosa by use of non-steroidal anti-inflammatory drugs. *Br J Pharmacol* 1975; 53:217.

46a. Malik AB: *Prostaglandins, Leukotrienes and Lung Fluid Balance* (symposium). *Fed Proc* 1985; 44:18–52.

47. Mathe AA: Prostaglandins and the lung, in Ramwell PW (ed): *The Prostaglandins*. New York, Plenum Press, 1977.

48. Meyers RF, Anthes JC, Casmer CJ, et al: Ex vivo effects of non-steroidal anti-inflammatory drugs on arachidonic acid metabolism in neutrophils from a reverse passive arthus reaction. *Fed Proc* 1984; 43:955.

49. McDonald JW, Ali M, Morgan E, et al: Thromboxane synthesis by sources other than platelets in association with complement-induced pulmonary leukostasis and pulmonary hypertension in sheep. *Circ Res* 1983; 52:1.

50. McGiff JC, Wong PYK: Compartmentalization of prostaglandins and prostacyclin within the kidney: Implications for renal function. *Fed Proc* 1979; 38:89.

51. McKean ML, Smith JB, Silver MJ: Formation of lysophosphatidylcholine by human platelets in response to thrombin: Support for the phospholipase A_2 pathway for the liberation of arachidonic acid. *J Biol Chem* 1981; 256:1522.

52. Moncada S, Vane JR: The role of prostacyclin in vascular tissue. *Fed Proc* 1979; 38:66.

53. Morganroth ML, Murphy RC, Voelkel NF: Diethylcarbamazine, a leukotriene synthesis blocker, blocks hypoxic pulmonary vasoconstriction. *Fed Proc* 1983; 42:303.

54. Muther RS, Potter DM, Bennett WM: Aspirin-induced depression of glomerular filtration rate in normal humans: Role of sodium balance. *Ann Intern Med* 1981; 94:317.

55. Ogletree ML, Brigham KL: Imidazole, a selective inhibitor of thromboxane synthesis, inhibits pulmonary vascular responses to endotoxin in awake sheep. *Am Rev Respir Dis* 1981; 123:247.

56. Olley PM, Coceani F, Rowe RD, et al: Clinical use of prostaglandins and prostaglandin synthetase inhibitors in cardiac problems of the newborn. *Adv Prostaglandin Thromboxane Res* 1980; 7:913.

57. Peterson DA, Gerrard JM, Rao GHR, et al: Reduction of ferric heme to ferrous by lipid peroxides: Possible relevance to the role of peroxide tone in the regulation of prostaglandin synthesis. *Prostaglandins Med* 1980; 4:73.

58. Piper P, Vane JR: The release of prostaglandin from lung and other tissues. *Ann NY Acad Sci* 1971; 180:363.

59. Pinckard RN, McManus LM, Hanahan DJ: Chemistry and biology of acetyl glyceryl ether phosphorylcholine (platelet activating factor). *Adv Inflamm Res* 1982; 4:147.

60. Radegran K, Papaconstantinou C: Prostacyclin infusion during cardiopulmonary bypass in man. *Thromb Res* 1980; 19:267.

61. Rittenhouse-Simmons S: Production of diglyceride from phosphatidylinositol in activated human platelets. *J Clin Invest* 1979; 63:580.

62. Robert A: Prostaglandins and the digestive system, in Ramwell PW (ed): *The Prostaglandins*. New York, Plenum Press, 1977.

63. Robinson HJ, Phares HF, Grassele OE: Prostaglandins synthetase inhibitors and infection, in Robinson HJ, Vane JR (eds): *Prostaglandin Synthetase Inhibitors*. New York, Raven Press, 1974.

64. Roth GJ, Majerus PW: The mechanism of the effect of aspirin on human platelets: I. Acetylation of a particular fraction protein. *J Clin Invest* 1975; 56:624.

65. Rybicki JP, Venton DL, LeBreton GC: The thromboxane antagonist, 13-aza-prostanoic acid, inhibits arachidonic acid-induced Ca^{2+} release from isolated platelet membrane vesicles. *Biochim Biophys Acta* 1980; 751:66.

66. Sekiya K, Okuda H, Arichi S: Selective inhibition of platelet lipoxygenase by esculetin. *Biochim Biophys Acta* 1982; 713:68.

67. Serhan CN, Lundberg U, Weissman G, et al: Formation of leukotrienes and hydroxy fatty acids by human neutrophils and platelets exposed to monoxodium urate. *Prostaglandins* 1984; 27:563.

68. Settipane GA: Aspirin and allergic diseases: A review. *Am J Med* 1983; 64(6A):102.

69. Smith WL, Lands WEM: Oxygenation of polyunsaturated fatty acids during prostaglan-

din biosynthesis by sheep vesicular gland. *Biochemistry* 1972; 11:3276.

70. Smith WL, Lands WEM: Oxygenation of unsaturated fatty acids by soybean lipoxygenase. *J Biol Chem* 1972; 247:1038.

71. Smith RJ, Sun FF, Iden SS, et al: An evaluation of the relationship between arachidonic acid lipoxygenase and human neutrophil degranulation. *Clin Immunol Immunopathol* 1981; 20:157.

72. Snapper JR, Ogletree ML, Hutchison AA, et al: Meclofenamate prevents increased resistance of the lung following endotoxemia in unanaesthetized sheep. *Am Rev Respir Dis* 1981; 123:200.

73. Stenson WF, Lobos E: Inhibition of thromboxane synthetase by sulfasalazine. *Biochem Pharmacol* 1983; 32:2205.

74. Szczeklik A, Gryglewski RJ, Czerniawska-Mysik G, et al: Aspirin, prostaglandins and bronchial asthma. *Adv Prostaglandin Thromboxane Res* 1980; 7:993.

9

Role of Prostacyclin, Thromboxane A$_2$, and Leukotrienes in Cardiovascular Function and Disease

Robert L. Zeid, B.S.

Robert R. Ruffolo, Jr., Ph.D.

Prostaglandins comprise a group of acidic lipids that are synthesized from 20-carbon polyunsaturated fatty acids (see chapter 8, ''Prostaglandins and Related Lipids''). Arachidonic acid (5,8,11,14-eicosatetraenoic acid) is the major precursor for most of the prostaglandins formed in humans and is commonly found as a key component of mammalian cell membranes. The release of arachidonic acid from membrane phospholipids by phospholipase A$_2$ can be activated by a variety of different stimuli[25, 54] and is considered to be the primary rate-limiting step in the synthesis of prostaglandins and related metabolites.

When mobilized from membrane stores, arachidonic acid is metabolized by either the lipoxygenase or the cyclo-oxygenase enzyme pathway (see chapter 7, ''Control of Organ Blood Flow''). Cyclo-oxygenase, also known as prostaglandin synthetase, metabolizes arachidonic acid into an unstable endoperoxide, prostaglandin G$_2$ (PGG$_2$), which is modified further by peroxidase to another endoperoxide, PGH$_2$. These endoperoxides are metabolized to either prostacyclin (via prostacyclin synthetase), thromboxane A$_2$ (via thromboxane synthetase), or other prostaglandins.

Metabolism of arachidonic acid through the lipoxygenase pathway forms leukotrienes. Unlike the cyclo-oxygenase enzyme, which is ubiquitous in the body, the lipoxygenase enzymes are not found in all tissues. Lipoxygenase has been identified in platelets,[34] leukocytes,[8] lung,[104] kidney,[19] monocytes,[79] peritoneal macrophages,[23] and the coronary vasculature.[83]

This chapter reviews the various effects of prostacyclin, thromboxane A$_2$, and the leukotrienes in relation to their activities in the cardiovascular system and their suspected roles in cardiovascular disorders.

PROSTACYCLIN

Effects of Prostacyclin on the Cardiovascular System and Vascular Smooth Muscle

Prostacyclin is a potent vasodilator in most mammalian species, including humans.[65] Prostacyclin also increases cardiac output, but appears to do so indirectly by decreasing afterload.[50] Infusion of prostacyclin in humans reduces coronary vascular resistance, increases coronary blood flow, and produces flushing of the skin, suggesting generalized systemic vasodilation.[85] The primary site of the vasodilator effects of prostacyclin is at the level of the smaller resistance vessels, and not the larger conduit vessels.

The formation of prostacyclin (and of thromboxane A$_2$) is blocked by aspirin and other cyclo-oxygenase inhibitors. Since cyclo-oxygenase inhibitors do not elevate blood pressure, it is believed that the basal production of prostacyclin does not contribute to vasodilation under normal physiologic conditions. However, in some hypoxic, inflammatory, or other pathologic states, a vasodilatory role of prostacyclin is probable.

Prostacyclin has been shown to inhibit vasoconstrictor responses elicited by nerve stimulation and by endogenous pressor hormones such as angiotensin II, epinephrine, and norepinephrine. Prostacyclin appears to antagonize neurogenic vasoconstriction by a postjunctional action on vascular smooth muscle rather than by inhibiting neurotransmitter (norepinephrine) release, since nerve-stimulated responses and responses to exogenously administered norepinephrine are inhibited to a similar extent. Furthermore, the responses to angiotensin II and norepinephrine are inhibited to a similar degree, suggesting that prostacyclin nonspecifically and functionally antagonizes hormone-induced vasoconstriction.[50]

The observation that "prostacyclin-like" substances are released spontaneously into the circulation and that prostacyclin is not inactivated in the lung suggests that prostacyclin may serve as a circulating hormone that could act in certain pathologic states to maintain the peripheral vascular bed in a dilated state.[32] Thus, there is an important difference between prostacyclin and other prostaglandins formed from arachidonic acid. Because prostacyclin is not inactivated by the pulmonary circulation, it is equipotent as a vasodilator when given intra-arterially or intravenously, whereas other prostaglandins such as prostaglandins E$_1$ and E$_2$ do not escape pulmonary metabolism and are much less active or inactive when given intravenously. Thus, circulating prostacyclin may produce a longer vasodilatory response owing to the fact that it escapes pulmonary inactivation.[50]

Prostacyclin is a potent activator of adenylate cyclase,[56] and this has been proposed to be the mechanism responsible for prostacyclin-induced vasodilation. Prostacyclin-mediated increases in cyclic adenosine monophosphate (cAMP) levels also inhibit phospholipase activity in platelets[55] and vascular endothelium,[9, 41] possibly indirectly by blocking the action of calcium.[9] Prostacyclin-mediated increases in cAMP can inhibit the basal production of prostacyclin, which suggests that prostacyclin has a negative feedback effect on its own synthesis.[56]

Effects of Prostacyclin on Platelet Aggregation

Prostacyclin is the most potent endogenous inhibitor of platelet aggregation, being 30-fold more potent than PGE$_1$ and 1,000-fold more potent than adenosine.[72, 73] The antiaggregatory effect of prostacyclin appears to result from elevated platelet cAMP levels.[106] At much higher concentra-

tions, prostacyclin also inhibits platelet adhesion. Basal levels are not sufficiently high to have a significant effect. However, local concentrations of prostacyclin may become high enough to inhibit platelet aggregation and thrombus formation under some circumstances. Whether in vivo levels of prostacyclin ever reach sufficient concentrations to inhibit platelet adherence to an injured blood vessel is less certain.

Renal Effects of Prostacyclin

Regulation of the renal circulation is complicated by the interplay between hormonal and neurogenic effects acting on vascular resistance, glomerular filtration rate, and renal blood flow. Involved in this delicate interplay are the renin-angiotensin system, catecholamines, prostaglandins, and the kallikrein-kinin system. Furthermore, the relative contribution of these factors may change in a variety of physiologic and pathologic states.

Prostacyclin is one of the most abundantly produced renal prostaglandins, primarily from arteriolar and glomerular sites. Renal cortical function, including renal blood flow and glomerular filtration rate, is modulated by cortical prostacyclin synthesis. Prostacyclin increases renal blood flow and antagonizes the renal pressor actions of angiotensin II and vasopressin (antidiuretic hormone). The natriuretic, kaliuretic, and diuretic actions of prostacyclin appear to be principally independent of the effects on renal blood flow and glomerular filtration rate, suggesting also a tubular action. Prostacyclin is formed in the renal cortex at sites of renin synthesis and storage, and also may modulate renin release.[87]

Prostacyclin formation also antagonizes the increased renal vascular resistance observed during periods of low sodium intake, reduced cardiac output, hypoxemic and ischemic renal states, and hepatic disease.[24] A number of studies suggest that prostacyclin has its greatest effect on renal function when circulating blood volume is reduced, and by blocking synthesis of prostacyclin, cyclo-oxygenase inhibition may exacerbate diminished renal function to the point of renal insufficiency.[24]

Another important effect of prostacyclin in the kidney is its interaction with vasopressin to increase urinary excretion of sodium and water. Numerous studies have shown that prostacyclin has diuretic and natriuretic effects.[28, 46] Furthermore, it has been shown in a variety of species, including humans, that cyclo-oxygenase inhibitors potentiate the hydro-osmotic effect of vasopressin on the renal tubule,[2, 7, 66] which suggests that prostacyclin may play a physiologic role in the renal tubule.[38]

It appears that renal function significantly depends on prostacyclin formation during low circulating volume, sodium depletion, low cardiac output, and several other pathologic states. These relatively hypovolemic or hypoperfused renal states reduce oxygen transport and impede renal function. In light of the enormous metabolic activity needed for normal countercurrent exchange of sodium, prostacyclin release may represent part of an "antihypoxic" response and be critical to maintaining normal renal function.

Systemic and Regional Hemodynamic Effects of Prostacyclin

Intra-arterial administration of prostacyclin produces an immediate decrease in mean arterial blood pressure secondary to a decrease in systemic vascular resistance. Cardiac output is significantly increased by prostacyclin, presumably as a direct consequence of the reduction in afterload.[50] Prostacyclin infusion is associated with increases in blood flow in coronary, renal, mesenteric, and hindquarter vascular beds.[50] These increases in regional blood flow produced by prostacyclin are secondary to decreases in the respective regional vascular resistances and are consistent with in vitro observations that prostacyclin produces direct arterial vasodilation in isolated strips prepared from the mesenteric, celiac, and coronary arteries.[50]

Prostacyclin also produces vasodilation in the pulmonary circulation. Prostacyclin infusion has been reported to reduce lobar arterial and small vein pressures without affecting left atrial pressure in normal animals. However, when pulmonary pressures are elevated, prostacyclin is associated with marked reductions in pulmonary vascular resistance. In fact, prostacyclin is the only product of the arachidonic acid cascade known to produce vasodilation in the pulmonary circulation.[50] It has been proposed that under resting conditions, the pulmonary vascular bed may be maintained in a dilated state by the production of prostacyclin in the lung.[50]

Effects of Prostacyclin on Local Blood Flow and Reactive Hyperemia

The function of the cardiovascular system over a dynamic range of activities and blood pressures depends to a large extent on the capacity of the peripheral vascular beds to autoregulate blood flow according to metabolic demands. Autoregulation of local blood flow is a complex interaction of central, local, and humoral factors, many of which are still unknown. One example is reactive hyperemia. Reactive hyperemia is not generally considered a true physiologic response but rather a maximal mobilization of the tissue's defenses against hypoxia. Cyclo-oxygenase inhibitors reduce both the maximum and the duration of the vasodilatory response after release of arterial occlusion,[68] and prostacylin has been implicated as a possible mediator of this response. Similar results have been observed in humans: total forearm reactive hyperemia seen after 5 minutes of arterial occlusion was reduced 50%–60% by indomethacin.[51, 75]

Relation of Prostacyclin to Cardiovascular Disease

Ischemic Heart Disease (Angina)

Given the vasodilatory and antiaggregatory properties of prostacyclin, there has been much interest in the possible relation of certain pathologic states to disorders in prostacyclin synthesis and/or release. The role of prostacyclin in ischemic heart disease, such as angina, coronary artery disease, or myocardial infarction, has been the target of many recent investigations.

Clinical trials with prostacyclin in patients with ischemic heart disease have been equivocal, showing inconsistent relief of anginal pain despite patients' low basal coronary prostacyclin levels on admission. Many studies have shown an improvement in some patients with angina when prostacyclin was infused.[65] Cyclo-oxygenase inhibitors have been shown to constrict coronary vessels and to decrease coronary blood flow in patients with ischemic heart disease, and to exacerbate the imbalance in the ratio between myocardial oxygen supply and demand. It seems likely that in patients with coronary artery disease, the endogenous release of prostacyclin in response to hypoxia may be part of a homeostatic mechanism to maintain adequate coronary perfusion.[26, 27]

The inconsistent effects of prostacyclin in patients with angina may be attributed in part to different patient selection criteria and to differences in the stage of the disease. Furthermore, the release of prostacyclin in response to myocardial ischemic episodes is dependent on local Po_2

levels, and the transient nature of ischemic attacks may not be of sufficient time duration to reduce oxygen tension below 47 mm Hg, a level that has been shown to stimulate prostacyclin synthesis.[105]

Myocardial Infarction

A number of animal studies have confirmed that infusion of prostacyclin significantly reduces infarct size and mortality following ligation of the left anterior descending coronary artery. Conversely, inhibitors of prostacyclin synthesis increase the size of experimental infarction zones.[59] The limiting effect of prostacyclin on infarct size may be related to its cytoprotective effects in the myocardium rather than to an antiaggregatory or coronary vasodilatory effect.[59, 86]

Prostacyclin infused within 6 hours of acute myocardial infarction reduced creatine phosphokinase release from the heart by 50% compared with that in control patients, suggesting that prostacyclin may also limit infarct size in humans.[40] Thus, although prostacyclin infusion may have variable effects in angina, it appears consistently effective in limiting the size of an acute myocardial infarction in animals and humans.[105]

Effects on Peripheral Vascular Disease

Disorders in prostacyclin synthesis and/or release may be important in the development of certain peripheral vascular diseases, such as chronic atherosclerotic occlusive disease, Buerger's disease, Raynaud's phenomenon, and idiopathic vasculopathy. Clinical studies have shown prostacyclin to be beneficial in distal arteriopathies associated with rest pain and ulceration.[65] Advanced peripheral vascular insufficiency responds well to prostacyclin infusion, and virtually all patients report relief of rest pain and healing of ischemic ulcerations. In these patients prostacyclin may be directly beneficial by augmenting local perfusion, since increases in blood flow to calf muscle have been observed. Studies in patients with a variety of distal arteriosclerotic disorders have demonstrated similar improvement.

THROMBOXANE A$_2$

Thromboxane A$_2$ (TXA$_2$), a potent vasoconstrictor and promoter of platelet aggregation, is a prostanoid also derived from arachidonic acid via the cyclo-oxygenase pathway. TXA$_2$ is synthe-

sized and released by activated platelets. However, other cells and tissues have the capacity to produce TXA$_2$; it has been found in polymorphonuclear leukocytes, macrophages, fibroblasts, spleen, iris, conjunctiva, lung, umbilical artery, pulmonary artery, and kidney.[106] TXA$_2$ may have adverse effects in patients with coronary artery disease because it strongly constricts the systemic vasculature and coronary arteries, and because it promotes platelet aggregation, all of which will exacerbate the existing imbalance between myocardial oxygen supply and demand. The pathophysiologic role of TXA$_2$ in the cardiovascular system remains undefined. Increased TXA$_2$ release has been seen in coronary artery vasospasm and pacing-induced angina.[63] Recently, TXA$_2$ (inferred by detection of its stable metabolite, TXB$_2$) has been found in peripheral venous samples taken from patients with evolving acute myocardial infarction. TXA$_2$ has been shown to promote the synthesis of prostacyclin in vascular smooth muscle.[36]

Effect of Thromboxane A$_2$ on Platelet Aggregation

Platelet aggregation is a multifactorial phenomenon that can be initiated by many humoral stimuli, including adenosine diphosphate (ADP), thrombin, epinephrine, arachidonic acid, and TXA$_2$. One common denominator of these proaggregatory agents is their ability to decrease platelet levels of cAMP.[106] Since the decrease in platelet cAMP can be abolished with thromboxane synthetase inhibitors, it may be the formation of TXA$_2$ by these agents that leads to the decrease in cAMP and subsequently to the induction of platelet aggregation. However, the concept that a decrease in cAMP is a significant factor in causing platelet aggregation has recently been questioned since a number of compounds that inhibit platelet adenylate cyclase do not promote platelet aggregation.[29]

TXA$_2$ plays an important and fundamental role in platelet function.[29] TXA$_2$ stimulates platelet granule centralization. The sequence of events appears to depend on calcium flux initiating phosphorylation of myosin light chain. The mechanism of TXA$_2$-induced stimulation of calcium flux, whether direct or indirect (via phosphoinositide breakdown), is uncertain. Furthermore, TXA$_2$ stimulates granule labilization, one of the essential steps in granule secretion. The biochemical sequence appears to require phosphorylation of critical intracellular proteins. The mechanism of TXA$_2$-induced phosphorylation, whether due to direct activation of protein kinase C or indirect via phosphoinositide breakdown and diglyceride production, is also uncertain.[29]

Platelet aggregation induced by arachidonic acid, prostaglandins H$_2$ and G$_2$, and collagen is accompanied by the further formation of TXA$_2$.[34, 78] Selective thromboxane receptor antagonists inhibit platelet aggregation induced by arachidonate, prostaglandin endoperoxides, and collagen, which suggests that TXA$_2$ generation may be a final common pathway leading to platelet aggregation for these substances.[43, 102, 106] The inhibition of arachidonate-induced platelet aggregation by thromboxane synthetase inhibitors could also result from diversion of prostaglandin endoperoxides to PGD$_2$, the latter being an inhibitor of platelet aggregation. However, since thromboxane synthetase inhibitors do not block platelet aggregation induced by the prostaglandin endoperoxides (i.e., PGG$_2$ and PGH$_2$), it is concluded that these compounds may also act directly on the same receptor as TXA$_2$.

Effects of Thromboxane A$_2$ on Coronary Circulation

TXA$_2$ is a potent coronary vasoconstrictor.[5, 12, 13, 16, 47, 48, 74, 101] The proaggregatory and vasoconstrictor properties of TXA$_2$ have been implicated in the etiology of several cardiovascular pathologies, such as myocardial ischemia,[15, 42, 53, 76, 96] variant angina, coronary vasospasm, myocardial infarction,[42, 44, 97] and sudden death syndrome.[58]

Renal Effects of Thromboxane A$_2$

TXA$_2$ release in the kidneys of young hypertensive rats is relatively high compared with the modest release observed in older hypertensive rats. This finding is consistent with the observation that increased TXA$_2$ production is seen in isolated glomeruli from hypertensive rats, and suggests further that a primary change resulting in increased renal glomerular TXA$_2$ synthesis may be a preliminary step leading to increased renal vascular resistance and subsequently to the development of hypertension.[52]

Role of Thromboxane A$_2$ in Cardiovascular Disorders

Ischemic Heart Disease

One minute after coronary artery occlusion in animals, levels of TXA$_2$ in the great cardiac vein effluent are elevated. This suggests that TXA$_2$ has a role in acute myocardial infarction. The known vasoconstrictive, platelet aggregatory, and cytolytic actions of TXA$_2$ may all contribute to myocardial damage following acute infarction.[57, 58] Following acute myocardial infarction there is generalized coronary vasoconstriction[39] that may result partly from TXA$_2$ released into the coronary circulation following platelet aggregation. Coronary venous blood obtained after experimenal coronary occlusion contracted strips of rabbit aorta and dog coronary artery, suggesting that it contained a vasoconstrictive substance.[99] Pretreatment of these animals with a cyclo-oxygenase inhibitor to block TXA$_2$ synthesis abolishes the constrictive effect of the coronary effluent. Furthermore, after experimental myocardial infarction, administration of a specific thromboxane synthetase inhibitor decreases infarction size.[91] Conversely, administration of a synthetic TXA$_2$ mimic will increase experimental infarct size.[95]

Several clinical studies have reported increased levels of circulating TXB$_2$, a stable metabolite and therefore biochemical marker of TXA$_2$, in patients with angina[42, 44, 53, 108] or coronary artery vasospasm.[15, 76] This finding confirms that platelet aggregation and arachidonic acid metabolism are increased in patients with ischemic heart disease, and has led to speculation that TXA$_2$ may have a causative role in this disease. Increased platelet aggregation and TXA$_2$ release in the coronary circulation during ischemic attacks has also been noted in several studies. Nonetheless, the importance of TXA$_2$ in angina remains controversial. Although increased TXB$_2$ has been demonstrated in pacing-induced angina, no beneficial effect of cyclo-oxygenase inhibitors has been demonstrated, which suggests that TXA$_2$ may not be the principal causative agent involved. However, aspirin therapy may be beneficial in unstable angina, highly suggestive of a role of TXA$_2$ in this pathology. Interestingly, the clinical efficacy of calcium channel blocking agents in coronary artery vasospasm may be related to their ability to block platelet aggregation and thus prevent the release of TXA$_2$ into the coronary circulation,[20] thereby eliminating TXA$_2$-induced coronary vasoconstriction.

Although clinical studies indicate that TXA$_2$ levels are elevated in patients with ischemic heart disease, additional factors also must be considered. The balance between prostacyclin and TXA$_2$ in these cardiovascular conditions appears to be a critical factor regulating coronary perfusion and myocardial dynamics. Higher ratios of prostacyclin:TXA_2 protect the myocardium and increase coronary blood flow, whereas lower ratios worsen ischemic heart disease by decreasing coronary blood flow[14] and unfavorably altering the ratio between myocardial oxygen supply and demand.

Endotoxin Shock

The role of TXA_2 in endotoxic shock has been documented in animals. TXA_2 has been implicated as a causative agent of cardiac and respiratory dysfunction during endotoxin shock. TXA_2 levels are elevated within 30 minutes of endotoxin challenge in animals, and this is presumed to be responsible for the observed pulmonary hypertension and thrombocytopenia. The increase in pulmonary vascular resistance and hypoxia observed in experimental endotoxic shock appears to be a direct consequence of the pulmonary vasoconstrictor effects of TXA_2, as well as of microemboli resulting from the aggregation of platelets in the pulmonary circulation, the latter also possibly induced by TXA_2. Studies with either thromboxane synthetase inhibitors[17] or thromboxane receptor antagonists[6] have shown markedly increased survival rates in animals, but only when administered before or with endotoxin. The mortality rate resulting from endotoxin challenge in animals is not significantly reduced when the thromboxane antagonist/synthetase inhibitor follows the endotoxin challenge, indicating that TXA_2 formation may be a causative factor in the early cascade of events leading to the hemodynamic sequelae of endotoxic shock.[17]

The hemodynamic effects mediated by TXA_2 in septic shock have been investigated in detail. As indicated previously, TXA_2 has been implicated as a mediator of pulmonary vasoconstriction during endotoxic shock.[93] High levels of TXA_2 in sepsis correlate with significantly elevated pulmonary artery pressure, pulmonary capillary wedge pressure, and lung lymph flow, and significantly decreased cardiac output. A significant increase in intrapulmonary shunting accompanies the hemodynamic changes induced by TXA_2. Inhibition of TXA_2 synthesis in septic shock with indomethacin, ibuprofen, or imidazole effectively attenuates the pulmonary vasoconstrictor response to endotoxin.

A strong correlation has been noted between increased plasma TXA_2 levels and decreased cardiac output, decreased stroke volume, and decreased left ventricular stroke work.[93] TXA_2-induced elevations in pulmonary vascular resistance preceded late decreases in mean arterial pressure. These interactions support the concept that, in sepsis, increased pulmonary vascular resistance limits the return of blood to the left side of the heart, with subsequent decrements in stroke volume, left ventricular stroke work, and cardiac output, followed by a late decline in mean arterial pressure.[93] Elevated plasma concentrations of TXA_2 appear to precede impaired cardiopulmonary function, a correlation which suggests that TXA_2 may be involved in the detrimental hemodynamic effects of early septicemia.[93] TXA_2 mediation of unstable hemodynamics may occur indirectly through increased pulmonary vascular resistance and/or by means of direct myocardial depression elicited by TXA_2.[27]

LEUKOTRIENES

Only recently have leukotrienes been identified and their structures elucidated. The major components of slow-reacting substance of anaphylaxis are leukotrienes C_4, D_4, and E_4; leukotriene C_4 is the most important component.[35, 90]

The leukotrienes are released in response to a variety of immunologic and nonimmunologic stimuli and have been demonstrated to be involved in contraction of bronchial smooth muscle, stimulation of vascular permeability, attraction and activation of leukocytes, and alteration of myocardial function. The leukotrienes are enzymatic derivatives of arachidonic acid formed via the lipoxygenase enzyme pathway and are synthesized in a variety of tissues and cell types, such as leukocytes, mastocytoma cells, macrophages, lung, kidney, and coronary vasculature.[45, 81, 107]

Not surprisingly, the synthesis and actions of the leukotrienes, prostacyclin, and TXA_2 show a direct interplay. The inhibitory effects of hydroperoxy fatty acids (HPETES), derived from the lipoxygenase pathway, on prostacyclin synthetase are well documented.[33, 70, 89, 103] In addition, the production of lipoxygenase products by endothelial cells may be a natural feedback inhibitor of prostacyclin synthesis.[31] Both LTC_4 and LTD_4 increase TXA_2 generation, as has been shown by the leukotriene-mediated release of TXA_2 from the guinea pig parenchyma. This effect may be due to activation of phospholipase A_2 by certain metabolites of the lipoxygenase pathway.[84]

Effects of Leukotrienes on Coronary Circulation

The leukotrienes C_4, D_4, and E_4 are potent mediators of coronary vasoconstriction and produce negative inotropic effects in a variety of species.[60, 69, 77, 84, 88, 100] Although the leukotriene-mediated negative inotropic response has been repeatedly demonstrated, it has not been conclusively established whether it results from a direct depressant effect on the myocardium or indirectly via coronary artery vasoconstriction.

Coronary artery vasoconstriction induced by LTC_4 is slower acting than that induced by LTD_4, but is much stronger. Cyclo-oxygenase inhibitors can reduce LTC_4-induced vasoconstriction by nearly 50% but do not affect LTD_4, indicating that LTC_4-induced coronary artery vasoconstriction may depend on the release of cyclo-oxygenase products, possibly TXA_2 (see Chapter 8). These observations are consistent with previous reports that TXA_2 is released from isolated guinea pig hearts by products of the lipoxygenase pathway.[1, 3, 4, 61, 64, 92]

Several studies have suggested that LTC_4 and LTD_4 may have direct depressant effects on the myocardium, independent of their effects on coronary blood flow. LTC_4 and LTD_4 decrease left ventricular systolic pressure and left ventricular contractility when perfused into guinea pig hearts.[100] Recently, direct depressant effects of LTC_4, LTD_4, and LTE_4 have been demonstrated in the isolated human pectinate muscle and the right ventricular papillary muscle of the guinea pig.[11] In isolated working guinea pig hearts, leukotriene-induced decreases in contractility were found to occur largely independently of the changes in coronary flow. It has been further shown that doses of angiotensin II producing coronary artery vasoconstriction equal to that seen with the leukotrienes have a smaller negative inotropic effect.[11] This suggests that the leukotrienes have a direct negative inotropic effect above and beyond that which may be attributed to compromised coronary blood flow.

LTD_4 has been shown to impair regional left ventricular systolic shortening independently of the reduction in coronary blood flow. Cyclo-oxygenase inhibitors do not antagonize the coronary artery vasoconstriction induced by LTD_4, indicating that TXA_2 is not produced. These results indicate that LTD_4 may have a negative inotropic effect on the myocardium, independent of coronary artery vasoconstrictive effects and of the release of cyclo-oxygenase products.[69]

It appears that at least part of the LTC_4-mediated effect on myocardial contractility and the coronary vasculature may be due to the release of TXA_2 into the coronary circulation. Recently it has been demonstrated that a selective thromboxane receptor end-organ antagonist inhibits the LTC_4-induced decrease in coronary blood flow.[10] Interestingly, the same thromboxane receptor antagonist was relatively more potent in antagonizing the negative inotropic effect of LTC_4 than in antagonizing the LTC_4-induced decrease in coronary blood flow, again suggesting that leukotrienes produce a negative inotropic effect that is independent of coronary artery vasoconstriction.[10] A recent study has shown that the negative inotropic effect of leukotrienes results from a reduction in calcium influx through the sarcolemmal membrane. This calcium channel blocking effect of the leukotrienes is inhibited by selective leukotriene receptor antagonists, suggesting the involvement of specific leukotriene receptors located in the myocardium.[37]

The dissociation of coronary blood flow from negative inotropy in the presence of a thromboxane receptor antagonist suggests that TXA_2 may partially mediate the negative inotropic effects of LTC_4. However, other possible explanations have been offered for this observed dissociation in the effects of leukotrienes on coronary artery blood flow and inotropy, including the existence of subpopulations of LTC_4 receptors in the coronary vasculature and cardiac muscle.[10]

Systemic Hemodynamic Effects of Leukotrienes

The systemic effects of leukotrienes on blood pressure vary with species and routes of administration. When LTC_4 and LTD_4 are administered intravenously to the guinea pig, there is an initial hypertensive response followed by a long-lasting hypotensive response.[22, 82] When the leukotrienes are given intra-arterially, the hypertensive phase is less marked and the hypotension is more prolonged. Cyclo-oxygenase metabolites may be involved in this leukotriene-mediated response, since inhibitors of the cyclo-oxygenase pathway have been shown to antagonize the hypertensive phase and shorten the duration of the hypotensive phase.

Injection of LTC_4 into the right atrium of

monkeys produces an acute rise in mean arterial pressure, pulmonary artery pressure, and right and left atrial pressures.[94] This initial pressor response results from an increase in both pulmonary and systemic vascular resistance, consistent with the known vasoconstrictive effects of LTC$_4$. Following the acute pressor response induced by LTC$_4$, there is a sustained hypotensive response characterized by a marked decrease in cardiac output and reductions in pulmonary artery pressure and right and left atrial pressures. This secondary hypotensive response is not the result of peripheral arterial vasodilation, since total peripheral vascular resistance actually increases further. It appears, therefore, that the sustained hypotensive response produced by LTC$_4$ results primarily from a reduction in cardiac output, possibly from altered cardiac dynamics secondary to coronary vasoconstriction,[84] or from a direct negative inotropic effect of LTC$_4$.[37] Furthermore, the LTC$_4$-induced pulmonary artery vasoconstriction that leads to increased pulmonary vascular resistance may limit left ventricular filling and thereby also contribute to the observed reduction in cardiac output. Additionally, reduced plasma volume resulting from LTC$_4$-induced increases in vascular permeability may also be a contributing factor and would account for the hemoconcentration (rise in hematocrit) observed after LTC$_4$ administration.[94] An identical hemodynamic profile for LTC$_4$ and LTD$_4$ has also been reported in rats following intravenous administration.[80]

Involvement of Leukotrienes in Human Disease States

Elevated leukotriene levels have been detected in sputum or lung lavage specimens from patients with asthma,[21] cystic fibrosis,[18] and neonatal hypoxemia with pulmonary hypertension.[98] In patients with adult respiratory distress syndrome (ARDS), LTD$_4$ levels and sometimes LTC$_4$ levels in lung edema fluid are significantly elevated.[67] Furthermore, the concentration of LTD$_4$ correlates highly with the ratio of protein concentration in the edema fluid, which suggests that LTD$_4$ might contribute to a fundamental abnormality in transcapillary permeability.[30, 66a]

The vasoconstriction produced by LTC$_4$ and LTD$_4$ in the coronary circulation of various species has led to speculation concerning their involvement in pathophysiologic conditions such as myocardial ischemia, angina, and coronary artery vasospasm. A lipoxygenase system exists in porcine coronary and pulmonary arteries, and these blood vessels can synthesize a leukotriene-like substance, which indicates that some species can generate leukotrienes locally in the coronary circulation.[83]

SUMMARY

Prostacyclin modulates vasoconstriction in the microvasculature resulting from circulating hormones and from enhanced neurogenic tone, and most likely participates in the reactive hyperemic response to hypoxia. Prostacyclin also acts on renal function, augmenting renal blood flow and sodium and water excretion and modulating the vasoconstrictive activity of angiotensin II. Furthermore, prostacyclin appears to be critical to the balance and modulation of hemostasis.

There is an enigmatic interplay between lipoxygenase and cyclo-oxygenase pathways that influences overt cardiovascular responses. The inhibitory action of lipoxygenase products on prostacyclin synthesis, the augmented response of leukotrienes induced (in certain cases) by cyclo-oxygenase inhibitors, the stimulatory effects of leukotrienes on cyclo-oxygenase products, and the stimulation of prostacyclin synthesis by TXA$_2$ and prostaglandin endoperoxides are all critical factors. Indeed, most of the products of the cyclo-oxygenase and lipoxygenase pathways appear to have a pathologic role, but the appearance of these substances in various cardiovascular and immunologic diseases is still subject to interpretation of cause or effect.

The primary sites of prostacyclin synthesis appear to be endothelial cells lining the pulmonary and systemic vasculature. The balance between prostacyclin and TXA$_2$ is a reflection of normal hemostasis and has profound effects on thrombus formation and endothelial repair. A perturbation in this balance has been proposed as a critical factor in the formation of overt thrombi as well as in alterations in cardiac function secondary to changes in coronary blood flow and myocardial contractility. Acutely, alterations in the balance between prostacyclin and TXA$_2$ could be etiologic for a number of ischemic cardiovascular events, such as coronary artery vasospasm, myocardial infarction, and angina. Chronically, an imbalance of this type might lead to coronary artery disease, ischemic heart disease, atherosclerosis, or peripheral vascular disorders.

Hypoxia, and the resultant local or systemic acidosis, is a common predisposing condition to inflammation. Although the exact relationship of prostacyclin release to hypoxia and vasodilation is still unknown, there is ample evidence to suggest that prostacyclin release may be part of a generalized "antihypoxic" response. In conclusion, the therapeutic potential of prostacyclin analogues, as well as of TXA_2 and leukotriene antagonists as antagonists to hypoxic-inflammatory processes, is just being realized.

Acknowledgment

The authors are indebted to Ms. Stephany Ruffolo for her assistance in the preparation of this manuscript.

REFERENCES

1. Allan G, Levi R: Thromboxane and prostacyclin release during cardiac immediate hypersensitivity reactions in vitro. *J Pharmacol Exp Ther* 1981; 217:157.
2. Anderson RJ, Berl T, McDonald KW, et al: Evidence for an in vivo antagonism between vasopressin & prostaglandins in the mammalian kidney. *J Clin Invest* 1975; 56:420.
3. Anhut H, Bernauer W, Peskar BA: Radioimmunological determination of thromboxane release in cardiac anaphylaxis. *Eur J Pharmacol* 1977; 44:85–88.
4. Anhut H, Peskar BA, Bernauer W: Release of 15-keto-13,14-dihydro-thromboxane B_2 and PGD_2 during anaphylaxis as measured by radioimmunoassay. *Naunyn Schmiedebergs Arch Pharmacol* 1978; 305:247.
5. Armstrong RA, Jones RL, Peesapati V, et al: Effect of the thromboxane receptor antagonist EP 092 on the early phase of endotoxin shock in the sheep. *Br J Pharmacol* 1984; 81:72P.
6. Ball HA, Parratt JR: Effects of new thromboxane receptor antagonist, AH23848, on the acute cardiopulmonary responses to *E. coli* endotoxin in cats. *Proc Br Pharm Soc* 1984; C51.
7. Berl T, Raz A, Wald H, et al: Prostaglandin synthesis inhibition and the action of vasopressin: Studies in man and rat. *Am J Physiol* 1977; 232:F529.
8. Borget P, Samuelsson B: Arachidonic acid metabolism in polymorphonuclear leukocytes: Effects of inophore A23187. *Proc Natl Acad Sci USA* 1979; 76:2143.
9. Brotherton AF, Hoak JC: Role of Ca^{+2} and cyclic AMP in the regulation of the production of prostacyclin by the vascular endothelium. *Proc Natl Acad Sci USA* 1982; 79:495–499.
10. Burke JA, Levi R, Gleason JG: Antagonism of the cardiac effects of leukotriene C_4 by compound SKF 88046: Dissociation of effects on contractility and coronary flow. *J Cardiovasc Pharmacol* 1984; 6(1):122.
11. Burke JA, Levi R, Guo Z-G, et al: Leukotrienes C_4, D_4, and E_4: Effects on human and guinea pig cardiac preparations in vitro. *J Pharmacol Exp Ther* 1982; 221:235.
12. Burke SE, DiCola G, Lefer AM: Protection of ischemic cat myocardium by CGS-13080, a selective potent thromboxane A_2 synthetase inhibitor. *J Cardiovasc Pharmacol* 1983; 5(5):842.
13. Casey L, Fletcher JR, Zmudka MI, et al: Prevention of endotoxin-induced pulmonary hypertension in primates by the use of a selective thromboxane synthetase inhibitor, OXY 1581. *J Pharmacol Exp Ther* 1982; 222(2):441.
14. Coker SJ, Parratt JR: Antiarrhythmic activity of the thromboxane antagonist AH23848 during canine myocardial ischemia and reperfusion. *Proc Br Pharm Soc* 1984; C52.
15. Chierchia S: Pathogenetic mechanisms of coronary vasospasm. *Acta Med Scand Suppl* 1982; 660:49.
16. Coleman RA, Humphrey PPA, Kennedy I, et al: Comparison of the actions of U-46619, a prostaglandin H_2-analogue with those of prostaglandin H_2 and thromboxane A_2 on some isolated smooth muscle preparations. *Br J Pharmacol* 1981; 73:773.
17. Cook JA, Wise WC, Halushka PV: Elevated thromboxane levels in the rat during endotoxic shock. *J Clin Invest* 1980; 65:227.
18. Cromwell O, Walport MJ, Morris H, et al: Identification of leukotrienes D and B in sputum from cystic fibrosis patients. *Lancet* 1981; 8236(2):164.
19. Currie M, Needleman P: Renal arachidonic acid metabolism. *Annu Rev Physiol* 1984; 46:327.
20. Dahl M, Uotila P: Thromboxane formation during blood clotting is decreased by verapamil. *Prostaglandins Leukotrienes Med* 1984; 13:217.
21. Dahlen S, Hansson G, Hedqvist P, et al: Allergen challenge of lung tissues from asth-

matics elicits bronchial contraction that correlates with the release of leukotrienes C_4, D_4, and E_4. *Proc Natl Acad Sci USA* 1983; 80:1712.

22. Drazen JM, Austen KF, Lewis DA, et al: Comparative airway and vascular activities of leukotrienes C-1 and D in vivo and in vitro. *Proc Natl Acad Sci USA* 1980; 77:4354.

23. Du JT, Foegh M, Maddox Y, et al: Human peritoneal macrophages synthesize leukotrienes B_4 and C_4. *Biochim Biophys Acta* 1983; 753:159.

24. Dunn MJ: Renal prostaglandins, in Klahr S, Massry SG (eds): *Contemp Nephrol* 1983; 2:145–193.

25. Flower RJ: Prostaglandins and related compounds, in Vane JR, Ferreira SH (eds): *Inflammation*. New York, Springer-Verlag, 1978, pp 374–422.

26. Friedman PL Brown EJ Jr, Gunther S, et al: Coronary vasoconstrictor effect of indomethacin in patients with coronary-artery disease. *N Engl J Med* 1978; 305:1171.

27. Friedman LW, Fitzpatrick TM, Bloom MF: Cardiovascular and pulmonary effects of thromboxane B_2 in the dog. *Circ Res* 1978; 44:748–751.

28. Fulgraff G, Brandenbusch G: Comparison of the effects of the prostaglandins A_1, E_2, and $F_{2\alpha}$ on kidney function in dogs. *Pflugers Arch* 1974; 349(1):9–17.

29. Gerrard JM: Prostaglandins and Leukotrienes: Blood and Vascular Cell Function, in Gerrard JM (ed): *Hematology*. New York, 1985, vol. 1, pp 77–106.

30. Goetzel EJ, Payan DG, Goldman DW: Immunopathogenetic roles of leukotrienes in human diseases. *J Clin Immunol* 1984; 4(2):79.

31. Greenwald JE, Bianchine JR, Wong LK: The production of the arachidonate metabolite HETE in vascular tissue. *Nature* 1979; 281:588.

32. Gryglewski RJ, Korbut R, Ogetkiewicz A, et al: Lungs as a generator of prostacyclin: Hypothesis on physiological significance. *Naunyn Schmiedebergs Arch Pharmacol* 1978; 304:45.

33. Ham EA, Egan RW, Soderman DD, et al: Peroxidase-dependent deactivation of prostacyclin synthetase. *J Biol Chem* 1979; 254:2191.

34. Hamberg M, Samuelsson B: Prostaglandin endoperoxides: Novel transformations of arachidonic acid in human platelets. *Proc Natl Acad Sci USA* 1974; 71:3400.

35. Hammarstrom S: Leukotrienes. *Annu Rev Biochem* 1983; 52:355.

36. Hassid A: Stimulation of prostacyclin synthesis by thromboxane A_2-like prostaglandin endoperoxide analogs in cultured vascular smooth muscle cells. *Biochem Biophys Res Commun* 1984; 123(1):21–26.

37. Hattori Y, Levi R: Negative inotropic effect of leukotrienes: LTC_4 and LTD_4 inhibit calcium dependent contractile responses in potassium-depolarized guinea pig myocardium. *J Pharmacol Exp Ther* 1984; 230(3):646–651.

38. Haylor J, Lote CJ: Renal function in conscious rats after indomethacin: Evidence for a tubular action of endogenous prostaglandins. *J Physiol* 1980; 298:371.

39. Hellstrom HR: Coronary artery stasis after induced myocardial infarction in the dog. *Cardiovasc Res* 1971; 5:371.

40. Henriksson P, Edhag O, Wennmalm A: Limitations of myocardial infarction with prostacyclin: A double-blind study, in Grycglewski R (ed): *Prostacyclin: Clinical Trials*. New York, Raven Press, 1985, pp 31–42.

41. Hopkins NK, Gorman RR: Regulation of endothelial cell cyclic nucleotide metabolism by prostacyclin. *J Clin Invest* 1981; 67:540–546.

42. Hoshida S, Ohmori M, Kuzuya T, et al: Augmented thromboxane A_2 generation and efficacy of its blockade in acute myocardial infarction. *Jpn Circ J* 1983; 47:1026.

43. Humphrey PPA, Lumley P: The effects of AH23848, a novel thromboxane receptor blocking drug, on platelets and vasculature. *Proc Br Pharm Soc* 1984; C50.

44. Ito T, Sikano M, Chen LS, et al: Effects of selective thromboxane A_2 synthetase inhibitor (OKY-1581, 046) in patients with angina pectoris and acute myocardial infarction. *Jpn Circ J* 1983; 47:896.

45. Jim K, Dunn M, Hassid A, et al: Lipoxygenase activity in rat renal glomeruli. *J Biol Chem* 1982; 257:10294.

46. Johnston HH, Herzog JP, Lauler OP: Effect of prostaglandin E_1 on renal hemodynamics, sodium and water excretion. *Am J Physiol* 1967; 213(4):939–946.

47. Jones RL, Smith GM, Wilson NH: The effects of a synthetic prostanoid EP 092 on in-

travascular platelet aggregation and broncho-constriction. *Br J Pharmacol* 1984; 81:100P.

48. Jones RL, Peesapati V, Wilson NH: Antagonism of the thromboxane-sensitive contractile systems of the rabbit aorta, dog saphenous vein and guinea pig trachea. *Br J Pharmacol* 1982; 76:423.

49. Kadowitz PJ, Chapnick B, Feigen LP, et al: Pulmonary and systemic vasodilator effects of the newly discovered prostaglandin, PGI_2. *J Appl Physiol* 1978; 45:408.

50. Kadowitz PJ, Lippton HL, McNamara DB, et al: Cardiovascular actions of the prostaglandins, in Antonaccio M (ed): *Cardiovascular Pharmacology*. New York, Raven Press, 1984, pp 453–474.

51. Kilbom A, Wennmalm A: Endogenous prostaglandins as local regulators of blood flow in man: Effect of indomethacin on reactive and functional hyperaemia. *J Physiol* 1976; 257:109.

52. Konieczkowski M, Dunn MJ, Hassid A: Glomerular synthesis of prostaglandins and thromboxane in spontaneously hypertensive rats. *Fed Proc* 1982; 41:1543.

53. Kuzuya T, Tada M, Hoshida S, et al: Excessive thromboxane A_2 generation could be a possible aggravating factor in unstable angina. *Circulation* 1983; 68:398.

54. Lapetina EG: Regulation of arachidonic acid production: Role of Phospholipase C and A_2. *Trends Pharmacol Sci* 1982; 3:115.

55. Lapetina EG, Schmitges CJ, Chandrabose K, et al: Cyclic adenosine $3',5'$-monophosphate and prostacyclin inhibit membrane phospholipase activity in platelets. *Biochem Biophys Res Commun* 1977; 76:828.

56. Larrue J, Dorian B, Daret D, et al: Role of cyclic AMP in the regulation of prostacyclin synthesis by cultured vascular smooth muscle cells. *Cyclic Nucleotide Res* 1984; 17:585–593.

57. Lefer AM, Okamatsu S, Smith EF, et al: Beneficial effects of a new thromboxane synthetase inhibitor in arachidonate-induced sudden death. *Thrombosis Res* 1981; 23:265.

58. Lefer AM, Smith JB, Nicolaou KC: Cardiovascular actions of two thromboxane A_2 analogs, in Hamar J, Szabo L (eds): *Cardiovascular Physiology: Microcirculation and Capillary Exchange*. Vol 7 in *Advances in Physiological Science*. New York, Pergamon Press, 1981, pp 91–98.

59. Lefer AM, Ogletree ML, Smith JB, et al:

Prostacyclin: A potentially valuable agent for preserving myocardial tissue in acute myocardial ischemia. *Science* 1978; 200:5.

60. Letts LG, Piper PJ: The actions of leukotrienes C_4 and D_4 on guinea pig isolated hearts. *Br J Pharmacol* 1982; 76:169.

61. Levi R, Allan G, Zavecz JH: Prostaglandins and cardiac anaphylaxis. *Life Sci* 1976; 18:1255.

62. Lewey RI, Wiener L, Smith JB, et al: Comparison of plasma concentrations of thromboxane B_2 in Prinzmetal's variant angina and classical angina pectoris. *Clin Cardiol* 1980; 2:404.

63. Lewey RI, Wiener L, Walinsky P, et al: Thromboxane release during pacing induced angina pectoris: Possible vasoconstrictor influence on the coronary vasculature. *Circulation* 1980; 61:1165.

64. Liebig R, Bernauer W, Peskar BA: Prostaglandin, slow-reacting substance and histamine release from anaphylactic guinea pig hearts and its pharmacological modification. *Naunyn Schmiedebergs Arch Pharmacol* 1975; 289:65.

65. Linet OI: Prostacyclin: A review of current clinical experience. *Postgrad Med* 1982; 72(6):105.

66. Lum GM, Aisenbrey GA, Dunn MJ, et al: In vivo effect of indomethacin to potentiate the renal medullary cyclic AMP response to vasopressin. *J Clin Invest* 1977; 59:8.

66a. Malik AB: *Prostaglandins, Leukotrienes, and Lung Fluid Balance* (symposium). *Fed Proc* 1985; 44:18–52.

67. Matthay MA, Eschenbacher WC, Goetzel EJ: Leukotrienes in the airway edema fluid of patients with the adult respiratory distress syndrome. *Clin Res* (in press).

68. Messina EJ, Weiner R, Kaley G: Arteriolar reactive hyperemia: Modification by inhibitors of prostaglandin synthesis. *Am J Physiol* 1977; 232:H571.

69. Michelassi F, Castorena G, Hill RD, et al: Effects of leukotrienes B_4 and C_4 on coronary circulation and myocardial contractility. *Surgery* 1982; 93:267.

70. Moncada S, Gryglewski RJ, Bunting S, et al: A lipid peroxide inhibits the enzyme in blood vessel microsomes that generates from prostacyclin endoperoxides the substance (prostaglandin X) which prevents platelet aggregation. *Prostaglandins* 1976; 12:715.

71. Moncada S, Vane JR: Unstable metabolites

of arachidonic acid and their role in haemostasis and thrombosis. *Br Med Bull* 1978; 34:129.

72. Moncada S, Vane JR: Discovery of prostacyclin—fresh insight into arachidonic acid metabolism, in Kharasch N, Fried J (eds): *Biochemical Aspects of Prostaglandins and Thromboxanes*. New York, Academic Press, 1977, pp 155–177.

73. Mullane KM, Dusting GJ, Salmon JA, et al: Biotransformation and cardiovascular effects of arachidonic acid in the dog. *Eur J Pharmacol* 1979; 54:217–228.

74. Nicolaou KC, Magolda RL, Smith JB, et al: Synthesis and biological properties of pinane-thromboxane A$_2$, a selective inhibitor of coronary artery constriction, platelet aggregation, and thromboxane formation. *Proc Natl Acad Sci USA* 1979; 76(6):2566.

75. Nowak J, Wennmalm A: A study on the role of endogenous prostaglandins in the development of exercise induced and post-occlusive hyperemia in human limbs. *Acta Physiol Scand* 1979; 106:365.

76. Ohmori M, Tada M, Kuzuya T, et al: Thromboxane A$_2$ as a precipitating factor in coronary arterial spasm of variant angina. *Circulation* 1983; 68(3):22.

77. Panzenbeck MJ, Kaley G: Leukotriene D$_4$ reduces coronary blood flow in the anesthetized dog. *Prostaglandins* 1983; 25(5):661.

78. Parise LV, Venton DL, Le Breton GC: Arachidonic acid-induced platelet aggregation is mediated by a thromboxane A$_2$/prostaglandin H$_2$ receptor interaction. *J Pharmacol Exp Ther* 1984; 228(1):240.

79. Pawlowski NA, Kaplan G, Hamill AL: Arachidonic acid metabolism by human monocytes. *J Exp Med* 1983; 158:393.

80. Pfeffer MA, Pfeffer JM, Lewis RA, et al: Systemic hemodynamic effects of leukotrienes C$_4$ and D$_4$ in the rat. *Am J Physiol* 1983; 244:H628.

81. Piper PJ: Formation and actions of leukotrienes. *Physiol Rev* 1984; 64(2):744–761.

82. Piper PJ, Samhoun MN, Tippins JR, et al: Pharmacological studies on pure SRS-A, and synthetic leukotrienes C$_4$ and D$_4$, in Piper PJ (ed): *SRS-A and Leukotrienes*. New York, John Wiley & Sons, Inc, 1981, pp 81–99.

83. Piper PJ, Letts LG, Galton SA: Generation of a leukotriene-like substance from porcine vascular and other tissues. *Prostaglandins* 1983; 25:591.

84. Piper PJ, Samhoun MN: Stimulation of arachidonic acid metabolism and generation of thromboxane A$_2$ by leukotrienes B$_4$, C$_4$, and D$_4$ in guinea-pig lung in vitro. *Br J Pharmacol* 1982; 77:267.

85. Pitt B, Shea MJ, Romson JL, et al: Prostaglandins and prostaglandin inhibitors in ischemic heart disease. *Annu Rev Med* 1983; 99:83–92.

86. Ribeiro LGT, Brandon TA, Hopkins DG, et al: Prostacyclin in experimental myocardial ischemia: Effects on hemodynamics, regional myocardial blood flow, infarct size and mortality. *Am J Cardiol* 1981; 47:835.

87. Rosenkranz B, Wilson TW, Seyberth H, et al: Prostaglandins and renal blood flow, in *Proceedings of the 8th International Congress of Nephrology*. Athens, 1981, pp 1045–1052.

88. Roth DM, Foster KA, Lefer AM: Coronary vascular responsiveness to non-eicosanoid vasoconstrictors in the perfused diabetic rat heart. *Res Commun Chem Pathol Pharmacol* 1984; 45(2):317–320.

89. Salmon JA, Smith DR, Flower RJ, et al: Further studies on the enzymatic conversion of prostaglandin endoperoxide into prostacyclin by porcine aorta microsomes. *Biochim Biophys Acta* 1978; 523:250–262.

90. Samuelsson B, Hammarstrom S, Murphy RC, et al: Luekotrienes and slow reacting substances of anaphylaxis (SRS-A). *Allergy* 1980; 35:375–381.

91. Schror K, Smith EF, Bickerton M, et al: Preservation of ischemic myocardium by pinane thromboxane A$_2$. *Am J Physiol* 1980; 238:H87–H92.

92. Schror K, Moncada S, Ubatuba FB, et al: Transformation of arachidonic acid and prostaglandin endoperoxides by the guinea pig heart: Formation of RCS and prostacyclin. *Eur J Pharmacol* 1978; 47:103.

93. Slotman GJ, Quinn JV, Burchard KW, et al: Thromboxane interaction with cardiopulmonary dysfunction in graded bacterial sepsis. *J Trauma* 1984; 24(9):803–810.

94. Smedegard G, Hedqvist P, Dahlen S-E, et al: Leukotriene C$_4$ affects pulmonary and cardiovascular dynamics in monkey. *Nature* 1982; 295:327.

95. Smith EF, Lefer AM, Aharony D, et al: Carbocyclic thromboxane A$_2$: Aggravation of myocardial ischemia by a new synthetic thromboxane A$_2$ analog. *Prostaglandins* 1981; 21(3):443.

96. Smith EF, Lefer AM, Smith JB: Influence of inhibition on the severity of myocardial ischemia in cats. *Can J Physiol Pharmacol* 1980; 58:294.

97. Spann JF: Changing concepts of pathophysiology, prognosis, and therapy in acute myocardial infarction. *Am J Med* 1983; 74:877.

98. Stenmark KR, James SL, Voelkel NF, et al: Leukotrienes C_4 and D_4 in neonates with hypoxemia and pulmonary hypertension. *N Engl J Med* 1983; 309:77.

99. Tanabe M, Terashita Z-I, Fijiwara S, et al: Coronary circulation failure and thromboxane A_2 release during coronary occlusion and reperfusion in anesthetized dogs. *Cardiovasc Res* 1982; 16:99.

100. Terashita Z-I, Fukui H, Hirata M, et al: Coronary vasoconstriction and PGI_2 release by leukotrienes in isolated guinea pig hearts. *Eur J Pharmacol* 1981; 73:357–361.

101. Toda N: Responses of human, monkey and dog coronary arteries *in vitro* to carbocyclic thromboxane A_2 and vasodilators. *Br J Pharmacol* 1984; 83:399.

102. Thomas M, Lumley P, Hornby EJ: A study to investigate the effects of a novel thromboxane receptor blocking drug AH 23848 on platelet aggregation *ex vivo* in man. *Proc Br Pharm Soc* 1984; C17.

103. Turk J, Wyche A, Needleman P: Inactivation of vascular prostacyclin synthetase by platelet lipoxygenase products. *Biochem Biophys Res Commun* 1980; 95:1628.

104. Walker JL: Interrelationships of SRS-A production and arachidonic acid metabolism in human lung tissue. *Adv Prostaglandin Thromboxane Res* 1980; 8:115–119.

105. Wennmalm A: Participation of prostaglandins in the regulation of peripheral vascular resistance, in Oates J (ed): *Prostaglandins and the Cardiovascular System*. New York, Raven Press, 1982, pp 303–331.

106. Whittle BJR, Moncada S: Prostacyclin-thromboxane interactions in hemostasis, in Antonaccio M (ed): *Cardiovascular Pharmacology*. New York, Raven Press, 1984, pp 519–534.

107. Winokur TS, Morrison AR: Regional synthesis of monohydroxy eicosanoids by the kidney. *J Biol Chem* 1981; 256:10221.

108. Yui Y, Hattori R, Takatsu Y, et al: Is increased coronary sinus thromboxane A_2 production a cause or result of vasospastic angina? *Circulation* 1983; 68(3):397.

PART 3 ——————   Cellular Oxygenation

10 _____ Oxygen Transport From Capillary to Cell

John B. Cone, M.D.

Adequate tissue oxygenation requires an intact microcirculation in addition to a well-functioning cardiopulmonary core. Clinical interest in the microcirculation has increased with the availability of techniques to assess local oxygenation and drugs that have selective microcirculatory effects. For discussions of the anatomy, physiology, and pharmacology of the microcirculation, we refer the reader to reviews published elsewhere.[7, 19] This chapter is limited to the transport of oxygen from the capillary to the cell.

The quantitative description of tissue oxygenation was pioneered by August Krogh in 1919.[11, 12] Although this early mathematical treatment has many shortcomings, it stands today as a useful tool for understanding the influence of many variables on tissue oxygenation. After studying the arrangement of capillaries in skeletal muscle, Krogh chose a cylinder of tissue with a capillary passing along its axis as his geometric model. Oxygen tension within the tissue was assumed to depend on the distance to the nearest capillary, the intercapillary distance (twice the radius of the "tissue cylinder"), the radius of the capillary, the tissue metabolic rate, and the diffusion coefficient of oxygen through the tissue. Two additional assumptions are inherent in this theory: that only radial, not longitudinal, oxygen pressure gradients contribute to tissue diffusion, and that adjacent capillaries are independent of one another. With this hypothesis, Krogh and the Danish mathematician Erlang developed the equation that bears their name:[11]

$$P_x = P_{O_2} - \frac{\dot{V}_{O_2}}{2K^2}\left(R^2 \ln \frac{x}{r} - \frac{x^2 - r^2}{2}\right)$$

(Eq. 10–1)

where P_x is the partial pressure of oxygen (P_{O_2}) at a point in the tissue at distance x from the capillary; R is the radius of the tissue cylinder and r the radius of the capillary; $\dot{V}_{O_2}$ is the tissue oxygen consumption; and K is a constant reflecting the oxygen solubility in tissue and the diffusion coefficient for oxygen. This equation predicts the radial oxygen diffusion gradient shown in Figure 10–1.

If we postulate a uniform tissue metabolic rate, the decline in oxygen content along the axis of the capillary will be linear. It follows from the oxyhemoglobin dissociation curve that the partial pressure will drop off more rapidly (see Fig 10–1). If we combine the linear and radial oxygen gradients to form a three-dimensional structure, the P_{O_2} isobars (points of equal oxygen tension) form cones with their apexes at the venous end of the capillaries. Equation 10–1 thus predicts that the earliest sites of tissue hypoxia will be those areas farthest from the venous ends of the capillaries ("deadly corners").

The Krogh-Erlang equation allows us to predict the results of changes in its several parameters. For a more detailed discussion of the predictive value of this approach it is valuable to use the experimentally determined values for parameters such as intercapillary distance and metabolic rate.[10] In general we can predict that the greater the intercapillary distance, the lower the diffusion coefficient; and the higher the metabolic rate, the greater the degree of tissue hypoxia and the steeper the radial diffusion curve of Figure 10–1. Conversely, in tissue with a low metabolic rate and small intercapillary distance, tissue P_{O_2} will closely approximate capillary oxygen tension.

Several investigators have shown experimentally that tissue P_{O_2} tracks arterial P_{O_2} in tissue that is well perfused with an acceptable hemoglobin concentration, whereas in poorly perfused tissue, the tissue P_{O_2} reflects perfusion.[2] To many, this may seem surprising, because of the widespread belief that tissue P_{O_2} is a function only of total oxygen delivery and that Pa_{O_2} greater than

153

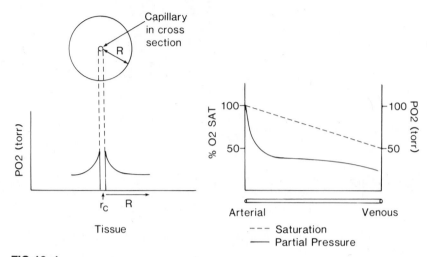

FIG 10–1.
Oxygen tension gradients around single capillary. (From Seisjo.[17] Reproduced by permission.)

80 torr has no benefit to the tissue. As we see from the predictions above, however, when oxygen delivery satisfies tissue oxygen needs, tissue Po_2 will follow Pa_{O_2}. Elevation of Pa_{O_2} to raise tissue Po_2 may be of value in tissues with ischemic or nonperfused areas, which depend on diffusion from adjacent tissue.

The Krogh-Erlang equation, in spite of its conceptual usefulness, has limitations that preclude its ability to quantitatively predict tissue oxygen tension. Just as oxygen is delivered along the path of the capillary, carbon dioxide produced in the tissue is taken up. As a result, pH decreases. Because of the Bohr effect, this drop in capillary pH causes a higher Po_2 at the venous end of the capillary. The difference is significant: venous Po_2 may be 40% higher than would otherwise occur.[19] Furthermore, the intercapillary distance may not be constant from arteriole to venule: it has been reported that the capillary density increases toward the venous end of the capillary.[19] These mechanisms may protect the "deadly corners." In those tissues containing myoglobin, there is a third protective mechanism. Myoglobin, like hemoglobin, reversibly binds oxygen. Myoglobin thus serves two functions. First, the oxygen bound to myoglobin at any time serves as a small but potentially important reservoir for the myocyte. Second, when oxygen is bound to myoglobin, its diffusion into the cell is facilitated; the diffusion coefficient for oxygen is effectively increased.

Many attempts have been made to extend the Krogh-Erlang equation by including additional parameters, such as those just described. However, these variations have been little more successful than Krogh's original model. The major weakness in all mathematical descriptions of the microcirculation is our inability to describe the geometry of the capillary bed. Capillaries do not consistently run in parallel and independently supply a single tissue cylinder. Even in striated muscle, the example studied by Krogh, the parallel arrangement does not persist during contraction.[4] Furthermore, the entire capillary bed does not seem to be perfused simultaneously. Experimental studies indicate that the microvascular beds are constantly "winking" open and closed.[17] These complicating factors have made an exact mathematical description of the microcirculation impossible. The Krogh-Erlang equation stands as a simple and suitable basis for conceptual considerations.

Inhomogeneous perfusion, shunting, and nonnutritive flow are important influences on tissue oxygenation. Although significant anatomical arteriovenous channels have not been demonstrated in normal tissue, significant shunting of highly diffusible gases such as oxygen may occur.[8] This diffusional shunting may occur between artery and vein or between capillary beds with countercurrent flow. Such shunts may be of clinical importance for two reasons. They may be of sufficient magnitude to compromise the oxygenation of the tissue. Furthermore, oxygen that bypasses the tissue elevates the venous oxygen content, which then misrepresents the tissue P_{O_2}. This may contribute to the discrepancy often seen between venous oxygen saturation and clinical assessment of the adequacy of tissue oxygenation.

Normally, local blood flow, oxygen demand, and oxygen delivery are closely coupled. However, strenuous exercise, vasodilator therapy, and perhaps other conditions may alter this coupling. Vasodilators may reduce resistance and increase flow to some capillary beds, resulting in a decreased flow and decreased oxygen consumption in adjacent beds.[13] In support of this is the observation that vasodilator infusions into isolated muscle can result in a loss of contractile force, which could indicate inadequate oxygenation.[6]

Changes in resistance at the microcirculatory level are difficult to interpret. In skeletal muscle only about 20% of the total vascular resistance is due to the capillaries. If the number of open capillaries is doubled and the intercapillary distance halved, the capillary resistance is also halved. The change in total vascular resistance may be only 10% and go undetected. However, as can be seen from equation 10–1, reducing the intercapillary distance by a factor of 2 notably increases tissue oxygen tension.

CLINICAL CORRELATION

In normal mammalian tissues oxygen consumption is independent of oxygen delivery over a wide range of values. Only when delivery is limited or metabolic demand increased does oxygen consumption correlate with delivery. In contrast, in some critically ill patients peripheral oxygen utilization is impaired such that oxygen consumption depends on oxygen delivery. This occurs in spite of a normal to high cardiac output and a high mixed venous oxygen level. This impairment of oxygen utilization has been reported in shock, trauma,[14] ARDS,[3] and sepsis.[9] In spite of the apparently good cardiac output and oxygen delivery ($\dot{D}_{O_2}$), this phenomenon suggests inadequate resuscitation. Although the mechanisms underlying these changes are not clearly established, the findings may be explained by a disturbance in microcirculation, according to the concepts presented earlier.

To resuscitate patients from shock, trauma, or sepsis, we often infuse a large volume of crystalloid solution, which results in tissue edema.

This soft tissue edema reduces tissue P_{O_2}.[2, 5, 18] The decrease is probably the result of increased intercapillary distance, although an alteration in the diffusion properties of the interstitial matrix has not been ruled out. Interstitial edema, when accompanied by an increase in interstitial pressure, may compromise capillary blood flow and $\dot{D}_{O_2}$. Patients resuscitated with large volumes of fluid have been shown to have increased circulating particulate matter and resulting microembolization.[15] This capillary occlusion may reduce capillary density and increase intercapillary distance.

Interstitial edema and endothelial cell edema with capillary occlusion are also associated with the reperfusion syndromes that accompany restoration of flow after severe ischemia.[1]

Each of these mechanisms may reduce tissue P_{O_2} and thus create a need for a higher oxygen level on the venous side of the capillary to oxygenate the expanded "deadly corners." To achieve adequate tissue oxygenation, a higher cardiac output and mixed venous oxygen tension are needed. The problem may be further complicated by ischemia distal to obstructed capillaries. The ischemic tissue may elaborate vasodilator substances such as hydrogen ion and adenosine, which diffuse to the still open capillaries, reducing their resistance and further compromising tissue oxygenation as discussed above.

To test each of these mechanisms under controlled conditions, Shah et al.[16] used the isolated canine hind limb as a model. They separately produced edema by massive crystalloid infusion, microembolization by polystyrene microspheres, and reperfusion syndrome by controlled hypotension. Interstitial edema decreased oxygen delivery but did not change oxygen utilization. However, in both microembolization and reperfusion, oxygen consumption was dependent on oxygen delivery when venous oxygen was normal or higher than normal.

Using their model to reproduce impaired peripheral oxygen utilization, Shah et al.[16] attempted to normalize oxygen utilization pharmacologically. The impaired oxygen utilization that followed reperfusion and microembolization was corrected by mannitol and imidazole, respectively.

While we have not yet defined the elements of tissue oxygenation in a satisfactory mathematical model, our understanding has continued to increase. The fundamental importance of partial pressure gradient as the driving force moving oxygen to the cell and the concept of deadly corners are important to consider clinically. High Pa_{O_2} may ameliorate the deadly corners; elevation of oxygen delivery may improve tissue oxygenation in states such as ARDS and sepsis. It seems likely that these and related microcirculatory dynamics are keys to the hemodynamic patterns we see clinically, and to appropriate therapy.

REFERENCES

1. Ames A, Wright RL, Kowada M: Cerebral ischemia, the no reflow phenomena. *Am J Pathol* 1968; 52:437–450.
2. Chang N, Goodson WH, Gottrup F, et al: Direct measurement of wound and tissue oxygen tension in postoperative patients. *Ann Surg* 1983; 197:470–478.
3. Danek KJ, Lynch JP, Wey JG, et al: The dependence of oxygen uptake on oxygen delivery in the adult respiratory distress syndrome. *Am Rev Respir Dis* 1980; 122:387–395.
4. Ellis CG, Potter RF, Groom AC: The Krogh cylinder geometry is not appropriate for modelling O_2 transport in contracted skeletal muscle. *Adv Exp Biol Med* 1983; 159:253–268.
5. Heughan C, Niinikoski J, Hunt TK: Effect of excessive infusion of saline solution on tissue oxygen transport. *Surg Gynecol Obstet* 1972; 135:257–260.
6. Hirvonen L, Korobkin M, Sonnenschein RR, et al: Depression of contractile force of skeletal muscle by intra-arterial vasodilatory drugs. *Circ Res* 1964; 14:525–535.
7. Kaley G, Altura BM (eds): *Microcirculation*. Baltimore, University Park Press, 1978.
8. Kampp M, Lundgren O, Nilsson NJ: Extravascular shunting of oxygen in the small intestine of the cat. *Acta Physiol Scand* 1968; 72:396–403.
9. Kaufman BS, Rackow EC, Falk JL: The relationship between oxygen delivery and consumption during fluid resuscitation of hypovolemic and septic shock. *Chest* 1984; 85:336–340.
10. Kety SS: Determinants of tissue oxygen tension. *Fed Proc* 1957; 16:666–670.
11. Krogh A (ed): *Anatomy and Physiology of Capillaries*. New Haven, Yale University Press, 1922.
12. Krogh A: The number and distribution of capillaries in muscles with calculations of the oxygen pressure head necessary for supplying the tissue. *J Physiol* 1919; 52:409–415.
13. Renkin EM: Transcapillary exchange in relation to capillary circulation. *J Gen Physiol* 1968; 52(suppl):96S–107S.
14. Rhodes GR, Newell JC, Shah DM, et al: Increased oxygen consumption accompanying increased oxygen delivery with hypertonic mannitol in adult respiratory distress syndrome. *Surgery* 1978; 84:490–497.
15. Saldeen T: The microembolization syndrome. *Microvasc Res* 1976; 11:227–259.
16. Shah DM, Newell JC, Saba TM: Defects in peripheral oxygen utilization following trauma and shock. *Arch Surg* 1981; 116:1277–1281.
17. Siesjö BK: *Brain Energy Metabolism*. New York, John Wiley & Sons, Inc, 1978.
18. Silver IA: The role of oxygen in some aspects of tissue repair, in Kessler M, Bruley T, Grunewald S (eds): *Oxygen Supply*. Baltimore, University Park Press, 1973, pp 294–296.
19. Weibel ER (ed): *The Pathway for Oxygen*. Cambridge, Mass, Harvard University Press, 1984.

11 _____ Cellular Oxygen Utilization

John B. Cone, M.D.

Sustained synthesis of high-energy compounds such as adenosine triphosphate (ATP) by the mitochondria is crucial to the survival of the cell. While numerous substrates are capable of providing reducing equivalents via the Krebs cycle to mitochondrial oxidative phosphorylation, only molecular oxygen is able to function as the terminal acceptor, in the process of which it is reduced to water. Since tissue stores of oxygen are minimal, adequate oxygen delivery to the cells is a major concern in the care of the critically ill. Although the importance of tissue oxygenation is universally recognized, the only tissue whose oxygenation is approached on a scientific basis clinically is the blood. This is not tunnel vision, but the result of a nearly total lack of nondestructive analytic techniques for monitoring the oxygenation and metabolism of other tissues. The usual approach is to monitor function and assume that if function is preserved, oxygen delivery is adequate. Although it may be true in many cases that normal function implies at least minimally adequate oxygenation, the converse is far from true. There are many causes of organ dysfunction unrelated to oxygen deficit. With the advent of newer techniques for assessing tissue oxygen metabolism in vivo, it becomes increasingly important for the critical care physician to have a basic understanding of the role of oxygen in the cell and the metabolic effects of altered oxygen metabolism, dysoxia.

The role of oxygen can be considered in terms of mitochondrial and nonmitochondrial oxygen metabolism. Mitochondrial oxygen utilization accounts for 80%–90% of total cellular oxygen consumption. This is the conventional role for oxygen, the provision of energy for the cell via oxidative phosphorylation. Less widely recognized and less well studied is the role of oxygen outside the mitochondria. Here oxygen participates in mixed-function oxidase reactions and is chemically incorporated into larger molecules. Although intramitochondrial and extramitochondrial oxygen consumption are undoubtedly interrelated in vivo, each will be considered independently here.

OXIDATIVE PHOSPHORYLATION

Oxidative phosphorylation, the process by which cellular oxygen consumption produces usable energy, is in fact two chemical reaction sequences that under normal circumstances are tightly coupled. Most of the energy used by the cell comes from ATP produced by the phosphorylation of adenosine diphosphate (ADP) to ATP, as shown in equation 11–1:

$$ADP + P_i + H^+ \rightleftharpoons ATP + H_2O, \Delta G = +7.3 \text{ kcal/mole} \qquad \text{(Eq. 11–1)}$$

where P_i is inorganic phosphate. This reaction obviously requires an exogenous source of energy if it is to proceed from left to right. Specifically, 7.3 kcal must be supplied for each mole of ATP synthesized.

The other component of oxidative phosphorylation is a sequence of reactions known as the respiratory or electron transport chain. This sequence of reactions takes reducing equivalents* from the Krebs cycle in the form of reduced nicotinamide adenine dinucleotide (NADH) and reduced flavin adenine dinucleotide (FADH) and reduces molecular oxygen to water. In the case of NADH, the free energy change that results is 53 kcal. As shown in Figure 11–1, this free energy change occurs in a series of steps, three of which are large enough to allow the synthesis of

___
*These reducing equivalents may be thought of as hydrogen ions, although in many cases it is electrons that are actually transported.

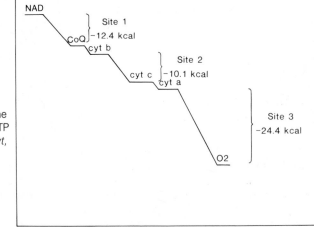

FIG 11–1.

Sites of free energy change in the respiratory chain, and sites of ATP synthesis. *CoQ,* coenzyme Q; *cyt,* cytochrome.

Free Energy Change in the Respiratory Chain
Showing the Sites of ATP Synthesis

ATP. These three steps are the sites of coupling of electron transport, and hence are the sites of oxygen consumption, to phosphorylation and the production of ATP. Under normal circumstances the three sites are closely coupled so that oxygen consumption does not continue if ADP and P_i are not available.

The respiratory chain can be thought of as a modification of Lehninger's hydraulic model, shown in Figure 11–2.[20, 27] In this model the water from the tap represents the flow of reducing equivalents or electrons supplied by the Krebs cycle. The level of water in each column represents the fraction of the corresponding member of the respiratory chain that is in the reduced form. The terminal valve is the amount of oxygen available. From this model we can draw several conclusions. If we turn off the outflow (as in anoxia) the level of water will rise in each column (a larger fraction of each member of the respiratory chain will be reduced). Conversely, if the terminal valve is open but the source is turned off (substrate deficiency, such as hypoglycemia), the level in each column will drop (more of the respiratory chain will be oxidized). Under normal conditions the flow through the system is not controlled by either inflow (substrate) or outflow (oxygen). Instead, the control points are the sites of

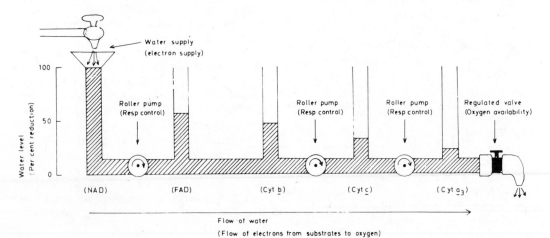

Flow of water
(Flow of electrons from substrates to oxygen)

FIG 11–2.

Hydraulic model of mitochondrial respiratory chain. (From Lehninger.[20] Reproduced by permission.)

coupling between oxidation and phosphorylation. These depend on the cellular metabolic rate, which is reflected by the concentration of ADP (represented by the three pumps shown in Fig 11–2).

If there is a sudden increase in pump activity without a change in the outflow valve then water will be drained from the column closest to the source and the level will rise toward the outflow. In terms of respiratory chain activity, an increase in energy expenditure and a resultant increase in ADP will decrease the reduction of the proximal carrier (NAD) and increase the reduction of the terminal member of the chain (cyt aa$_3$).

Most clinicians are aware of the importance of cellular ATP, but the electron transport component of oxidative phosphorylation has received little attention. The individual members of the respiratory chain have optical properties that differ depending on whether they are in reduced form (NADH) or oxidized form (NAD). These properties are the basis of much of the noninvasive monitoring of tissue oxygenation, to be discussed in a subsequent chapter.

As can be seen from this analogy, the level of tissue oxygenation, the energy state of the tissue, and the level of reduction/oxidation of members of the respiratory chain are closely interrelated. To assess the adequacy of cellular oxygenation, then, we can measure either the partial pressure of oxygen in the cell, the high-energy phosphate available in the cell, or the relative reduction levels of key members of the respiratory chain. Each of these techniques is discussed in greater detail in chapter 12, "Monitoring of Tissue Oxygenation."

The partial pressure of oxygen (Po$_2$) in arterial blood needed to preserve various functions when blood flow is not compromised is known with reasonable accuracy (Table 11–1). The corresponding requirements at the cellular level are less clear. There are several indices that can be used to quantify the need for oxygen by a specific reaction or reaction sequence. The concentration of oxygen at which the first measurable decrease in reaction rate occurs, called the critical Po$_2$, can be used. A second approach, of value in noninvasive optical monitoring, is the level of oxygen that produces the half-maximal reduction level. The third and the most widely used index, the rate constant (Km), is that partial pressure of oxygen required to sustain half-maximal reaction rates. As a carryover from in vitro enzyme kinetics, most of the available data on the sensitivity of various reactions to oxygen are expressed as Km values (Table 11–2).

Although mitochondrial oxidative phosphorylation is unquestionably the major mechanism of cellular oxygen consumption and is vital to cell survival, it may not be the system most sensitive to oxygen deprivation. Many in vitro studies suggest that the level of oxygenation needed to sustain oxidative phosphorylation is minimal. The most recent data obtained from isolated mitochondria suggest that the Km is 0.07 torr,[3] and the critical Po$_2$ is 6.5 torr.[16] Although recent studies have raised questions regarding the direct application of in vitro mitochondrial data to in vivo situations,[17] this should not detract our attention from other important reactions, which may be even more sensitive to hypoxia.

Oxygen participates in a number of biosynthetic, degradative, or detoxifying oxidations, some of which may be more sensitive to hypoxia than oxidative phosphorylation.[14] Among these lesser known oxygen-dependent enzyme systems, oxygen may serve as an electron acceptor, in a manner similar to its role in the respiratory chain, or it may be chemically inserted into an organic substrate, usually in the form of a hydroxyl group (OH).

Of particular interest is a group of reactions catalyzed by enzymes, known as mixed-function

TABLE 11–1.

Events Associated With Decreased Pa$_{O_2}$

Pa$_{O_2}$ (torr)	EVENT
65	Increased ventilation
55	Impaired short-term memory
50	Increased lactate production
40–50	Loss of judgment
30	Unconsciousness
20–25	High-energy phosphates unchanged

TABLE 11–2.

Oxygen Affinities of Selected Enzyme Systems

ENZYME	Km (torr)
Prolyl hydroxylase	42
Tryptophan hydroxylase	37
Tyrosine hydroxylase	7.6
Cytochrome aa	0.07

oxidases. As the name implies, these reactions utilize oxygen both as an electron acceptor and to hydroxylate the substrate. The general form of such reactions is:

$$AH + BH_2 + O_2 \rightleftharpoons AOH + B + H_2O$$
(Eq. 11–2)

Obviously the substrate AH has been hydroxylated. The reducing agent BH_2 serves as the electron donor, and one oxygen is reduced to water. In most biologically significant mixed-function oxidase reactions this source of electrons is either NADH or nicotinamide adenine dinucleotide phosphate (NADPH). For example, the rate-limiting steps in the synthesis of the catecholamines dopamine and epinephrine and the indolamine serotonin are mixed-function oxidases (tyrosine and tryptophan hydroxylase).[8, 9] Because mixed-function oxidases are more sensitive to hypoxia than is oxidative phosphorylation, alterations in catecholamine synthesis may occur early in hypoxia, prior to alterations in energy metabolism.

Oxygen may also serve as a substrate for another class of enzymes, known as dioxygenases or oxygen transferases, in reactions such as:

$$AH_2 + O_2 \rightleftharpoons A(OH)_2 \quad \text{(Eq. 11–3)}$$

Dioxygenases of clinical importance include prolyl and lysyl hydroxylase, which are required for the synthesis of collagen.[15, 29] Hydroxyproline and hydroxylysine found in collagen are not directly incorporated into the protein molecule. Instead, selected prolyl and lysyl residues in the molecule are hydroxylated with α-ketoglutarate and molecular oxygen in the presence of ascorbic acid. In the absence of this hydroxylation, the stable triple helix of collagen does not form.

The best-known pathologic state resulting from deficient hydroxylation of proline and lysine in collagen is scurvy. In the absence of ascorbic acid as a reducing agent, the hydroxylation does not occur. Although not conclusive, the data of Niinikoski,[24] which show decreased and defective collagen synthesis in the wounds of hypoxic subjects, support the existence of an "oxygen-deficiency scurvy."

Two additional oxygen-dependent systems merit attention by the critical care physician. The microsomal fraction of hepatic and adrenal cells contains a complex electron transport chain, whose terminal component is cytochrome P-450, and a mixed-function oxidase system.[26] The source of reducing equivalents for this system is NADPH. The reduced form of cytochrome P-450 reacts with molecular oxygen and any of a number of substrates with the result that one oxygen is reduced to water while the other is incorporated into the substrate. This substrate hydroxylation plays an essential role in the synthesis of cholesterol, the conversion of cholesterol to steroid hormones and bile acids, and many other critical biosynthetic reactions. The cytochrome P-450 system is also very important in the detoxification of foreign substances such as drugs. The introduction of hydroxyl groups provides sites of conjugation (i.e., of glucuronidation or sulfation) and in general increases the water solubility of the molecule.

The phagocytes contain the last of the oxygen-consuming systems to be discussed here.[1, 2] The respiratory burst that follows phagocytosis is not associated with oxidative phosphorylation and ATP synthesis, as was once thought. Rather, NADPH oxidase catalyzes the single electron reduction of molecular oxygen to the highly active superoxide (O_2^-):

$$2O_2 + NADPH \xrightarrow{\text{NADPH OXIDASE}} 2(O_2^-) + NADP^+ + H^+$$
(Eq. 11–4)

This superoxide production initiates a number of pathways that result in the release of other active oxygen forms such as singlet oxygen ($^1O_2$) and hydroxyl radicals (OH·) as well as hydrogen peroxide. Active oxygen participates, via several mechanisms, in the intracellular killing of certain bacteria.

Although neutrophils are capable of normal chemotaxis and phagocytosis in an anaerobic environment, the importance of this oxidative burst is best illustrated by the result of its absence. The congenital condition known as chronic granulomatous disease results from absence of the enzyme NADPH oxidase.[14] Without this enzyme the increase in oxygen consumption normally seen after phagocytosis does not occur. This condition is manifested by severe pyogenic infections, which are difficult to treat and slow to heal in spite of appropriate antibiotic treatment. Patients with chronic granulomatous disease are very susceptible to *Staphylococcus aureus* infections and infection by Enterobacteriaceae, including *E. coli*, *Pseudomonas, Klebsiella, Proteus,* and others.[1] This aspect of chronic granulomatous disease is not unlike problems frequently encountered in the critically ill patient. Severe infections with similar organisms that resist seemingly appropriate therapy are a major cause of death in patients with poor oxygenation or poor tissue perfusion. The role of tissue oxygenation in severe infections in the critically ill remains speculative. However, there are data to suggest that infections of superficial wounds and tissue oxygenation are related.[19]

TISSUE HYPOXIA

Inadequate delivery of oxygen to the tissues may result from hypoxemia (inadequate arterial oxygen content) or ischemia (inadequate blood flow), or a combination of the two. Several mechanisms exist to protect tissue oxygenation, including redistribution of local blood flow and shifts in the oxyhemoglobin dissociation curve. When tissue oxygenation cannot be maintained by these mechanisms, critical biochemical alterations occur within the cell.

The first manifestations of inadequate oxygenation occur in metabolically active organs such as the brain and the heart rather than in less metabolically active organs such as resting skeletal muscle. Although failure of oxygenation is usually thought of in terms of failure of energy metabolism, the earliest signs of hypoxia (see Table 11–1) occur prior to any change in tissue high-energy phosphates.[28] As discussed earlier, many extramitochondrial enzyme systems are quite sensitive to oxygen deprivation, and alterations in their function (neurotransmitter synthesis, etc.) may account for many of these abnormalities.

The response to hypoxia/ischemia differs among organs depending on their metabolic rate and the availability of substrates (creatine phosphate, glucose, glycogen) capable of sustaining ATP levels anaerobically. Although there are tissue-specific differences, certain generalizations can be made. In the absence of oxygen the mitochondrial pyridine nucleotides (NAD, NADP) remain reduced, as do cytochromes such as cyt aa$_3$. Differences in the optical properties of these compounds between the oxidized and reduced states are important in the monitoring of cellular oxygen metabolism, to be discussed in a subsequent section. The mitochondrial redox state is a major determinant of the rate of flux through the Krebs cycle. Thus, as lack of oxygen causes a rise in the NADH/NAD ratio, flux through the Krebs cycle slows.

With the progressive failure of oxidative phosphorylation to meet the energy needs of the cell, the continued hydrolysis of ATP results in the buildup of ADP, P$_i$, and AMP. These compounds are powerful modulators of the regulatory enzymes of anaerobic glycolysis, with the result that glucose consumption rises during the initial fall in oxygen consumption. This increase in glycolytic rate may reach tenfold in ischemic human cerebral cortex.[18] Pyruvate production via this accelerated glycolysis is therefore poorly matched to a decrease in pyruvate consumption by a slowed TCA system. Although glycolysis does not require the presence of oxygen, it does require a method of oxidizing the NADH produced back to NAD. This is accomplished via the lactate dehydrogenase (LDH) reaction.

$$\text{Pyruvate} + \text{NADH} \underset{\text{LDH}}{\rightleftharpoons} \text{Lactate} + \text{NAD}^+$$

$$(\text{Eq. } 11\text{--}5)$$

Since the lactate dehydrogenase reaction is reversible, an accumulation of lactate can inhibit not only this reaction but also glycolysis, owing to lack of NAD$^+$. Of interest is the correlation between the lactate formed and the preinsult levels of glucose and glycogen. This close correlation suggests that the magnitude of tissue acidosis may be varied within wide limits by manipulating carbohydrate availability.[21] That increased tissue lactate concentrations are an early biochemical indicator of tissue hypoxia/ischemia and occur before any change in high-energy phosphate levels[12, 13, 22] demonstrates that glycolysis, though inefficient, does provide a degree of bioenergetic reserve.

Electrically excitable tissues (brain, heart, skeletal muscle) also have another anaerobic source of ATP. Creatine phosphate (PCr) present in these tissues can support ATP levels via the creatine kinase reaction:

$$\text{PCr} + \text{ADP} + \text{P}_i \rightleftharpoons \text{Cr} + \text{ATP} \quad (\text{Eq. } 11\text{--}6)$$

Both the presence of ADP and tissue acidosis shift equilibrium toward ATP. Thus, relatively little change occurs in ATP levels until PCr is largely depleted.

Another reaction capable of yielding ATP anaerobically is the adenylate kinase reaction:

$$\text{ADP} + \text{ADP} \rightleftharpoons \text{ATP} + \text{AMP} \quad (\text{Eq. } 11\text{--}7)$$

However, this reaction depletes the cellular adenine nucleotide pool, since many of the degradation products of AMP are diffusible and may be lost to the tissue.[10, 23]

OXYGEN-DERIVED FREE RADICALS

No discussion of cellular oxygen metabolism today is complete without some mention of oxygen-derived free radicals. Only a brief overview of the formation of these radicals and their potential role in clinical medicine will be given here. Several recently published reviews cover the subject in greater depth.[5, 6, 11]

Most chemical compounds are surrounded by clouds of paired electrons with oppositely directed spins. This is a relatively stable arrangement. In contrast, the free radical has a lone, unpaired electron with its spin unopposed in the outer shell. This is a highly unstable and violently reactive chemical species.

Although molecular oxygen has a paired complement of electrons, it behaves in many of its chemical reactions as two free radicals bonded together, a biradical. Under normal conditions virtually all of the oxygen consumed by the cell is tetravalently reduced, as in the four-electron reduction of oxygen to water by the respiratory chain. However, 1%–2% of the oxygen "leaks" by with one-, two-, or three-electron reduction to yield superoxide (O_2^-), hydrogen peroxide (H_2O_2), or hydroxyl radical (OH^-), respectively. Oxygen-derived free radicals undoubtedly participate in beneficial processes, such as intracellular killing of bacteria, but it is their harmful effects that have attracted the most attention. Such active forms of oxygen have been implicated in the tissue damage seen in a variety of pathologic processes, including pulmonary oxygen toxicity, radiation injury, ischemia/reperfusion syndromes, inflammation, and cancer, and in aging. Oxygen free radicals provide a number of potentially harmful tissue responses, such as increased capillary permeability and damage to cell membranes. The mechanisms of free radical damage are incompletely understood but much attention has focused on the peroxidation of polyunsaturated fatty acids within the phospholipid structure of membranes. This peroxidation may alter elements of the membrane that are essential to either structural or functional integrity. These reactions occur partially through the direct attack of activated oxygen and secondarily from lipid fragmentation products, which are also active oxidizing agents. This chain reaction phenomenon is characteristic of free radical–induced processes and allows them to exert an influence out of proportion to their concentration in the tissue. Normal tissues possess a multilevel system that affords them protection from this lipid peroxidation.[7] The first line of defense is enzymatic. The enzymes superoxide dismutase and catalase keep concentrations of superoxide and hydrogen peroxide low. The second line of defense is provided by such naturally occurring free radical scavengers as tocopherol, ascorbic acid, and β-carotene. The final mechanism, also enzymatic, is glutathione peroxidase, which detoxifies the lipid peroxides produced to limit the chain reaction. Despite the level of interest in the free radicals in biologic systems, they are almost never studied directly. Their minute tissue concentrations and short half-life make direct measurement in biologic systems extremely difficult. Our meager understanding of oxygen free radicals in medicine is derived from such indirect indicators as the disappearance of free radical scavengers and the formation of lipid peroxidation fragments.

The lack of direct measurement techniques and limited understanding have not prevented therapeutic trials based on free radical pathology. Experimental therapies have largely attempted to copy the body's endogenous defense against free radicals. The superoxide dismutase, catalase, and free radical scavengers such as tocopherol have been administered alone or in combination.[25] The result of such therapies at this time is unclear. In some models they provide significant protection whereas in others there is no benefit.

CONCLUSION

Oxygen is crucial to the function and ultimately the survival of mammalian cells. Most cellular oxygen consumption occurs in the mitochondria, where a complex system known as the respiratory chain transports reducing equivalents from the TCA cycle to molecular oxygen, reducing it to water. The energy released in this process is coupled to the syntheses of ATP. Although this system of oxidation phosphorylation is critical to the cell, it is not the system most sensitive to oxygen deprivation. Systems such as neurotransmitter synthesis and toxin degradation appear to be more sensitive and may account for the earliest manifestations of oxygen deprivation. Oxygen deprivation leads to a progressive shift in the redox state of the cell and the eventual failure of oxidative phosphorylation to meet the energy needs of the cell. In an attempt to compensate, anaerobic glycolysis may increase as much as tenfold, but eventually its own byproducts inhibit further ATP production. Oxygen is essential, but in excess or in the presence of injury it may lead to the accumulation of highly destructive oxygen free radicals. The precise role of oxygen free radicals in the pathogenesis of critical illness remains unknown.

REFERENCES

1. Babior BM: Oxygen-dependent microbial killing by phagocytes. *N Engl J Med* 1978; 298:659–668, 721–725.
2. Bagioline M: Phagocytes use oxygen to kill bacteria. *Experientia* 1984; 40:906.
3. Bienfait HF, Jacobs JMC, Slater EC: Mitochondrial oxygen affinity as a function of redox and phosphate potential. *Biochim Biophys Acta* 1975; 376:446.
4. Bloch K: Oxygen and biosynthetic patterns. *Fed Proc* 1962; 21:1058.
5. Bulkley GB: The role of oxygen free radicals in human disease processes. *Surgery* 1983; 94:407.
6. Butterfield JD, McGraw CP: Free radical pathology. *Stroke* 1978; 9:443.
7. Chance B, Boveris A: Hyperoxia and hydroperoxide metabolism, in Robin ED (ed): *Extrapulmonary Manifestations of Respiratory Disease.* New York, Marcel Dekker, 1978, pp 185–237.
8. Davis JN, Carlsson A: The effect of hypoxia on monoamine synthesis, levels and metabolism in rat brain. *J Neurochem* 1973; 21:783.
9. Davis JD, Carlsson A, MacMillan V, et al: Brain tryptophan hydroxylation: Dependence on arterial oxygen tension. *Science* 1973; 182:72.
10. Deuticke B, Gerlach E, Dierkesmann R: Über freier Nucleotide in Herz, Skeletmuskel, Gehirn und Leber der Ratte bei Sauerstoffmangel. *Pflugers Arch Ges Physiol* 1966; 292:239.
11. Dormandy TL: An approach to free radicals. *Lancet* 1983; 2:1010.
12. Gurdjian ES, Stone WE, Webster JE: Cerebral metabolism in hypoxia. *Arch Neurol Psychiatry* 1944; 54:472.
13. Gurdjian ES, Webster JE, Stone WE: Cerebral constituents in relation to blood gases. *Am J Physiol* 1949; 156:149.
14. Hohn DC, Rehrer RI: NADPH oxidase deficiency in x-linked chronic granulomatous disease. *J Clin Invest* 1975; 55:707.
15. Hutton JJ, Tappel AL, Udenfriend S: Cofactor and substrate requirements of collagen proline hydroxylase. *Arch Biochem Biophys* 1967; 118:231.
16. Jöbsis FF: Oxidative metabolism at low P_{O_2}. *Fed Proc* 1972; 31:1404.
17. Jöbsis FF, Lamanna JC: Kinetic aspects of intracellular redox reactions, in Robin ED (ed): *Extrapulmonary Manifestations of Respiratory Disease.* New York, Marcel Dekker, Inc, 1978, pp 63–106.
18. Kirsch WM, Leitner JW: Glycolytic metabolites and co-factors in human cerebral cortex and white matter during complete ischemia. *Brain Res* 1967; 4:358.
19. Knighton DR, Halliday D, Hunt TK: Oxygen as an antibiotic. *Arch Surg* 1984; 119:199.
20. Lehninger AL: *Bioenergetics.* Menlo Park, Calif, WA Benjamin, 1973.
21. Lowry OH, Passonneau JV: The relationship between substrates and enzymes of glycolysis in brain. *J Biol Chem* 1964; 239:31.
22. MacMillan V, Siesjö BK: Brain energy metabolism in hypoxemia. *Scand J Clin Lab Invest* 1972; 30:127.
23. McIlwain H: Regulatory significance of the release and action of adenine derivatives in cerebral systems. *Biochem Soc Symp* 1972; 36:69.
24. Niinikoski J: Oxygen and wound healing. *Clin Plast Surg* 1977; 4:361.
25. Novelli GP, de Gaudio AR: Oxygen free radicals in shock states, in Lewis DH, Haglund U (eds): *Shock Research.* New York, Elsevier, 1983, pp 31–42.
26. Omura T, Sato R, Cooper CY, et al: Function of cytochrome P-450 of microsomes. *Fed Proc* 1965; 24:1181.
27. Siesjö BK: *Brain Energy Metabolism.* New York, John Wiley & Sons, Inc, 1978.
28. Siesjö BK, Nordström CH: Brain metabolism in relation to oxygen supply, in Jöbsis FF (ed): *Oxygen and Physiological Function.* Dallas, Professional Information Library, 1977, pp 459–479.
29. Stryer L: *Biochemistry,* ed 2. San Francisco, WH Freeman, 1981.

12   Monitoring of Tissue Oxygenation

John B. Cone, M.D.

The goal of monitoring is not to replace close observation by skilled professionals, but to detect significant changes earlier than they can be detected by the human senses—early enough to allow therapeutic intervention. A major portion of our monitoring and data collection effort in the intensive care unit (ICU) involves assessment of oxygen transport and metabolism. Virtually all of our attention is devoted to bulk transport variables such as total oxygen delivery or metabolic variables such as total body oxygen consumption. Accordingly our therapy is directed toward improving cardiac output and blood oxygen content. Implicit in this approach is the assumption that the human body is homogeneous and remains so despite illness. Although that assumption is universally recognized as invalid, our approach to monitoring has been necessitated by our inability to accurately assess regional or local oxygenation. As technical advances move from the laboratory to the bedside, it becomes increasingly clear that not only are the various organ systems perfused and oxygenated differently, but also, apparently homogeneous tissues such as the liver may be inhomogeneously oxygenated under pathologic circumstances.[37] This uneven distribution has long been recognized in experimental models and assumed to apply to humans, but only recently have clinically applicable techniques become available to monitor the oxygenation of isolated organs or tissues.

Tissue oxygen content reflects the balance between oxygen supply and demand. Available techniques can measure its three components—perfusion, oxygen utilization, and oxygen content—either regionally or locally. Exactly what information is either necessary or useful clinically remains unknown.

Inherent in the structure of the microvasculature is an inhomogeneous distribution of oxygen within the tissue. Therefore the choice of monitoring technique depends not only on the variable of interest but also on the volume of tissue monitored. For example, to determine the fraction of tissue with a partial pressure of oxygen less than a critical value (e.g., 5 torr), one must sample multiple microscopic sites. In contrast, if one wishes to know the mean partial pressure of oxygen in a macroscopic volume of tissue, such as a skin flap, then a technique that sums over many microvascular units is appropriate.

TISSUE OXIMETRY

If oxygen delivery and utilization were uniform then mixed venous oxygen pressure would accurately reflect tissue oxygenation.[5] However, there are common pathologic conditions, such as vascular occlusive disease and chronic liver disease, in which a normal mixed venous oxygen pressure may belie severe local ischemia. This has led to the use of venous oxygen values obtained by selective catheterization of critical organs such as the brain.[12] These techniques undoubtedly provide a specificity lacking with the use of mixed venous oxygen but still may not reliably reflect tissue oxygenation in conditions in which microvascular regulation is disturbed, such as sepsis, loss of autoregulation from injury, microembolism, or certain pharmacologic manipulations.[39] Although unproven, it is logical that a direct knowledge of the oxygenation of vital organs would be clinically useful.

The most direct approaches to the measurement of tissue oxygen have involved variations of the oxygen electrode. These include the increasingly popular transcutaneous oxygen sensors, the multiwire surface electrodes of the Dortmund type, and various deep-tissue electrode configurations. All of the devices have in common the circuit shown in Figure 12–1. The oxygen elec-

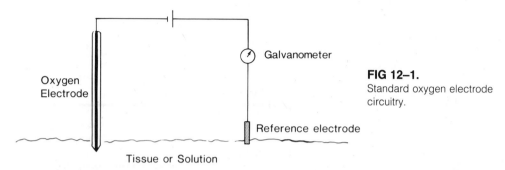

FIG 12–1.
Standard oxygen electrode circuitry.

trode (Fig 12–2) is an electrochemical system consisting of a platinum electrode immersed in the solution of interest and connected to a suitable voltage source. The circuit is completed through a sensitive galvanometer connected to a nonpolarizable reference electrode. When the circuit is polarized, oxygen is reduced at the platinum electrode, creating a current proportional to the partial pressure of oxygen. Thus the oxygen electrode is an oxygen-consuming system and care must be taken that the attempt at measurement does not significantly alter the system being measured.

The most widespread use of oxygen electrodes, other than for ex vivo blood gas analysis, is in the transcutaneous oxygen sensors.

Transcutaneous Oxygen Tension (TCO$_2$)

Under normal physiologic conditions the oxygen tension at the skin surface (TCO$_2$) is close to zero. However, if the skin beneath the oxygen electrode is heated to 42°–45° C the barrier to diffusion is reduced, capillary flow is increased, and TCO$_2$ approaches Pa$_{O_2}$. This technique was initially used to monitor Pa$_{O_2}$ in neonates and subsequently was extended to adults. As experi-

ence accumulated it became obvious that factors other than Pa$_{O_2}$ influenced TCO$_2$. In theory, TCO$_2$ is a measure of the tissue oxygen content of the skin[28] and as such is a balance between oxygen delivery and use. If we assume that the metabolic rate of the skin remains constant (although abnormal because of heating) and that other factors do not disturb local flow, then TCO$_2$ should be a function of cardiac output, hemoglobin concentration, and local vasomotor tone, in addition to Pa$_{O_2}$. This is in fact the case. TCO$_2$ ranges from 80%–90% of Pa$_{O_2}$ under *optimal* circumstances to less than P$\bar{v}_{O_2}$ in the presence of shock or ischemia.[45] This failing of the transcutaneous oxygen sensor as a Pa$_{O_2}$ monitor has actually increased its value. In the absence of sepsis, a normal or high TCO$_2$ indicates that a patient's cardiorespiratory status is adequate and reduces the need for invasive monitoring. The use of transcutaneous oximetry to monitor whole body oxygen delivery will not be discussed in greater depth here. The subject has been extensively reviewed elsewhere.[45]

Local Surface Oximetry

While transcutaneous oximetry is widely used clinically to assess systemic oxygen transport, it

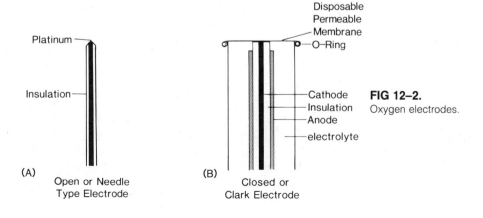

FIG 12–2.
Oxygen electrodes.

(A) Open or Needle Type Electrode

(B) Closed or Clark Electrode

is also the logical starting point for measurement of local or regional oxygenation. It is in this role that the oxygen electrode offers information not readily available from standard invasive hemodynamic monitoring techniques.

Peripheral vascular occlusive disease offers a nearly ideal situation for the evaluation of regional oximetry techniques. Both the patient and the pathologic process are stable, the bulk oxygen transport variables are within acceptable limits, and the tissue being studied can be easily isolated for study by other, established techniques.

The interpretation of local tissue oxygenation data is simplified if local effects can be distinguished from systemic effects. In the case of peripheral vascular disease this can be accomplished to some degree by looking at the regional perfusion index (RPI) proposed by Hauser and Shoemaker.[18] The RPI is the ratio of oxygen tension at the site of interest and oxygen tension at a site presumed free of local pathology. For example, the extremities may be compared with the anterior chest wall in an attempt to correct for the effects of the cardiopulmonary disease so often seen in association with peripheral vascular disease.

Tissue oximetry has been found highly reliable in the diagnosis of lower extremity ischemia when exercise values are compared with values obtained at rest. Normal subjects demonstrate no significant drop in RPI with exercise. Transcutaneous oximetry has been compared with noninvasive vascular diagnostic techniques, with mixed results. Its advocates find it superior to the Doppler techniques; others have shown no clear advantage.

Certain aspects of vascular disease are not so clearly defined, such as claudication, in which resting oxygenation is adequate but pain results from the inability to meet the increased oxygen demands of exercise. Diabetic microvascular disease combined with large-vessel occlusive disease often presents a confusing picture, which may be further complicated by the sensory changes accompanying diabetic neuropathy. Transcutaneous oximetry has been reported to be superior to other noninvasive techniques in this setting.[17] In spite of the array of tests available, choosing the optimal level for amputation still retains an element of guesswork. A recent report indicates that transcutaneous oximetry can discriminate without overlap between healing and nonhealing levels.[23] Transcutaneous oxygen sen-

sors have also been reported to be useful in monitoring oxygen delivery to tissue flaps[1] and reimplanted limbs.[30]

Although peripheral vascular occlusive disease and the resulting tissue hypoxia may appear to have little relevance for the critical care physician, they serve to illustrate and validate a technique, which may then be applied to tissues of more obvious concern such as the liver, the kidney, and the brain. Kram and Shoemaker have recently reported the use of a miniature version of the transcutaneous oxygen sensor on the surfaces of viscera exposed at the time of surgery.[27] They demonstrated that the visceral surface Po_2 closely paralleled Pa_{O_2} and TCo_2 over a range of oxygen tensions as long as perfusion was maintained. During periods of reduced flow, visceral surface Po_2 tracked TCo_2 but not Pa_{O_2}, indicating that like TCo_2, visceral surface Po_2 is an indicator of net tissue oxygenation. Abrupt and appropriate changes in surface Po_2 followed manipulation of organ vasculature. The investigators were also able to correctly predict the viability of a questionably ischemic gastrointestinal anastomosis.

Although devices such as these may not be suitable for placement in the ICU, they can be placed at the time of surgery in much the same way that left atrial lines and epicardial pacing wires are placed during cardiac surgery.

Multiwire Surface Electrodes

Even the smallest of the conventional surface oxygen sensors (such as the one just described for use on viscera) records the mean Po_2 over a field 1–2 mm in diameter. This obviously represents a summation over a large number of capillary units. As long as any changes in oxygen delivery are homogeneous this mean value appears to be representative of the adequacy of tissue oxygenation. However, when changes in oxygen delivery are inhomogeneous and perhaps nonnutritive, then a single mean value may not reflect a portion of the tissue that is hypoxic.

Kessler and Lübbers have modified the surface electrode concept in order to address the problem of inhomogeneous oxygenation.[25] In their assembly 8 to 16 platinum wires (diameter 15 μ) are isolated from each other in an enclosed electrode. Each wire electrode measures the oxygen tension in a hemispheric field of 20–25 μ radius, permitting a determination at points between two single capillaries. Multiple measurements are made over a surface; the Po_2 values are stored and subsequently expressed as a histogram (Fig 12–3). Such histograms obtained under normal conditions demonstrate a wide range of Po_2 values in a bell-shaped distribution about some mean value. This mean is typically lower than the venous Po_2 of the tissue in question. This is presumed to be the result of nonnutritive or shunted blood flow at the microcirculatory level. There is some evidence to suggest that this shunted oxygen can be redistributed to provide nutritive flow as a reserve or protective mechanism in tissue hypoxia. Tissue hypoxia may result from either a homogeneous decrease in oxygen delivery to the tissue (either a total body reduction such as in hemorrhage or a regional but homogeneous reduction such as in vascular occlusion) or a microcirculatory derangement such that microscopic regions within the tissue are ischemic despite normal or supranormal overall blood flow and high venous Po_2. Each form of tissue hypoxia produces a characteristic Po_2 histogram (see Fig

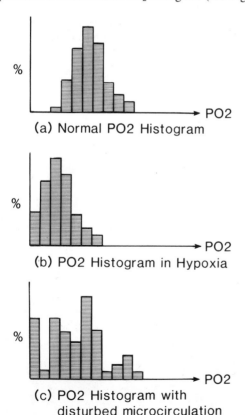

(a) Normal PO2 Histogram

(b) PO2 Histogram in Hypoxia

(c) PO2 Histogram with disturbed microcirculation

FIG 12–3.
Typical Po_2 histograms.

12–3). With a homogeneous reduction in oxygenation the oxygen is symmetrically left-shifted but relatively undistorted, whereas a microcirculatory defect may severely distort the shape of the curve.

The multiwire surface electrode is in limited clinical use as a monitor of tissue oxygenation in both the ICU and the operating room. The conditions to which it has been applied are quite similar to those discussed earlier for transcutaneous and single electrode surface sensors. The multiwire electrodes have been applied to skeletal muscle (via a small skin incision) in ICU patients to monitor overall oxygen transport.[39] It has been claimed that in conditions such as hypovolemia, the Po_2 histogram changes earlier than does any of the standard monitoring indicators.[24] The multiwire system has also been applied to visceral surfaces intraoperatively to evaluate renal allograph function,[41] hepatic oxygenation after portacaval anastomosis,[6] and the results of vascular surgery.[19]

Although the multiwire system would appear to offer information not available from systems that measure only mean Po_2, this additional information must be paid for in more complex technology and interpretation. Is the Po_2 histogram superior to a mean tissue Po_2? This question cannot be answered from the available data. The two systems have not been compared in a simultaneous test. One can speculate that in homogeneous processes they would provide comparable information. However, it seems reasonable to assume that in circumstances involving a disturbance in the microcirculation, such as the microembolism of trauma and sepsis, and reperfusion syndromes, the Po_2 histogram would offer valuable additional information, particularly for quantifying the effectiveness of therapy.

If further specificity or localization is necessary, needle microelectrodes are available that allow the determination of oxygen tension at precise locations, such as intracellularly.[48] These techniques are sufficiently tedious and complex that they remain research tools and will not be discussed further.

The oldest technique for the determination of tissue oxygen tension involves the placement of a hollow, freely permeable wire mesh chamber in the tissue. The chamber fills with fluid in equilibrium with the tissue. This fluid is then aspirated for ex vivo gas analysis on a standard blood gas analyzer. Niinikoski and Hunt[33] have modified this technique to make it clinically applicable. The surgically implanted chamber is replaced by Silastic tubing, which can be inserted via a large-bore needle, minimizing the effects of local trauma. This tubing, which is freely permeable to oxygen, is attached to impermeable tubing, which enters and exits the skin. The tubing is then filled with anaerobic saline and allowed to equilibrate with the surrounding tissues. The saline is then flushed from the tubing and the P_{O_2} measured on an ordinary blood gas analyzer. This technique obviously determines an average P_{O_2} over a large cylinder of tissue and cannot detect areas of inhomogeneity. Although this technique has been applied to the same problems as the devices discussed above, it has had its greatest impact when placed in surgical incisions. Chang and associates[11] have clearly shown the importance of oxygen in wound infections and wound healing using this technique.

MASS SPECTROSCOPY

The oxygen electrode forms the heart of virtually all clinical oxygen sensors, both in vitro and in vivo. However, another approach is available and may offer advantages in selected circumstances. Mass spectroscopy (MS) utilizes one of several techniques for separating and quantitating molecules of gas on the basis of molecular weight. The spectrometer can be considered a black box capable of measuring the quantity of gas with a molecular weight of 32. In physiologic systems this is equivalent to measuring the amount of molecular oxygen present. The mechanics of tissue oximetry with mass spectroscopy are remarkably similar to those of the oxygen electrode. The system may be applied as a surface sensor or as a needle placed in the deeper tissues. In contrast to electrode techniques, in which oxygen moves in an externally applied electrical field, in MS the diffusion gradient is created with a vacuum pump. Although it may appear that we have further complicated the business of oximetry by replacing a galvanometer with a mass spectrometer, MS does have its advantages. It is not limited to gases of a single molecular weight. Most units can simultaneously measure two, three, or ten different compounds. The applications of MS to tissue oximetry are identical to those of the oxygen electrode and therefore will not be discussed here. However, certain potential applications of

MS may place it in a favorable position relative to the oxygen electrode for future use. The ability of MS to measure local carbon dioxide tension may allow the assessment of local tissue metabolic rate.[29] With further refinement of the technique it should be possible to study local metabolism in even greater detail by administering substrates such as glucose amino acids and fatty acids, labeled with the nonradioactive isotope ^{13}C, and following their metabolism as marked by the production of $^{13}CO_2$.[46]

The principles of tissue oximetry represent a generalization of blood gas analysis and interpretation, and as such, tissue oximetry is the logical starting point in understanding tissue oxygenation.

MONITORING OXYGEN DELIVERY (PERFUSION)

The second major determinant of tissue oxygenation is local oxygen delivery, which is discussed in chapter 10, "Oxygen Transport from Capillary to Cell." The third is oxygen metabolism.

MONITORING TISSUE OXYGEN METABOLISM

Clinical analysis of oxygen metabolism is not so well developed or so straightforward as the measurement of tissue oxygen tension. In contrast to tissue oximetry, which has a single variable of interest (P_{O_2}), oxygen metabolism has a multitude of variables that might be useful in clinical medicine.

As pointed out in chapter 11, "Cellular Oxygen Utilization," one of the earliest biochemical changes in hypoxia is increased lactate production. Several investigators have attempted to correlate serum lactate levels with the severity of the hypoxic insult, but without consistent success. This lack of correlation was explained in 1957 by Huckabee[21] on the basis of the lactate dehydrogenase (LDH) equilibrium reaction:

$$\text{Pyruvate} + \text{NADH} \underset{\text{LDH}}{\rightleftharpoons} \text{Lactate} + \text{NAD}^+$$

(Eq. 12–1)

As oxidation of NADH by molecular oxygen falls off, oxidation of NADH by the LDH reaction provides NAD^+ to allow continued glycolysis.

But, in contrast to the other reduction-oxidation reactions, the LDH reaction is a dead end. Lactate, unable to enter into another reaction, accumulates and eventually inhibits further oxidation of NADH. However, as seen in equation 12–2, lactate concentration is influenced by factors other than the relative reduction state of the NAD-NADH couple.

$$[Lactate] = [Pyruvate] \times K \times \frac{[NADH]}{[NAD]}$$
(Eq. 12–2)

Thus, the relative reduction state of NADH/NAD within the cell should be reflected by the ratio of lactate to pyruvate (L/P). Huckabee proposed the term "excess lactate" for lactate that could not be explained on the basis of changes in [pyruvate], and thus reflected anaerobic metabolism. This technique has been widely used both experimentally and clinically to reflect the degree of hypoxia and the contribution of anaerobic glycolysis.[3, 47]

Because LDH is a cytoplasmic enzyme, it may not reliably reflect the level of oxygenation present within the critical region of the cell, the mitochondria. By analogy with the LDH system, the intramitochondrial reduction state has been studied using the β-hydroxybutyrate dehydrogenase (HBDH) system,[43] which is present within mitochondria (equation 12–3):

Acetoacetate + NADH
$$\underset{\text{HBHD}}{\rightleftharpoons} \text{β-hydroxybutyrate} + NAD^+$$
(Eq. 12–3)

Thus, by equation 12–4, the ratio of β-hydroxybutyrate to acetoacetate should reflect the mitochondrial reduction state:

$$\frac{NADH}{NAD} = K \times \frac{[\text{β-hydroxybutyrate}]}{[\text{Acetoacetate}]}$$
(Eq. 12–4)

Both techniques have disadvantages. First, they are indirect and require assumptions that may not be valid under all pathologic circumstances. Second, although they may be used regionally they are primarily bulk or whole-body techniques.

Cellular energy production may be broken down into components: glycolysis and oxidative phosphorylation. Oxidative phosphorylation may be further separated into respiration and high-energy phosphate synthesis. Under physiologic conditions all three components are tightly coupled so that a system that monitored one component would provide reliable information about all. However, in pathologic states close coupling is often lost, particularly between glycolysis and oxidative phosphorylation. Although the technology exists today to nondestructively analyze each component in situ, this field is so primitive that we do not know which parameters may be clinically useful.

The vast technological arrays available today make it impossible to discuss all the techniques for measuring some aspect of oxygen metabolism. Three techniques will be presented to illustrate the range of possibilities. Optical techniques enable continuous monitoring of the redox state of tissue, and ^{31}P NMR can measure the levels of high-energy phosphates in the tissue. Positron emission tomography can be used to measure several aspects of energy metabolism, but we will limit our discussion to its use in measuring glycolytic rate.

Optical Monitoring

The fraction of each member of the respiratory chain that is in its reduced form reflects both local metabolic rate and oxygen availability (see chapter 11, "Cellular Oxygen Utilization"). Serendipitously, many members of the chain have significantly different optical properties in the reduced and oxidized states. These differences allow nondestructive analysis of the redox state in situ. Although several members of the electron transport system have been used in this manner, we will concentrate on two. The compensated fluorometry method of Chance and associates,[10] which allows the quantitation of NADH, and the transmission infrared technique of Jöbsis,[22] which measures the amount of oxidized cytochrome aa₃ (cyt aa₃), will be used to illustrate the concepts.

Chance and colleagues developed a fluorometer based on the principle that the reduced form, NADH, fluoresces in tissue at 450 nm when excited by incident light at 366 nm. Interpretation of the fluorescence signal is complicated because changes in blood flow and local blood volume can cause artificial changes.[26] Part of the excitation light is scattered by the red cells and reflected by vessel walls and cell membranes. Therefore the reflected light is measured along with the fluorescence and a corrected fluorescence is derived. This corrected fluorescence has been shown to reflect the mitochondrial redox state with little or no contribution from cytoplasmic NADH.[34]

Although this technique has been applied to multiple organs, including the heart, the liver, and skeletal muscle, the most extensively studied tissue is cerebral cortex. Using reflectance fluorometry it is possible to show shifts in the reductive state of the tissue while cellular metabolism is maintained.[38] This may allow us to identify a "margin of safety" in tissue oxygenation rather than waiting for function to fail.

Using this technique it is possible to study the effects of therapeutic intervention at the cellular level. When superficial temporal artery (STA) to middle cerebral artery (MCA) anastomosis was first introduced for the treatment of cerebral ischemia, there was considerable skepticism concerning its benefit at the cellular level. Although blood flow could be shown to increase, many dismissed this as nonnutritive, and hence worthless, flow. Using intraoperative reflectance fluorometry, Austin and co-workers[4] were able to demonstrate an increased level of brain NADH oxidation with flow through an STA-MCA anastomosis and thus improved cellular oxygenation.

Surface reflectance fluorometry allows excellent spatial (1 mm) and temporal (1 sec) resolution. Thus it can be used to study microheterogeneities in tissue perfusion and also rapidly changing phenomena.[9] However, it is not without drawbacks. The surface of interest must be exposed surgically. Because of the high degree of light scattering and absorption, the method can be used to study only the most superficial 1 mm of an organ. This is not a serious limitation in a relatively homogeneous organ, such as the liver, but it compromises the usefulness of fluorometry in many sites.

In the 700–1,300 nm range of the near infrared spectrum, incident light may penetrate several centimeters of biologic tissues. The terminal member of the electron transport chain, cyt aa_3, is a metalloprotein with an absorption peak within this window. This absorption peak is present only for oxidized cyt aa_3, disappearing as the enzyme is reduced. The fortuitous superimposition of these optical properties led to the development of a technique known as near infrared spectroscopy (niroscopy) to noninvasively assess the intracellular oxygenation. Oxidized cyt aa_3 has an absorption peak with a broad maximum (820–840 nm) that disappears on reduction. Reduced hemoglobin has an absorption peak at 760 nm that disappears with oxygenation. These two facts, combined with the tissue penetration of these wavelengths, allow determination of the intravascular and the intracellular oxygenation. As pointed out earlier, this distinction may be of critical importance in areas of disturbed microcirculation. In such regions the cells may be ischemic while well-oxygenated blood bypasses them via nonnutritive channels.

Because of the critical dependence of nervous tissue on oxygenation, niroscopy has been applied primarily to the brain. Fiber optic light guides bring the incident light to one side of the head while another fiber optic bundle applied to the opposite side of the head delivers the transmitted light to a photon detector and counter. The technique can be applied completely noninvasively. By using the appropriate wavelengths for oxidized cyt aa_3, reduced hemoglobin, and a reference wavelength one can assess intracellular oxygenation, hemoglobin saturation, and tissue blood volume.

This technique has been applied to humans to demonstrate the reduced blood volume and relative intracellular ischemia that accompanies voluntary hyperventilation. This capability has great potential value in patients with increased intracranial pressure (ICP). Standard care of such patients has included hyperventilation to lower ICP, but we cannot currently assess the point at which hyperventilation does more harm by reducing perfusion than it does good by reducing ICP. In animal models, niroscopy appears to be able to make that distinction.[36]

Nuclear Magnetic Resonance

In recent years nuclear magnetic resonance (NMR) imaging has emerged from the basic science laboratory and entered clinical medicine with great fanfare. However, the spectacular images produced by NMR scanners [now called magnetic resonance (MR) imagers] are not our concern. NMR spectroscopy, although based on the same physical principles, is capable of quantitative chemical analysis of tissues in situ.

NMR is based on the fact that many atomic nuclei have a property called spin which is analogous to the angular momentum of a child's top. When a spinning particle such as the nucleus is placed in an external magnetic field it will align either with or against the field (intermediate configurations are not possible because of quantum mechanical restrictions). To flip the alignment of a nucleus from parallel with the field to antiparallel requires that the nucleus absorb a photon of precisely the resonance frequency, ω, of that nucleus. The resonance or Larmor frequency is defined by equation 12–5:

$$\omega = \gamma H_0 \qquad \text{(Eq. 12–5)}$$

where γ denotes the gyromagnetic moment, an inherent property of each nucleus, and H_0 denotes the externally applied magnetic field. Once the nucleus has flipped to an antiparallel alignment it is unstable and will decay to its original, parallel alignment and emit a photon identical to the one it absorbed. The number of emitted photons, the signal strength, is proportional to the number of nuclei present that have the same resonance frequency. Since the frequencies of interest are in the radio frequency range, an NMR spectroscope consists of a magnet and a radio frequency transmitter and receiver.

If the only factors that influenced the resonance frequency were the gyromagnetic moment and the external field, then we would be able to quantify the total number of a given type of nucleus but would lack information about its chemistry. Fortunately the value of NMR spectroscopy is further enhanced by the chemical shift phenomenon. Equation 12–5 predicts that all nuclei of a given isotope will have the same resonance frequency when placed in a magnetic field, H_0. However, a nucleus that is present as part of a larger molecule or structure is influenced not only by the externally applied H_0 but also by small local magnetic fields produced by the surrounding cloud of electrons. Thus the resonance frequency is more accurately written as:

$$\omega = \gamma \, (H_0 + H_{local}) \qquad \text{(Eq. 12–6)}$$

For example, adenosine triphosphate (ATP) contains three phosphorus nuclei, each in a slightly different chemical environment. Thus each phosphorus nucleus has a slightly different resonance frequency and the NMR spectrum of ATP has three peaks. Chemical shifts are usually measured relative to an arbitrary reference compound. It is then possible to identify a peak by its frequency shift away from a reference peak and to quantify the signal by measuring the area under a peak. The chemical shift determined in this manner is obviously a function of the external magnetic field, which makes it difficult to com-

pare results obtained on differing systems. To standardize chemical shift terminology and eliminate the dependence on external field strength, a dimensionless parameter δ is defined:

$$\delta = \frac{\omega - \omega_r}{\omega_r} \times 10^6 \qquad \text{(Eq. 12–7)}$$

where ω is the resonance frequency of the peak of interest and ω_r is the resonance frequency of the arbitrary reference peak. δ is expressed in parts per million (ppm) because the resonance frequency is in megahertz, whereas the magnitude of the shift is only a few hertz.

In theory any nucleus that has spin is suitable for NMR spectroscopy. To date, however, only three have had significant impact in the nondestructive monitoring of tissue metabolism: ^1H, ^{13}C, and ^{31}P. ^{31}P and ^1H have the advantage that they represent virtually 100% of the naturally occurring isotopes of hydrogen and phosphorus. ^{13}C, on the other hand, makes up less than 2% of the naturally occurring carbon. Therefore, most ^{13}C studies must follow the administration of ^{13}C-labeled substrate.

Until a few years ago the largest sample that could be analyzed in a high-resolution NMR magnet was 10–20 mm, which essentially precluded anything more than isolated tissues and perfused organs. Today magnets of sufficient size, although expensive, are available for in vivo animal and human studies.

^{31}P NMR offers a simple spectrum and direct application to oxygen metabolism. In most biologic tissues the phosphorus compounds present in sufficient concentration for NMR analysis (approximately 1mM) are ATP, phosphocreatine, inorganic phosphate, and various sugar phosphates. In addition, because the chemical shift of inorganic phosphate (P_i) is very sensitive to intracellular pH, pH also can be followed and gives a measure of the anaerobic metabolism. In order to be consistent with our previous examples we will use the ^{31}P NMR spectra of the brain to illustrate the capabilities of in vivo NMR.

In vivo ^{31}P NMR of the brain requires the application of a radio frequency surface coil to the head.[2] (This serves as the antenna for both the excitation pulse and the emitted signal.) The head and surface coil are then placed in the bore of a high-field, superconducting magnet. Such a technique has been described in detail for rabbits,[14] dogs,[20] and humans.[8] A complex spectrum is generated that may require computer curve fitting to analyze, but the peak areas enable one to quantify ATP, phosphocreatine, and P_i. In animal studies, in which the NMR results can be verified biochemically, the results obtained with NMR are reliable.[31]

Figure 12–4 illustrates the use of ^{31}P NMR in monitoring oxygen metabolism. This shows the sequential ^{31}P NMR spectra of a dog made progressively hypoxic by lowered F_{IO_2}. Concomitant EEG and hemodynamic studies (not shown) can be done to show the correlation between metabolism and function. As expected, the first changes seen are the shift to the right of P_i consistent with intracellular acidosis and anaerobic glycolysis. Subsequently phosphocreatine falls and P_i increases, with preservation of ATP. Deterioration of ATP is a late event, occurring for

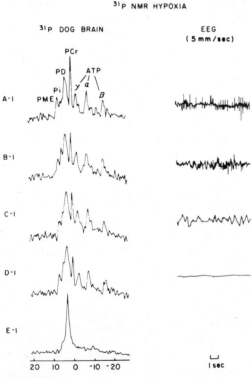

FIG 12–4.
Serial ^{31}P nuclear magnetic resonance spectra and EEG of dog brain during the course of progressive hypoxia. The spectrum is dominated by inorganic phosphate *(Pi)* with shoulders in the phosphomonoester *(PME)* and phosphodiester *(PD)* region. There was no net loss of phosphorus signal. *PCr,* phosphocreatine. (From Hilberman et al.[20] Reproduced by permission.)

the most part after loss of function, as shown by EEG. Systems such as this allow close correlation between metabolism and function, which may provide answers to some of the cause versus effect questions in pathophysiology.[31] NMR also allows relatively good (on the order of 1 minute) time resolution of bioenergetic events.

The capabilities of in vivo NMR are not limited to those shown here. Several systems have been studied extensively: skeletal muscle,[13] myocardium,[16] and others. These and other uses of ^{31}P NMR and the capabilities of ^1H NMR and ^{13}C NMR are discussed in detail elsewhere.[7, 40]

Positron Emission Tomography

Positron emission tomography (PET) allows one to follow and quantify the distribution of labeled tracers without tissue destruction. PET has been adapted to a wide range of in vivo metabolic studies, including oxygen utilization and fatty acid metabolism. A description of the details of PET and the full range of its uses is beyond the scope of this chapter but has been reviewed elsewhere.[35, 44] The basic principles of PET and its application to the measurement of local tissue metabolic rate for glucose in the brain will be presented here.

The positron is a particle of antimatter, an antielectron. In spite of its name, PET does not depend directly on the detection of positrons. Because of the high density of electrons in tissue, the positron travels only a short distance in tissue before colliding with an electron. This collision results in the complete annihilation of the positron-electron pair and the production of two identical γ-rays, 180 degrees apart. It is this simultaneously emitted pair of γ-rays that is counted in the detector. The difference between PET and the traditional nuclear medicine techniques is that it relies on the simultaneous detection of the γ-ray pair, annihilation coincidence detection. This technique serves as an electronic collimator. When a photon strikes a detector it is not counted unless the opposite detector is activated simultaneously. Therefore the only γ-rays seen by the detector pair are those emitted along the axis of that pair of detectors. In contrast, a standard gamma camera requires bulky mechanical shielding to localize the source of a photon. Since much of the emitted radiation is absorbed in these mechanical collimators, the system is inherently inefficient. A tightly packed circular array of detectors using annihilation coincidence detection can be as much as 100 times more efficient than the traditional systems.

An important factor in the use of PET in biologic systems is the availability of positron-emitting isotopes of such elements as carbon 11, nitrogen 13, and oxygen 15, whose incorporation into biologic compounds does not alter the behavior of the system. Labeling compounds with the usual γ-ray emitters, such as technetium 99, often alters cellular transport and may disturb critical chemical reactions.

In keeping with the earlier comments about isotope choice, the logical approach to the study of glucose metabolism would seem to be labeling glucose with carbon 11. Unfortunately, glucose is converted to carbon dioxide and cleared from the tissue so rapidly that this is not feasible. In 1977 Sokoloff and colleagues[42] reported the use of the glucose analogue ^{14}C-2-deoxyglucose to measure local cerebral metabolic rate for glucose using autoradiography. To convert this to a nondestructive technique, Reivich and associates[38] chose the positron-emitting isotope fluorine 18 and the chemical glucose analogue 2-(^{18}F)-fluoro-2-deoxyglucose (FDG). Fluorine 18 has the appropriate size and reactivity to allow its substitution for hydrogen in many organic compounds. Although such substitution appears to cause minimal perturbation, it cannot be assumed to be a perfect mimic. Further, both the Sokoloff and PET methods depend on the assumption that the glucose analogues are taken up by the cells and phosphorylated normally. However, the analogues cannot proceed further through glycolysis and therefore they accumulate, allowing detection. There are naturally a number of rate constants that must be determined experimentally to compensate for the substitution of FDG for glucose.

The FDG method of quantifying the local metabolic rate for glucose remains controversial. Although the data from normal volunteers seem valid, the behavior of the rate constants in pathologic states such as ischemia continues to be debated.[15]

Although PET has proved valuable in analyzing the biochemical changes associated with physiologic functions of the brain, we are primarily interested in its capabilities in cerebral ischemic/hypoxic conditions. It appears that a single study such as metabolic rates for glucose may incompletely characterize an area of tissue hypoxia. In the early period following a stroke in humans there is an uncoupling of glucose utilization and local blood flow. Glucose uptake is less impaired than perfusion, a situation compatible with ischemia and enhanced anaerobic glycolysis. In later, stable infarcts, glucose metabolism and blood flow are both decreased and recoupled. Such studies have led to the speculation that nonfunctional but salvageable tissue may be distinguished from irreversibly damaged tissue. Trials are under way to test this hypothesis.

SUMMARY

Recent advances in technology afford the capability of nondestructively assessing all the components of tissue energy metabolism. Now the clinician and the basic scientist must cooperate to determine which of these factors are useful to a basic understanding of the pathophysiology and which are useful in the clinical management of the seriously ill patient.

As with most recent advances in medical science we are faced here with increasing cost and complexity. For a new test to be worthwhile it must do one of two things: (1) give standard information in a better way, for example faster, safer, or cheaper, or (2) give new and useful information. Without question the techniques discussed in this chapter fail to meet the first requirement. They do give new information, but it remains for those of us who care for the critically ill to determine scientifically how useful this information is.

REFERENCES

1. Achauer B, Black KS, Litke DK: Transcutaneous PO in flaps: A new method of survival prediction. *Plast Reconstr Surg* 1980; 65:732.

2. Ackerman JJH, Grove TH, Wong GG, et al: Mapping of metabolites in whole animals by ^{31}P-NMR using surface coils. *Nature* 1980; 283:167.

3. Allen SHG, Rahm R, Shal DM: Metabolic alterations in trauma: Lactate and pyruvate levels after aortic surgery. *Circ Shock* 1983; 11:13.

4. Austin G, Jutzy R, Chance B, et al: Noninvasive monitoring of human brain oxidative metabolism, in Dutton PL (ed): *Frontiers of Biological Energetics II*. New York, Academic Press, 1978, pp 1445–1456.

5. Birman H, Haq A, Hew E, et al: Continuous monitoring of mixed venous oxygen saturation

in hemodynamically unstable patients. *Chest* 1984; 86:753.

6. Broelsch C, Höper J, Kessler M: Oxygen supply to the cirrhotic liver following various portocaval shunt procedures. *Adv Exp Med Biol* 1978; 94:633.

7. Burt CT, Koutcher JA: Multinuclear NMR studies of naturally occurring nuclei. *J Nucl Med* 1984; 25:237.

8. Cady EB, Dawson MJ, Hope PL, et al: Noninvasive investigation of cerebral metabolism in newborn infants by phosphorus nuclear magnetic resonance spectroscopy. *Lancet* 1983; 1:1059.

9. Chance B: A noninvasive biochemical assay and imaging of animal and human tissues by optical and nuclear magnetic resonance techniques. *Proc Am Philosoph Soc* 1983; 127:1.

10. Chance B, Cohen P, Jöbsis F, et al: Intracellular oxidation-reduction sites in vivo. *Science* 1962; 137:499.

11. Chang N, Goodson WH, Gottrup R, et al: Direct measurement of wound and tissue oxygen tension in postoperative patients. *Ann Surg* 1983; 197:470.

12. Cruz J, Miner ME, Allen SJ: Modulating cerebral oxygen delivery in coma following acute diffuse brain injury. *Soc Neurosci Abst* 1984; 10:542.

13. Dawson J, Gadian DG, Wilkie DR: Contraction and recovery of living muscles studied by ^{31}P nuclear magnetic resonance. *J Physiol (Lond)* 1977; 267:703.

14. Deply DT, Gordon RE, Hope PI, et al: Noninvasive investigation of cerebral ischemia by phosphorus nuclear magnetic resonance. *Pediatrics* 1982; 70:310.

15. Fox JL: PET scan controversy aired. *Science* 1984; 244:143.

16. Gadian DG, Hoult DI, Radda GK, et al: Phosphorus nuclear magnetic resonance studies on normoxic and ischemic cardiac tissue. *Proc Natl Acad Sci USA* 1976; 73:446.

17. Hauser CJ, Klein SR, Mehringer M, et al: Superiority of transcutaneous oximetry in noninvasive vascular diagnosis in patients with diabetes. *Arch Surg* 1984; 119:690.

18. Hauser CJ, Shoemaker WC: Use of a transcutaneous PO_2 regional perfusion index to quantify tissue perfusion in peripheral vascular disease. *Ann Surg* 1983; 197:337.

19. Hauss J, Schönleben K, Spiegel U, et al: Measurements of local oxygen pressure in skeletal muscle of patients suffering from disturbances of arterial circulation. *Adv Exp Med Biol* 1978; 94:419.

20. Hilberman M, Subramanian H, Haselgrove J, et al: In vivo time resolved brain phosphorus nuclear magnetic resonance. *J Cerebr Blood Flow Metab* 1984; 4:334.

21. Huckabee WE: Relationships of pyruvate and lactate during anaerobic metabolism. *J Clin Invest* 1958; 37:244.

22. Jöbsis FF: Noninvasive infrared monitoring of cerebral and myocardial oxygen sufficiency and circulatory parameters. *Science* 1977; 198:1264.

23. Katsamouris A, Brewer DC, Megerman J, et al: Transcutaneous oxygen tension in selection of amputation level. *Am J Surg* 1984; 147:510.

24. Kessler M, Hoper J, Krumme BA: Monitoring of tissue perfusion and cellular function. *Anesthesiology* 1976; 45:184.

25. Kessler M, Lübbers DW: Aufbau und Anwendungs möglichkeiten verschiedener PO_2-Electroden. *Pflugers Arch Ges Physiol* 1966; 291:82.

26. Kovach AGB, Dora E, Eke A, et al: Effects of microcirculation on microfluorometric measurements, in Jöbsis FF (ed): *Oxygen and Physiological Function*. Dallas, Professional Information Library, 1977, pp 111–132.

27. Kram HB, Shoemaker WC: Method of intraoperative assessment of organ perfusion and viability using a miniature oxygen sensor. *Am J Surg* 1984; 148:404.

28. Lübbers DW: Theoretical basis of the transcutaneous blood gas measurements. *Crit Care Med* 1981; 9:721.

29. Magovern GJ, Flaherty JT, Kanter KR, et al: Assessment of myocardial protection during global ischemia with myocardial gas tension monitoring. *Surgery* 1982; 92:373.

30. Matsen FA, Bachy AW, Wyss CR, et al: Transcutaneous PO_2: A potential monitor of the status of replanted limb parts. *Plast Reconstr Surg* 1980; 65:732.

31. Meyer R, Kushmerick JJ, Brown TR: Application of ^{31}P-NMR spectroscopy to the study of striated muscle metabolism. *Am J Physiol* 1982; 242:C1.

32. Moon RB, Richards JH: Determination of intracellular pH by ^{31}P magnetic resonance. *J Biol Chem* 1973; 248:7276.

33. Niinikoski J, Hunt TK: Measurement of wound oxygen with implanted silastic tube. *Surgery* 1972; 71:22.

34. O'Connor JJ: Origin of labile NADH tissue fluorescence, in Jöbsis FF (ed): *Oxygen and Physiological Function*. Dallas, Professional Information Library, 1977, pp 90–99.

35. Phelps ME, Schelbert HR, Mazziotta JC: Positron computed tomography for studies of myocardial and cerebral function. *Ann Intern Med* 1983; 98:339.

36. Proctor HJ, Cairns C, Fillipo D, et al: Brain metabolism during increased intracranial pressure as assessed by niroscopy. *Surgery* 1984; 96:273.

37. Quistorff B, Chance B, Takeda H: Two and three dimensional redox heterogeneity of rat liver effects of anoxia and alcohol on the lobular redox pattern, in Dutton PL (ed): *Frontiers of Biological Energetics II*. New York, Academic Press, 1978, pp 1487–1497.

38. Reivich M, Kuhl D, Wolf A, et al: The (^{18}F) fluorodeoxyglucose method for the measurement of local cerebral glucose utilization in man. *Circ Res* 1979; 44:127.

39. Schönleben K, Hauss JP, Spiegel U, et al: Monitoring of tissue Po_2 in patients during intensive care. *Adv Exp Med Biol* 1978; 94:593.

40. Shulman RG, Brown TR, Ugurbil K, et al: Cellular application of ^{31}P and ^{13}C nuclear magnetic resonance. *Science* 1979; 205:160.

41. Singagowitz E, Golsong M, Halbfass HJ: Local tissue Po_2 in kidney surgery and transplantation. *Adv Exp Med Biol* 1978; 94:721.

42. Sokoloff L, Reivich M, Kennedy C, et al: The (^{14}C)-deoxyglucose method of the measurement of local cerebral glucose utilization. *J Neurochem* 1977; 28:897.

43. Tanaka J, Kamiyama Y, Sata T, et al: Pathophysiology of hemorrhagic shock: A role of arterial ketone body ratio as an index of anoxic metabolism of the liver in acute blood loss. *Adv Shock Res* 1981; 5:11.

44. Ter-Pogossian MM, Raichle ME, Sobel BE: Positron emission tomography. *Sci Am* 1980; 243:171.

45. Tremper KK, Shoemaker WC: Transcutaneous oxygen monitoring of critically ill adults with and without low flow shock. *Crit Care Med* 1981; 9:706.

46. Weaver JC: Continuous monitoring of volatile metabolites by mass spectrometer, in Cohen JS (ed): *Noninvasive Probes of Tissue Metabolism*. New York, John Wiley & Sons, 1982, pp 25–47.

47. Weil MH, Afifi AA: Experimental and clinical studies on lactate and pyruvate as indicators of the severity of acute failure (shock). *Circulation* 1978; 41:989.

48. Whalen WJ: Recent experiences with an intracellular oxygen electrode. *Prog Respir Res* 1969; 3:158.

PART 4 _____ Clinical
Evaluation
of Oxygen
Transport

13 Assessment of Systemic Oxygen Transport

James V. Snyder, M.D.

The foundation of supportive care of the critically ill patient is sustaining adequate transport of oxygen relative to need. Our practical first concern is for the net effect. Are the tissues getting sufficient oxygen, or not? We can often ascertain on clinical grounds that oxygen transport, both overall and in distribution, is sufficient for tissue needs. For example, a patient admitted with chest pain who is later alert, with normal vital signs and no symptoms, can justifiably be denied invasive monitoring. No laboratory data are more confirming of the adequacy of oxygen transport than is the demonstration of normal function. Normal function provides no quantitation and indicates nothing about any reserve that might be present, but it clearly ensures sufficient and adequately distributed oxygen transport. Other circumstances require more specific information—the adequacy of reserve, for example. If positive end-expiratory pressure (PEEP) is required to splint open the lung, will a decrease in cardiac output be tolerated or necessitate therapy?

It is worth noting that major errors occur frequently even when experienced clinicians estimate cardiac output on the basis of physical examination both of patients with a wide variety of problems and of others appearing well (see chapter 14, "Invasive Hemodynamic Assessment Compared with Clinical Evaluation").[10] *Physicians responsible for the care of patients in intensive care can correctly estimate the range of cardiac output or wedge pressure (WP) in less than 50% of their patients.* Further documentation of high or low total body flow says little about

whether it is distributed appropriately, whether it is adequate to meet the needs of the moment, or whether it is optimal. The need for this critical information is used to justify invasive monitoring, but quantitative assessment also has significant problems (see chapter 15, "Technical Problems in Data Acquisition"). The evaluation of overall systemic oxygen transport is discussed in this chapter. The emphasis is on components of the cardiopulmonary profile, but the reliable value of clinically observing function should be kept in mind.

THE USE OF CHALLENGES

Short of observing perfectly normal functions of all tissues, there is no way in clinical medicine to confirm that oxygen transport is adequate for current needs. The documentation of normal or high mixed venous oxygen tension ($P\bar{v}_{O_2}$) or cardiac output or any other index of cardiovascular performance does not ensure the absence of hypoxia, and values of each index that are usually associated with ischemia may in fact support normal function. Therefore, it is not possible to ascertain whether obtundation or poor renal function in a critically ill patient is due to insufficient perfusion simply by "collecting a profile." Fodder should not be confused with answers.

Rather than seek data that are quantitative but not directive, it is often more instructive to challenge the patient's physiology in various ways and observe the response. A patient with normal blood pressure but a decrease in urine output that may be due to covert blood loss or sepsis is an example. The responsiveness of the heart to increased preload may be easily and rapidly assessed at the bedside. Sudden elevation of the legs shifts venous blood from the legs into the abdomen, resulting in a transient increase in venous return. This increase in preload may be reflected in an increase in central venous pressure (CVP) or WP, and if cardiac output increases, in mean arterial pressure (MAP) as well. Elevating the legs also increases impedance to blood flow in the legs, and this increase in vascular resistance can contribute to the rise in MAP. Still, an increase in MAP from a sudden elevation of the legs suggests that a similar increase in MAP can be expected from intravascular volume loading. Thus a hypotensive patient in whom MAP increases with leg elevation deserves a volume challenge. No rise in MAP on leg elevation may indicate an inadequate volume shift, cardiac failure, or loss of peripheral vasomotor tone. In hypovolemic states, venoconstriction may deplete leg vein capacitance, minimizing the volume shift. This will be manifested by little or no increase in CVP. In cardiac failure, increases in preload may not increase cardiac output; thus, CVP and/or WP will increase without a resulting increase in MAP. Likewise, if cardiac function is normal but peripheral vasomotor tone is reduced, then increases in cardiac output associated with leg elevation may not increase MAP. However, in these conditions $S\bar{v}_{O_2}$ and $P\bar{v}_{O_2}$ should transiently increase and if monitored will document such a condition. Application of military antishock trousers provides a similar but more aggressive challenge as a change in position.[17]

If CVP or WP is lower than normal in a hypoperfused patient, it is usually appropriate to administer volume to raise that pressure. However, if CVP or WP is normal or high, challenging with volume may still be indicated—because a higher than normal preload may be necessary, because systemic vascular resistance (SVR) is excessively increased from hypovolemia and will not decrease until volume is adequate, or because neither CVP nor WP is a reliable indicator of preload. The presence of ventricular failure can be accounted for by observing the response to a sustained increase in airway pressure as described below. In the absence of ventricular failure, the risk of inducing pulmonary edema by administering volume to a patient whose WP is elevated (or unknown) is real but is only a calculated risk and not an absolute contraindication. Other risks in the same calculation are the complications of ongoing hypovolemia. Because hypovolemia enhances the probability of acute renal failure, the duration and risk of which are greater than in well-managed hydrostatic pulmonary edema, a trial of incrementally increased intravascular volume may be warranted in spite of the normal or high preload indicator. The increments may be continued until the deteriorating variable, in this case urine output, has improved or until the filling pressure has been elevated (by 5 torr, for example) for 2 hours without improvement. Worsening of pulmonary function or pulmonary edema may necessitate an increase in airway pressure but does not necessarily mean that volume administration must be stopped. On the other hand, elevating the filling pressure for 2 hours is usually sufficient to improve a low urine output when hypovolemia is an important factor. New pulmonary dysfunction with no improvement in spontaneous urine output indicates failure of the trial. Infusions may be stopped and administration of a chemical diuretic or even phlebotomy should be considered. This aggressive approach to volume administration commonly is justified in septic patients, as in case 13–1.

In other cases we have continuously restrained fluid administration in spite of oliguria. Patients with poor ventricular function after acute myocardial infarction or cardiac surgery are common examples. After an initial trial in which WP may be raised as high as 30 torr (in chronic ventricular failure) without improvement, fluids may be restricted in spite of urine output as low as 20–30 ml/hour. If urine osmolality remains high, renal perfusion may still be sufficient, and stable serial creatinine levels confirm that impression. Creatinine levels are misleading only when creatinine is diluted by massive fluid administration and in acute renal failure, when it overestimates renal function. Myocardial function commonly improves after 2 or 3 days in such patients, and renal function rarely is lost.

Concern that applying PEEP will retard venous return does not always necessitate pulmonary arterial catheter insertion. The filling of the venous capacitance bed can be estimated by applying a sustained increase in pressure to the airways of intubated patients. In the absence of very stiff lungs, no drop in arterial pressure during or after the increase in airway pressure indicates that the patient is probably not hypovolemic and that increasing PEEP is not likely to severely reduce venous return.

Hemodynamic Effect of Lung Inflation

Straining against a closed glottis (Valsalva maneuver) normally causes arterial pressure to change in a classic fashion, as shown in Figure 13–1,A. Because the main components of the underlying physiology of this arterial pressure response are understood, variations in it can be analyzed to gain useful insights regarding the state of contractility and circulating blood volume.[43] The response normally consists of an immediate increase in arterial pressure equal to the increase in pleural pressure. This increase is followed by a progressive decrease in stroke volume and a change in arterial pulse pressure as the obligatory decrease in venous return finally reaches the left ventricle (LV). On release from the strain phase with its associated sudden decrease in pleural pressure, arterial pressure immediately decreases. The fall in cardiac output during the latter part of the strain phase elicits reflex sympathetic output that increases vasomotor tone such that on re-

lease, when there is a marked increase in venous return, both stroke volume and arterial pressure rise above baseline. This postrelease increase in arterial pressure is called "overshoot."

When cardiac function is reduced, the increase in arterial pressure due to increased pleural pressure is still apparent, but the heart is unable to increase stroke volume much above baseline, and the overshoot phenomenon is lost. This is illustrated in Figure 13–1,B. The decrease in stroke volume is less prominent than normal, showing the decrease in venous return to be less pronounced in congestive heart failure states. When pleural pressure returns to normal on release, the surge in venous return is not associated with an overshoot of arterial pressure, which suggests that the ventricle is incapable of a greater response.

When ventricular function is severely compromised, a classic square wave response to the Valsalva maneuver can be seen (Fig 13–1,C). After the initial increase in arterial pressure, failure of the arterial pressure pulse to decrease suggests that venous return was not significantly lowered or that changes in preload do not affect stroke volume, which further suggests that the venous capacitance reservoirs are sufficiently

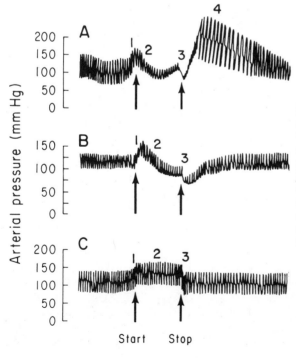

FIG 13–1.
Arterial pressure responses during the Valsalva maneuver. **A,** normal sinusoidal arterial pressure response; systolic arterial pressure rises transiently *(1)*, falls below baseline as positive ITP is maintained *(2)*, drops further with release of strain *(3)*, and then overshoots *(4)*. **B,** overshoot response in arterial pressure is absent. **C,** square wave arterial pressure response. (From Zema et al.[42] Reproduced by permission.)

filled that venous return is not influenced by the increase in pleural pressure. On release from the strain, neither a fall nor an overshoot of arterial pressure is seen.

To simulate a Valsalva maneuver in the intubated, uncooperative patient, one can use sustained manual hyperinflation to assess cardiovascular response. The application of sustained high pressure to the airway is different from the Valsalva maneuver in that the increase in intrathoracic pressure is greater than the intra-abdominal pressure, and pulmonary vascular resistance is more likely to be increased because lung volume increases. However, observations comparable to those described above can still be made, although none of the following have been confirmed or quantified to a satisfactory degree.

The increase in pleural pressure due to manual hyperinflation can be estimated by the initial change in CVP or WP. The immediate increase in arterial pressure should be the same as the immediate increase in venous pressure, although it is usually not as accurately seen, owing to the difference in scales used. The effect of increased airway pressure on venous return is better reflected in changes in stroke volume than in arterial pressure because the arterial pressure is sustained by the increase in pleural pressure. The absence of an overshoot in arterial pressure and the failure of arterial pressure to decline (the classic square wave response) suggest that the intravascular volume status is relatively high and that the ventricle is operating on a flat portion of the ventricular function curve. That is, the patient is in congestive heart failure. The normal decline in arterial pressure associated with an increase in airway pressure is not of predictive value since it can be seen in both normal and hypovolemic conditions.

$P\bar{v}_{O_2}$ AS AN INDICATOR

The most reliable single physiologic indicator for monitoring the overall balance between oxygen supply and demand is mixed venous oxygen tension ($P\bar{v}_{O_2}$). This view is not held widely and needs some defense. The two practical components of the defense will show that $P\bar{v}_{O_2}$ is the only index that reflects all the components of the oxygen supply/demand-release relationship and that $P\bar{v}_{O_2}$ is also the index least subject to tech-

nical artifacts in a sophisticated world highly sensitive to "garbage in, garbage out."

Logical Basis for Partial Pressure versus Content of Oxygen as an Indicator

The primary force that moves oxygen from the capillary into the cell is the partial pressure gradient. Oxygen diffusion is in direct proportion to capillary P_{O_2} minus the P_{O_2} at the site of consumption. Capillary P_{O_2} at any point reflects arterial oxygen content, local blood flow, and local oxygen uptake. End-capillary P_{O_2} reflects the balance among these factors, and mixed venous P_{O_2} is simply a flow-weighted mixture of the end-capillary P_{O_2} throughout the body; as such, it is the best indicator of the oxygen supply/demand balance in perfused tissues.[12, 24]

Empirical Basis for $P\bar{v}_{O_2}$ as an Indicator

The physiologic significance of $P\bar{v}_{O_2}$, compared with venous oxygen content or saturation or other components of oxygen supply or demand, is demonstrated in the various responses to leftward shift of the oxyhemoglobin dissociation curve, reviewed in chapter 1, "Oxygen Transport: The Model and Reality." There are multiple examples of tissue hypoxia related to lower venous P_{O_2} even when venous saturation is unchanged or higher. $P\bar{v}_{O_2}$ also reflects systemic supply/demand imbalance when the dissociation curve is normal. In studies of orthotopic cardiac prosthesis implantation, $P\bar{v}_{O_2}$ indicated changes in cardiac output earlier than did mixed venous saturation ($S\bar{v}_{O_2}$) or content ($C\bar{v}_{O_2}$) or arteriovenous oxygen content difference ($C(a-\bar{v})_{O_2}$).[34] In assessing the adequacy of oxygen transport, monitoring of $P\bar{v}_{O_2}$ was also superior to monitoring of $S\bar{v}_{O_2}$, total flow, and $C(a-\bar{v})_{O_2}$ in patients during cardiopulmonary bypass.[34] These experiments led to the conclusion that even continuous measurement of cardiac output would not be as valid an indication of the adequacy of tissue perfusion as $P\bar{v}_{O_2}$ in patients with marginal myocardial reserve. As described by Stanley and Isern-Amaral, "The reason is that cardiac output reflects only the ability of the heart and vascular system to move a certain volume of blood in a given time period and does not take into consideration the adequacy of that pumped blood to meet tissue metabolic needs. In animals who cannot increase cardiac output but yet sustain increases in tissue oxygen requirements, as from a rise in body temperature or shivering, monitoring the cardiac output will detect an unchanged cardiac output but not an imbalance of oxygen requirements and supply. However, $P\bar{v}_{O_2}$ or $S\bar{v}_{O_2}$ monitoring quickly reveals such imbalances and allows treatment to be initiated earlier, before dangerous degrees of anaerobic metabolism and metabolic acidosis occur."[34] (p 458)

In 20 patients with severe cardiac or pulmonary disease, or both, $P\bar{v}_{O_2}$ correlated better with both hyperlactatemia and survival than did cardiac output or partial pressure of oxygen in arterial blood (Pa_{O_2}) (Fig 13–2). A $P\bar{v}_{O_2}$ below 28 torr was usually associated with hyperlactatemia and was always associated with death in this study.[18]

In dogs, the lactate production threshold for $P\bar{v}_{O_2}$ was 27 whether caused by arterial hypoxemia, low cardiac output, or a combination of these variables (Fig 13–3).[30] These observations suggest that when vasoregulation is intact there is a threshold value, or critical $P\bar{v}_{O_2}$, of about 28 torr, below which anaerobic metabolism is usually manifest as an increase in blood lactate. In states of depressed myocardial function the correlation of $P\bar{v}_{O_2}$ with lactic acidosis has been better than the correlation of any other index, including cardiac output.

There is also support for a second critical $P\bar{v}_{O_2}$ threshold at about 20 torr, below which tissue function is progressively disturbed. For example, the $P\bar{v}_{O_2}$ at maximal exercise capacity is remarkably consistent at about this level in patients with normal hemoglobin, with acute anemia, and with chronic anemia[40] and in most patients with chronic obstructive pulmonary disease.[26, 37] This degree of consistency was not seen in unstressed (nonexercising, anemic, but otherwise healthy) individuals.[40] This suggests that exercise can induce vasoregulatory changes that are unnecessary at rest. The critical threshold for $P\bar{v}_{O_2}$ below which gross metabolic dysfunction is likely may be lower in chronic hypoxia. This may be due to enzymatic adaptation in the hypoxic state,[27] to an increase in capillary density,[36] or to enhanced microvasoregulation.[7, 8]

All this discussion suggests that metabolic activity is "normal" and oxygen consumption in ml/min ($\dot{V}_{O_2}$) is stable when perfusion is above a certain threshold (that which results in a $P\bar{v}_{O_2}$ of 28 torr when vasoregulation is intact) and abnormal below that point. However, it is important to recognize that metabolic changes do occur at higher levels of perfusion, such as when $P\bar{v}_{O_2}$ is greater than 28 torr, and only become more grossly evident at that threshold. For example, increased production of lactate by some tissues (as might be detected by monitoring muscle pH)

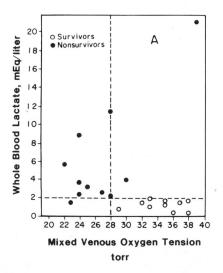
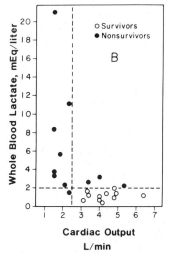

FIG 13–2.

Relation between blood lactate and $P\bar{v}_{O_2}$ **(A)** and cardiac output **(B)** in patients with cardiac failure. *Horizontal dashed line* at 2 mEq/L represents upper limit of normal lactate concentration. *Vertical dashed line* represents $P\bar{v}_{O_2}$ = 28 torr, suggested as a "critical level." (From Kasnitz et al.[18] Reproduced by permission.)

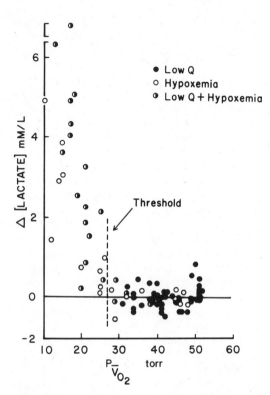

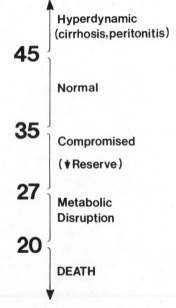

FIG 13–3.
Relation between $P\bar{v}_{O_2}$ and changes in blood lactate concentration in dogs with hypoxemia or low cardiac output. Threshold $P\bar{v}_{O_2}$ for increased lactate concentration is 27 torr. At elevated blood lactate concentrations, points for low Pa_{O_2} lie to left (at a lower $P\bar{v}_{O_2}$) of those for combined low cardiac outputs plus hypoxemia. (From Simmons et al.[30] Reproduced by permission.)

crease in $P\bar{v}_{O_2}$ reflects a decrease in the ratio of overall oxygen transport to demand in perfused tissues. In most circumstances, anaerobic metabolism and other signs of tissue dysfunction are evident when $P\bar{v}_{O_2}$ is below 28 torr. The difference between the observed $P\bar{v}_{O_2}$ and 28 torr allows approximation of the reserve oxygen transport relative to the current demand in perfused tissues. A Po_2 higher than 35 torr reliably indicates that overall oxygen transport is adequate for the current needs of the tissues represented. These observations lead to a simplistic concept of $P\bar{v}_{O_2}$ as an indicator of the adequacy of tissue oxygenation (Fig 13–4). Because diffusion of oxygen to the cell depends on the Po_2 gradient, and because gas solubility changes with temperature, the $P\bar{v}_{O_2}$ should be corrected to body temperature to reflect the in vivo $P\bar{v}_{O_2}$.

That $P\bar{v}_{O_2}$ reflects all the components of the oxygen supply/demand-release balance in perfused tissues is the source of its value but also the reason why detailed analysis is not simple. In straightforward cases $P\bar{v}_{O_2}$ decreases with cardiac output or hemoglobin, and increases with effective therapy. Table 1–1 in chapter 1, "Oxygen

might be compensated for by increased lactate consumption by heart, kidney, and liver.[4] The threshold $P\bar{v}_{O_2}$ value of 28 torr actually marks the level of metabolic change that is no longer fully compensated for (in terms of arterial lactate levels) rather than the onset of tissue hypoxia. In most conditions, $\dot{V}o_2$ remains stable when oxygen delivery ($\dot{D}o_2$) varies above this level. Disturbance of this threshold by edema or vascular obstruction–impaired vasoregulation is discussed later.

Interpretation of $P\bar{v}_{O_2}$

$P\bar{v}_{O_2}$ is normally about 40 torr. As long as tissue perfusion is adequate to support aerobic metabolism everywhere, any compromise of oxygen transport or increase in oxygen consumption causes $P\bar{v}_{O_2}$ to decrease. Without exception, a de-

FIG 13–4.
Simplistic analysis of $P\bar{v}_{O_2}$. In practice it must be recalled that unperfused tissue is not represented, and that this is an average value. A $P\bar{v}_{O_2}$ of 40 torr might represent normal oxygen supply/demand, or myocardial failure in a vasodilated septic patient.

Transport: The Model and Reality,'' gives the impression that the multiple components of oxygen transport and consumption are related in a simple algebraic sum, as in the following illustration. If administration of PEEP causes Pa_{O_2} to increase from 100 to 200 torr at the same FI_{O_2} without other change in therapy, it is very likely that pulmonary function (venous admixture) has been improved significantly and that arterial oxygen saturation and content have been increased by about 5% (see Fig 1–4). If at the same time cardiac index were reduced by 5%, $C(a-\bar{v})_{O_2}$ would increase, because more oxygen would be extracted from the lower blood flow. Because oxygen content of arterial blood (Ca_{O_2}) was increased the same amount as $C(a-\bar{v})_{O_2}$ increased, the oxygen supply/demand balance and the $P\bar{v}_{O_2}$ would not change. If cardiac index were depressed 10% instead of 5%, $S\bar{v}_{O_2}$ would drop about 5%, and $P\bar{v}_{O_2}$ would decrease accordingly. Measuring individual components of the oxygen supply/demand relationship without considering the overall balance may be misleading. The correspondence of $P\bar{v}_{O_2}$ with any one of its determinants is like the relation of a child's height to its father's: the mother's height, the child's age and nutritional status, and other determinants affect height as well, and its correlation with any one of these determinants will be poor.

When cardiac index is depressed so severely that perfusion of some tissues is lost, analysis becomes more complex.

CASE 13–1.—An 83-year-old man who developed respiratory distress after hip surgery had the cardiopulmonary profile shown in Table 13–1. A chest x-ray film showed a right lower lobe infiltrate. There was increased pulmonary shunt (Qs/Qt), "adequate" filling pressure, and subnormal cardiac performance, along with a somewhat greater than normal oxygen consumption. The near-normal cardiac index and increased $C(a-\bar{v})_{O_2}$ were not sufficient to compensate for the high $\dot{V}_{O_2}$, and loss of reserve in the system was shown by the $P\bar{v}_{O_2}$ of 32 torr. Blood was transfused to the patient, he was mechanically ventilated, and PEEP was increased. Shunting subsequently was decreased, but the cardiac index deteriorated markedly (see Table 13–1, column 2).

Discussion.—Marked imbalance in the oxygen supply/demand in perfused tissues is apparent in the $P\bar{v}_{O_2}$ of 23 torr after PEEP was increased. However, the threat to the patient was more severe than that suggested by the $P\bar{v}_{O_2}$, as the car-

TABLE 13–1.

Cardiopulmonary Response to Aggressive Application of PEEP (Case 13–1)*†

PARAMETER	PROFILE 1	PROFILE 2	PROFILE 3
PEEP (cm H_2O)	5	20	5
MAP (torr)	65	58	70
WP (torr)	14	25	18
CVP (torr)	18	16	NA
CI (L/min/m²)	3.2	1.2	2.9
FI_{O_2}	.5	.5	.45
Pa_{O_2} (torr)	95	81	122
$P\bar{v}_{O_2}$ (torr)	32	23	34
$\dot{V}_{O_2}$ (ml/min/m²)	179	113	203
$\dot{Q}va/\dot{Q}t$	.15	.05	.04

*From Snyder et al.[33] Reproduced by permission.
†Pulmonary function improved but venous return was so compromised as to cause tissue hypoxia. Pulmonary function remained excellent after PEEP was reduced, suggesting that a more transient elevation of airway pressure might have given the same result, without significant depression of cardiac function. NA, not available; CI, cardiac index; WP, wedge pressure.

diac index and the oxygen consumption show. Although the $\dot{V}_{O_2}$ of 110/min/m² is within normal limits, the 38% drop in oxygen consumption made it apparent that oxygen provision was inadequate. Even a 68% increase in $C(a-\bar{v})_{O_2}$ is insufficient to compensate for the reduction in cardiac index. Recall that by the Fick relation, $\dot{V}_{O_2}$ is the product of cardiac output and Ca_{O_2}. If $\dot{V}_{O_2}$ is constant, a reduction in one multiplier to 3/4 requires an increase in the other by 4/3, or in this case, a reduction in cardiac output to 37% is fully compensated for only by an increase in $C(a-\bar{v})_{O_2}$ of 1/.37, or 270%. That extraction being impossible, $\dot{V}_{O_2}$ must drop.

The influence of PEEP on cardiac output varies with pulmonary compliance; more compliant lung allows greater change in pleural pressure when airway pressure is increased. A limited infiltrate on the chest x-ray film and the relatively low shunt seen in the first study suggest that pulmonary compliance may be close to normal; this increases the probability that an increase in PEEP will depress venous return. We could also question the increase in PEEP in this patient on the basis that the high $D(a-a)_{O_2}$ was due largely to low $P\bar{v}_{O_2}$, and little to pulmonary disease. The relative maintenance of arterial pressure during this dramatic drop in blood flow exemplifies the danger of monitoring systemic arterial pressure for change in cardiac output.

The Influence of Loss of Vasoregulation

Although $P\bar{v}_{O_2}$ always indicates oxygen supply/ demand for perfused tissues, the use of $P\bar{v}_{O_2}$ to mark a *threshold* for oxygen transport, below and above which anaerobic metabolism is and is not manifest, depends on intact, consistent vasoregulation and no significant edema. The loss or compromise of vasoregulation or the presence of edema does not change the value of $P\bar{v}_{O_2}$ as an indicator of overall oxygen supply/demand for perfused tissues, but it does negate the critical threshold.

Several modifiers of vasoregulation have important effects: (1) Changing cutaneous vasoregulation to control heat dissipation[16, 28] and changing renal blood flow in response to various stimuli both have significant influence on oxygen transport variables. (2) The vasoregulating response varies with different compromises of oxygen transport. (3) The classic stress response may be superimposed on local control. (4) Vasoregulation can be quite distorted in disease states.

The components of cardiac output that normally are subject to considerable influence other than local metabolic regulation are the blood flows to the skin and to the kidneys.[29] Neurohumoral response by the hypothalamus to elevated core temperature may dilate cutaneous vessels, causing a significant drop in SVR and decreasing ventricular preload as the enlarged capacitance of skin vessels is filled. If cardiac output is limited, blood flow to vital tissues, such as ischemic brain or working respiratory muscles, may be compromised as flow is "stolen" for the function of heat reduction. Yet cardiac output and $P\bar{v}_{O_2}$ might be unchanged or increased and $C(a-\bar{v})_{O_2}$ lowered. Changes in the renal blood flow may also be confusing. A decrease in cardiac output and in $P\bar{v}_{O_2}$ would have a different implication when caused by a decrease in return of highly oxygen-saturated renal blood flow, due to a chemical change, than when caused by blood loss. Monitoring $C(a-\bar{v})_{O_2}$ or $\dot{V}_{O_2}$ would not distinguish this difference sensitively, either.

Vasoregulation is distorted by various disease states. It is limited whenever there is anatomical vascular compromise (severe systemic atherosclerosis, cerebral or coronary vasospasm, arterial embolism) and becomes abnormal whenever vascular beds are pathologically dilated, as in cerebral hyperperfusion following ischemic insults,[21] in inflammatory hyperperfusion,[1] and in cirrhosis[22] and sepsis. A rise in $P\bar{v}_{O_2}$ may be the first noticeable sign of sepsis, and a higher than normal $P\bar{v}_{O_2}$ is associated with lactic acidosis almost as predictably as is a low $P\bar{v}_{O_2}$. In systemic sepsis there is risk of inadequate perfusion to many tissues at the same time that cardiac output, $C(a-\bar{v})_{O_2}$, and $P\bar{v}_{O_2}$ values suggest adequate oxygen transport. The overperfusion of some beds more than compensates for the low perfusion of other tissues in effect on cardiac output, $C(a-\bar{v})_{O_2}$, and $P\bar{v}_{O_2}$, and the drop in oxygen consumption is often not great enough to identify inadequate perfusion of a small vascular bed. This circumstance emphasizes that cardiac output, $C(a-\bar{v})_{O_2}$, $P\bar{v}_{O_2}$, and oxygen consumption are only net figures; they contribute information relative to overall oxygen supply/demand, but give no specific information about local events. The analysis of $P\bar{v}_{O_2}$ must therefore include the recognition that mixed venous blood contains no efflux from nonperfused tissues, that severely hypoxic tissues are underrepresented, and that perfusion of some vascular beds in excess of the normal reserve "artifactually" elevates $P\bar{v}_{O_2}$. Thus, a septic patient with adequate volume repletion might initially have a $P\bar{v}_{O_2}$ greater than 45 torr. A later decrease in $P\bar{v}_{O_2}$ to 38 torr might be due to the onset of some compromise of $\dot{D}_{O_2}$ such as ventricular failure, as a result of which some adequately perfused vascular beds might become underperfused, or the decrease in $P\bar{v}_{O_2}$ might instead be due to resolution of the septic process with a decrease in hyperperfusion of dilated vessels. Such a critical distinction can be difficult to make, and it is usually impossible to make from hemodynamic data alone.

There is an obvious flaw in applying this algebraic concept of oxygen transport and consumption to conditions in which vasoregulation is impaired, as in some patients with liver cirrhosis or sepsis. Under these circumstances, local physiology is often dissociated from *all* indicators of overall function, and although changes in cardiac output, $C(a-\bar{v})_{O_2}$, and $P\bar{v}_{O_2}$ are likely to reflect relative improvement or deterioration, absolute correlations are unreliable. It is important to realize this flaw in all whole-system monitoring approaches. If, for example, blood flow to an extremity or a visceral organ is abruptly stopped by emboli, there may be no change in any commonly available systemic monitoring index unless the device happens to be sensing via that tissue. Tissue that is not perfused is not represented in

$P\bar{v}_{O_2}$, and vascular obstructions must be quite large to be directly evident in monitored cardiac output or $\dot{V}_{O_2}$.

CASE 13–2.—A 68-year-old man with renal failure and severe peripheral vascular disease underwent resection of an abdominal aortic aneurysm. After recovering from anesthesia, he experienced pain in his right leg, which became mottled and colder than the left. Progressive metabolic acidosis required the infusion of several hundred mEq of bicarbonate over 6 hours. He was returned to the operating room for insertion of an arteriovenous fistula and for additional attempts to remove vascular obstructions from the right leg. Initial evaluation on his return to the ICU showed an increased bicarbonate and pH even though no bicarbonate had been administered since he left the ICU. Initial enthusiasm about his improved condition was dampened by continued observation of the right leg. It became apparent that severely compromised flow to the leg had been sufficient to return metabolic acids to the systemic circulation, creating the need for bicarbonate administration. That flow had now stopped, and the ischemia was no longer clinically apparent in the systemic circulation.

OTHER OXYGEN SUPPLY/ DEMAND COMPONENTS AS INDICATORS OF OXYGEN TRANSPORT ADEQUACY

While these complex changes in sepsis and cirrhosis make analysis of $P\bar{v}_{O_2}$ difficult in many patients, the problems in assessing the adequacy of a patient's hemodynamic status using other components of oxygen transport and consumption are comparable or worse. Abnormal cardiac output, hemoglobin concentration, and Pa_{O_2} commonly contribute to deficient transport, but their measurement is both insufficient and inefficient. Cardiac output reflects hyperperfused as well as hypoperfused beds and reflects only supply, not demand.

$C(a-\bar{v})_{O_2}$ is valuable in that it varies inversely with the ratio of oxygen transport to oxygen consumption when the compromise is not severe. However, severe inadequacies are not fully reflected in $C(a-\bar{v})_{O_2}$, as demonstrated in case 13–1. In fact, a patient with very severe anemia or a left-shifted dissociation curve might have tissue hypoxia (appropriately reflected in low $P\bar{v}_{O_2}$) when $C(a-\bar{v})_{O_2}$ is still less than normal.

$S\bar{v}_{O_2}$ approximates $P\bar{v}_{O_2}$ in monitoring value and implication in most cases.[20, 36] However, the superiority of $P\bar{v}_{O_2}$ is apparent when shifts in the oxyhemoglobin dissociation curve induce lower $P\bar{v}_{O_2}$ and organ dysfunction while $S\bar{v}_{O_2}$ remains unchanged (reviewed in chapter 1, "Oxygen Transport: The Model and Reality"). Also, $S\bar{v}_{O_2}$ is commonly less available than $P\bar{v}_{O_2}$. In spite of these limitations, the continuous measurement of $S\bar{v}_{O_2}$ improves the monitoring of some unstable patients. This is reviewed in a following section and in chapter 16, "Mixed Venous Oximetry." The oxygen utilization coefficient is defined as the ratio of oxygen consumption to oxygen delivery ($\dot{V}_{O_2}/\dot{D}_{O_2}$), which can also be expressed as $C(a-\bar{v})_{O_2}/Ca_{O_2}$.[36] It does consider the demand and supply in oxygen economics, but because $\dot{V}_{O_2}$ can be pathologically reduced owing to nonperfusion of some tissues, the ratio may be normal in severe shock. As reviewed in chapter 16, the oxygen utilization coefficient has the same meaning as the reciprocal of $S\bar{v}_{O_2}$ but is more complicated to determine.

In most patients, $\dot{V}_{O_2}$ is an insensitive indicator because change is minimal until all compensatory mechanisms have been exhausted and because the $\dot{V}_{O_2}$ itself varies with many factors. We have found the principal value in measuring $\dot{V}_{O_2}$ to be in demonstrating the adequacy of cardiac output during the treatment of shock and in detecting artifactual cardiac output measurements. When intravenous infusion of volume to a patient in shock has quickly resulted in higher cardiac output and $\dot{V}_{O_2}$, we assume that hypoxic tissues are being better perfused and that the increase in blood flow is beneficial. That $\dot{V}_{O_2}$ will increase simply because of increased cardiac work must be taken into account. Increased activity of non-ATP oxidase systems is another possible cause of confusion.[8] Monitoring $\dot{V}_{O_2}$ to titrate therapy has other complications. Our experimental laboratory data helped elucidate some of the reasons for the insensitivity of $\dot{V}_{O_2}$ in this application.[9] In primates receiving a large infusion of *E. coli*, $\dot{V}_{O_2}$ decreased only when cardiac output was decreased (and increased dramatically when shivering occurred). However, even after controlling for noncirculatory influences on $\dot{V}_{O_2}$ such as shivering and hyperventilation,[19] interpretation of our $\dot{V}_{O_2}$ values is difficult. Sepsis places metabolic demands on the organism, the satisfaction of which increases $\dot{V}_{O_2}$. Consequently, even an elevated $\dot{V}_{O_2}$ could be consistent with impairment of oxidative metabolism, since the $\dot{V}o_2$ might have been even greater without the impairment. As the stress and dysfunction of shock progress, the measured $\dot{V}o_2$ might be decreased, normal, or increased, depending on the algebraic sum of the changes mentioned. Another factor weighing against the use of $\dot{V}o_2$ as a monitoring tool is the ability of heart and voluntary muscle to function during strenuous activity under an oxygen debt as great as 40 ml/kg of muscle tissue,[13] in contrast to the limited tolerance of visceral organs to oxygen debt. Hence, the implications of depression of $\dot{V}o_2$ from compromise of somatic perfusion may be quite different from the implications of depression of $\dot{V}o_2$ caused by change in visceral perfusion. When $\dot{V}o_2$, calculated from cardiac output and $C(a-\bar{v})o_2$, seems inappropriately high or low for the observed clinical condition, we suspect artifactual cardiac output measurement is a common cause.

Despite these complexities, measuring $\dot{V}o_2$ has unique value when metabolic vasoregulation is impaired. When loss of vasoregulation distorts the significance of all other indices, valid documentation that an increase in $\dot{D}o_2$ is accompanied by an increase in $\dot{V}o_2$ (more than that caused by increase in cardiac work) strongly suggests that tissue oxygenation has been meaningfully improved.

PLASMA LACTIC ACID AS AN INDICATOR OF OXYGEN TRANSPORT

Lactate concentrations are subject to interpretation difficulties also. Circulatory failure is associated with increased lactate production.[39] However, lactic acidemia can result from alkalemia-induced increases in red blood cell glycolysis[31, 35] or decreased liver lactate metabolism[25] (which can in itself reflect circulatory failure for one organ) or be due to the increase in lactic acid incurred by vigorous muscular exercise (including rigors and seizures). Furthermore, the "washout" of hypoperfused tissue can increase blood lactate levels during fluid resuscitation when perfusion is actually improving.[9, 39]

In addition to nonspecificity, insensitivity of lactic acidemia to tissue hypoxia has been found experimentally.[30] Nonetheless, lactate concentration is clinically useful as an index of the severity of hemodynamic insufficiency.[6]

QUANTITATION OF OXYGEN TRANSPORT ADEQUACY

Numeric estimates of the adequacy of oxygen transport are the consumable oxygen coefficient and the reserve oxygen transport coefficient. The *consumable oxygen coefficient* is $(C\bar{v}o_2 - C_{20}O_2)/Cao_2$, where $C_{20}O_2$ is the calculated content of blood at a Po_2 of 20 torr.[5] It specifies the proportion of total oxygen transport that has not been but could be consumed, based on the assumption that a $P\bar{v}o_2$ of 20 torr indicates the lower limit of oxygen available to the tissues.

We prefer our calculated index, *reserve oxygen transport (ROT) coefficient* (Fig 13–5), which specifies the proportion of total oxygen transport that is in aerobic reserve. The ROT is the additional oxygen that could be consumed per minute until $P\bar{v}o_2$ reached 28 torr, since blood lactate levels tend to increase when $P\bar{v}o_2$ is at or below 28 torr. The ROT coefficient is the ratio of ROT to total $\dot{D}o_2$.

Both ROT and the consumable oxygen index quantify oxygen reserve on the basis of all the overall factors involved in oxygen physiology. According to the ROT concept, when $P\bar{v}o_2$ is 28 torr there is no ROT, but if vasoregulation is intact (including no vascular obstruction) and edema is not significant, arterial oxygen transport is still sufficient to fully satisfy tissue needs without manifest metabolic disruption. Any increase in needs or decrease in oxygen transport is likely to be associated with clinical signs of tissue hypoxia. In contrast, when $P\bar{v}o_2$ is 20 torr all theoretically possible oxygen extraction has occurred (except for poorly understood states of chronic adaption to hypoxia).[27] Both of these quantitative approaches can be applied regionally or to organ perfusion when the appropriate venous sampling is possible. However, both approaches suffer from one having to assume that the $\dot{V}o_2$ present, even if depressed, specifies the demand to which the supply should be compared. Indeed it is that very case, depressed $\dot{V}o_2$, that proves difficult for analysis by any means except maneuvers to increase oxygen transport in order to find out if the increased $\dot{D}o_2$ will support increased $\dot{V}o_2$, and even then the change in $\dot{V}o_2$ may only be a manifestation of increased cardiac work. Assessing the relation between short-term changes in $\dot{V}o_2$ and $\dot{D}o_2$, as described in chapter 5, "Patterns of

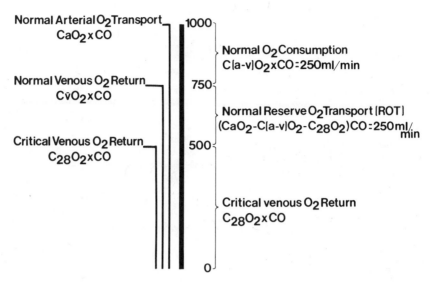

FIG 13–5.
Components of oxygen transport, with emphasis on reserve oxygen transport *(ROT)* as the difference between actual venous oxygen return and oxygen re- turn when $P\bar{v}_{O_2}$ = 28 torr. (From Snyder and Carroll.[32] Reproduced by permission.)

Hemodynamic Response,'' may prove to be more insightful than simpler approaches.

SHORTCUTS IN ASSESSMENT

Shortcuts can improve efficiency, cut costs, speed interim diagnosis, and improve the titration of care. However, because most shortcuts entail assumptions, they are dangerous if the assumptions are not kept in mind as possible sources of error. Using $P\bar{v}_{O_2}$ to assess all the components of oxygen supply/demand is a shortcut. The use of challenges, such as increasing airway pressure to assess preload, might be considered a shortcut. The calculation of pulmonary venous admixture is only a representation of the degree of V/Q mismatch, as is pulmonary deadspace measurement. Perhaps least appreciated is the concise information available from sequential pairs of arterial and mixed venous P_{O_2} values. And the most abused and misleading shortcut might be the assumption that Pa_{O_2} represents either pulmonary function or tissue oxygenation. Additional shortcuts are available in knowing the time needed for stabilization after effecting a change in therapy, in looking for common events first, and in the physician's observing the patient while drawing blood samples.

Arterial Oxygen Tension

Interpretation of Pa_{O_2} without knowledge of $F_{I_{O_2}}$ is limited to the assurance that saturation is probably high if Pa_{O_2} is over 60 torr. The alveolar-arterial P_{O_2} gradient ($P(A-a)_{O_2}$) is commonly derived after approximating alveolar P_{O_2} as $F_{I_{O_2}} \times P_B - 47 - Pa_{CO_2}/0.8$ (P_B indicating barometric pressure) and then using alveolar P_{O_2} to estimate the pulmonary shunt as equal to 1% for each 20 torr gradient when $F_{I_{O_2}}$ = 1.0. Equating the $P(A-a)_{O_2}$ gradient with intrapulmonary shunt assumes $C(a-\bar{v})_{O_2}$ to be normal. This is commonly incorrect, of course, and can lead to grossly inappropriate therapy.[38] When oxygen content of mixed venous blood ($C\bar{v}_{O_2}$) is higher than assumed, the pulmonary function is worse than is indicated by the calculation from $P(A-a)_{O_2}$. If $C\bar{v}_{O_2}$ is lower, the more severely desaturated blood passes through the shunt or low V/Q lung regions and causes arterial desaturation, and the estimated venous admixture is then worse than actual pulmonary function.

CASE 13–3.—A 37-year-old woman underwent aortic and mitral valve replacement and tricuspid annuloplasty. When fully awake 36 hours after surgery she repeatedly became dyspneic and anxious when ventilatory support was diminished. The cause was initially considered to be pulmonary failure because Pa_{O_2} was 96 while she was receiving an FI_{O_2} of .45, and she was hemodynamically stable. However, a Po_2 value from a catheter in the superior vena cava was 23 torr, suggesting that most of the increase in $P(A-a)_{O_2}$ was due to venous hypoxia. A more detailed study showed $P\bar{v}_{O_2}$ to be 26 torr, Ca_{O_2} to be 13.1 ml/dl, $C\bar{v}_{O_2}$ to be 7.1 ml/dl, and venous admixture to be only 8%.

Thus, in the interpretation of Pa_{O_2}, venous oxygenation is pertinent as well as FI_{O_2}. Assessment of the venous oxygen level is particularly important when cardiac output is likely to vary from normal or to change. This is illustrated further in the following section on Po_2 pairs.

The primary effect on Pa_{O_2} of changing FI_{O_2} can be measured within 10 minutes in patients without obstructive lung disease and within 30 minutes in patients with chronic lung disease.[41]

Po_2 Pairs

The Po_2 values in simultaneously drawn samples of arterial and mixed venous blood provide independent information about systemic oxygenation and pulmonary function. As discussed in earlier chapters, when $P\bar{v}_{O_2}$ is less than 35 torr, there is always less than normal oxygen transport relative to demand. When $P\bar{v}_{O_2}$ is less than 28 torr, there is minimal or no reserve left, even when vasoregulation is intact. Higher values of $P\bar{v}_{O_2}$ always reflect a higher than normal oxygen transport to demand ratio in perfused tissues, but tissue hypoxia may still be present because of vascular obstruction or vasoderegulation. The $P\bar{v}_{O_2}$ represents all tissues in proportion to their flow; nonperfused tissues are not represented. The addition of a Pa_{O_2} value to this interpretation merely indicates whether arterial hypoxemia is contributing significantly to any venous hypoxia. Because Po_2 pairs are more often available and reliable than other variables, reviewing examples of the use of Po_2 pairs in evaluating systemic oxygenation can be valuable.

Example 13–1 $P\bar{v}_{O_2}$ of 40 torr; Pa_{O_2} of 100 torr

The interpretation is normal oxygen supply/demand in perfused tissues. Note that distribution of perfusion may be severely altered, and tissues with no perfusion are not represented. Arterial blood is almost fully saturated unless there is a very severe rightward shift in the oxyhemoglobin dissociation curve or abnormal hemoglobin is present.

Example 13–2 $P\bar{v}_{O_2}$ of 30 torr; Pa_{O_2} of 70 torr

Obviously the oxygen transport is significantly compromised. The decrease in $S\bar{v}_{O_2}$ is about 20%. ($P\bar{v}_{O_2}$ of 30 torr is approximately equal to $S\bar{v}_{O_2}$ of 53 if the dissociation curve is normal.) Half of this drop in $S\bar{v}_{O_2}$ is due to a decrease in Sa_{O_2} of about 10%. The other 10% drop in $S\bar{v}_{O_2}$ is probably not due to anemia because arteriovenous content and saturation differences are not usually affected by anemia. The severity of venous hypoxia is therefore due to some combination of increase in oxygen consumption and decrease in cardiac output, or to a severe leftward shift of the dissociation curve.

Example 13–3 $P\bar{v}_{O_2}$ of 30 torr; Pa_{O_2} of 500 torr

Obviously the patient is receiving a high FI_{O_2}, and oxygen transport is severely compromised. Is the high Pa_{O_2} of value to the patient? If we knew that hemoglobin was 10 gm/dl and the dissociation curve was normal, we could calculate $C\bar{v}_{O_2}$ to equal $S\bar{v}_{O_2}$ (53%) $\times$ oxygen-carrying capacity (10 gm/dl $\times$ 1.36 ml O_2/gm), or about 7.2 ml/dl. If Pa_{O_2} were reduced to normal and no other changes occurred, both Ca_{O_2} and $C\bar{v}_{O_2}$ would be reduced by (400 $\times$ 0.03 ml/dl), or 1.2 ml/dl. $C\bar{v}_{O_2}$ would be reduced to 6.0 ml/dl, which would be .44 $\times$ capacity, or $S\bar{v}_{O_2}$ = .44; and $P\bar{v}_{O_2}$ would be about 25 torr. The chance of tissue hypoxia would clearly be increased by this change, and Pa_{O_2} should therefore be maintained at this high value until oxygen transport can be improved in some other way.

Example 13–4 $P\bar{v}_{O_2}$ of 50 torr; Pa_{O_2} of 80 torr

Oxygen transport in perfused tissues is greater than normal. This is not significantly influenced by a minor decrease in arterial saturation. Nothing can be said about arterial oxygen content because that depends so much on hemoglobin concentration. Pulmonary venous admixture is not as low as suggested by the Pa_{O_2}, regardless of the $F_{I_{O_2}}$, as seen when the high $P\bar{v}_{O_2}$ is taken into account.

Assessment of Pulmonary Function by P_{O_2} Pairs

As summarized in the section on Pa_{O_2} and illustrated by case 13–3, the analysis of lung function depends on assessment of venous oxygen content. However, although accurate calculation of pulmonary venous admixture requires calculation of arterial and venous oxygen content with the accuracy of a research laboratory, significant changes in pulmonary function usually can be appreciated by looking at changes in arterial and mixed venous P_{O_2} pairs. In this approach it is assumed the dissociation curve does not change between sequential measurements. When Pa_{CO_2} changes (or other changes that shift the dissociation curve) take place, interpretation is made more cautiously. It should be clear that pulmonary function is improved when the P_{O_2} pair

$$\begin{bmatrix} P\bar{v}_{O_2} \text{ of 40 torr} \\ Pa_{O_2} \text{ of 100 torr} \end{bmatrix}$$ changes, following the addi-

tion of PEEP, to $\begin{bmatrix} P\bar{v}_{O_2} \text{ of 40 torr} \\ Pa_{O_2} \text{ of 200 torr} \end{bmatrix}$. It might

take an extra moment to understand that the change from

$$\begin{bmatrix} P\bar{v}_{O_2} \text{ of 40 torr} \\ Pa_{O_2} \text{ of 100 torr} \end{bmatrix} \text{ to } \begin{bmatrix} P\bar{v}_{O_2} \text{ of 50 torr} \\ Pa_{O_2} \text{ of 100 torr} \end{bmatrix}$$ indi-

cates a deterioration in pulmonary function. A change from

$$\begin{bmatrix} P\bar{v}_{O_2} \text{ of 40 torr} \\ Pa_{O_2} \text{ of 100 torr} \end{bmatrix} \text{ to } \begin{bmatrix} P\bar{v}_{O_2} \text{ of 30 torr} \\ Pa_{O_2} \text{ of 100 torr} \end{bmatrix}$$ is an

improvement (again in lung function; systemic oxygenation is worse). Intuitively, the lung is not functioning as effectively if it receives blood with more oxygen and cannot at the same time increase the arterial P_{O_2}. When Pa_{O_2} is unchanged or lower and $P\bar{v}_{O_2}$ is higher, venous admixture is greater. When Pa_{O_2} is the same or increased and $P\bar{v}_{O_2}$ is lower, venous admixture is less.

Thus, P_{O_2} pairs can provide information on both systemic oxygen transport and pulmonary function. Consider the following result of increasing PEEP:

Example 13–5 $P\bar{v}_{O_2}$ of 35 torr, Pa_{O_2} of 80 torr with no PEEP; $P\bar{v}_{O_2}$ of 27 torr, Pa_{O_2} of 180 torr following the addition of 15 cm H_2O PEEP; other variables, such as $F_{I_{O_2}}$, are constant.

Severely depressed oxygen transport is evident in the lower $P\bar{v}_{O_2}$. We can see that the improvement in pulmonary function suggested by the elevation of Pa_{O_2} is a marked improvement when we realize that the elevation occurs in spite of a decrease in $P\bar{v}_{O_2}$.

The analysis is more complicated if the arterial and venous P_{O_2} both change in the same direction, as in the following change from the addition of PEEP:

Example 13–6 $P\bar{v}_{O_2}$ of 34 torr, Pa_{O_2} of 60 torr without PEEP; $P\bar{v}_{O_2}$ of 39 torr, Pa_{O_2} of 90 torr after addition of 10 cm H_2O PEEP.

Both arterial and venous P_{O_2} improved, but do the changes represent primarily improved pulmonary function or cardiac output? Initially, it could appear that improvement in cardiac output caused $P\bar{v}_{O_2}$ (and $C\bar{v}_{O_2}$) to rise, which appeared as higher Pa_{O_2}, with no change in venous admixture. Or the pulmonary function might have been dramatically improved, the subsequent increase in Sa_{O_2} simply causing an equal increase in $S\bar{v}_{O_2}$, with no change in cardiac output. The point can be discriminated by comparing the changes in saturation and invoking the Fick relation. The change in Pa_{O_2} from 60 to 90 torr represents a change in Sa_{O_2} of almost 10%, and the change in saturation in the venous range is about 2%/1 torr P_{O_2}, or in this case, also about 10%. Therefore, the increase in $S\bar{v}_{O_2}$ is the same as the increase in arterial saturation. By the Fick relation, $\dot{V}_{O_2}$ = cardiac output $\times$ $C(a-\bar{v})_{O_2}$. We can use saturation instead of content unless hemoglobin is dramatically changed between measurements, and if we assume that $\dot{V}_{O_2}$ is not different between these two measurements, then the difference between arterial and venous saturation should change inversely with cardiac output. Because Sa_{O_2} and $S\bar{v}_{O_2}$ change the same percentage, $C(a-\bar{v})_{O_2}$ was the same and cardiac output was probably the same, and the changes seen were due primarily to lower venous admixture.

A common error is to look only at Pa_{O_2} after removal of PEEP, and to assume that an unchanged value indicates no deterioration in venous admixture. The next sequence illustrates another likely possibility.

Example 13–7 $P\bar{v}_{O_2}$ of 38 torr, Pa_{O_2} of 100 torr with 10 cm H_2O PEEP; $P\bar{v}_{O_2}$ of 43 torr, Pa_{O_2} of 100 torr after reducing PEEP to 5 cm H_2O.

The increase in $S\bar{v}_{O_2}$ with no change in Sa_{O_2} indicates that cardiac output increased after removal of PEEP. The failure of Pa_{O_2} to increase despite an increase in $S\bar{v}_{O_2}$ shows an increase in venous admixture that was compensated for, in terms of Pa_{O_2}, by an increase in cardiac output and $C\bar{v}_{O_2}$.

Finally, consider the effect of nitroprusside administration to a hypertensive patient with bibasilar atelectasis shown by chest x-ray film and high SVR after coronary artery bypass grafting.

Example 13–8 $P\bar{v}_{O_2}$ of 30 torr, Pa_{O_2} of 180 torr prior to nitroprusside;

$P\bar{v}_{O_2}$ of 40 torr, Pa_{O_2} of 80 torr with nitroprusside.

Systemic oxygen transport is markedly improved, as shown by the increase in $P\bar{v}_{O_2}$ despite a drop of a few percentage points in Sa_{O_2}. The increase in venous admixture is due to suppression of hypoxic pulmonary vasoconstriction in atelectatic lung and is more apparent when the higher $P\bar{v}_{O_2}$ is considered in addition to the lower Pa_{O_2}. The implications of change in Po_2 pairs are listed in Table 13–2.

Response Time and Mixed Venous Oximetry

Prompt feedback is essential to effective analysis and titration of therapy. The most immediate return of information is continuous, such as mixed venous oximetry. For example, the advantage and optimal settings of balloon counterpulsation and of atrial pacing are immediately apparent in Figure 13–6. The goal of a fluid challenge is to increase not preload but oxygen transport, which is achieved more directly by monitoring of $S\bar{v}_{O_2}$ than of WP (Fig 13–7). PEEP may be increased to 20 cm H_2O within minutes without impairment of oxygen transport, or minimal changes may depress tissue oxygenation immediately; either response may be apparent in the $S\bar{v}_{O_2}$ (Fig 13–8). Similarly, changing from assisted to intermittent mandatory ventilation may increase venous return and $S\bar{v}_{O_2}$ (Fig 13–9), or a frail patient may be intolerant of breathing spontaneously, especially

TABLE 13–2.

Common Implications of Arterial and Venous Po_2 Changes*

BLOOD GAS VALUE	IMPLICATIONS
Unchanged Pao_2 and ↑ $P\bar{v}_{O_2}$	↑ $\dot{Q}va/\dot{Q}t$ and ↑ CI
↑ Pa_{O_2} and unchanged or ↓ $P\bar{v}_{O_2}$	↓ $\dot{Q}va/\dot{Q}t$
↓ Pa_{O_2} and unchanged or ↑ $P\bar{v}_{O_2}$	↑ $\dot{Q}va/\dot{Q}t$
↑ Pa_{O_2}	↓ $\dot{Q}va/\dot{Q}t$; ↑ $P\bar{v}_{O_2}$ (usually ↑ CI); or large ↓ Pa_{CO_2}
↓ Pa_{O_2}	Reverse of above
No change in Pa_{O_2}	No change or multiple changes in physiology, e.g., ↓ $\dot{Q}va/\dot{Q}t$ and ↓ CI after an increase in PEEP

*From Snyder and Carroll.[32] Reproduced by permission.

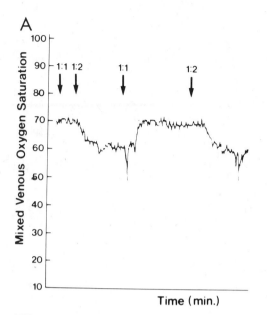

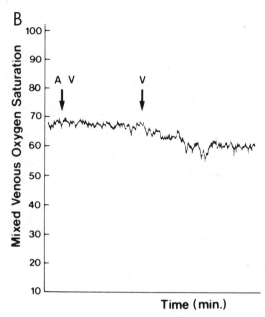

FIG 13–6.

A, effect of changing frequency of counterpulsation from 1:1 (counterpulsation with each heart beat) to 1:2 (counterpulsation with every other heart beat) on S$\bar{v}_{O_2}$. When only one oxygen supply component is altered, the relation with S$\bar{v}_{O_2}$ is linear. The cardiac out- put can therefore be estimated to rise by one third when the frequency is increased. **B,** comparison of temporary pacing in atrioventricular *(AV)* mode vs. ventricular *(V)* mode (rate constant) on S$\bar{v}_{O_2}$. (From Gore et al.[14] Reproduced by permission.)

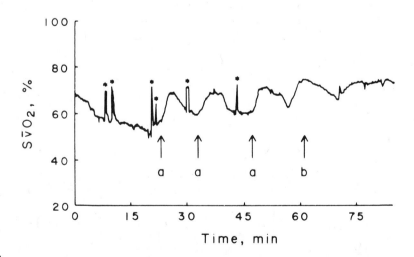

FIG 13–7.

Effect of successive 100-ml intravenous boluses of lactated Ringer's solution (arrows labeled *a*) to reverse downward trend in S$\bar{v}_{O_2}$, and subsequent maintenance of normal S$\bar{v}_{O_2}$ by increased rate of infusion of same solution (arrow *b*). The increase in S$\bar{v}_{O_2}$ from about 50% to 75% suggests that oxygen transport doubled in 60 minutes. *Indicates catheter balloon inflated to measure pulmonary wedge pressure. (From Baele et al.[2] Reproduced by permission.)

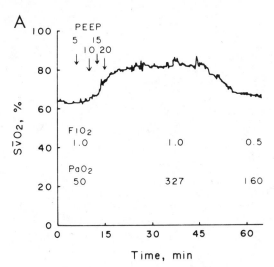

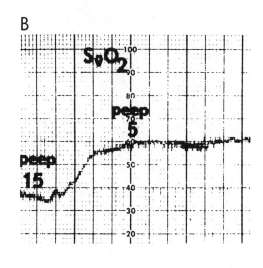

FIG 13–8.

A, S$\bar{v}_{O_2}$ values in a patient who was receiving 100% oxygen and who had an arterial oxygen tension of 50 torr. At the same time S$\bar{v}_{O_2}$ was approximately 62%. There was little change when 5 cm H$_2$O PEEP was added to the ventilator circuitry. There was a small increase in saturation when 10 cm H$_2$O was added, and an even more marked increase with 15 and 20 cm H$_2$O PEEP. A decrease in the inspired oxygen fraction to 0.5 produced an S$\bar{v}_{O_2}$ of approximately 65% and an arterial oxygen tension of 160 torr. Thus, in this patient, PEEP of 20 cm H$_2$O permitted a de-

crease of administered oxygen to 50%, and these changes were accomplished safely in less than 1 hour. (From McMichan.[23] Reproduced by permission.)
B, continuous recording of S$\bar{v}_{O_2}$ in 25-year-old man with neurogenic pulmonary edema receiving 15 cm H$_2$O of PEEP to establish P$_{O_2}$ of 84 torr. Initial S$\bar{v}_{O_2}$ was 38%, indicating inadequate oxygen delivery. With reduction of PEEP to 5 cm H$_2$O, venous return and cardiac output recovered promptly, increasing S$\bar{v}_{O_2}$ to 60%. (From Fahey et al.[11] Reproduced by permission.)

FIG 13–9.

The increase in S$\bar{v}_{O_2}$ with change from assisted ventilation *(A/C)* to intermittent mandatory ventilation *(IMV)* probably reflects an intravascular volume that is appropriate for low airway pressure support but suboptimal for use of higher airway pressure. (From McMichan.[23] Reproduced by permission.)

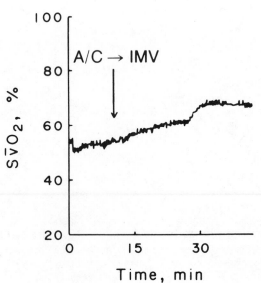

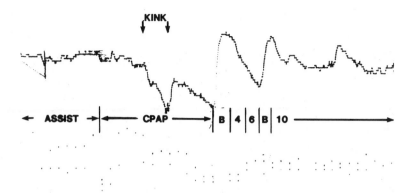

FIG 13–10.

A 58-year-old woman, 48 hours after laparotomy for peritonitis and systemic sepsis, was hemodynamically stable and appeared rested on assisted ventilation. $S\bar{v}_{O_2}$ deteriorated within 15 minutes after change to CPAP using a demand-valve system. Improvement after obstruction of the tracheal tube was relieved *(KINK)* was brief; by then she was using accessory muscles of respiration vigorously but oxygen transport remained inadequate. Vigorous assistance of ventilation by bag-valve unit *(B)* restored $S\bar{v}_{O_2}$ to above baseline. Deterioration recurred on demand valve IMV (rates/min indicated as *4* and *6*) and remained acceptable only after restoration by manual ventilation, then increasing the IMV rate to 10/min.

with a demand-valve system, and require greater mechanical support (Fig 13–10).

The rapid response of $S\bar{v}_{O_2}$ to changes in Sa_{O_2} allows effective monitoring of continuous positive airway pressure treatment (Fig 13–11). Titration of short-acting inotropic drug therapy is facilitated by $S\bar{v}_{O_2}$ monitoring because of the same responsiveness (Fig 13–12). If continuous mixed venous oximetry is not available to them, well-oriented and least dependent physicians carry sterile heparinized syringes to draw samples for analysis; appropriately diplomatic ones also manage not to alienate the stat lab personnel in their efforts to provide good patient care.

Common Phenomena Happen More Often

The most common cause of an abrupt decrease in Pa_{O_2} in a stable, mechanically ventilated patient seems to be mucus plugging, which is diagnosed presumptively and treated by changes in position, vigorous sighing, coughing, and so on. Alternative causes such as pulmonary embolism, pulmonary edema, or a drop in cardiac output are entertained when mucus is not obtained or vital signs change. An increase in peak pressure might indicate a mucus plug, pulmonary edema, bronchial intubation, or pneumothorax. A rise in pulmonary artery pressure could indicate pneumo-

CPAP Mask Off

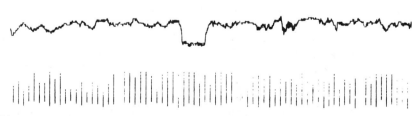

FIG 13–11.

Continuous record of $S\bar{v}_{O_2}$ in 61-year-old man with pulmonary edema. Treatment included high-flow oxygen delivered via CPAP mask. Removal of mask for 5 minutes resulted in prompt decrease in $S\bar{v}_{O_2}$. We cannot tell from the tracing whether the improvement is because of lower venous admixture, improved cardiac output, or simply a higher $F_{I_{O_2}}$. (From Fahey et al.[11] Reproduced by permission.)

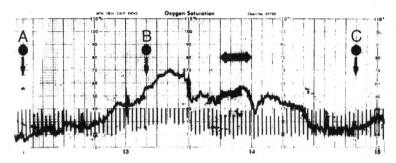

FIG 13–12.
$S\bar{v}_{O_2}$ tracing in a patient with severe cardiomyopathy. At point *A*, cardiac output was 1.8 L/min and $S\bar{v}_{O_2}$ was 17%. Amrinone (75 mg) was given orally immediately after *A*. At point *B* (60 minutes later), cardiac output was 2.9 L/min and $S\bar{v}_{O_2}$ was 53%. At point *C* (160 minutes after *A*), cardiac output was 1.9 L/min and $S\bar{v}_{O_2}$ was 24%. The dramatic effect would probably be missed by discontinuous monitoring, and adjustment of dosage would be less efficient. (From Birman et al.[3] Reproduced by permission.)

thorax. An increase in Pa_{CO_2} may be due to pulmonary embolism or hypovolemia, which may be shown by the associated increase or decrease, respectively, in pulmonary artery pressure and CVP. Venous hypoxia as a cause of arterial hypoxia is suggested by clinical signs of hypoperfusion and is confirmed by demonstrating a lower $P\bar{v}_{O_2}$.

SUMMARY

In summary, normal organ function is a more reliable indicator of the adequacy of perfusion than any hemodynamic variable. When more information about oxygen supply/demand is needed, $P\bar{v}_{O_2}$ is the single most reliable monitor of all the components of that balance. However, $P\bar{v}_{O_2}$ tells nothing about unperfused tissues or the distribution of perfusion. Monitoring of $S\bar{v}_{O_2}$ is comparably useful because it can be monitored continuously, and because its algebraic relations with changes in hemoglobin, Sa_{O_2}, cardiac output, and $\dot{V}_{O_2}$ are straightforward. Similar quantitative interpretation of $P\bar{v}_{O_2}$ requires more familiarity with the dissociation curve, but the $P\bar{v}_{O_2}$ provides a more reliable assessment of the reserve oxygen supply. As opposed to routine collection and analysis of "profiles," it is often more useful to assess cardiopulmonary status by cautiously applying stress, as by a change in position, volume administration, or drug therapy, and observing the response.

REFERENCES

1. Albrecht M, Clowes GHA Jr: The increase of circulatory requirements in the presence of inflammation. *Surgery* 1964; 56:158.
2. Baele PL, McMichan JC, Marsh HM, et al: Continuous monitoring of mixed venous oxygen saturation in critically ill patients. *Anesth Analg* 1982; 61:513.
3. Birman H, Haq A, Hew E, et al: Continuous monitoring of mixed venous oxygen saturation in hemodynamically unstable patients. *Chest* 1984; 86:753.
4. Breivik H, Grenvik A, Millen E, et al: Normalization of low arterial CO_2 tension during mechanical ventilation. *Chest* 1973; 63:525.
5. Bryan-Brown CW, Baek SM, Makabali G, et al: Consumable oxygen: Availability of oxygen in relation to oxyhemoglobin dissociation. *Crit Care Med* 1973; 1:17.
6. Cady LD Jr, Weil JH, Afifi AA, et al: Quantitation of severity of critical illness with special reference to blood lactate. *Crit Care Med* 1973; 1:75.
7. Cain SM: Oxygen delivery and uptake in dogs during anemic and hypoxic hypoxia. *J Appl Physiol* 1977; 42:228.
8. Cain SM: Review: Supply dependency of oxygen uptake in ARDS—Myth or reality? *Am J Med Sci* 1984; 28:119.
9. Carroll G, Snyder J: Hyperdynamic severe intravascular sepsis depends on fluid administration in cynomolgus monkeys. *Am J Physiol* 1982; 243:R131–R141.

10. Del Guercio LRM, Cohn JD: Monitoring operative risk in the elderly. *JAMA* 1980; 243:1350.

11. Fahey PJ, Harris K, Vanderwarf C: Clinical experience with continuous monitoring of mixed venous oxygen saturation in respiratory failure. *Chest* 1984; 86:748.

12. Farber MO, Daly RS, Strawbridge RA, et al: Steroids, hypoxemia, and oxygen transport. *Chest* 1979; 75:451.

13. Finch CA, Lenfant C: Oxygen transport in man. *N Engl J Med* 1972; 286:407.

14. Gore JM, Sloan K: Use of continuous monitoring of mixed venous saturation in the coronary care unit. *Chest* 1984; 86:757.

15. Henry W, West G, Wilson R: A comparison of oxygen uptake between a high continuous flow constant positive airway pressure (CPAP) system and a demand breath CPAP system by use of the Beckman metabolic measurement. *Respir Care* 1983; 28:1273.

16. Ilabaca PA, Ochsner JS, Mills NL: Positive end-expiratory pressure in the management of the patient with a postoperative bleeding heart. *Ann Thorac Surg* 1980; 30:281.

17. Jastremski MS, Beney KM: Military antishock trouser (MAST): Application as a reversible fluid challenge in patients on high PEEP. *Chest* 1984; 85:595.

18. Kasnitz P, Druger GL, Yorra F, et al: Mixed venous oxygen tension and hyperlactatemia. *JAMA* 1976; 236:570.

19. Khambatta HJ, Sullivan SF: Effects of respiratory alkalosis in oxygen consumption and oxygenation. *Anesthesiology* 1973; 38:53.

20. Krauss XH, Verdouw PD, Hugenholtz PG, et al: On line monitoring of mixed venous oxygen saturation after cardiothoracic surgery. *Thorax* 1975; 30:636.

21. Lassen NA: The luxury-perfusion syndrome. *Lancet* 1966; 2:113.

22. Martini GA, Baltzer G, Arndt H: Some aspects of circulatory disturbances in cirrhosis of the liver, in Popper H, Schaffner F (eds): *Progress in Liver Diseases*. New York, Grune & Stratton, 1972, 231.

23. McMichan JC: Continuous monitoring of mixed venous oxygen saturation, in Schweiss JF (ed): *Continuous Measurement of Blood Oxygen Saturation in the High Risk Patient*. San Diego, Beach International, Inc, vol 1, 1983.

24. Mithoefer JC: Indications for oxygen therapy in chronic obstructive pulmonary disease. *Am Rev Respir Dis* 1974; 110:S35.

25. Parrot JR, Ledingham I McA: Pathophysiology of shock, in Ledingham I McA (ed): *Shock*. Amsterdam, Excerpta Medica, 1974, p 17.

26. Raffestin B, Escourrou P, Legrand A, et al: Circulatory transport of oxygen in patients with chronic airflow obstruction exercising maximally. *Am Rev Respir Dis* 1984; 125:426–431.

27. Robin E: Of men and mitochondria: Coping with hypoxic dysoxia. *Am Rev Respir Dis* 1980; 122:517.

28. Rowell LB: The distribution of blood flow and its regulation in humans, in Loeppky JA, Riedesel ML (eds): *Oxygen Transport to Human Tissues*. New York, Elsevier/North-Holland, 1982, pp 113–124.

29. Shepherd AP, Granger HJ, Smith EE, et al: Local control of tissue oxygen delivery and its contribution to the regulation of cardiac output. *Am J Physiol* 1973; 225:747–755.

30. Simmons DH, Alpas AP, Tashkin DT, et al: Hyperlactatemia due to arterial hypoxemia or reduced cardiac output, or both. *J Appl Physiol* 1978; 45:195.

31. Smith TC: Carbon dioxide and anesthesia: Respiratory circulatory and metabolic effects, in Hersey SG (ed): *Refresher Courses in Anesthesiology*. Philadelphia, The American Society of Anesthesiologists, Inc, 1976, vol 4, p 125.

32. Snyder JV, Carroll GC: *Tissue Oxygenation: A Physiologic Approach to a Clinical Problem*. *Curr Probl Surg* 1982, vol 19.

33. Snyder JV, Carroll GC: *Mechanical Ventilation: Physiology and Application*. *Curr Probl Surg* 1984, vol 21.

34. Stanley TH, Isern-Amaral J: Periodic analysis of mixed venous oxygen tension to monitor the adequacy of perfusion during and after cardiopulmonary bypass. *Can Anaesth Soc J* 1974; 21:454.

35. Takano N: Effects of CO_2 on O_2 transport, O_2 uptake, and blood lactate in hypoxia of anesthetized dog. *Respir Physiol* 1970; 10:38.

36. Tenney SM, Mithoefer JC: The relationship of mixed venous oxygenation to oxygen transport: With special reference to adaptations to high altitude and pulmonary disease. *Am Rev Respir Dis* 1982; 125:474.

37. Vu-Dinh M, Lee HM, Dolan GF, et al: Hypoxemia during exercise in patients with chronic obstructive pulmonary disease. *Am Rev Respir Dis* 1979; 120:787.

38. Wagner PD: Recent advances in pulmonary gas exchange. *Int Anesthesiol Clin* 1977; 15:81.

39. Weil MH, Afifi AA: Experimental and clinical studies on lactate and pyruvate as indicators of the severity of acute circulatory failure (shock). *Circulation* 1970; 41:989.

40. Woodson RD, Wills RE, Lenfant C: Effect of acute and established anemia on oxygen transport at rest, submaximal and maximal work. *J Appl Physiol* 1978; 44:36.

41. Woolf CR: Arterial blood gas levels after oxygen therapy (letter). *Chest* 1976; 69:808.

42. Zema MJ, Restivo B, Sos T, et al: Left ventricular dysfunction: Bedside Valsalva maneuver. *Br Heart J* 1980; 44:560–569.

43. Zema MJ, Masters AP, Margouleff D: Dyspnea: The heart or the lungs? Differentiation at bedside by use of the simple Valsalva maneuver. *Chest* 1984; 85:59.

14

Clinical Evaluation Compared With Invasive Hemodynamic Assessment

Paul R. Eisenberg, M.D., M.P.H.

Daniel P. Schuster, M.D.

Pulmonary arterial and systemic arterial catheterization have dramatically altered the care of critically ill patients by allowing frequent or continuous measurement of various hemodynamic variables. However, since these invasive techniques carry some degree of morbidity, the relative sensitivity and specificity of noninvasive compared with invasive hemodynamic evaluation is an important issue. The clinician must determine whether the findings of repeated physical examination, together with corroborative data obtained by the measurement of urine output, laboratory, and/or radiographic studies, accurately reflect cardiovascular function and organ perfusion. Ideally, invasive hemodynamic monitoring should be used only if the information obtained would improve patient outcome. However, since there is little evidence concerning the influence of invasive monitoring on outcome, the decision must instead be based on the presumption that invasive hemodynamic assessment improves the accuracy of diagnostic and therapeutic decisions. The accuracy of noninvasive hemodynamic assessment is the subject of this chapter.

ASSESSMENT OF CARDIOVASCULAR FUNCTION

Since the introduction of the flow-directed pulmonary arterial catheter, invasive hemodynamic monitoring has become a routine part of caring for critically ill patients.[13, 19] Despite its widespread use, the indications for and benefits of pulmonary arterial catheterization remain controversial. Until recently, surprisingly few studies have appeared that compare the information obtained by pulmonary arterial catheterization with that obtained by noninvasive assessment.

The specificity of clinical signs, and especially of a ventricular gallop sound (S_3), to indicate congestive heart failure and left ventricular end-diastolic pressure over 15 torr in patients with coronary artery disease was documented by Harlan and associates in 1977.[15] In their initial retrospective study of patients with acute myocardial infarction, Forrester et al.[9] compared data obtained from pulmonary arterial catheterization with that obtained from physical examination. They found a high correlation between measured hemodynamic values and their clinical impression of the hemodynamic state. Specifically, the finding of a third heart sound or of signs of peripheral hypoperfusion was associated with a wedge pressure (WP) of greater than 18 torr and a cardiac index (CI) of less than 2.2 L/min/m^2, respectively, in more than 80% of their patients. In addition, their clinical evaluation was predictive of the correct combination of these variables in approximately 70% of patients. From such data, the concept of well-defined hemodynamic subsets of patients with acute myocardial infarction emerged. Forrester et al. suggested that identification of the appropriate subset had prognostic importance, since the highest mortality was associated with the presence of both a WP above 18 torr and a CI below 2.2 L/min/m^2.

In contrast to this initial experience, a subsequent prospective study of patients with acute myocardial infarction by the same group showed that the correlation between physical findings and hemodynamic values was poor.[25] In this later series, despite a careful physical examination and review of a chest radiograph, cardiologists were unable to correctly predict whether WP would be greater or less than 18 torr more than 68% of the time (or only 36% more often than would be expected by chance alone). In patients with acute myocardial infarction who did not survive, estimated wedge pressure was correct only 9% more frequently than was expected by chance. Similarly, 30% of patients with a WP above 18 torr did not have pulmonary crackles, while in 35% of patients with a WP of less than 18 torr pulmonary crackles were present. A third heart sound occurred in 50% of patients regardless of whether WP was greater or less than 18 torr. Thus, these authors concluded that the presence of pulmonary crackles or S_3 in the early hours of a transmural infarction was neither sensitive nor specific for the accurate assessment of cardiovascular function or in-hospital mortality.

In patients with septic shock, the lack of specificity and sensitivity of the clinical examination was appreciated even before the introduction of bedside hemodynamic monitoring. In a study by Bell and Thal,[3] little correlation was found between the CI and clinical signs of peripheral perfusion (skin temperature, sensorium, and urine output). These authors found that cold skin did not reliably predict a depressed CI, and that in some patients oliguria was associated with a normal CI.

Similarly, two recent prospective studies have documented the inability of physicians to predict hemodynamic variables on the basis of clinical evaluation in most critically ill patients. In one of these studies,[6] a critical care team of attending physicians, fellows, and residents, using clinical findings, was unable to accurately predict values for several hemodynamic variables (WP, CI, right atrial pressure, and pulmonary artery pressure) more than 50% of the time. More important, treatment (either drug or titration of fluid therapy) was changed in 48.4% of the patients after catheterization. We designed a similar study[7] in which the primary physician (a second- or third-year medical resident) was asked to predict the WP, cardiac output, systemic vascular resistance, and right atrial pressure within a range of values, before catheterization. In addition, the presumed diagnosis and plan for therapy were recorded and compared with therapy actually given during the 8 hours after catheterization. Just as in the previous study, we found that physicians were unable to correctly predict values for the hemodynamic variables more than 33%–50% of the time (depending on the variable) (Fig 14–1). After catheterization, planned therapy was altered in 58% of patients; in 30% a therapy that was not anticipated prior to catheterization was initiated. As might be expected, planned therapy was altered somewhat more often when predictions of WP were incorrect. However, alterations occurred even when predictions were correct, which suggests that other information obtained by catheterization influenced therapeutic decisions (Fig 14–2). When subgroups of patients were analyzed by whether the indication for catheterization was hypotension or impaired oxygenation, no difference in the ability to predict the hemodynamic data emerged.

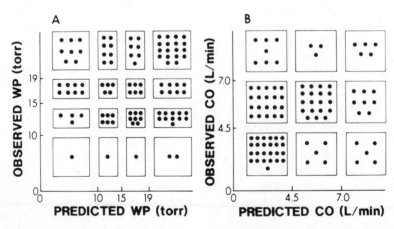

FIG 14–1.
Relation between observed and predicted hemodynamic values for **(A)** wedge pressure (WP) ($n = 102$) and **(B)** cardiac output (CO) ($n = 97$). Each *box* represents the range in which predictions were made.

Each *circle* represents a prediction. The rate of correct predictions was 30% for WP and 51% for CO. (From Eisenberg et al.[7] Reproduced by permission.)

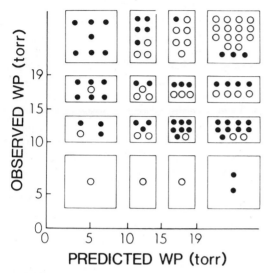

FIG 14–2.

Relation between alterations in therapy and accuracy of predicting the wedge pressure (WP). *Boxes* indicate a range of values, as in Figure 14–1. The distribution of values is the same as in Figure 14–1. *Open circles* indicate there was no change in planned therapy after catheterization. *Closed circles* indicate instances when planned therapy was changed. (From Eisenberg et al.[7] Reproduced by permission.)

In a study of patients with pulmonary edema, Fein et al.[8] found that a clinical diagnosis of permeability pulmonary edema was more likely to be verified by pulmonary arterial catheterization (85%) than was a diagnosis of cardiogenic pulmonary edema (62%). Classification into either one of these groups was based on whether the WP was greater than 18 torr (indicative of cardiogenic pulmonary edema) or less than 18 torr (permeability edema). Overall, 69% of predictions were correct, a rate similar to that observed in the two studies just discussed, in which less selected populations were studied.[6, 7]

Connors et al.[6] considered the level of training of the physician making the assessment. They found no difference between predictions made by the attending staff and fellows and those made by residents and medical students. Thus, the ability to predict the hemodynamic state apparently is not significantly enhanced by the experience of the physician. This surprising and perhaps sobering finding is not an endorsement of pulmonary arterial catheterization for all critically ill patients, since we suspect that the greatest impact of the experienced physician is in helping decide

in whom and when the procedure is most appropriate. This important factor has not been studied.

In summary, several recent studies have documented that pulmonary artery catheterization provides hemodynamic information that cannot be accurately derived from the physical examination, routine laboratory studies, or the chest radiograph. These studies did not consistently identify any subgroup in which the accuracy of the clinical evaluation was as good as that based on pulmonary arterial catheterization. In addition, therapy was often altered as a result of the additional information provided by this procedure.

The reasons for discrepancies between clinical assessment and the results of pulmonary arterial catheterization are not clear but are often attributed to the lack of specificity that clinical findings have when there is multiorgan system involvement in acutely ill patients. For example, whatever the diagnostic value of an S_3 gallop in chronically ill patients may be, its specificity is diminished if hypovolemia or tachycardia is present or if cardiac auscultation is difficult. Similarly, the interpretation of pulmonary crackles is difficult because adventitial sounds emanating from small airways and alveoli (as in pulmonary edema) are difficult to distinguish from sounds in larger airways (due to secretions) or from ventilator noise. Even when the crackles indicate increased extravascular lung water, the etiology may be cardiogenic or noncardiogenic. Furthermore, the lack of specificity and sensitivity of the physical examination is even more apparent when examination findings are used as an end point for titration of therapy. For example, the development of pulmonary crackles or an S_3 gallop is not likely to be either a sensitive indicator or a desirable end point of intravascular volume resuscitation.

Despite the ability of pulmonary arterial catheterization to provide accurate hemodynamic data, the potentially serious complications associated with this technique must always be considered. These include complications from central venous catheterization (e.g., pneumothorax), infection, venous thrombosis, arrhythmias, pulmonary artery rupture, and death. The latter two complications are infrequent (< 1%). However, the report by Fein et al.[8] of three deaths in 70 catheter insertions underscores the need for thoughtful consideration of the indications for catheterization in each case.

ASSESSMENT OF LUNG WATER

Accurate measurement of lung water is a recent addition to the database that can be obtained using pulmonary arterial and systemic arterial catheterization. The technique most commonly used is the double indicator dye dilution technique.[17, 20] This method utilizes a thermal indicator (diffusible) to measure total lung water and indocyanine green dye (nondiffusible) to measure intravascular water. Iced indocyanine green dye is injected into the right atrium and the thermal and dye curves are measured through a specially designed, thermistor-tipped femoral arterial catheter. The difference in the mean transit times of the two curves is multiplied by the cardiac output to arrive at a measure of lung water. Several investigators have found the technique accurate in animal studies when compared with gravimetric measurement of lung water.[17] A few initial clinical studies suggest that this measurement may provide additional information to that provided by the WP and the chest radiograph.[2, 27] For example, Sivak et al.[27] found that although initial chest radiographs could be used to predict an abnormal elevation of lung water in 64% of patients, changes in lung water were predicted only 42% of the time. In patients with severe trauma, Baudendistel et al.[2] found that a normal chest x-ray film correlated well with a normal lung water measurement. However, 47 of 70 (67%) lung water measurements did not correlate with a concurrent (± 5 hours) radiographic assessment of the amount of lung water. In another study changes in the quantity of lung water were not predicted by the WP or by colloid osmotic pressure gradient.[30] Initial data from one study[24] suggest that the lung water measurement may be used, instead of WP, as an end point for titration of vasoactive drugs and fluid therapy without adverse outcome. However, until more definitive data are available, the utility of routinely measuring extravascular lung water in critically ill patients remains uncertain.

RECENT ADVANCES IN NONINVASIVE ASSESSMENT OF CARDIAC FUNCTION

Noninvasive assessment of cardiac function has improved significantly with the availability of radionuclide ventriculography,[29] two-dimensional echocardiography,[21] and recently, Doppler echocardiography.[16] The radionuclide techniques are further described in chapter 18, "Functional Imaging of the Critically Ill Patient." The echocardiographic techniques estimate left ventricular systolic function and wall motion abnormalities. Although two-dimensional echocardiography is probably less accurate in estimating global function, it does have the advantage of permitting frequent examinations. Therefore changes in left ventricular function can be monitored over time. However, neither technique is suitable at present for continuous monitoring or for titrating therapy. Doppler echocardiography is used primarily to determine flow across the cardiac valves. Both regurgitant and stenotic lesions can be defined and intracardiac shunts can be identified.[16] Cardiac output can also be determined by Doppler echocardiography,[18] but this use requires higher quality echocardiographic imaging than is often possible in most critically ill adult patients.

MEASUREMENT OF ARTERIAL PRESSURE

Invasive monitoring of the arterial blood pressure is commonly used in the care of critically ill patients. However, the indications for intra-arterial monitoring are controversial. Appropriate uses might include (1) to monitor persistent hypotension, (2) to titrate vasoactive agents, (3) to resolve discrepancies between auscultated blood pressure and other findings from the physical examination, (4) to continuously monitor blood pressure, and (5) to minimize patient discomfort and nursing time when multiple arterial blood gas determinations are necessary.[12, 13, 19] Complications have been reported in as many as 5%–15% of catheterizations, but serious complications are less common.[12, 22, 23, 26] Common problems include local bleeding and catheter bacterial colonization; more serious complications include peripheral embolization, systemic infection, arteriovenous fistulas, and arterial thrombosis.

Intra-arterial monitoring of blood pressure can also be inaccurate, of course. Most often this will be due to errors in calibration or failure to properly level the transducer.[11] When compared with auscultated blood pressure, the intra-arterial systolic pressure is often higher because of resonance in the monitoring system. Proper damping of monitoring equipment can minimize this problem, as reviewed in chapter 15, "Technical Problems in Data Acquisition." In general, the mean arterial pressure is less prone to error and variation than are systolic and diastolic values. Studies comparing the intra-arterial measurement of blood pressure with values determined by auscultation in normotensive patients have found varying degrees of correlation, perhaps in part related to the technique of measurement. In hypotensive patients accurate monitoring of blood pressure usually requires either intra-arterial or Doppler measurements.

Arterial catheterization can be particularly useful in patients who appear hypotensive on auscultation but who still have adequate organ function. For example, consider the patient in whom the titration of pressors is based on auscultated blood pressure. An inaccurate underestimation of blood pressure by auscultation in this instance might lead to inappropriate titration of pressor therapy. A clue to such inaccuracy might be the lack of evidence for organ hypoperfusion, such as obtundation or low urine output.

Recently the availability of Doppler ultrasound techniques has provided another means for noninvasively measuring blood pressure in hypotensive patients; a device that allows for repeated Doppler measurements is now available as well.[1] Several studies have found an excellent correlation with intra-arterial measurements in both normotensive and a limited number of hypotensive patients.[5, 14, 28] In a series of patients studied by Buggs et al.,[5] Doppler-measured blood pressure correlated well ($r = .98$) with intra-arterial measurements in 44 acutely ill adult patients, most of whom were hypotensive. However, in an experimental model, Doppler and intra-arterial measurements of blood pressure did not agree as intravascular volume was decreased by more than 30%.[14] Unfortunately, data from a large number of critically ill patients, which might identify those patients in whom Doppler-determined blood pressure is accurate, have not been reported. Thus, experience is too limited at present to recommend this technique as an alternate means of rapid and continuous blood pressure monitoring in hypotensive patients.

CONCLUSIONS

Despite the apparently increased accuracy of pulmonary arterial catheterization and other invasive means of hemodynamic measurement compared with most noninvasive techniques, there are still no data to suggest that the information they provide changes outcome. Until such data are available it is reasonable to conclude that carefully acquired hemodynamic data will be accurate and may direct the physician toward the most appropriate therapy, thereby improving patient outcome.

REFERENCES

1. Aaslid R, Brubakk AO: Accuracy of an ultrasound Doppler servo method for noninvasive determination of instantaneous and mean blood pressure. *Circulation* 1981; 63:753–754.
2. Baudendistel L, Shields JB, Kaminski DL: Comparison of double indicator thermodilution measurements of extravascular lung water with radiographic estimation of lung water in trauma patients. *J Trauma* 1982; 22:983–988.
3. Bell H, Thal A: The peculiar hemodynamics of septic shock. *Postgrad Med* 1970; 48:106–114.
4. Bruner JMR, Krenis LJ, Kunsman JM, et al: Comparison of direct and indirect methods of measuring blood pressure: Parts 1–3. *Med Instrum* 1981; 15:11–21, 97–101, 182–188.
5. Buggs H, Johnson PE, Gordon LS, et al: Comparison of systolic arterial blood pressure by transcutaneous Doppler probe and conventional methods in hypotensive patients. *Anesth Analg* 1973; 52:776–778.
6. Connors AF, McCaffree DR, Gray BA: Evaluation of right heart catheterization in the critically ill patient without myocardial infarction. *N Engl J Med* 1983; 308:263–267.
7. Eisenberg PR, Jaffe AS, Schuster DP: Clinical evaluation compared with pulmonary artery catheterization in the hemodynamic assessment of critically ill patients. *Crit Care Med* 1984; 12:549–553.
8. Fein AM, Goldberg SK, Walkenstein MD: Is pulmonary artery catheterization necessary for the diagnosis of pulmonary edema? *Am Rev Respir Dis* 1984; 129:1006–1009.
9. Forrester JS, Diamond G, Chatterjee K, et al: Medical therapy of acute myocardial infarction by application of hemodynamic subsets: Parts 1–2. *N Engl J Med* 1976; 295:1356–1362, 1404–1413.
10. Funderburk CF, Paulshock C, Yu PN: Validation of the thermal-dye method of measuring lung water: Patient studies. *Crit Care Med* 1980; 8:752–759.

11. Gardner RM: Direct blood pressure measurement: Dynamic response requirements. *Anesthesiology* 1981; 54:227–236.

12. Gardner RM, Schwartz R, Wong HC, et al: Percutaneous indwelling radial artery catheters for monitoring cardiovascular function. *N Engl J Med* 1974; 290:1227–1231.

13. Goldenheim PD, Kazemi H: Cardiopulmonary monitoring of critically ill patients: Part 2. *N Engl J Med* 1984; 311:776–780.

14. Harken AH, Smith RM: Aortic pressure versus Doppler-measured peripheral arterial pressure. *Anesthesiology* 1973; 38:184–186.

15. Harlan WR, Oberman A, Grimm R, et al: Chronic congestive heart failure in coronary artery disease: Clinical criteria. *Ann Intern Med* 1977; 86:133–138.

16. Hatle L, Angelsen B: *Doppler Ultrasound in Cardiology.* Philadelphia, Lea & Febiger, 1982.

17. Lewis FR, Elings VB, Hill SL, et al: The measurement of extravascular lung water by thermal-green dye indicator dilution. *NY Acad Sci* 1982; 384:394–409.

18. Lewis JF, Kuo LC, Nelson JG, et al: Pulsed Doppler echocardiographic determination of stroke volume and cardiac output: Clinical validation of two new methods using the apical window. *Circulation* 1984; 70:425–431.

19. Matthay MA: Invasive hemodynamic monitoring in critically ill patients. *Clin Chest Med* 1983; 4:233–249.

20. Noble WH, Kay JC, Maret KH, Caskanette G: Reappraisal of extravascular lung thermal volume as a measure of pulmonary edema. *J Appl Physiol* 1980; 48:120–129.

21. Parisi AF, Moynihan PF, Folland FD: Echocardiographic evaluation of left ventricular function. *Med Clin North Am* 1980; 64:61–81.

22. Pinilla JC, Ross DF, Martin T, et al: Study of the incidence of intravascular catheter infection and associated septicemia in critically ill patients. *Crit Care Med* 1983; 11:21–25.

23. Puri VK, Carlson RW, Bander JJ, et al: Complications of vascular catheterization in the critically ill. *Crit Care Med* 1980; 8:495–499.

24. Schuster DP, Babcock D, Gurley R, et al: Extravascular lung water versus wedge pressure measurements in the management of critically ill patients (abstract). *Am Rev Respir Dis* 1985; 131:158.

25. Shell WE, DeWood MA, Peter T, et al: Comparison of clinical and hemodynamic state in the early hours of transmural myocardial infarction. *Am Heart J* 1982; 104:521–528.

26. Singh S, Nelson N, Acosta I, et al: Catheter colonization and bacteremia with pulmonary and arterial catheters. *Crit Care Med* 1982; 10:736–739.

27. Sivak ED, Richmond BJ, O'Donavan PB, et al: Value of extravascular lung water measurement versus portable chest x-ray in the management of pulmonary edema. *Crit Care Med* 1983; 11:498–501.

28. Stegall HF, Kardon MB, Kemmerer WT: Indirect measurement of arterial blood pressure by Doppler ultrasonic sphygmomanometry. *J Appl Physiol* 1968; 25:793–797.

29. Thrall JH, Pitt B, Brady TJ: Radionuclide wall motion study and ejection fraction in clinical practice. *Med Clin North Am* 1980; 64:99–117.

30. Tranbaugh RF, Elings VB, Christensen J, et al: Determinants of pulmonary interstitial fluid accumulation after trauma. *J Trauma* 1982; 22:820–826.

15 Technical Problems in Data Acquisition

Loren D. Nelson, M.D.

James V. Snyder, M.D.

In the overwhelming majority of patients sustaining trauma or undergoing major surgery, cardiopulmonary status (i.e., oxygen transport balance) may be adequately assessed by clinical determination of pulse rate, blood pressure, urine output, and mentation. However, clinical assessment of oxygen transport variables in critically ill patients may be unreliable and misleading (see chapter 14, "Invasive Hemodynamic Assessment Compared With Clinical Evaluation").[18, 26] In these patients pulmonary artery catheterization may be the only source of an adequate database.

The database required for the interpretation, diagnosis, and treatment of oxygen transport imbalance encompasses knowledge of the patient's clinical course and status as well as of measured and derived variables.[53] As the data used for decision-making become more abstract (values are derived from other measurements) or more technical (new or unfamiliar instrumentation is used), the validity of the data is increasingly suspect. Unfortunately, digital readouts and computer printouts imply to many people both precision and accuracy of the measurement, and blind trust may be placed in values displayed in these fashions. The computer acronym GIGO (garbage in, garbage out) applies to patient monitoring as well. *It is the responsibility of the critical care physician to understand both the technology used for measurements and the implications of "bad" data when assessing the derived oxygen transport indices.*

Perhaps the greatest errors in clinical hemodynamic monitoring are to believe erroneous values correct and to presume a close correlation between a measured variable and a more fundamental aspect of physiology. Physicians commonly fall into the trap of assuming that central venous pressure (CVP) or wedge pressure (WP) really does reflect ventricular preload, or that arterial blood pressure reflects blood flow, and we neglect other powerful but often unmeasured determinants of those variables.

This chapter reviews the technical problems of acquiring data regarding oxygen transport in critically ill patients. Specifically, the "necessary and sufficient" database for the assessment of oxygen transport, the technical aspects of each measurement, and the potential pitfalls are reviewed.

OXYGEN TRANSPORT DATABASE

Our first concern is the sufficiency of oxygen transport relative to demand. This relationship is shown most clearly in end-organ function and secondarily by indicators such as venous oxygen values and blood lactate levels. A detailed database is needed only when a decision is made to monitor more closely. It must be emphasized that most of the hemodynamic data available ignore nonperfused tissues, and most systems of analysis presume that metabolic regulation of flow is intact. When all tissues are perfused and vasoregulation is normal, the weaknesses of the hemodynamic analysis approach are only the presumptions and technical errors to be discussed here. However, it should be kept in mind that to assess problems associated with loss of perfusion and with vasoderegulation, we remain heavily dependent on assessment of tissue function and on measurement of oxygen consumption. The database necessary for oxygen supply/demand analysis includes the variables required for the calculation of oxygen delivery to the tissues (supply) and of oxygen consumption by the tissues (demand) (Table 15–1). These determining factors may be divided into three areas: cardiac output,

TABLE 15–1.

Indicators Used to Assess Oxygen Transport

VARIABLE (ABBREVIATION)	NORMAL RANGE	UNITS	SOURCE
Oxygen delivery ($\dot{D}o_2$)	800–1,800	ml/min	Derived
Cardiac output (CO)	Varies (BSA)	L/min	Measured indirectly
Arterial oxygen content (Ca_{O_2})	16–22	ml/dl	Derived
Hemoglobin (Hb)	10–15	gm/dl	Measured directly
Arterial oxygen saturation (Sa_{O_2})	Varies ($F_{I_{O_2}}$)	(fraction)	Measured directly
Arterial oxygen tension (Pa_{O_2})	Varies ($F_{I_{O_2}}$)	torr	Measured directly
Oxygen consumption ($\dot{V}o_2$)	180–280	ml/min	Derived/measured
Arterial-venous oxygen content difference $C(a-\bar{v})_{O_2}$	3–5.5	ml/dl	Derived
Venous oxygen saturation ($S\bar{v}_{O_2}$)	0.68–0.78	(fraction)	Measured directly
Venous oxygen tension ($P\bar{v}_{O_2}$)	35–45	torr	Measured directly
Oxygen utilization coefficient (O_2UC)	0.22–0.33	(fraction)	Derived

arterial oxygen content, and venous oxygen content.

The measurement of cardiac output is of prime importance in the evaluation of disturbances in oxygen transport balance. Cardiac output is one of the two variables used to calculate both oxygen delivery and oxygen consumption and is also one of the hemodynamic indices most commonly affected by critical illness. Cardiac output is the product of heart rate and mean stroke volume. Stroke volume is determined by preload, afterload, and contractility. Evaluation of each of these variables will be discussed in detail later in this chapter.

Arterial oxygen content (Ca_{O_2}) is determined by the hemoglobin concentration, the arterial oxygen saturation (Sa_{O_2}), and, to a small degree, the arterial oxygen tension (Pa_{O_2}). Oxygen delivery ($\dot{D}o_2$) is the product of cardiac output times arterial oxygen content ($\dot{D}o_2 = CO \times Ca_{O_2} \times 10$.

Venous oxygen content ($C\bar{v}_{O_2}$) is determined by the hemoglobin concentration, the venous oxygen saturation ($S\bar{v}_{O_2}$), and, to a very small degree, the venous oxygen tension ($P\bar{v}_{O_2}$). The great importance of venous blood gas analysis is discussed in chapter 16, "Mixed Venous Oximetry." Suffice it to say here that $C\bar{v}_{O_2}$ is used to calculate the volume of oxygen returned to the heart from the peripheral tissues (oxygen return $= CO \times C\bar{v}_{O_2} \times 10$). Tissue oxygen consumption as calculated using the Fick equation is equal to oxygen delivery minus oxygen return ($\dot{V}o_2 =$

$\dot{D}o_2 - O_2$ return, or $\dot{V}o_2 = CO \times 10 \times [Ca_{O_2} - C\bar{v}_{O_2}]$).

Measurement of cardiac output and calculation of Ca_{O_2} and $C\bar{v}_{O_2}$ allow calculation of all of the oxygen transport variables and thereby provide the necessary and sufficient database for evaluation of the adequacy of overall oxygen transport through perfused tissues.

TECHNICAL ASPECTS OF OXYGEN CONTENT CALCULATION

The volume of oxygen contained in the blood is dependent on that bound to hemoglobin and that dissolved in the plasma:

$$Ca_{O_2} =$$

$$\underset{\text{(Bound)}}{(Hb \times 1.39 \times Sa_{O_2})} + \underset{\text{(Dissolved)}}{(0.003 \times Pa_{O_2})}$$

(Eq. 15–1)

Normally the dissolved fraction is of little clinical importance, but as hemoglobin concentration decreases and oxygen tension increases, the dissolved fraction becomes more significant.

Hemoglobin Concentration

Accurate measurement of the hemoglobin concentration is important for the calculation of oxygen content. The hemoglobin concentration may be measured in blood samples sent for blood gas analysis, but large errors (up to 19%) may result because of variance in the volumes of anticoagulant and blood.[33] Standard volume blood samples with standard amounts of anticoagulant should eliminate this source of error.

Oxygen Tension

Oxygen tension is most commonly measured using a Clark electrode. Although use of this type of electrode is subject to many kinds of error,[17] modern blood gas analyzers use internal electronic checks and automatic calibrations to minimize most analysis errors. The use of appropriate quality control materials in the laboratory is important, but not yet a uniform practice.[36] Certain gases, notably nitrous oxide and halothane, may interfere with Clark electrode measurements and cause significant apparent increases in the oxygen tension.[23]

Sampling and transport of blood are the most common sources of error in oxygen tension analysis. Oxygen tension can be changed by air bubbles or cellular metabolism.[50] The use of plastic rather than glass syringes does not cause a clinically significant change in gas tensions if analysis is prompt.[28] Cellular metabolism may cause a decrease in oxygen tension and pH and an increase in carbon dioxide tension. Significant changes can occur in hyperleukocytic blood if samples are not promptly processed. Submersion of the sampling syringe in ice water will reduce cellular metabolism and improve the accuracy of the analysis.[17]

Oxygen Saturation

The relation between oxygen tension and saturation may be altered by a shift in the oxyhemoglobin dissociation curve or by the presence of abnormal hemoglobin. Carboxyhemoglobin or methemoglobin will cause a reduction in the hemoglobin available to carry oxygen. The content of oxygen available for metabolic processes may then be significantly less than that calculated from oxygen tension, even if a shift in the dissociation curve is taken into account. It is therefore advisable to identify and measure abnormal hemoglobin fractions, or to estimate their impact on available oxygen as the difference between measured Sa_{O_2} and 1.0 when Pa_{O_2} is 150 torr or greater. Measured methemoglobin values may be artifactually high in patients receiving Intralipid, and perhaps other intravenous fat preparations.[69]

In the absence of abnormal hemoglobin, since the oxyhemoglobin dissociation curve is nearly flat at high oxygen tension (> 100 torr), Sa_{O_2} may be estimated from the tension measurement using a nomogram. Even large shifts in the dissociation curve have little effect on saturation in this part of the curve. However, at low oxygen tension the dissociation curve is quite steep, and a change in the position or shape of the curve may have a significant effect on the saturation value. The position of the dissociation curve may be estimated by comparing $P\bar{v}_{O_2}$ and $S\bar{v}_{O_2}$ with a standard dissociation curve, or by using the same values to calculate the in vivo P50 (see Appendix 15–1).

Blood oxygen content also may be measured directly by a modification of the Van Slyke manometric technique or with commercially available oxygen-sensitive fuel cell techniques.[1] These are technically more demanding and perhaps less efficient than currently available cooximeters.

TECHNICAL ASPECTS OF HEMODYNAMIC MEASUREMENTS

While hemodynamic measurements per se are not used to define the adequacy of oxygen transport, they are important in identifying therapeutic maneuvers most likely to improve oxygen transport. This section briefly reviews the technical requirements for valid hemodynamic measurements and examines in some detail how improper measurements may adversely affect patient care.

Arterial Catheterization

Arterial catheterization provides safe and convenient access to the left side of the circulation both for the measurement of mean arterial pressure (MAP) (used in the calculation of the derived hemodynamic indices of systemic vascular resistance and left ventricular work) and for the analysis of arterial blood gases (used for the calculation of Ca_{O_2}, oxygen delivery, oxygen consumption, and arterial-venous oxygen content difference). The influence of insertion site on the resulting arterial waveform is illustrated in Figure 15–1. Details of indications, insertion techniques, advantages and disadvantages of each site, contraindications, and potential complications are discussed in the references.[14, 53]

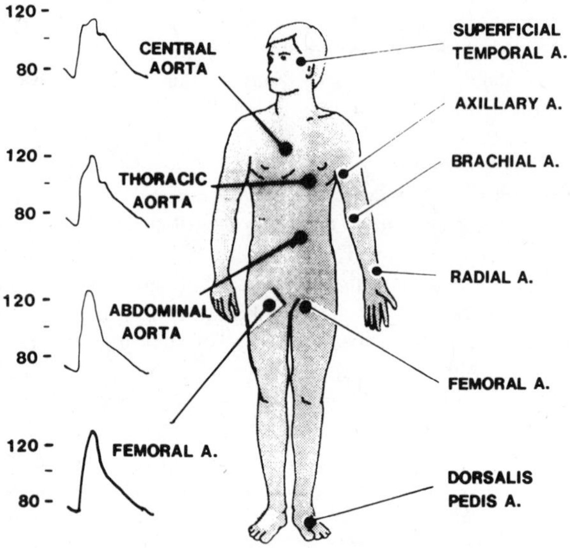

FIG 15–1.
Right, common sites for arterial catheterization. *Left,* the waveforms obtained at the locations indicated while a Millar transducer tip catheter is pulled from the central aorta to the femoral artery. The change in waveform is greater in more distal arteries. Deriving physiologic conclusions from the features of arterial waveforms is made difficult by this anatomy-dependent variation in waveform. (Waveforms courtesy of Barry F. Uretsky, M.D.)

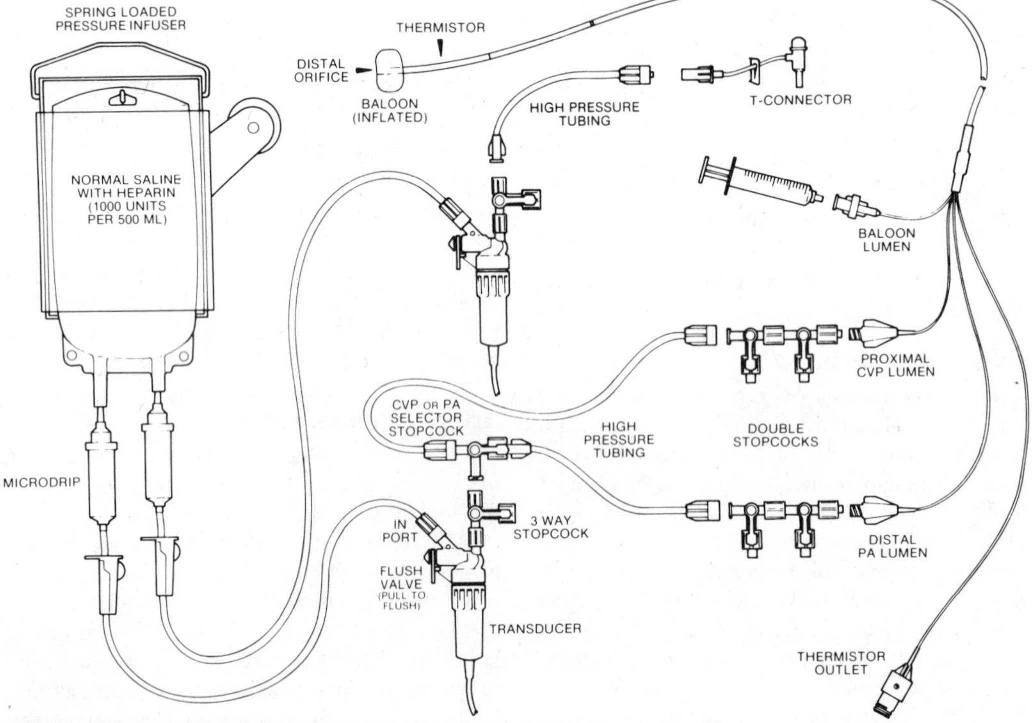

FIG 15–2.
Hemodynamic monitoring for a patient with inadequate oxygen transport may include both arterial and pulmonary arterial catheterization. The required components are shown here. See text for details.

Central Venous Catheterization

Indications for central venous catheterization are fluid administration, parenteral nutrition, drug therapy, repetitive blood sampling, measurement of CVP, and pulmonary artery (PA) catheterization. The technical details and complications associated with the use of different sites are described in detail elsewhere.[53]

CVP reflects the ability of the right ventricle (RV) to discharge the volume load presented to it. However, since the functional capability of the two ventricles can differ, CVP can differ greatly from left ventricular (LV) filling pressure. This is especially true during times of rapid changes in function. Because of this, PA catheterization has generally replaced CVP measurement as a means of assessing the therapeutic response to interventions aimed at improving oxygen transport in critically ill patients.[51, 53]

Electronic Pressure Monitoring Systems

A clinical pressure monitoring system comprises three component groups: the intravascular catheter, connecting tubing, and flush system; the electromechanical transducer; and the electronic amplifier and display (Fig 15–2). Its appropriate use requires proper selection and integration of these components and an understanding of the limitations that remain inherent.

The Monitoring Catheter

As illustrated in Figure 15–1, the accurately transduced systemic arterial waveform varies at different catheterization sites. In addition the dynamic response of the catheter and connecting tubing used clinically alters the waveform of the pressure that is transmitted through them. Even perfect transmission of the waveform from the catheter may still yield a waveform different from that obtained by an intravascular transducer (Fig 15–3). Therefore, waveform analysis must be performed with caution because both the timing and the absolute values may be distorted. In addition, correctly transmitted waveforms vary widely in contour, so that manipulation of resonance and damping to obtain a "proper" waveform may induce further distortion rather than improve the reproduction. Superimposed on this complex state are problems with the dynamic response characteristics of the monitoring system.[32] These can be evaluated and often minimized, as related in the following section. While a waveform that appears to be satisfactory does not ensure that the dynamic response characteristics of the monitoring system are acceptable, a markedly

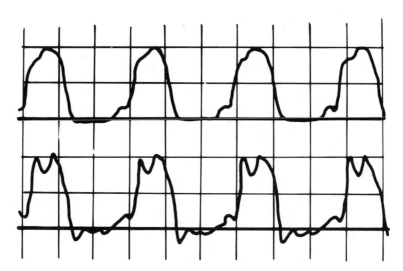

FIG 15–3.
Effect of 7-F thermodilution catheter on a pressure waveform. A column of fluid was subjected to a pressure wave, which was monitored by a Millar catheter pressure transducer, model PC-350, placed in the column of fluid *(top)*, and by an identical pressure transducer via a thermodilution catheter *(bottom)*. The differences in waveform are due to resonance from transmission through the PA catheter. (Comparison performed courtesy of Millar Catheter, Inc.)

blunted or hyperdynamic waveform should alert the clinician to the possibility of unacceptable dynamic response characteristics. However, because of the many sources of distortion, considerable caution is appropriate in interpreting pressure waveforms even when the external monitoring system is optimal.

The External Monitoring System

Currently available electronic portions of the system can detect amplitude changes to a frequency of 20–30 Hz (cycles per second). This is necessary to detect significant harmonics of the fundamental frequencies of 2–3 Hz, or the equivalent of a heart rate of 120–180 beats per minute.

The electromechanical pressure transducer converts mechanical energy in the form of a pressure change into an electrical signal. For more than 20 years this has been done clinically using a semirigid diaphragm strain gauge connected as one limb of a Wheatstone bridge. As the diaphragm is distorted by the pressure change the Wheatstone bridge becomes unbalanced, altering the voltage measured across the bridge. The voltage change is then converted into an analogue of pressure, which is displayed on a cathode ray tube. This system must be balanced electronically, zeroed to ambient atmospheric pressure, and calibrated mechanically with a known pressure.[74] Since there is physical movement of the fluid in the connecting tubing toward the transducer (producing the distortion of the diaphragm), the accuracy of the measurement (the distortion of the waveform) is dependent on the elasticity of the system, the mass of the fluid column, and the friction created by the catheter and tubing resistance.[32]

A new generation of solid-state disposable pressure transducers recently has become available. The devices appear to be extremely accurate and stable over time. Although the elimination of balancing, mechanical calibration, and fluid movement in the transducer has diminished the potential for contamination and error in measurement, occasional mechanical confirmation of accurate calibration seems prudent.

Calibration using air compressed by a mercury manometer is often used but has caused arterial air infusion and death when patients were not securely isolated from the system used for calibration. A safer method of calibration uses the static column of fluid in the pressure transmission tubing opened to atmospheric pressure

and positioned at two points a known vertical distance apart. The zero point is set at the lower position and the gain control is then adjusted so that the monitor displays the pressure difference to the second position of the tubing tip. A convenient distance is chosen, such as 67 cm, which corresponds to a pressure change of 50 torr (1.34 cm H_2O = 1 mm Hg [torr]).[14]

Reference Points

All pressure monitoring transducers must be zeroed to ambient pressure at the anatomical reference point selected for the particular measurement. The anatomical landmark chosen is invariably a compromise since the reference points for the various measurements differ by several centimeters in different individuals and in different positions. None of the central circulation reference points commonly used can be located reliably using surface anatomy.[74]

Dynamic Response Characteristics

The dynamic response of the monitoring system depends on the characteristics of the conducting tubing as well as on the characteristics of the catheter and transducer. The dynamic response of a system is described by the two physical characteristics of natural frequency and damping coefficient. The natural frequency describes how fast the system oscillates and the damping coefficient describes how quickly it comes to rest.[32] Both of these characteristics can be measured using the simple techniques described in Appendix 15–2.

For practical purposes the natural frequency of a system is fixed by the physical characteristics of the intravascular catheter and the tubing to the transducer. The greater the length of the system, the lower the natural frequency will be. As the natural frequency of the system decreases, approaching the frequencies generated by the biologic system being studied, resonance may occur, resulting in harmonic amplification. In an underdamped system this can result in a great overestimation of the true pressure change (a marked increase in the displayed systolic pressure and a decrease in the displayed diastolic pressure).

This phenomenon may be better understood by considering a musical instrument such as a flute. When air passes over the mouthpiece a number of low-amplitude (inaudible) frequencies are generated, causing the column of air in the instrument to oscillate. The flutist may change

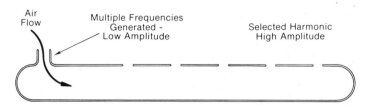

Air Flow

Multiple Frequencies Generated - Low Amplitude

Selected Harmonic High Amplitude

"Natural" Frequency ↓ With ↑ Length

FIG 15–4.
The mechanism for underdamping that results in "harmonic amplification" may be understood by considering the changes in natural frequency of a flute that can be selected by the musician. As the functional length of the instrument increases the natural frequency decreases, allowing the production of audible (higher amplitude) tones at harmonic frequencies to the inaudible tones generated at the mouthpiece. See text for discussion.

the natural frequency of the instrument by changing the functional length of the air column, thereby producing high-amplitude (audible) tones at harmonic frequencies to those produced at the mouthpiece (Fig 15–4). In a physiologic monitoring system harmonic amplification produces artifactually large fluctuations in the recorded pressure changes.

At the other end of the spectrum is the problem of overdamping. A common cause of overdamping is the presence of small air bubbles in the fluid pathway of the monitoring system. Since

the gas bubbles are compressible, their volume decreases with increased pressure. The result of the decrease in volume is a decrease in the fluid movement displacing the transducer diaphragm. The result is a smaller voltage change across the Wheatstone bridge and a smaller displayed pressure change (Fig 15–5).

Because of the very slow response time of the digital display, only mean pressure values of stable waveforms are reliable. Examination of the waveform display at times may yield a clue to artifacts produced by inappropriate damping. An

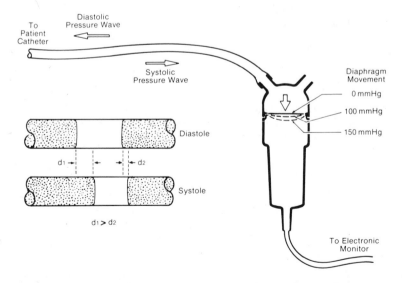

FIG 15–5.
Overdamping of a pressure wave occurs most commonly because compressible gas bubbles are present in the fluid-filled pathway from the intravascular catheter to the electromechanical transducer. Compression of the gas during periods of increasing pressure results in decreased displacement of the transducer diaphragm. The systolic and diastolic pressures tend to converge toward the mean pressure.

overdamped waveform may have a slower rate of rise to systolic pressures and fall to diastolic pressures, blunting of the pressure peak, and often loss of the dicrotic notch. The result of overdamping is that the systolic and diastolic pressures tend to converge toward the mean, making variables derived from these numbers uninterpretable. For example, the heart rate-systolic pressure product (an index of myocardial oxygen consumption) would be artifactually decreased and the coronary perfusion pressure [diastolic blood pressure minus left ventricular end-diastolic pressure (LVEDP)—a determinant of myocardial oxygen delivery] would be artifactually increased if the arterial pressure tracing were overly damped. This situation may lead the clinician into believing that the myocardial oxygen consumption/oxygen delivery balance is better than it actually is.

Similarly, an underdamped system usually cannot be detected from the digital pressure display. The first clue to underdamping may be a marked discrepancy between sphygmomanometer systolic pressure and the arterial line systolic pressure values. Since underdamping may allow harmonic amplification of pressure changes (sometimes referred to as "ringing"), the electronically displayed systolic pressure will be significantly higher than that obtained by blood pressure cuff. Again, examination of the pressure waveform may be helpful. An underdamped waveform may have narrow, high, peaked systolic curve with a low but prominent dicrotic notch. The very narrow peak indicates that very little (if any) flow occurs during this time. Discrepancy between pressures obtained from sphygmomanometry and arterial catheterization raises the question of which is accurate. Unfortunately, it remains unclear what correctly transduced intra-arterial pressures and carefully obtained Korotkoff sound pressures mean. Even when obtained carefully they are not related in a reliable fashion, and the characteristic that is generally sought, flow, is not better reflected by either. An artifactually high measured systolic pressure may give the clinician a false sense of security that a borderline low blood pressure is "adequate" when the true pressure is lower. Conversely, an artifactually high systolic pressure may lead to overtreatment of "hypertension" that is the result of the method of measurement.

Damping artifact may be minimized by using as short a length of low-compliance connecting tubing and as few additional components as possible, achieving a proper dome-to-transducer interface, and meticulously eliminating air bubbles from the dome and tubing.[32] If underdamping continues in spite of these suggestions, damping may be induced by using a short segment of high-compliance tubing[14] or a commercially available damping device (Accudynamic, Sorenson Research Co., Salt Lake City, Utah).[32] The electronic mean pressure is affected little by the dynamic response of the system. Recording the mean pressure, rather than systolic and diastolic pressures, will minimize dynamic response artifact.[7]

Pulmonary Artery Catheterization

Bedside PA catheterization has provided a quantum leap in the physiologic information available for assessing oxygen transport balance in critically ill patients.[14] The technical details of insertion and the potential complications are discussed elsewhere.[14, 53, 77] Directly measured variables include PA systolic, diastolic, and mean pressures; CVP; PA occlusion pressure or WP; and cardiac output. With the addition of systemic blood pressure data, a multitude of derived variables reflecting cardiac function and vascular tone can be calculated. With the analysis of arterial and mixed venous oxygen content all of the derived oxygen transport variables can also be calculated (see Table 15–1). Because so much information is available from the catheter and because errors of omission may be made, an organized approach to the collection, analysis, and review of data is essential. The use of a hand-held programmable calculator or microcomputer will simplify the calculations and present the data in a logical format.[15] (Programming for the Hewlett-Packard HP-41 series of calculators is available at a reasonable cost from Joseph M. Civetta, M.D., Department of Surgery, University of Miami School of Medicine, P.O. Box 016960 (R-44), Miami, FL 33101. Program suggestions for many other calculator and microcomputer systems are available from the Society of Critical Care Medicine, P.O. Box 3158, Anaheim, CA 92803.) These devices can be programmed to alert the clinical team to abnormalities in both measured and derived variables to minimize the risk of not detecting a value outside of defined physiologic limits.

The task, however, is not simply to interpret this mass of data. The task is to identify erroneous data, disregard questionable data, and keep in mind the assumptions underlying the interpretation of each value. Finally, it is essential to integrate the cardiopulmonary data with clinical observations to explain the patient's status and determine appropriate therapy.

Pulmonary Artery Catheter Positioning

Proper positioning of the PA catheter is essential to accurate measurements. A catheter that is too proximal in the PA may not occlude flow sufficiently to yield a pressure that reflects that of the left atrium. On the other hand, a catheter tip that is too distal may cause aspiration of pulmonary capillary blood rather than mixed venous (PA) blood. A distal catheter is also more prone to WP measurement errors induced by local pulmonary factors than is a proximal catheter, where a greater total area of pulmonary vasculature may be occluded for the pressure measurement. More important, a catheter that is too distal creates a potentially dangerous situation for the patient in that if the occluding balloon is inflated to its maximum, it may produce sufficient pressure on the PA wall to cause rupture.[35]

Finally, measurement conditions must be standardized for each patient. Because changes in body position can affect both preload and afterload, the patient should be in the same position for each measurement. This position should be a customary position for the patient. The use of an arbitrary position, such as supine, for measurements when the patient is not routinely in that position may be inappropriate. Changes in activity or emotional state of the patient may affect intravascular pressure, cardiac output, oxygen consumption, and arterial and venous blood oxygen contents. Since critical illness represents a nonsteady state,[16] the timing of measurements must be carefully coordinated so that measurements used to calculate the derived variables are as simultaneous as possible.[74]

Measurement of Cardiac Output

The assessment of cardiac output is fundamental to the assessment of oxygen transport. Clinical estimation of cardiac output is unreliable.[18, 26] Thermodilution measurement of cardiac output has been shown to be safe, reliable, and reproducible in a variety of critically ill patient populations.[31, 44, 79] However, methodologic and technical errors may still occur.

Thermodilution is one form of indicator dilution technique used to measure an unknown volume of fluid. If a known volume of an indicator (dye, radionuclide, or thermal) at a known concentration (counts per minute, temperature) is injected into an unknown volume, the unknown volume may be calculated by measuring the new concentration (counts per minute or temperature) of the indicator in the new volume:

$$V_1 \times C_1 = V_2 \times C_2 \quad \text{(Eq. 15–2)}$$
$$V_2 = \frac{V_1 \times C_1}{C_2}$$

where V_1 denotes the volume of indicator solution, C_1 denotes the concentration (etc.) of indicator, V_2 denotes the volume to be measured, and C_2 denotes the final concentration (etc.).

To measure cardiac output as a volume of blood per unit of time, it is necessary to integrate the change in blood temperature produced by a bolus of cold solution over a known period of time. Cardiac output is inversely proportional to the area under the temperature change curve produced by the injection. Factors that produce a larger temperature change curve (colder indicator solution, larger indicator volume, or lower cardiac output) cause the computer to calculate a lower cardiac output value.

The measurement of cardiac output by thermodilution is based on a modification of the Stewart-Hamilton equation:[76]

$$CO = \frac{VI \times (TB - TI) \times SI \times CI \times K \times 60}{SB \times CB \times \int_0^\infty TB\,(t)\,dt}$$

$$\text{(Eq. 15–3)}$$

where $K = (Tb - Tm)/(Tb - Ti)$, CO is the cardiac output (L/min), VI is the volume of injectate (ml), TB is the temperature of right atrial blood (degrees), TI is the temperature of delivered injectate (degrees), SI is the specific gravity of the injectate, CI is the specific heat of the injectate, SB is the specific gravity of blood, CB is the specific heat of blood, Tb is the temperature of blood (degrees), Tm is the mean temperature of the delivered injectate (degrees), and Ti is the injectate temperature prior to injection (degrees).

The measurement of cardiac output by the thermodilution technique therefore depends on the injectate volume and delivered temperature, the specific gravity and specific heat of both blood and injectate, the patient's blood tempera-

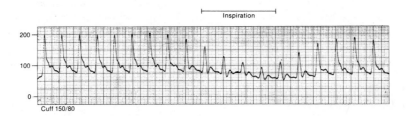

FIG 15–6.

A dramatic decrease in both diastolic pressure and pulse pressure during mechanical ventilation may oc- cur because of decreases in left ventricular stroke volume in hypovolemic patients.

ture, and the measured temperature change caused by the injectate bolus.

The ratios of specific gravities and specific heats of injectate to those of blood are essentially constant within physiologic ranges if the same type of injectate solution is used. Even large variations in hematocrit affect measured cardiac output by less than 1%.[2]

Because PA blood temperature varies during the ventilatory cycle, the baseline temperature for the thermal curve, from which cardiac output is calculated, varies according to the phase of ven- tilation at which the measurement is initiated.[88] Although this effect may be small during unla- bored spontaneous ventilation,[3] calculated cardiac output in dogs was shown to vary by 36% on this basis alone during intermittent positive pressure breathing (IPPB).[88] The variation can be tem- pered or eliminated in some thermodilution car- diac output devices if the baseline temperature is

sampled during one or more ventilatory cycles before the indicator is injected. The device will determine the mean PA blood temperature and use this value in the calculation of cardiac output.

Unrelated to this temperature change artifact, there may be a true change in stroke volume at different phases of the ventilatory cycle. This may be seen as a variation in pulse pressure with ventilation since the area under the pulse curve is proportional to that particular stroke volume (Fig 15–6).[83] The variation in pulse pressure and stroke volume may be due to changing beat-to- beat intervals, as in sinus arrhythmia, and to car- diopulmonary interactions, described in chapter 21, ''Hemodynamic Effects of Artificial Ventila- tion.'' Because blood flow varies with the venti- latory cycle, the timing of indicator injections rel- ative to ventilation is of importance. The data shown in Figure 15–7 are from observations in a mechanically ventilated dog. The cardiac curve

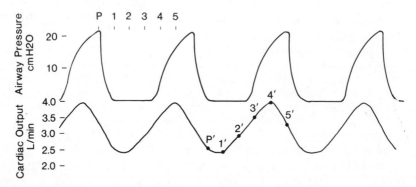

FIG 15–7.

Changes in airway pressure cause changes in car- diac output as measured during controlled mechani- cal ventilation at 10 breaths per minute in dogs. This graph is reconstructed from sequential measure- ments of cardiac output using injections of indicator spaced 1 minute apart at the time of peak airway pressure and at 1-second intervals after peak airway pressure has been reached. Primes indicate the car- diac output measurement made by injecting indicator at the second of peak airway pressure. Because the time between indicator injection and measurement of cardiac output varies, there is no moment of the ven- tilatory cycle at which indicator injection can be used reliably to determine mean cardiac output.

was compiled from data collected over several minutes, and the phase relation between airway pressure (AWP) and change in cardiac output (or the time between injection and critical temperature change at the thermistor) is not known exactly, and is arbitrary in the figure. The cardiac output data points are averages of three or four measurements, and the line is drawn by eye. If the relation between AWP and cardiac output change were exactly as shown and were fixed, we could predict that indicator injections made 5 seconds after peak AWP would closely estimate the mean cardiac output. Injection at any other time would be highly reproducible, but would not equal the mean. However, the phase relation between AWP and change in cardiac output is not fixed, nor is the time between the moment of injection and the moment that flow is actually measured constant. This continuous variation in cardiac output occurs in humans with ventilatory rates as low as 10/min, and at a rate of 6/min, the period of stable output is brief and the flow during the stable period is higher than the mean cardiac output (Fig 15–8). As a result, we are restricted in our timing of indicator injections.

When the mechanical expiratory pause is prolonged during intermittent mandatory ventilation (IMV less than 3/min) and spontaneous breathing is quiet, injections made synchronous with peak AWP will probably reflect a relatively stable cardiac output during the ensuing 20 seconds. The depression of cardiac output that occurs with each mechanical breath will not be reflected, but its inclusion would be unlikely to lower the mean significantly, and so measurements initiated at this moment of the ventilatory cycle are likely to be reproducible as well as a reasonable reflection of the mean value.

However, when inspiration is mechanically assisted at a rate higher than 4/min, injection of indicator at the same moment of the ventilatory cycle risks repeated sampling of the peak or nadir value of the changing cardiac output, as would injections made 1 and 4 seconds after peak in Figure 15–7.[75] Therefore, when mechanical ventilation is provided at a rate higher than 3/min, injections should be made randomly or at equal intervals throughout the respiratory cycle in order to sample appropriately the variation in flow. The resulting data are more likely to have a wide scatter than when injections are made at the same moment of the ventilation cycle, but the mean value is more likely to reflect the average cardiac output.

Variations in the injectate volume cause a linear error in the measured cardiac output value

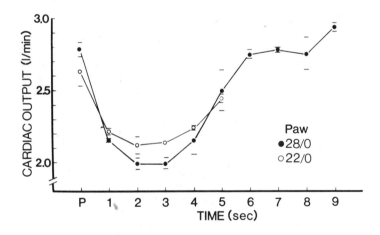

FIG 15–8.
Effect of changing airway pressure *(Paw)* on thermodilution cardiac output determinations. Cardiac output varies throughout the ventilatory cycle. *P* represents the results of thermodilution cardiac output determinations obtained when the thermal indicator was injected at the peak inspiratory pressure provided to the patient by a mechanical ventilator. The subsequent points show mean values of cardiac output obtained from injections made 1 to 9 seconds after peak pressure was achieved. *Closed circles* indicate data obtained when the mechanical ventilatory rate was 10 breaths per minute; *open circles* indicate data obtained when the ventilatory rate was 6 breaths per minute. Peak and end-expiratory airway pressures measured at the two ventilatory rates are shown on the right.

(smaller volumes of injectate cause a spurious increase in the estimated cardiac output). Mechanical injection devices may diminish variations in measured cardiac output values due to changes in injectate volume[24] and operator errors.[54]

Another potential source of error in the thermodilution measurement of cardiac output is variation in injectate temperature.[43, 67] When iced injectate is used as the thermal indicator, warming of the solution begins as soon as the sample is drawn into the injection syringe. At normal room temperature a 5- to 10-ml sample warms at about 1° C every 28 seconds, and faster if hand contact is allowed.[61] An experienced operator may take 15–20 seconds to draw the solution, check the volume, connect the syringe, turn the appropriate stopcocks, and inject the solution. If the injection is timed to a particular phase of the mechanical ventilatory cycle, 10–30 seconds more (at slow rates of IMV) may elapse before injection. A 1° C increase in injectate temperature above that registered by the thermodilution computer will cause a 3%–6% artifactual increase in measured cardiac output. This results in an error of 6%–12% if the delay prior to injection is 30–60 seconds.[61]

Several attempts have been made to address the problem of variable injectate temperature. Probes placed in the ice baths used to cool the injectate will indicate to the computer what the temperature of the injectate was at the time of aspiration—if the probe is not inadvertently removed from the ice bath. A new in-line thermistor probe measures the temperature of the injectate as it enters the PA catheter (Fig 15–9).

Using room temperature injectate is technically simple and yields results similar to those obtained using iced injectate.[27, 71, 72, 75] When specific patient subgroups with high and low cardiac output, blood pressure, or body temperature were reviewed, no significant difference was found between measured cardiac output values obtained using room-temperature and iced injectate.[51] Although room-temperature injectate is less susceptible to temperature change induced by delays in injection, it can still be warmed significantly by handling. A given temperature change will cause more than twice the error caused by a

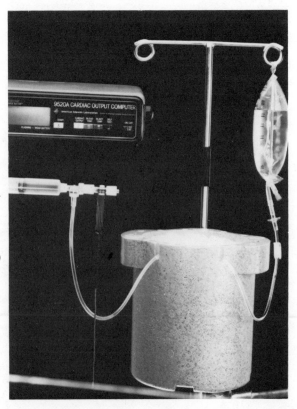

FIG 15–9.
A commercially available closed system for the delivery of ice-temperature indicator for thermodilution cardiac output determinations. This system has a thermistor that measures the injectate temperature as it enters the pulmonary arterial catheter. (Courtesy of American-Edwards Laboratories, Division of American Hospital Supply Corp., Irvine, CA 92714.)

similar degree of warming of iced injectate. Warmer rooms, hypothermic patients, and small injectate volumes result in lower doses of indicator and potentially greater artifact.

Several suggestions can be made to avoid pitfalls in the thermodilution measurement of cardiac output. The measurement should be made with the patient in as close to a stable condition as possible. Appropriate sedation may be given for pain or agitation to minimize variation from increased activity. Multiple measurements should be made. Usually four or five evenly spaced injections are made. The initial injection is only to "cool the catheter" and the value is discarded. A closed injection system will reduce the incidence of bacterial colonization of the injectate.[56] Care must be taken to ensure that the correct calculation constant (K) is entered into the computer and the correct volume of indicator is injected. The injections must be smooth and completed within 4 seconds. However, the rate of injection (within reason) may not be as important as the constancy of the injection. When inexperienced operators must make the injections, an automatic injection device may improve the reproducibility of the measurement.[54] Finally, room-temperature injectate yields results statistically similar to those obtained with iced injectate and is considerably easier to use.

VARIABLES AFFECTING CARDIAC OUTPUT

As was discussed in chapter 5, four factors determine cardiac output: heart rate, preload, afterload, and contractility. This section examines in detail the measurement and assessment of these variables.

Heart Rate

The measurement of heart rate in critically ill patients is usually done electronically from a continuously recorded electrocardiogram (ECG). Depending on the gain control setting for the electronic circuit, the digital display may count artifacts such as pacemaker spikes, abnormal T waves, or stray electrical activity as "beats." As is the case with all bedside digital readouts, correlation with both the displayed waveform and findings from the physical examination of the patient is essential. The disconnection of a sensing electrode has resulted in more than one patient's

being treated inappropriately for ventricular fibrillation or asystole! Most heart rate monitoring systems allow an input from an arterial pressure signal, instead of the ECG, so that the heart rate monitor can be used in situations where extraneous electrical activity (such as electrocautery) may interfere with recording of the ECG. This may also be applied when ECG abnormalities cause spurious heart rate readings.

Ventricular Preload

Ventricular preload is defined by the muscle fiber length of the ventricle prior to systole.[65] The end-diastolic fiber length determines the end-diastolic volume of the ventricle. For a given compliance, the end-diastolic volume is proportional to the end-diastolic pressure. In the absence of mitral valve disease, LVEDP is equal to left atrial pressure (LAP), and in most clinical situations PA occlusion pressure or WP is equal to LAP. In a very roundabout manner, WP serves as a guide to LV preload if these assumptions are valid for a particular patient. In clinical terms, WP is used to indicate the balance between the volume presented to the LV and its functional capability. There are technical and physiologic problems with this usage.

Catheter Position

Ideally, at least 75% of the maximum volume of the balloon (about 1.25 ml in a 1.5-ml balloon) should be needed to produce a change in configuration from PA waveform to WP waveform. Failure to obtain a venous tracing may be due to balloon rupture. An intact balloon will tend to evacuate spontaneously into the syringe. The act of inflating the PA balloon may be lethal if appropriate precautions are not taken. The most common cause of disaster has been PA rupture. This is almost invariably avoided if it can be ascertained that the waveform present represents the PA waveform prior to balloon inflation. *The PA balloon should never be inflated if there is any possibility of a distal migration of the PA tip into a wedge position.*

Failure to obtain a WP tracing by inflation of an intact balloon will occasionally respond to removal of positive end-expiratory pressure (PEEP). The WP tracing is usually retained when PEEP is reapplied. Discontinuing a continuous flush of fluid through the distal lumen of the PA catheter should result in a prompt fall of the recorded pressure, assuring free runoff via the dis-

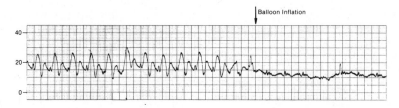

FIG 15–10.
Pulmonary artery pressure tracing showing the characteristics of a satisfactory wedge pressure after balloon inflation. Note brief depressions of both PA and WP tracings, indicating spontaneous inspiration. See text for discussion.

tal pulmonary circulation. Blood withdrawn from a catheter in the "wedge" position in a normal lung should yield blood saturated with oxygen and with a carbon dioxide tension lower than or equal to that of arterial blood. This may not occur if the catheter tip lies in a lung segment with poor ventilation. Obtaining a sample of true pulmonary capillary blood may require a 30- to 40-ml aspirate. Finally, deflation of the balloon should result in prompt restoration of the PA tracing.[60, 78]

Waveform

The PA waveform as obtained routinely in critically ill patients is highly susceptible to reso-

nance artifact. Figure 15–10 illustrates resonance problems common in the recording of PA pressure. Note that an immediately postsystolic nadir in the tracing is lower than the end-diastolic (immediately presystolic) value. In Figure 15–10 the brisk 3-mm upward presystolic deflection is probably another artifact of resonance, although it could reflect left atrial contraction.[63] Damping sufficient to remove these artifacts is likely to lower significantly the apparent systolic pressure of 26 torr. The diastolic value of 14 torr is less likely to be changed.

If AWP exceeds capillary pressure distal to the PA balloon (West zone I or II), the fluid pathway between the wedged catheter and the left

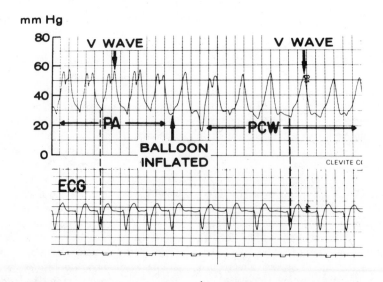

FIG 15–11.
V waves may elevate mean WP value. The catheter may appear not to wedge, but careful examination of a simultaneous ECG tracing reveals that systolic pressure wave is occurring later in the cardiac cycle by retrograde transmission through the pulmonary capillary circulation. This demonstrates the importance of determining WP from a strip recording rather than from the digital readout. In this example the change in the waveform from a double to a single peak is also helpful. (From Buchbinder and Ganz.[8] Reproduced by permission.)

atrium may be interrupted, causing WP pressure to be falsely high.[40] This is unlikely when WP and PEEP differ, and especially if WP is lower.[70]

When the balloon is slowly inflated the waveform should promptly change to a characteristic atrial waveform with a lower amplitude change and a decrease in mean pressure (see Fig 15–10). WP should always be lower than mean PA pressure and usually equal to or lower than PA diastolic pressure. PA end-diastolic pressure and mean LAP have been reported to be the same or lower than LVEDP in patients with coronary artery disease or angina pectoris.[63]

If mitral regurgitation is suspected or if V waves are present (Fig 15–11) on the WP tracing, the diastolic value of the WP tracing is probably a better reflection of LAP than is the mean WP. However, even large V waves are not diagnostic of mitral insufficiency. If mitral valve stenosis is suspected on the basis of history, physical examination findings, or chest radiograph, then WP may be higher than LVEDP, but no relation is reliable and adequacy of filling is better determined by response to therapeutic challenge than by pressure measurement.

Transmural Pressure

Ventricular preload is determined by ventricular filling pressure, which is the transmural ventricular end-diastolic pressure, rather than the absolute (relative to atmosphere) pressure. That is, the volume of the ventricle at end-diastole is determined by LVEDP minus pleural pressure. Any change in pleural pressure alters the interpretation of LVEDP, and therefore WP. We can usually ignore the pleural pressure and transmural pressure gradient because pleural pressure is both low and constant at about − 3 torr. Measuring pleural pressure is cumbersome, and the value of esophageal pressure as a substitute is limited when the

pressure is positive since it is transmitted poorly through the esophagus. When pleural pressure is not measured it is important to estimate likely changes and to time measurements so that the pleural pressure is least altered and most predictable. In Figure 15–10, the 1-second fluctuations in PA waveform are minor artifacts that are due to spontaneous inspiration by the patient. The slight increase after each inspiration probably represents a mild expiratory strain by the patient. After balloon inflation, the appearance of a negative deflection in the WP tracing of similar duration and magnitude provides additional assurance of a valid WP reading. Expiratory efforts, tachypnea, prolonged exhalation, or other evidence of respiratory straining are all evidence of respiratory muscle effort causing change in pleural pressure and absolute WP.[12, 57, 64] Estimation of the effect of pleural pressure and therefore estimation of ventricular filling pressure is reliable only when the respiratory muscle effort is minimal, as evidenced by minimal fluctuation between inspiratory and expiratory WP (Fig 15–12; see also Fig 15–10). Except for the effect of PEEP, ventricular filling pressure can usually be estimated by achieving a relaxed end-expiratory state, which may occur after manual hyperventilation, sedation, or the pharmacologic paralysis of intubated patients.[62, 68]

Several other factors change pleural pressure to an unpredictable degree in critically ill patients. The most widely recognized of these is PEEP. Depending on pulmonary compliance, up to 65% of PEEP may be transmitted to the pleural space.[13] Therefore, the absolute WP may be elevated by 0%–65% of PEEP while LV filling pressure is actually decreased. For example, PEEP of 20 cm H_2O may cause pleural pressure to be unchanged or increased up to 12 cm H_2O, or 9 torr, and LV filling pressure may be 0–9 torr lower

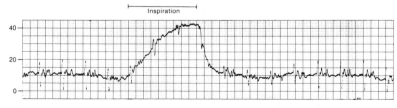

FIG 15–12.
Increases in airway pressure that are transmitted to the pulmonary vasculature may cause marked increases in the observed wedge pressure (WP). Tracing was obtained via a pulmonary artery catheter with the balloon inflated. During the positive pressure ventilator breath (lasting approximately 1.8 seconds) there is an increase in the observed WP, while transmural WP and ventricular preload actually decrease.

than is indicated by WP at resting end-exhalation. Obviously, true LV preload may be grossly overestimated.[32, 45] Removal of PEEP allows an increase in venous blood return and other hemodynamic changes, which can alter WP measurement.[84] Also, acute loss of lung volume may increase venous admixture and cause arterial hypoxemia, which may affect pulmonary vascular tone and further alter WP.[25] However, the immediate "pop-off" WP after an abrupt disconnection from PEEP does seem to reflect LV filling pressure before significant hemodynamic destabilization, especially when filling pressure is low.[11] The nadir of WP during resting end-exhalation immediately after disconnection of PEEP reflects LV filling pressure during PEEP in dogs both with normal lungs and with pulmonary edema (Fig 15–13). Since the time of disconnection is short, pulmonary dysfunction is minimal. Hypoxemia that may occur is usually quickly reversible.[22]

Patients with air trapping, hepatorenal syndrome, or placed in military antishock trousers (MAST suits) may also have significant changes in pleural pressure. Air trapping increases functional residual capacity (FRC) and pleural pressure and, secondarily, the absolute value of CVP and WP. However, the increase in pleural pressure is greater than that in CVP and WP, and therefore transmural filling pressure (ventricular preload) is decreased.[59]

Hepatorenal syndrome is diagnosed in the presence of liver failure when urine findings are those typical of hypovolemia in the presence of adequate intravascular volume. However, the adequacy of intravascular volume is usually judged by the absolute RV or LV filling pressure. Elevation of the diaphragm by ascites and the presence of pleural effusions will increase pleural pressure, resulting in a lower ventricular filling pressure than normal for any given absolute value of CVP or WP.

MAST application might similarly increase pleural pressure and cause absolute pressures to rise more than would be a valid reflection of filling pressures or preload.

In summary, the measurement of WP as an indicator of LV preload is based on a number of assumptions that are not valid in all clinical circumstances. When the electronic monitoring system is properly balanced and calibrated, the dynamic response characteristics are optimal, the catheter tip position is correct, a patent fluid-filled pathway to the left atrium is present, and the measurement is made at the correct time in the ventilatory cycle, the finding of a low WP indicates that LAP is also low. However, in the same clinical situation the finding of a high WP must be viewed with suspicion because of the many potential sources of artifact that will cause WP to overestimate both absolute and transmural LAP.

Regrettably, the correlation between WP and LVEDV in patients with sepsis or cardiac disease is weak, even in patients not receiving PEEP.[9] Reasons for this poor correlation include differences in ventricular compliance and the influence of atrial contraction on LVEDP.[63] The atrial kick may elevate LVEDP 10 or even 20 torr above mean WP. It seems likely that correlation between changes in WP and LVEDV would be better in individual patients, especially in the absence of myocardial ischemia.

Cardiac Function

Ventricular function should be distinguished from contractility. The function of the ventricle is to provide sufficient blood flow for tissue needs,

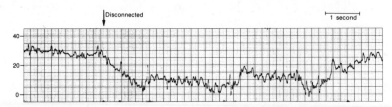

FIG 15–13.
The "pop-off" wedge pressure[11] is the nadir occurring after transient disconnection from mechanical ventilatory support. This is a wedge pressure (WP) tracing obtained from a patient receiving PEEP at 32 cm H_2O. While PEEP is on, WP is 30 torr. Within 1 second of disconnection of PEEP, WP falls to about 6 torr, but that low point is due to a spontaneous inspiration, as can be judged from the rest of the tracing. The delayed but progressive increase in venous return is shown by the rise in WP, at the next end-exhalation, to 13 torr.

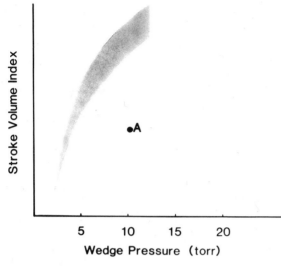

FIG 15–14.

Ventricular function curve. By comparison with the normal *(shaded)* area, stroke volume index (SVI) is seen to be depressed *(A)*. However, the depression may be due to a marked depression of contractility or a high afterload. Heart rate and body size are accounted for when SVI is used instead of cardiac output on this vertical axis, but this still does not distinguish among the different causes of depressed ventricular function.

whereas contractility is one of the four principal determinants of ventricular function (the others are heart rate, preload, and afterload). Plotting cardiac output against WP provides an indication of the adequacy of cardiac function relative to the function expected for that filling pressure (Fig 15–14). However, cardiac output may be depressed due to any combination of low heart rate, increase in afterload, and depressed contractility. Heart rate is taken into account by using stroke volume on the vertical axis, and heart rate and afterload are incorporated by using stroke work (SW) instead of stroke volume. Thus, plotting the work done by the ventricle for each beat against an estimate of preload and comparing that point with a normal range is a more useful means of assessing ventricular function in the intensive care unit (ICU).

Work is equal to force times distance and, when fluids are involved, pressure change times volume. The LV stroke work (LVSW) is often indexed for body surface area (BSA):

$$LVSWI = \frac{(CO/HR) \times (MAP - WP)}{BSA} \times 0.0136$$

$$(Eq.\ 15\text{--}4)$$

Plotting SWI against WP is a common and

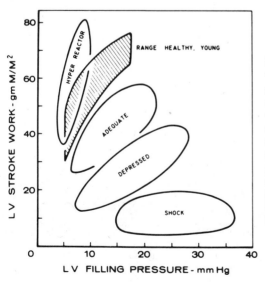

FIG 15–15.

Ventricular function curve. Because an estimate of systemic resistance to flow is included in the calculation of LV stroke work index (LVSWI), ventricular function can be usefully estimated on this diagram. Catecholamine levels should be considered. Data in the adequate range indicate severe depression of function if obtained from a patient manifesting stress or receiving exogenous epinephrine. (From Sodeman WA, Sodeman TM (eds): *Pathologic Physiology: Mechanisms of Disease.* Philadelphia, WB Saunders Co, 1974. Reproduced by permission.)

FIG 15–16.

Descending limb of the Starling curve. If a patient with severe ventricular dysfunction (point *1*) is given a volume challenge and then has a lower SWI with a higher WP (point *2*), it is tempting to conceive of a "descending limb" to the Starling curve *(dashed line)*. However, it is more accurate to refer to the diagram as a ventricular function curve (VFC), and to recognize that loading conditions are changed and VFC is depressed *(arrow)*, and that a second *(lower)* curve should be drawn to explain the second data point. The same change in data could be due to a decrease in contractility, a decrease in diastolic compliance, or a significant increase in wall tension. (Figure and text completed in consultation with Barry F. Uretsky, M.D.)

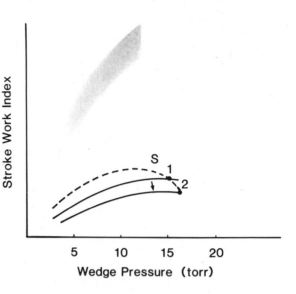

useful means of evaluating ventricular function, as well as changes in function such as are related to alterations in contractility (Fig 15–15). However, there are several problems with this use. First, constructing "curves" by manipulating one of these components and connecting the plotted data points may be simplistic because of the degree of interaction between the incorporated variables. For example, if volume loading in a patient with severe LV dysfunction is associated with a further decline in SW and an increase in WP, it is common to refer to this as a movement down the descending limb of the Starling curve. However, there is little evidence for a descending limb in isolated muscle preparations unless the muscle fiber is stretched so severely that myocyte disruption occurs. It is probably more valid to draw separate curves for each of the data points (Fig 15–16). As the term ventricular function curve indicates, drawing a line for each data point suggests a change in ventricular function; but the change may not be due to a change in intrinsic contractility. There are at least three possible mechanisms for the change in ventricular function, which can be distinguished by using both pressure-volume and force-volume diagrams for the LV (Fig 15–17).

Thus, plotting SW and WP against normal curves is an appropriate use of data currently available in the ICU, but the underlying physiology is often better understood if it is considered in terms of the LV pressure-volume or force-volume relation.

Left Ventricular Afterload

Ventricular afterload refers to factors that determine the velocity of shortening of ventricular muscle fibers during systole.[41] In clinical terms these factors are those that contribute to the impedance of blood flow from the ventricle. Factors that impede blood flow include the mass and viscosity of blood, compliance of the ventricle, distensibility of the great vessels, and the major determinant of vascular runoff, arteriolar tone. Of these factors the only ones that can be changed significantly in the clinical situation are vascular tone and blood viscosity, both of which are included in the calculated systemic vascular resistance (SVR). Although it is not physiologically correct to speak of afterload in terms of SVR, it is clinically useful to relate changes in SVR to changes in LV afterload.

Systemic Vascular Resistance

Arterial tone varies over time as well as in response to therapies. In an attempt to define either baseline arterial tone or the response to therapy in a given patient, the arterial resistance must be determined. Resistance (R) can be defined as the relation between driving pressure (P) and flow (Q), such that:

$$R = P/Q \qquad \text{(Eq. 15–5)}$$

The driving pressure or pressure gradient for arterial flow is the central arterial pressure minus some appropriate downstream pressure. Tradi-

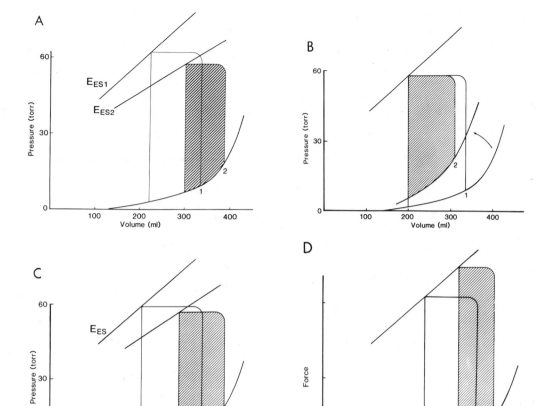

FIG 15–17.

Alternative mechanisms to the descending limb of the Starling curve. **A,** lower intrinsic contractility. Various factors such as ischemia, acidosis, or negative inotropic agents can decrease contractility. Despite higher end-diastolic pressure and volume (*2* compared with *1*), stroke volume (distance moved along x axis) is less. The end-systolic pressure-volume relation (E_{ES}), which usually reflects contractility, is shifted to the right. **B,** lower diastolic compliance. The possibility that end-diastolic volume decreases in spite of a higher filling pressure is diagramed. This situation would arise if the left ventricle became "stiffer" or less compliant *(arrow),* as it might with ischemia. In contrast to a descending limb of a Starling curve, the sarcomere length at point *2* may actually be less than at point *1*. **C,** higher afterload due to increased wall tension: pressure-volume diagram. After sarcomere length is maximal in the intact heart, further volume loading may increase wall tension, which is a measure of afterload. When this occurs a great rise in developed tension is required to develop the same pressure. Because more of the ventricular force is expended in isometric contraction, less remains for ejection.[46] As a result, stroke volume is

less. If arterial tone does not increase sufficiently to compensate for the lower cardiac output, arterial pressure drops (as shown). When this change is diagramed as a pressure-volume relation (as shown in **C**), the end-systolic pressure-volume relation (E_{ES}) is shifted to the right. If E_{max} is taken to reflect contractility, as in **A** and **B**, then intrinsic contractility is depressed. However, the stroke volume and pressure generated are actually lower because afterload (tension) is higher; contractility may be unchanged. This artifact is corrected when force or tension is used instead of pressure. **D,** higher afterload due to increased wall tension: pressure-force diagram. The same situation as in **C** can be seen to involve no change in contractility when force is plotted instead of pressure.[86] Starting from the higher preload and afterload, because more work must be done (higher tension must be generated) to raise ventricular pressure to open the aortic valve, less volume can be ejected. The end-systolic force-volume relation does not change. The force-volume relation is less easily understood on an intuitive basis, but is a more reliable indicator of contractility. (Figures and text completed in consultation with Barry F. Uretsky, M.D.)

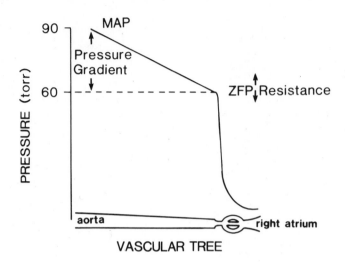

FIG 15–18.

Vascular waterfall. Flow is related to the pressure gradient between mean arterial pressure *(MAP)* and the zero-flow pressure *(ZFP)*. Arteriolar resistance, ZFP, and cardiac output could all change significantly with no change in MAP or central venous pressure (CVP). Volume loading increases flow by raising MAP and the pressure gradient. Changes in CVP have no primary effect on LV output and are not normally a major determinant of SVR. (Figure and discussion constructed in consultation with Michael R. Pinsky, M.D.)

tional calculation of SVR as arteriovenous pressure difference divided by cardiac output presupposes both that resistance throughout the circulatory tree is linear (independent of pressure or flow) and that the appropriate downstream pressure to flow out of the heart is CVP. Unfortunately, neither of these assumptions is correct. Since most of the resistance to blood flow rests in the small arteries and arterioles,[80] resistance in the circulatory tree is not linear, and as a result there is a waterfall effect (Fig 15–18).

As discussed in chapter 4, "Control of Cardiac Output by the Circuit," the downstream pressure for calculating arterial resistance is related to arterial sphincter tone. Briefly, blood vessels are normally filled with blood under pressure. As the tone of the smooth muscle in arterioles increases, the vessel tends to constrict, narrowing its lumen. If the intraluminal pressure falls below some critical pressure, the tone of the vessel's smooth muscle will exceed the pressure of the intraluminal blood and the vessel will collapse despite the continued presence of a positive luminal pressure. The pressure at which a vessel will spontaneously collapse is the zero-flow pressure (ZFP). As vascular tone increases ZFP increases, and as vascular tone decreases ZFP falls. The area of the sphincter is the edge of the waterfall (Fig 15–18). Flow over the waterfall is dependent on the upstream pressure (MAP) and the pressure at the edge of the waterfall (ZFP), but independent of how far the water falls over the ledge (venous pressure).

Arteriolar constriction creates vascular "waterfalls" in most of the systemic vasculature, including coronary, renal, cerebral, and skeletal muscle beds. Since ZFP is a function of local bed arteriolar tone, the pressure gradient for arterial blood flow in different vascular beds can be quite different despite a common MAP (see Fig 7–4 in chapter 7, "Control of Organ Blood Flow"). Collectively, however, these vascular beds establish total arterial resistance and can be thought of as defining a mean arteriolar tone that would cause blood flow to stop if MAP were to abruptly decrease below this value. Many factors affect arterial tone and thus ZFP. At present it is unclear how they interact in complicated disease states such as septic shock and end-stage liver disease. Nonetheless, on the basis of these concepts the arterial pressure-flow relation seen with bleeding and transfusion in an intact animal preparation (Fig 15–19) is more comprehensible. As can be appreciated from this graph, as cardiac output falls, MAP falls, but proportionately less and not to the CVP value. This initial pressure/flow (P/Q) relation along the arterial resistance curve is defined by the resistance to arterial flow (slope of

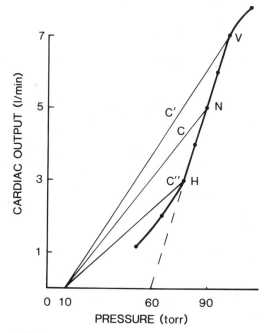

FIG 15–19.
Conventional versus conceptual systemic vascular resistance. The normal arterial pressure-flow relationship has a zero-flow pressure (ZFP) of about 60 torr. If MAP is 90 torr and cardiac output is 5 L/min (point N), resistance is 90 − 60 (torr)/5 (L/min), or 6 torr/L/min. When CVP is used as downstream pressure, resistance (slope C) would be calculated as (90 − 10)/5, or 16 torr /L/min. Arteriolar tone, reflected in changes in ZFP, could vary significantly with no change in MAP, CVP, or calculated resistance. On the other hand, volume administration to point V would be accompanied by a decrease in calculated resistance (slope C′) when no change in tone had occurred, and hemorrhage to point H may be accompanied by no real change in resistance, whereas resistance calculated in the conventional manner (slope C″) would be much higher. (Figure and discussion constructed in consultation with Michael R. Pinsky, M.D.)

P/Q) and the closing pressure of the arterioles (ZFP). The linear extrapolation of the data intersects the pressure axis at ZFP. The slope of this line is a better approximation of arterial tone than is the slope of a line through the venous pressure.

In practice, ZFP for a regional vascular bed (which is not necessarily reflective of the entire systemic circulation) may be appreciated by noting the pressure in the artery sustained momentarily after arterial inflow is obstructed. ZFP in the arm of a patient with a radial artery catheter

in place can be estimated by abruptly occluding arterial inflow (Fig 15–20). It is not appropriate to calculate systemic resistance on the basis of this crude estimate of ZFP because the observed ZFP applies only to the forearm, and because repeated or prolonged occlusion causes a postischemic dilation, but we can at least appreciate the imprecision of the customary approach.

Traditional measurement of SVR does tell us about gross directional changes in tone as estimated by changes in cardiac output and MAP. However, the inaccuracy of the estimate can lead to misinterpretation of the results of therapeutic interventions. For example, changes in cardiac output that are due to intravascular volume change may have no change in arterial tone (movement between points V and H in Fig 15–19), although resistance as routinely estimated is significantly altered. On the other hand, arteriolar tone could be dramatically decreased with no change in calculated resistance. This would occur if nitroprusside were to cause a shift to the right of point N in Figure 15–19. When we see a decrease in calculated SVR at the same time that cardiac output is increased by dobutamine, we can recognize the potential for this being an artifact of the measurement technique.

When LV function is impaired, increases in SVR may significantly reduce cardiac output.[41] Pharmacologic reduction of SVR with vasodilators may restore cardiac output to baseline values provided that intravascular volume is maintained by the infusion of fluid. Since mechanoreceptors, which are the sensors governing the homeostasis of the cardiovascular system, are pressure responsive, hypotension is uncommon when appropriate doses of vasodilators are used in normovolemic patients.[30] However, ascertainment of normovolemia in a stressed patient with elevated ventricular filling pressures due to constricted capacitance and arterial beds is unreliable.

Therefore PA catheterization is usually indicated when vasodilators are used intravenously to improve cardiac output. Vasodilators may improve cardiopulmonary function in the patient with a failing heart by several mechanisms. By lowering SVR, the ejection fraction (EF) may be increased, resulting in an increase in stroke volume and augmented blood flow to the organs. Second, an increase in EF will result in a decrease in end-systolic volume, leading to a decrease in end-diastolic volume, end-diastolic pressure, LAP, and finally pulmonary capillary

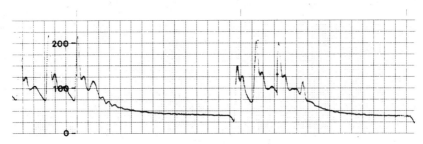

FIG 15–20.
Zero-flow pressure (ZFP) in the forearm. Abrupt oc-clusion of the brachial artery in a patient with a radial artery catheter allows estimation of ZFP in the forearm to be 35–50 torr.

pressure (i.e., a reduction in "backward fail-ure").[30] Third, vasodilator therapy may improve the myocardial oxygen transport balance because less work is required when impedance to flow is reduced and because the smaller ventricle is more efficient.[49] Since coronary blood flow is depen-dent on diastolic blood pressure, normovolemia is important to prevent decreases in diastolic pres-sure during vasodilator therapy. In addition, if cardiac output improves, $S\bar{v}_{O_2}$ may increase, causing improved arterial oxygenation even though pulmonary function has not changed. If pulmonary function improves with the decrease in pulmonary capillary pressure, oxygenation may improve to an even greater degree, further augmenting myocardial oxygen delivery.

TECHNICAL ASPECTS OF OXYGEN CONSUMPTION MEASUREMENTS

So far we have dealt with the supply side of the oxygen supply/demand balance. Traditional thinking has been that oxygen delivery is more important than consumption because interven-tions designed to improve oxygen delivery are readily available and interventions designed to al-ter oxygen consumption ($\dot{V}_{O_2}$) have not been shown to improve patient outcome. It has also been assumed by some that $\dot{V}_{O_2}$ in a sedated pa-tient at rest is relatively constant. Finally, $\dot{V}_{O_2}$ has been difficult to measure in critically ill pa-tients by methods other than the Fick equation.

Alterations in $\dot{V}_{O_2}$ are common in critically ill patients. Injury, sepsis, shock, open wounds, alterations in adrenergic nervous system activity related to stress, changes in environmental tem-perature, activity, agitation, fluctuations in body temperature, shivering, and endocrine disorders have all been shown to alter $\dot{V}_{O_2}$ significantly (see chapter 2, "Oxygen Consumption").[19] De-creases in $\dot{V}_{O_2}$ (perhaps caused by marked reduc-tions in oxygen delivery) are associated with in-creased mortality.[87] It is unclear whether or not manipulations of $\dot{V}_{O_2}$ will alter patient outcome, but it is clear that when oxygen delivery does not meet tissue oxygen demand, mortality is high.[40] An important use of $\dot{V}_{O_2}$ measurements is to as-sess the adequacy of resuscitation. Because of all of these facts there has been renewed interest in the measurement of $\dot{V}_{O_2}$ in critically ill patients.

The most commonly used method of esti-mating $\dot{V}_{O_2}$ in patients with a PA catheter in place is by the Fick equation:

$$\dot{V}_{O_2} = CO \times C(a-\bar{v})_{O_2} \times 10 \quad \text{(Eq. 15–6)}$$

This calculation requires the accurate measure-ment of cardiac output and arterial-venous oxy-gen content difference. The calculation of $C(a-\bar{v})_{O_2}$ requires the measurement of hemoglo-bin concentration, Sa_{O_2}, Pa_{O_2}, $S\bar{v}_{O_2}$, and $P\bar{v}_{O_2}$. Since there is a small but real error in each mea-surement and since it is not possible clinically to measure all of these variables simultaneously, the variance between Fick calculations of $\dot{V}_{O_2}$ and direct measurement of $\dot{V}_{O_2}$ is as much as 25%.[55, 89]

Because of the shortcomings in calculations of $\dot{V}_{O_2}$ using the Fick equation in non-steady-state, critically ill patients, other methods to es-timate $\dot{V}_{O_2}$ have been devised. Either open or closed systems are used. The closed systems use some form of volumetric spirometer (Fig 15–21) connected to a closed ventilator circuit with an in-line carbon dioxide absorber. The rate of de-crease in volume of oxygen in the gas-tight cir-

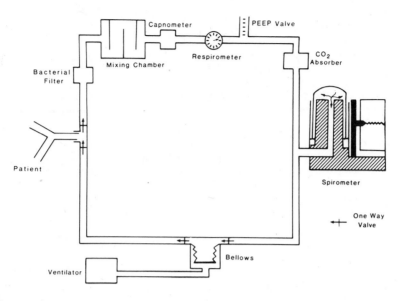

FIG 15–21.

Schematic diagram of a "closed" system device used to calculate oxygen consumption in critically ill patients. (From Bartlett et al.[5] Reproduced by permission.)

cuit is equal to the oxygen uptake of the patient.[5] This method of measurement requires that there be no gas leak, and that accurate measurements of volume change can be made. A commercial system of this design is expected to be available shortly (Metabolic Analyzer MRM 6000, Waters Instruments, Inc., Rochester, Minn.). Another closed system technique for the measurement of $\dot{V}O_2$ calculates the rate at which oxygen must be added to the circuit to maintain either a constant volume in the circuit or a constant oxygen con-

centration. When exhaled carbon dioxide is completely absorbed, the rate at which oxygen is added will equal the rate at which it is being consumed.[85] Again, any gas leak will cause major changes in $\dot{V}O_2$ values.

Open and semiopen systems for the measurement of $\dot{V}O_2$ have also been devised. These systems usually require analysis of both inspired and expired gas concentrations and either the expired minute volume from the patient (in the semiopen system) or the flow of gas through the analyzers

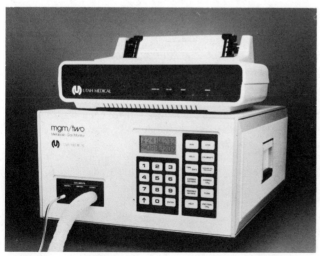

FIG 15–22.

Metabolic gas monitor capable of measuring both oxygen consumption and carbon dioxide production in critically ill patients receiving mechanical ventilatory support. (Reproduced by permission of Utah Medical Products, Midvale, Utah.)

(in the open system). The open system works well for metabolic studies in patients who tolerate breathing room air in a head canopy.[4] The problem has been making these measurements in patients with deficient oxygen transport who need mechanical ventilation and supplemental oxygen. New technology (Fig 15–22) is now available that allows $\dot{V}O_2$ and carbon dioxide production to be measured continuously in critically ill patients requiring mechanical ventilatory support.[85]

While serial measurements of $\dot{V}O_2$ may provide great insight into the problems of oxygen transport balance in critically ill patients, these measurements are fraught with potential technical errors. Fluctuations in the inspired oxygen fraction of as little as 0.005 may cause a 25% error in the measured $\dot{V}O_2$.[6] In addition, the random error of the measurement increases at high (> 0.60) oxygen fractions.[82] High flows of inspired gases may dilute expired gas concentrations and may further increase measurement errors if valving systems are not used to divert inspired gas from the collection system. The valving systems themselves may increase the work of breathing and increase $\dot{V}O_2$. The interfaces between patient, ventilator, and gas monitor must be carefully matched. With so many potential sources of error it is essential that any technique used to measure $\dot{V}O_2$ in critically ill patients be carefully validated.[20] Finally, it must be recognized that a single-point measurement may not reflect the $\dot{V}O_2$ over time since relatively minor stimuli may cause quite profound changes in $\dot{V}O_2$ during the measurement.[21]

NONINVASIVE MONITORING OF OXYGEN TRANSPORT BALANCE

Since virtually all forms of invasive monitoring are potentially morbid, it is desirable to use these monitors selectively in patients who in fact have an abnormal oxygen transport balance. Noninvasive screening techniques to identify such patients would be a significant advance in patient care. While noninvasive means to estimate blood pressure[58] and cardiac output[38] are available today, the devices have major shortcomings when applied to critically ill patients who may have oxygen transport imbalance. Noninvasive measurement of blood pressure is intermittent rather than continuous and is notoriously inaccurate in hypotensive patients with abnormal vascular resis-

tance. Furthermore, oxygen transport assessment requires frequent measurements of arterial oxygenation and acid-base status, available reliably only from arterial blood gas analysis. Similarly, although noninvasive measurement of cardiac output may be accurate by some techniques, without information about filling pressures and vascular resistance, therapy to improve cardiac output by modifying preload, afterload, and contractility would be by trial and error. Finally, the most important information regarding the adequacy of oxygen transport depends on mixed venous blood gas analysis (see chapter 16), which requires PA catheterization.

Two techniques developed to evaluate "oxygenation" noninvasively have been demonstrated to correlate with Pa_{O_2} during normal flow states but to decrease disproportionately to Pa_{O_2} in hypoperfusion states. Both transcutaneous Po_2[81] and transconjunctival Po_2[29] show this characteristic and therefore may be noninvasive indicators of adequate oxygen transport when the values are normal and may indicate that more invasive monitoring is needed when the values are abnormal.

With present technology, noninvasive hemodynamic and oxygenation monitors are usually limited to use as screening tools to detect patients who need further invasive monitoring.

CONCLUSIONS

The technology of monitoring oxygen transport indicators in critically ill patients is evolving rapidly. As new technologies become available, clinicians must fully understand the theoretical background and practical application of the measurements. The measurements must be carefully validated clinically and the data must be interpreted in physiologic terms rather than responded to by rote. Absolute values are not as important as trends and the rate of change in variables. Continuous monitoring of oxygen transport indicators may provide an early warning that will allow intervention before tissue hypoperfusion has caused permanent organ damage. With serial measurements, therapeutic trials may be undertaken to determine the (often unpredictable) optimal patient care. Serial measurements will also help detect the potentially adverse effects that therapy to improve the function of one organ system may have on another. Finally, the clinical correlation of multiple measured variables requires the skill and experience of a dedicated health care team. Placement of monitoring devices and acquisition of data should not delay therapy but should proceed concomitantly with therapy. It is only with precise and complete data that optimal therapy directed toward specific physiologic goals can be accomplished.

Acknowledgments

We thank J. Robert Boston, Ph.D., Presbyterian University Hospital, University of Pittsburgh, and Reed Gardner, M.D., Latter Day Saints Hospital, University of Utah, for their expert advice and comments on the pressure monitoring portions of this chapter.

REFERENCES

1. Adams L, Cole PV: A new method for the direct estimation of oxygen content of whole blood. *Cardiovasc Res* 1975; 9:443–446.
2. Andreen M: Computerized measurement of cardiac output by thermodilution: Methodological aspects. *Acta Anaesthesiol Scand* 1974; 18:297–305.
3. Armengol J, Man GCW, Balys AJ, et al: Effects of respiratory cycle on cardiac output measurements: Reproducibility of data enhanced by timing the thermodilution injections in dogs. *Crit Care Med* 1981; 9:852–854.
4. Arturson G: Continuous oxygen uptake determinations. *Acta Anaesthesiol Scand* 1978; 70:137–143.
5. Bartlett RH, Dechert RE, Mault JR, et al: Measurement of metabolism in multiple organ failure. *Surgery* 1982; 92:771–779.
6. Browing JA, Linberg SE, Turney SZ, et al: The effect of a fluctuating FiO2 on metabolic measurements in mechanically ventilated patients. *Crit Care Med* 1982; 10:82–85.
7. Bruner JMR, Krenis LJ, Kunsman JM, et al: Comparison of direct and indirect methods of measuring arterial blood pressure: Parts I, II, and III. *Med Instrum* 1981; 15:11–21, 97–101, 182–188.
8. Buchbinder N, Ganz W: Hemodynamic monitoring: Invasive techniques. *Anesthesiology* 1976; 45:146.
9. Calvin JE, Driedger AA, Sibbald WJ: Does the pulmonary capillary wedge pressure predict left ventricular preload in critically ill patients? *Crit Care Med* 1981; 9:437–443.
10. Carroll GC, Snyder JV: Hyperdynamic severe intravascular sepsis depends on fluid administration in cynomolgus monkey. *Am J Physiol* 1982; 243:R131–R141.
11. Carter RS, Snyder JV, Pinsky MR: Estimating left ventricular filling pressure during PEEP: Use of nadir wedge pressure following airway disconnection. *Am J Physiol* 1985; 249:H770–776.
12. Cengiz M, Crapo RO, Gardner RM: The effect of ventilation on the accuracy of pulmonary artery and wedge pressure measurements. *Crit Care Med* 1983; 11:502–507.
13. Chapin JC, Downs JB, Douglas ME, et al: Lung expansion, airway transmission, and positive end-expiratory pressure. *Arch Surg* 1979; 114:1193–1197.
14. Civetta JM: Invasive catheterization, in Shoemaker WC, Thompson WL (eds): *Critical Care: State of the Art.* Fullerton, Calif, Society of Critical Care Medicine, 1980, vol 1, section B.
15. Civetta JM: Cardiopulmonary calculations: A rapid, simple, and inexpensive technique (abstract). *Intensive Care Med* 1977; 3:208.
16. Civetta JM: Critical illness: The non-steady state. *Surg Forum* 1972; 23:153–155.
17. Cole PV: Bench analysis of blood gases, in Spence AA (ed): *Respiratory Monitoring in Intensive Care.* New York, Churchill Livingstone, 1982.
18. Connors AF, McCaffree DR, Gray BA: Evaluation of right heart catheterization in the critically ill patient without acute myocardial infarction. *N Engl J Med* 1983; 308:263–267.
19. Cuthbertson DP: Alterations in metabolism following injury: Parts I and II. *Injury* 1980; 11:175–189, 286–303.
20. Damask MC, Weissman C, Askanazi J, et al: A systematic method for validation of gas exchange measurements. *Anesthesiology* 1982; 57:213–218.
21. Damask MC, Askanazi J, Weissman C, et al: Artifacts in measurement of testing energy expenditure. *Crit Care Med* 1983; 11:750–752.
22. DeCampo T, Civetta JM: The effect of short-term disconnection of high-level PEEP in patients with acute respiratory failure. *Crit Care Med* 1979; 7:47–49.
23. Dent JG, Nettar KJ: Errors in oxygen tension analysis caused by halothane. *Br J Anaesth* 1976; 48:195–197.
24. Dizon CT, Gezari WA, Barash PG, et al:

Hand-held thermodilution cardiac output injector. *Crit Care Med* 1977; 5:210–212.

25. Downs JB, Douglas ME: Assessment of cardiac filling pressures during continuous positive pressure ventilation. *Crit Care Med* 1980; 8:285–290.

26. Eisenberg PR, Jaffe AS, Shuster DP: Clinical evaluation compared to pulmonary artery catheterization in the hemodynamic assessment of critically ill patients. *Crit Care Med* 1984; 12:549–553.

27. Elkayam U, Berkley R, Azen S, et al: Cardiac output by thermodilution technique: Effect of injectate's volume and temperature on accuracy and reproducibility in the critically ill patient. *Chest* 1983; 84:418–422.

28. Evers W, Racz GB, Levy AA: A comparative study of plastic (polypropylene) and glass syringes in blood gas analysis. *Anesth Analg* 1972; 51:92–97.

29. Fatt I, Deutsch TA: The relation of conjunctival Po_2 to capillary bed Po_2. *Crit Care Med* 1983; 11:445–448.

30. Forrester JS, da Luz PL, Chatterjee K: Peripheral vasodilatation in low cardiac output states. *Surg Clin North Am* 1975; 55:531–544.

31. Forrester JS, Ganz W, Diamond G, et al: Thermodilution cardiac output determination with a single flow-directed catheter. *Am Heart J* 1972; 83:306–311.

32. Gardner RM: Direct blood pressure measurement: Dynamic response requirements. *Anesthesiology* 1981; 54:227–236.

33. Gast LR, Scacci R, Miller WF: The effect of heparin dilution on hemoglobin measurement from arterial blood samples. *Respir Care* 1978; 23:149–154.

34. Geer RT: Interpretation of pulmonary artery wedge pressure when PEEP is used. *Anesthesiology* 1977; 46:383–384.

35. Hannan AT, Brown M, Bigman O: Pulmonary artery catheter-induced hemorrhage. *Chest* 1984; 85:128–131.

36. Hansen JE, Stone ME, Ong ST, et al: Evaluation of blood gas quality control and proficiency testing materials by tonometry. *Am Rev Respir Dis* 1982; 125:480–483.

37. Hughes JMB, Glazier JB, Maloney JC, et al: Effect of lung volume on the distribution of blood flow in man. *Respir Physiol* 1968; 4:58–72.

38. Huntsman LL, Stewart DK, Barnes SR, et al: Noninvasive Doppler determinations of cardiac output in man: Clinical validation. *Circulation* 1983; 67:593–602.

39. Kane PB, Askanazi J, Neville JF, et al: Artifacts in the measurement of pulmonary artery wedge pressure. *Crit Care Med* 1978; 6:36–38.

40. Krasnitz P, Druger GL, Yorra F, et al: Mixed venous oxygen tension and hyperlactatemia: Survival in severe cardiopulmonary disease. *JAMA* 1976; 236:570–574.

41. Lappas DG, Fahmy NR: The heart, in Burke JF (ed): *Surgical Physiology*. Philadelphia, WB Saunders Co, 1983.

42. Lefcoe MS, Sibbald WJ, Holliday RL: Wedged balloon catheter angiography in the critical care unit. *Crit Care Med* 1977; 7:449–453.

43. Levett JM, Replogle RL: Thermodilution cardiac output: A critical analysis and review of the literature. *J Surg Res* 1979; 27:392–404.

44. Levine BA, Sirinek KR: Cardiac output determinations by thermodilution technique: The method of choice in low flow states. *Proc Soc Exp Biol Med* 1981; 167:279–283.

45. Lozman J, Powers SR, Older T, et al: Correlation of pulmonary wedge and left atrial pressures: A study in the patient receiving positive end expiratory pressure ventilation. *Arch Surg* 1974; 109:270–277.

46. MacGregor DC, Covell JN, Mahler F, et al: Relations between afterload, stroke volume, and descending limits of Starling's curve. *J Appl Physiol* 1974; 227:884–890.

47. Mammana RB, Hiro S, Levitsky S, et al: Inaccuracy of pulmonary capillary wedge pressure when compared to left atrial pressure in the early postsurgical period. *J Thorac Cardiovasc Surg* 1982; 84:420–425.

48. Marland AM, Glauser FL: Significance of the pulmonary artery diastolic-pulmonary wedge pressure gradient in sepsis. *Crit Care Med* 1982; 10:658–661.

49. Mason DT: Afterload reduction and cardiac performance. *Am J Med* 65:106–124, 1978.

50. Mueller RG, Lang GE, Beam JM: Bubbles in samples for blood gas determinations. *Am J Clin Pathol* 1976; 65:242–249.

51. Nelson LD: Monitoring and measurement in shock, in Barrett J, Nyhus LM (eds): *Treatment of Shock: Principles and Practice,* ed 2. Philadelphia, Lea & Febiger, 1986.

52. Nelson LD, Anderson HB: Patient selection for iced vs. room temperature injectate for

thermodilution cardiac output determinations. *Crit Care Med* 1985; 13:182–184.

53. Nelson LD, Civetta JM: Surgical intensive care and perioperative monitoring, in Monaco AP, Jones RS, Ebert P, Simmons R (eds): *Textbook of Surgery*. New York, Macmillan Publishing Co, 1986.

54. Nelson LD, Houtchens BA: Automatic vs manual injections for thermodilution cardiac output determinations. *Crit Care Med* 1982; 10:190–192.

55. Nelson LD, Houtchens BA, Westenskow DR: Oxygen consumption and optimal PEEP in acute respiratory failure. *Crit Care Med* 1982; 10:857–862.

56. Nelson LD, Martinez O, Anderson HB: The incidence of positive cultures in open versus closed thermodilution injectate delivery systems. *Crit Care Med* 1986; 14:291–293.

57. O'Quin R, Marini JJ: Pulmonary artery occlusion pressure: Clinical physiology, measurement, and interpretation. *Am Rev Respir Dis* 1983; 128:319–325.

58. Paulus DA: Noninvasive blood pressure measurement. *Med Instrum* 1981; 15:91–94.

59. Pepe PE, Marini JJ: Occult positive end-expiratory pressure in mechanically ventilated patients: The auto-PEEP effect. *Am Rev Respir Dis* 1982; 126:166–170.

60. Pierson DJ, Hudson LD: Monitoring hemodynamics in the critically ill. *Med Clin North Am* 1983; 67:1343–1360.

61. Powner DJ: Thermodilution technique for cardiac output. *N Engl J Med* 1975; 293:1210–1211.

62. Quintana E, Sanchez JM, Serra C, et al: Erroneous interpretation of pulmonary capillary wedge pressure in massive pulmonary embolism. *Crit Care Med* 1983; 11:933–935.

63. Raimtoola SH: Left ventricular end-diastolic and filling pressures in assessment of ventricular function. *Chest* 1973; 63:858–860.

64. Rice DW, Awe RJ, Gaasch HW, et al: Wedge pressure measurement in obstructive lung disease. *Chest* 1974; 66:628–632.

65. Ross J.: Role of vasodilator therapy, in Karliner JS, Gregoratos G (eds): *Coronary Care*. New York, Churchill Livingstone, 1981.

66. Roy R, Powers SR, Feustel PJ, et al: Pulmonary wedge catheterization during positive end expiratory pressure ventilation in the dog. *Anesthesiology* 1977; 46:385–390.

67. Runciman WB, Isley AH, Roberts JG: An evaluation of thermodilution cardiac output measurement using the Swan-Ganz catheter. *Anaesth Intensive Care* 1981; 9:208–220.

68. Schuster DP, Seeman MD: Temporary muscle paralysis for accurate measurement of pulmonary artery occlusion pressure. *Chest* 1983; 84:593–597.

69. Sehgal LR, Sehgal HL, Rosen AL, et al: Effect of Intralipid on measurement of total hemoglobin and oxyhemoglobin in whole blood. *Crit Care Med* 1984; 12:907–909.

70. Shatsby DM, Dauber IM, Pfister S, et al: Swan-Ganz catheter location and left atrial pressure determine the accuracy of the wedge pressure when positive end expiratory pressure is used. *Chest* 1981; 80:666–670.

71. Shellock FG, Riedinger MS: Reproducibility and accuracy of using room-temperature vs. ice-temperature injectate for thermodilution cardiac output determinations. *Heart Lung* 1983; 12:175–176.

72. Shellock FG, Riedinger MS, Bateman TM, et al.: Thermodilution cardiac output in hypothermic post-cardiac surgery patients: Room vs. ice temperature injectate. *Crit Care Med* 1983; 11:668–670.

73. Sodeman WA, Sodeman TM (eds): *Pathologic Physiology: Mechanisms of Disease*. Philadelphia, WB Saunders Co, 1974.

74. Snyder JV, Carroll GC: Tissue oxygenation: A physiologic approach to a clinical problem. *Curr Probl Surg* 1982; 19:649–719.

75. Snyder JV, Powner DJ: Effects of mechanical ventilation on the measurement of cardiac output by thermodilution. *Crit Care Med* 1982; 10:677–682.

76. Sorensen MB, Bille-Brahe NE, Engel HC: Cardiac output measurement by thermal dilution: Reproducibility and comparison with dye dilution technique. *Ann Surg* 1976; 183:67–72.

77. Sprung CL (ed): *The Pulmonary Artery Catheter: Methodology and Clinical Applications*. Baltimore, University Park Press, 1983.

78. Sprung CL, Rackow EC, Civetta JM: Direct measurements and derived calculations using the pulmonary artery catheter, in Sprung CL (ed): *The Pulmonary Artery Catheter: Methodology and Clinical Applications*. Baltimore, University Park Press, 1983.

79. Stetz CW, Miller RG, Kelly GE, et al: Reliability of the thermodilution method in the determination of cardiac output in clinical prac-

tice. *Am Rev Respir Dis* 1982; 126:1001–1004.

80. Sylvester S, Gilbert RD, Traystman RJ, et al: Effects of hypoxia on the closing pressure of the canine systemic arterial circulation. *Circ Res* 1981; 49:980–987.

81. Tremper KK, Shoemaker WC: Transcutaneous oxygen monitoring of critically ill adults, with and without low flow shock. *Crit Care Med* 1981; 9:706–709.

82. Ultman JS, Bursztein S: Analysis of error in the determination of respiratory gas exchange at varying FiO2. *J Appl Physiol* 1981; 50(1):210–216.

83. Warner HR, Swan HJC, Connally DC, et al: Quantitation of beat-to-beat changes in stroke volume from the aortic pulse contour in man. *J Appl Physiol* 1953; 5:495.

84. Weisman IM, Rinaldo JE, Rogers RM: Positive end-expiratory pressure in adult respiratory failure. *N Engl J Med* 1982; 307:1381–1384.

85. Westenskow DR, Cutler CA, Wallace WD: Instrumentation for monitoring gas exchange and metabolic rate in critically ill patients. *Crit Care Med* 1984; 12:183–187.

86. Wilson JR, Reichek N, Dunkman WB, et al: Effect of diuresis on the performance of the failing left ventricle in man. *Am J Med* 1980; 70:234–239.

87. Wilson RF, Christensen C, LeBlanc LP: Oxygen consumption in critically ill surgical patients. *Ann Surg* 1972; 176:801–804.

88. Woods M, Scott RN, Harken AH: Practical considerations for the use of a pulmonary artery thermister catheter. *Surgery* 1976; 79:469–475.

89. Zeirler KL: Theory of the use of arteriovenous concentration differences for measuring metabolism in steady and nonsteady states. *J Clin Invest* 1962; 40:2111–2125.

APPENDIX 15–1
CALCULATION OF IN VIVO P50

The Hill equation may be used to estimate the in vivo oxygen tension that will produce 50% saturation of hemoglobin (P50) and thereby indicate shifts in the oxyhemoglobin dissociation curve. Although newer equations have been introduced, we believe Hill's equation is the most reliable and applicable and uses constants with the greatest empirical verification. The equation is:

$$S\bar{v}_{O_2} = \frac{\left(\dfrac{P_{O_2}}{P50}\right)^n}{1 + \left(\dfrac{P_{O_2}}{P50}\right)^n}$$

The value of n is defined empirically as 2.65. Using venous blood, once $S\bar{v}_{O_2}$ and $P\bar{v}_{O_2}$ are determined, P50 can be calculated as follows:

$$S\bar{v}_{O_2} = \frac{\left(\dfrac{P\bar{v}_{O_2}}{P50}\right)^{2.65}}{1 + \left(\dfrac{P\bar{v}_{O_2}}{P50}\right)^{2.65}}$$

Rearranging terms:

$$P50 = \text{anti-ln}\left(\frac{\ln\left(\dfrac{S\bar{v}_{O_2}}{(1 - S\bar{v}_{O_2})}\right)^{-2.65\,(\ln\,P\bar{v}_{O_2})}}{-2.65}\right)$$

APPENDIX 15–2

The dynamic response characteristics of a pressure monitoring system may be assessed at the patient's bedside by performing a "fast flush." With the intravascular catheter connected to the pressure monitoring system and the pressure being recorded on a strip recorder, the flush device used to maintain catheter patency is opened to the flush position. The valve is then suddenly closed and the amplitude ratio and cycle length between the first two pressure oscillations are measured. The natural frequency of the system is equal to the speed of the recording paper divided by the wavelength of the oscillations:

Natural frequency (f_n)

$$= \frac{\text{Paper speed (mm/sec)}}{\text{Cycle length (mm)}}\;\text{Hz}$$

The damping coefficient is determined by the amplitude ratio of the first two oscillation waves:

$$\text{Damping coefficient} = \frac{-\ln\left(\dfrac{A_2}{A_1}\right)}{\sqrt{\pi^2 + \left(\ln\left(\dfrac{A_2}{A_1}\right)\right)^2}}$$

(Eq. 15–A1)

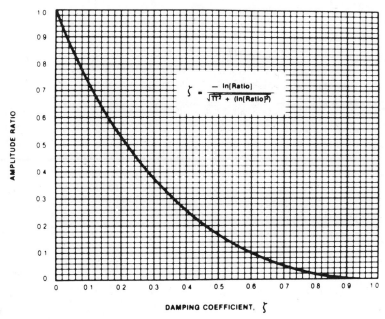

$$\zeta = \frac{-\ln(\text{Ratio})}{\sqrt{\Pi^2 + (\ln(\text{Ratio})^2)}}$$

FIG 15–A1.
Graphic solution for equation 15–A1. (From Gardner.[32]
Reproduced by permission.)

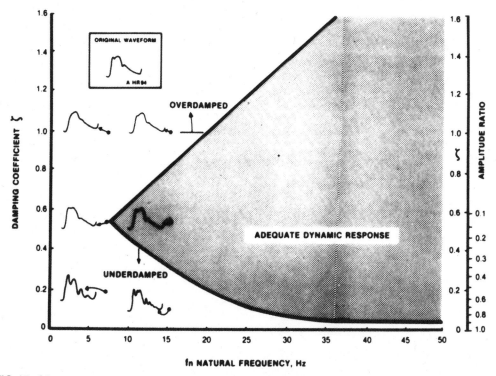

FIG 15–A2.
For a typical arterial waveform this plot shows the ranges of damaging coefficients and natural frequencies that do not distort the pressure waveform *(stippled area)*. For the underdamped region *(lower left)* the pressure waveform has overshoot (increase in systolic pressure) and "ringing," while for the overdamped region *(upper area)* there is loss of fine detail in the waveform, as well as a decrease in systolic pressure. (From Gardner.[32] Reproduced by permission.)

Where A_1 is the amplitude of the first oscillation wave (mm) and A_2 is the amplitude of the second oscillation wave. The graphic solution of equation 15–A1 is shown in Figure 15–A1.

Both the damping coefficient and natural frequency calculations have practical application in the care of critically ill patients.[32] As can be seen from Figure 15–A2, virtually all systems with a natural frequency below about 8 Hz are unacceptable for clinical hemodynamic monitoring, and nearly all systems with a natural frequency above 30 Hz are acceptable clinically. Between 8 and 30 Hz, calculation of the damping coefficient will aid in the evaluation of the dynamic response of the monitoring system. At natural frequencies above 15 Hz, damping coefficients from 0.4 to 0.8 usually result in an adequate dynamic response. Damping coefficients below 0.1 always produce an underdamped (resonant) response; those above 1.0 nearly always produce an overdamped response at the natural frequency of most monitoring systems.

Methods to minimize pressure monitoring artifact resulting from inadequate dynamic response characteristics are discussed in the text.

16 _____ Mixed Venous Oximetry

Loren D. Nelson, M.D.

Mixed venous blood gas analysis may be considered the cornerstone for assessing the adequacy of global oxygen transport. This chapter examines the rationale for and technical aspects of mixed venous blood gas analysis, the use of continuous venous oximetry in critically ill patients, and the application of venous oximetry in patient management.

RATIONALE FOR VENOUS BLOOD GAS ANALYSIS

To serve as a clinically important basis for the assessment of oxygen transport, mixed venous blood gas analysis must delineate a physiologically important variable that is capable of responding rapidly to changes in the patient's condition. The measurement should be readily available and should provide a quantitative estimate of the degree of the oxygen transport deficit. Ideally, the measurement would also provide the clinician with both therapeutic and prognostic information. This section reviews the definition and physiologic determinants of mixed venous oxygen content and examines the relative contributions of oxygen saturation and tension to the calculation of oxygen content.

Definition of Mixed Venous Blood

Theoretically, mixed venous blood may be defined as the mixture of all blood that has traversed the capillary beds capable of extracting oxygen. Specifically excluded is blood that has not traversed these capillary beds, such as blood that has passed through intracardiac or peripheral left-to-right shunts.[11] The theoretical definition is important to remind the clinician that left-to-right shunts may make the interpretation of mixed venous blood gas results more difficult. While appropriate blood sampling from the central veins

and heart chambers will detect significant intracardiac left-to-right shunts, peripheral shunting and maldistribution of perfusion will have an effect on mixed venous blood gas results that is not predictable from the clinical evaluation of the patient.

In practical terms, mixed venous blood is a flow-weighted mixture of all blood that has traversed the systemic vascular beds of the body. This venous effluent is thoroughly mixed so that the oxygen saturation is a flow-weighted representation of blood with different oxygen saturations from different vascular beds. Therefore, samples of blood from the proximal pulmonary artery have the unique property of reflecting the total body balance between oxygen delivery and oxygen consumption of perfused tissues. Analysis of mixed venous blood may play a key role in the assessment of oxygen transport in critically ill patients.

Determinants of Mixed Venous Oxygen Content

Mixed venous oxygen content is determined by the variables of the Fick equation. The Fick equation (Eq. 16–1) relates cardiac output, tissue oxygen consumption, and the arterial-venous oxygen content difference. In equations 16–2 through 16–5 below, the variables are rearranged to solve for venous oxygen content. Equations 16–6 through 16–9 solve for venous oxygen saturation.

$$\dot{V}_{O_2} = CO \times C(a-\bar{v})_{O_2} \times 10$$
$$\text{[divide by } CO \times 10] \quad \text{(Eq. 16–1)}$$

$$\dot{V}_{O_2}/(CO \times 10) = C(a-\bar{v})_{O_2}$$
$$\text{[definition of } C(a-\bar{v})_{O_2}] \quad \text{(Eq. 16–2)}$$

$$\dot{V}_{O_2}/(CO \times 10)$$
$$= Ca_{O_2} - C\bar{v}_{O_2} \text{ [subtract } Ca_{O_2}] \quad \text{(Eq. 16–3)}$$

235

$$\dot{V}_{O_2}/(CO \times 10) - Ca_{O_2}$$
$$= -C\bar{v}_{O_2} \text{ [divide by } -1] \qquad \text{(Eq. 16–4)}$$

$$C\bar{v}_{O_2} = Ca_{O_2} - [\dot{V}_{O_2}/(CO$$
$$\times 10)] \text{ [divide by } Ca_{O_2}] \qquad \text{(Eq. 16–5)}$$

$$C\bar{v}_{O_2}/Ca_{O_2} = 1 - \dot{V}_{O_2}/(CO \times 10$$
$$\times Ca_{O_2}) \text{ [definition of } \dot{D}_{O_2}] \qquad \text{(Eq. 16–6)}$$

$$C\bar{v}_{O_2}/Ca_{O_2} = 1 - \dot{V}_{O_2}/\dot{D}_{O_2}$$
$$\text{[definition of } O_2 \text{ content]} \qquad \text{(Eq. 16–7)}$$

$$C\bar{v}_{O_2}/Ca_{O_2} = S\bar{v}_{O_2}/Sa_{O_2}$$
$$\text{[substitution of saturation]} \qquad \text{(Eq. 16–8)}$$

$$S\bar{v}_{O_2} = 1 - \frac{O_2 \text{ consumption}}{O_2 \text{ delivery}} \text{ [if } Sa_{O_2} = 1]$$
$$\qquad \text{(Eq. 16–9)}$$

In the above equations, $\dot{V}_{O_2}$ represents tissue oxygen consumption (ml/min), CO is cardiac output (L/min), $C(a - \bar{v})_{O_2}$ represents arterial-venous oxygen content difference (ml O_2/dl blood), Ca_{O_2} represents arterial oxygen content (ml O_2/dl blood), $C\bar{v}_{O_2}$ represents mixed venous oxygen content (ml O_2/dl blood, 10 is the conversion factor from L to dl, and $\dot{D}_{O_2}$ represents O_2 delivery (ml O_2/min). Equation 16–9 assumes the Sa_{O_2} to be 1.0.

Therefore, the determinants of venous oxygen content include the principal components of oxygen supply and demand: oxygen consumption, cardiac output, hemoglobin concentration, and arterial oxygen saturation. Because dissolved oxygen does not contribute significantly to oxygen content in most cases, $S\bar{v}_{O_2}$ effectively reflects changes in all these components.

The oxyhemoglobin dissociation curve defines the relationship between oxygen saturation and tension. Saturation is determined by the physiologic principles described above, and tension is determined by the position and shape of the curve. Several factors are known to alter the position of the curve. Increases in blood temperature, carbon dioxide tension, hydrogen ion concentration, 2,3-diphosphoglycerate (2,3-DPG), intracellular sodium, and hemoglobin concentration all cause a decrease in the affinity of hemoglobin for oxygen.[7] These factors shift the oxyhemoglobin dissociation curve to the right and improve oxygen unloading at the tissue level. This change is characterized by an increase in P50 (the partial pressure of oxygen that results in 50% saturation of hemoglobin). On the other hand, hypothermia, hypocarbia, alkalosis, ane-

mia, and decreases in 2,3-DPG and intracellular sodium lower the P50, shift the curve to the left, and inhibit peripheral oxygen unloading. A 2-mm Hg shift in P50 may affect oxygen availability to the tissue as much as a 1.12 L/min change in cardiac output.[34]

Importance of Venous Oxygen Tension

Venous oxygen content (and therefore saturation) is determined by the variables in the Fick equation. Venous oxygen tension ($P\bar{v}_{O_2}$) is determined by these same factors and the position of the oxyhemoglobin dissociation curve. The effects of interventions aimed at improving oxygen unloading may be evaluated only when both of these parameters are measured[20] (see chapter 1 for a discussion of the effect of the oxyhemoglobin dissociation curve on tissue oxygenation).

The association between marked venous hypoxemia ($P\bar{v}_{O_2} < 27$ mm Hg) and lactic acidosis, and the high mortality resulting from lactic acidosis[13, 29] were discussed in chapter 3. While a precise relationship between $S\bar{v}_{O_2}$ and lactic acidosis has not been reported, the probability of tissue hypoxia increases when $S\bar{v}_{O_2}$ falls below 0.55, and reserve oxygen transport is likely to be compromised when $S\bar{v}_{O_2}$ is less than 0.60. Indeed, in a small study of patients with traumatic shock, the importance of sustained venous desaturation was emphasized by the fact that four of four patients whose $S\bar{v}_{O_2}$ increased to above 0.60 with resuscitative efforts survived, whereas five of six patients whose $S\bar{v}_{O_2}$ failed to increase above 0.60 died.[12]

ANALYSIS OF VENOUS BLOOD GASES

The first concern regarding the analysis of venous blood gases is obtaining a proper sample. Samples of venous blood representing flow from multiple vascular beds may be obtained from the central veins, the right atrium or ventricle, or the pulmonary artery (PA) (Table 16–1). However, the correlation between central venous and PA oxygen saturation is not satisfactory for the clinical use of central venous oxygen saturation as an estimate of true mixed venous saturation. Local variations in blood flow and oxygen consumption cause superior vena cava (SVC) and inferior vena cava (IVC) values to differ from each other and from the true mixed venous value. In addition, the relative distribution of flow varies with dis-

TABLE 16–1.

Average % Oxygen Saturation and Range of
Saturations in Various Locations in the Central
Circulation*

SOURCE	OXYGEN SATURATION (%)	
	MEAN	RANGE
Systemic artery	97.3	(95–99)
Inferior vena cava	83.0	(76–88)
Superior vena cava	76.8	(66–84)
Right atrium	79.5	(72–86)
Right ventricle	78.5	(64–84)
Pulmonary artery	78.4	(73–85)
Pulmonary artery wedge	98.2	(90–100)

*Measured in 26 healthy volunteers breathing room
air.[2] Variation between superior and inferior vena cava
samples represents differences in blood flow and oxygen consumption of the different vascular beds.

ease states commonly found in critically ill patients. In fact, while IVC saturation normally exceeds that of the PA, the redistribution of renal
and mesenteric blood flow that occurs during
shock causes a reversal of the relative saturations,
making the PA blood have a higher saturation
than IVC blood (Fig 16–1). The relative saturations of SVC and PA blood change in the opposite manner.[16]

Other investigators have considered the use
of central venous blood in place of PA blood for
the calculation of the derived parameters of arterial-venous oxygen content difference and intra-

pulmonary shunt fraction in certain patients admitted to intensive care units (ICUs).[32] They
conclude, however, that "the exact numerical
value of mixed venous blood samples can only
be measured from blood collected from the PA
itself." In fact, meaningful information can be
obtained from central venous oxygen tension or
saturation measurements. Very low values reliably indicate a severe compromise of oxygen
transport, and high values indicate that transport
in perfused tissues is not depressed relative to
need. However, the correlation with the oxygen
supply/demand relation is not as high as when
mixed venous values are used, and using sequential central venous values to monitor for change
in oxygen transport clearly is unreliable.

The major problem with using central venous blood to estimate mixed venous oxygenation
is that the patients in whom the value is most
crucial for therapeutic decisions are the same patients in whom the central venous values are least
likely to represent a true mixed sample.[24]

PITFALLS IN PULMONARY ARTERIAL BLOOD GAS ANALYSIS

"Contamination" of mixed venous blood with
arterialized pulmonary capillary blood is an important potential source of error in the evaluation
of oxygen transport problems.[28] If a significant

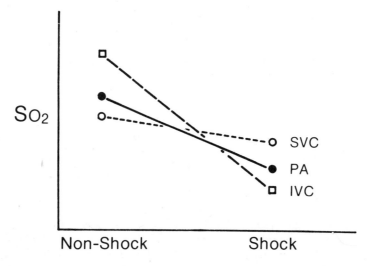

FIG 16–1.
Relationship between superior *(SVC)* and inferior *(IVC)* vena cava blood oxygen saturation (So₂) and pulmonary artery *(PA)* saturation reverses in the shock state.

portion of the vessel lumen is occluded by the catheter or adherent clot so that inflow of mixed venous blood is slower than the sample aspiration rate, blood from the PA distal to the catheter may be sampled. If this blood has been exposed to ventilated alveoli, gas exchange may have occurred, causing a false increase in the oxygen tension and saturation of the sample. This will result in large errors in the derived values of arterial-venous oxygen content difference, intrapulmonary shunt fraction, oxygen consumption, and oxygen utilization ratio.

One clue to help identify an arterialized sample is the finding of higher than expected venous oxygen content. Unfortunately the measurement of mixed venous oxygen saturation or tension is performed because we are clinically unable to estimate accurately these values and therefore usually cannot reliably expect a given value. Sampling errors are not predictable, and normal values of venous oxygen saturation do not rule out sample contamination with pulmonary capillary blood.[31]

It has also been suggested that evaluation of the venous carbon dioxide tension (Pv_{CO_2}) may be helpful to identify an arterialized sample. Pv_{CO_2} must be higher than Pa_{CO_2} but the difference is dependent on carbon dioxide production, cardiac output, the carbon dioxide dissociation curve, the degree of venous hypoxemia, and the ventilation-perfusion balance in the lung. When blood is sampled from vessels perfusing ventilated lung segments, the P_{CO_2} of venous blood contaminated with pulmonary capillary blood may be equal to or less than that of arterial blood. However, if the alveoli are poorly ventilated (low ventilation to perfusion ratio), Pv_{CO_2} will approach that of mixed venous blood and cannot be used to distinguish the sample from one contaminated with pulmonary capillary blood.[28]

Inspection of the pressure waveform may help identify a wedged or partially wedged catheter tip. This is useful and should be performed prior to aspirating blood for gas analysis. Since the waveform cannot be displayed during the sampling, it should be inspected immediately after the sample is obtained and before the catheter is flushed, as flushing might move it from a wedge position. Also, it is the practice in some ICUs to observe carefully the catheter balloon volume required to occlude the pulmonary artery for "wedge" pressure measurements. If the minimal volume required for occlusion approaches

the maximum volume of the balloon, a proximal position of the catheter tip is assured. Proper catheter positioning is more important than withdrawal rates to avoid aspiration of arterialized samples.[19]

Rapid or forceful aspiration of a blood sample through a high-resistance PA catheter may be associated with the formation of many small gas bubbles in the syringe. If there is no leak in the aspirating system, these bubbles are formed because dissolved gases in the blood are subjected to high negative pressure. Gentle aspiration should prevent bubble formation. Manually tapping the syringe will usually cause unavoidable bubbles to coalesce so that they may be expelled from the tip of the syringe.

The same cautions regarding sampling technique for arterial blood should be observed when sampling mixed venous blood. A small volume (1–2 ml) of blood should be obtained anaerobically in a heparinized syringe and any gas bubbles should be expelled. The volume of heparin should be appropriate for the volume of the sample. One hundred units (0.1 ml of 1,000 units/ml) will adequately anticoagulate a 2-ml blood sample and will not significantly affect the pH of the sample.[27] The syringe should be capped with a gas-tight closure and processed immediately. If the analysis is delayed more than a few minutes the sample should be placed on ice to reduce cellular metabolism, which may alter the test results.

Finally, while calculated saturation values may be acceptable for arterial blood samples, measured saturation values are desirable for venous samples. Arterial saturation values are often at the flat portion of the oxyhemoglobin dissociation curve and therefore are little affected by changes in the position of the curve. Venous saturation values, on the other hand, are usually on the steep portion of the curve where small changes in P50 may make major changes in a value calculated from a nomogram. Since the derived values of arterial-venous content difference, intrapulmonary shunt fraction, oxygen consumption, and oxygen utilization ratio are dependent on an accurate calculation of venous oxygen content, the major determinant of venous content, $S\bar{v}_{O_2}$, must be accurately measured. In a study conducted in our surgical ICU we found that venous saturation values estimated from the venous Po_2, even when corrected for patient temperature and pH, were significantly lower than those mea-

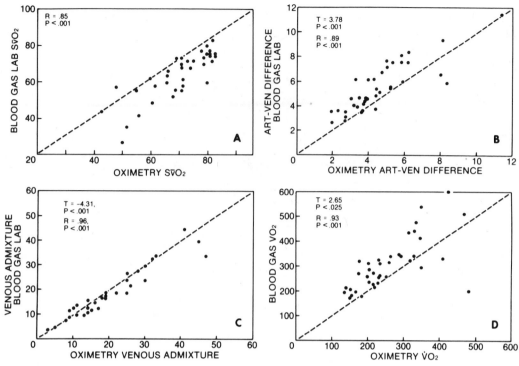

FIG 16–2.
Mixed venous oxygen saturation ($S\bar{v}_{O_2}$) calculated from oxygen tension, as measured by an automated blood gas analyzer, is significantly lower than that measured by reflection cooximetry in these critically ill patients **(A).** Since venous saturation is a major determinant of venous oxygen content, the derived parameters of arterial-venous oxygen content difference (*art-ven difference,* **B**) and oxygen consumption ($\dot{V}_{O_2}$, **D**) are significantly increased, and venous admixture **(C)** is significantly decreased when calculated venous saturation values are used.

sured by cooximetry. As illustrated in Figure 16–2, derived values were significantly altered.

CONTINUOUS VENOUS OXIMETRY

Rationale for Continuous Oximetry

The "non-steady-state" nature of critical illness[4] has taught specialists in the field that real-time measurements may yield a wealth of information on patient status that is unavailable from intermittent measurements. An example is real-time monitoring of cardiac rhythm in patients with suspected myocardial infarction, in whom detection of transient arrhythmias may allow early therapy and improve survival.[3, 9] Real-time monitoring of intravascular pressures, temperature, urine output, and drug infusion rates have certainly improved the accuracy and reduced the time required for these procedures, and perhaps have improved patient care.

A fiber optic catheter and processor suitable for continuous analysis of blood oxygen saturation at the bedside was available clinically in 1972. The spectrophotometer and processor were significantly improved in 1977, and the fiber optics were incorporated into a flow-directed pulmonary artery catheter in 1981 (Fig 16–3). The catheter design and handling characteristics were improved in early 1982, and popularity of the catheter has increased steadily.[26]

Since $S\bar{v}_{O_2}$ reflects the overall balance between oxygen supply and demand, many ICUs use this parameter to evaluate the adequacy of oxygen transport.[22] Because a decrease in $S\bar{v}_{O_2}$ may indicate inadequate oxygen transport, continuous monitoring of the value may be desirable in patients with acute cardiopulmonary disease. It will not identify the cause for the inadequate ox-

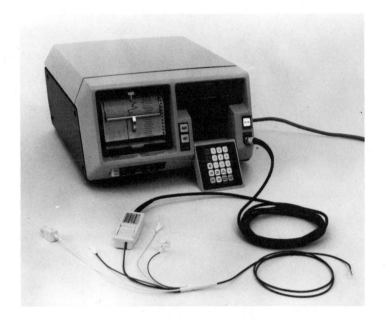

FIG 16–3.
The PA catheter, optical module, oximetry processor, and continuous recorder for mixed venous oximetry are commercially available for clinical applications in the operating room or intensive care unit. (Courtesy of Oximetrix, Inc., Mountain View, Calif.)

ygen transport, but rather will bring to attention any change in the major components of oxygen supply or demand, and will do so without delay and with few false alarms. The cause of the alarm is often apparent in clinical context, but may require further hemodynamic and/or laboratory evaluation.

Technical Considerations

Systems currently available for continuous in vivo venous oximetry are based on the principle of reflection spectrophotometry. Traditional in vitro oximetry uses transmission spectrophotometry, in which a source producing multiple wavelengths of light is directed through a blood sample. The relative attenuation of the different wavelengths is measured to calculate the ratio of oxyhemoglobin to total hemoglobin in the sample (Fig 16–4). This ratio is the fraction of hemoglobin saturated with oxygen (i.e., in venous blood, the $S\bar{v}_{O_2}$).

Reflection spectrophotometry is similar in that multiple (three) wavelengths of light are passed through fiber optic bundles in an intravascular catheter. The light is reflected from red blood cells flowing by the end of the catheter to another fiber optic bundle which returns the light to a photodetector sensitive to the different wavelengths. The relative reflectance of total hemoglobin and oxyhemoglobin are calculated to yield the

FIG 16–4.
Conventional bench cooximetry uses the principle of transmission spectrophotometry. (Courtesy of Oximetrix, Inc., Mountain View, Calif.)

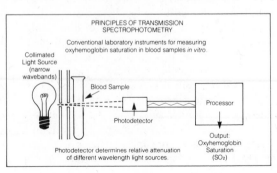

PRINCIPLES OF TRANSMISSION
SPECTROPHOTOMETRY

Conventional laboratory instruments for measuring
oxyhemoglobin saturation in blood samples *in vitro*.

Collimated
Light Source
(narrow
wavebands)

Blood Sample

Photodetector

Processor

Output:
Oxyhemoglobin
Saturation
(SO_2)

Photodetector determines relative attenuation
of different wavelength light sources.

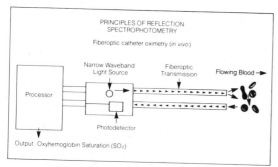

FIG 16–5.
The continuous in vivo oximeter uses the principle of reflection spectrophotometry. (Courtesy of Oximetrix, Inc., Mountain View, Calif.)

fraction of hemoglobin saturated with oxygen (Fig 16–5).

The clinical application of reflection spectrophotometry requires blood flow past the fiber optic transmission bundles. For mixed venous oximetry this means that the PA catheter must be properly positioned in the proximal portion of the vessel. Distal migration of the catheter may cause a reduction in blood flow or allow the tip to come into contact with a vessel wall (especially at a bifurcation). The result may be an erroneous saturation measurement. Catheter tip position may be ensured most easily by carefully observing the pressure tracing and measuring the balloon volume required to achieve an occluded pressure

tracing. The currently available system for continuous mixed venous oximetry may be calibrated by in vitro standardization prior to insertion into the PA, and in vivo by obtaining a mixed venous blood sample and measuring $S\bar{v}_{O_2}$ with a bench cooximeter and entering this value into the processor. If the system was properly warmed up prior to standardization and monitoring was not interrupted by turning off the machine or disconnecting the catheter from the optical module, it is remarkably stable and holds its calibration for at least 24 hours.[1] If for any reason the measurement is suspected of being in error, the system may be recalibrated by the in vivo method without interrupting monitoring.

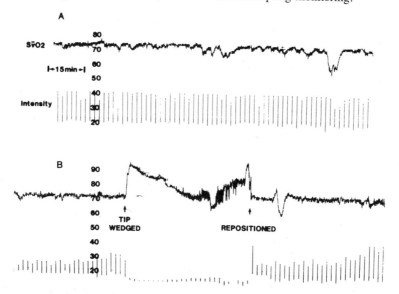

FIG 16–6.
A strip chart recording from a hemodynamically stable patient demonstrates small variations in the continuously measured $S\bar{v}_{O_2}$. The vertical bars represent the intensity signal from light returned from the fiber optic catheter **(A).** When the pulmonary artery catheter tip migrates distally it may lodge against the wall of a smaller pulmonary vessel. This often results in an abrupt increase in the $S\bar{v}_{O_2}$ value recorded and a diminution of the intensity signal **(B).** Repositioning of the catheter tip will correct the artifactual values.

The intensity of the light received by the optical module is also monitored by the system (Fig 16–6). A decrease in the intensity will alert the operator that the saturation being displayed may be in error. This may occur if the tip of the catheter comes in contact with a vessel wall or if fibrin is deposited over the fiber optics. Once the catheter position is confirmed the intensity signal may be readjusted to the proper level to compensate for fibrin deposition. A low-intensity alarm must be corrected before considering the saturation measurement to be reliable.[23]

Relationship to Other Physiologic Parameters

The saturation measured by catheter oximetry correlates to a high degree with values obtained by in vitro oximetry (Fig 16–7). Hemoglobin concentration, body temperature, and cardiac output do not affect the accuracy of the system; variance due to drift is less than 1% per day.[1]

The continuous venous oximetry system has been established as an accurate indicator of venous oxygen saturation. The question remains how to interpret and utilize the new on-line information. To answer these questions we began a series of investigations to examine our use of continuous venous oximetry in critically ill patients in the surgical ICU at Jackson Memorial Hospital, Miami.

To establish an understanding of the meaning of changes in $S\bar{v}_{O_2}$ in critically ill patients we first looked for correlations between $S\bar{v}_{O_2}$ and the individual determinants of $S\bar{v}_{O_2}$ from the Fick equation. When arterial oxygen content was maintained at a high level (by transfusion of blood to keep the hemoglobin concentration at or above 10 gm/dl and pulmonary support with supplemental oxygen and positive end-expiratory pressure ventilation to keep arterial oxygen saturation above 0.95 when possible), there was no correlation between $S\bar{v}_{O_2}$ and either arterial saturation or tension (Fig 16–8).

In 1978 De La Rocha et al. reported a statistically significant correlation between $S\bar{v}_{O_2}$ and cardiac output in children undergoing surgical correction of congenital heart defects.[5] Four years later Waller et al. noted the correlation to be considerably lower in adults being anesthetized for coronary artery bypass surgery.[33] These authors concluded that "this correlation . . . is not so strong that clinically reliable quantitative infer-

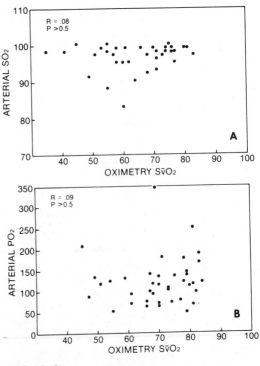

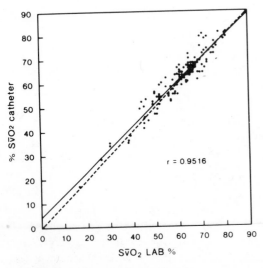

FIG 16–7.
Paired venous blood samples analyzed by in vivo and in vitro oximetry show a high degree of correlation. (Modified from Baele et al.,[1] by permission.)

FIG 16–8.
There is no statistical relationship between either arterial saturation (S_{O_2}, **A**) or tension (P_{O_2}, **B**) and venous oxygen saturation ($S\bar{v}_{O_2}$) when arterial saturation is maintained at a relatively high level (>0.90).

ences [regarding cardiac output] can be made from the $S\bar{v}_{O_2}$ changes alone.'' Later in 1982 Jamieson et al. reported ''no fixed relation'' of $S\bar{v}_{O_2}$ to any variable of myocardial function in adult patients being anesthetized for cardiac surgery.[10] Finally, in our own study, we found a low but statistically significant correlation between $S\bar{v}_{O_2}$ and cardiac output (Fig 16–9,A).[22] These data emphasize that $S\bar{v}_{O_2}$ is determined by multiple factors, any combination of which can disrupt the balance between oxygen supply and demand. Because it is multifactorial, $S\bar{v}_{O_2}$ cannot be expected to correlate closely with any one of the oxygen supply/demand variables. Thus, correlations between $S\bar{v}_{O_2}$ and Sa_{O_2}, cardiac output, oxygen delivery, and oxygen consumption are poor (Fig 16–9,B and C). However, correlation of $S\bar{v}_{O_2}$ and all of the components acting at once

(oxygen utilization), as suggested in equation 16–9, is clear (Fig 16–9,D).

Clinical Utility of Continuous $S\bar{v}_{O_2}$

Continuous venous oximetry may have utility either as an assurance to the clinician of relative cardiopulmonary stability or as an indicator of the need for further clinical assessment. Martin et al. concluded in 1973 that ''a rapidly falling $S\bar{v}_{O_2}$ was ominous and usually preceded a major cardiovascular complication such as severe hypotension or cardiac arrest.'' The decrease in $S\bar{v}_{O_2}$ usually preceded the disaster by 2 to 10 minutes, but it is not clear from the paper whether interventions at this time were able to alter the outcome.[17] The suggestion remains that changes in $S\bar{v}_{O_2}$ may precede hemodynamic events and therefore may provide an early warning that additional infor-

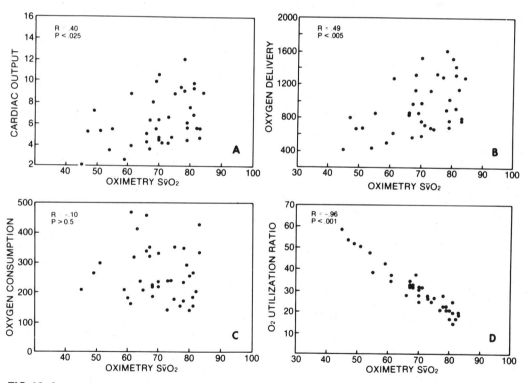

FIG 16–9.
The correlation between cardiac output and venous oxygen saturation ($S\bar{v}_{O_2}$) in critically ill patients is low **(A).** Similarly, the correlations between oxygen delivery **(B)** and oxygen consumption **(C)** and $S\bar{v}_{O_2}$ are low. These observations suggest that changes in $S\bar{v}_{O_2}$ occur because of factors other than any *single* determinant of the oxygen supply/demand balance. When the overall balance of oxygen supply and de- mand (the oxygen utilization ratio) is plotted against $S\bar{v}_{O_2}$ a high degree of inverse correlation is evident **(D),** suggesting that continuously measured $S\bar{v}_{O_2}$ may provide an "on-line" indication of the oxygen supply/demand balance. However, these data must be interpreted cautiously because of the potential for mathematical coupling errors in the statistical analysis (see text).

mation (cardiac output and arterial oxygen content) is needed.[35]

Economics of Continuous Venous Oximetry

A major concern today with health care professionals is the rising cost of new technology. While new devices may appear to improve patient care at the bedside, it is usually difficult to prove that outcome is significantly altered. Because of this, decisions regarding the purchase of new monitoring devices may be made on the basis of potential cost savings to the hospital. At this time the continuous oximetry catheter (Shaw Opticath, Oximetrix, Inc., Mountain View, Calif.) has a list price of $175. The list price of a typical PA catheter without fiber optics for oximetry (Swan-Ganz PA catheter, American-Edwards Laboratories, Santa Ana, Calif.) is $85. To be cost-saving to the hospital, the $90 cost difference must be compensated by reductions in other patient care costs possible with the use of the oximetry catheter.

The most obvious potential cost savings would be a reduction in the number of blood gas analyses performed in patients with the oximetry catheter. A study of continuous umbilical arterial oximetry in neonates demonstrated a 37% decrease (from 35 to 22) in the average number of blood samples drawn for gas analysis during the first 48 hours after catheterization.[15] In a study of adults with respiratory or cardiac failure the average number of arterial blood gas analyses during the initial 48 hours of therapy was 10.3 in patients without continuous venous oximetry and 6.3 in patients with the device.[8] This was a statistically significant reduction. Since a "normal" $S\bar{v}_{O_2}$ does not rule out a low arterial P_{O_2} and since arterial blood gas analysis is used to evaluate ventilation (Pa_{CO_2}) and acid-base status (pH), factors that (except at the extremes of physiologic ranges) do not affect $S\bar{v}_{O_2}$, in our own study we were not able to decrease the number of arterial samples obtained from critically ill, traumatized, and postoperative patients. However, we did note a significant decrease in the number of venous blood gas samples obtained (average, 4.9 samples during the first 48–72 hours of the study) and a decrease in the number of times that cardiac output was measured (savings of 2.5 measurements in the first 48–72 hours). The charge to the patient for a blood gas analysis is $50. The charge for the measurement of cardiac output and the calculation of the derived parameters is $45.

This resulted in a net decrease in charges to the patient of more than $250 over the 3 days of the study. While we were unable to determine the true cost to the hospital of a blood gas analysis, the estimated total operational cost of the blood gas laboratory at the Presbyterian-University Hospital of Pittsburgh is $19 per sample.

While the actual cost-effectiveness of continuous venous oximetry will vary with the patient population, the costs and charges of the individual hospital, and the standard medical practice of the ICU, the real utility may be to eliminate unnecessary blood gas and hemodynamic measurements in stable patients and to alert the clinical team to the need for additional measurements if an imbalance of oxygen consumption and delivery develops (i.e., a change in $S\bar{v}_{O_2}$).[22]

Application of Continuous Venous Oximetry to Patient Care

The normal value for $S\bar{v}_{O_2}$ is about 0.75 and the usual acceptable range is 0.68–0.77.[18] Values above this range indicate an increase in oxygen delivery relative to consumption (i.e., a decreased utilization ratio) and are associated with cirrhosis, the hyperdynamic phase of sepsis, peripheral left-to-right shunting, cellular poisoning such as cyanide toxicity (rare), marked arterial hyperoxia, or a technical malfunction of the system. The two most common technical problems in our experience have been advancement of the catheter tip into the wedge position (see Fig 16–6,B) and occasionally a calibration error.

Normal or high values (see Fig 16–10,A) do not ensure that the oxygen supply and demand balance is satisfactory. The use of venous oximetry to assess the balance between oxygen supply and demand is dependent on "intact and consistent vasoregulation."[30] Systemic end-capillary oxygen content reflects the local balance between arterial content, local blood flow, and local oxygen consumption. Mixed venous content (or saturation) is a "flow-weighted" mixture of all of the end-capillary oxygen contents of the body and as such is the best available index of the whole body oxygen supply-demand balance.[30] Since this is a "flow-weighted" average, a high-blood-flow, low-oxygen-extracting organ (such as the kidney) will have a greater effect on the mixed venous value than will a relatively low-blood-flow, high-oxygen-extracting organ (such as the myocardium). In no way does a normal venous oxygen saturation determined from renal vein

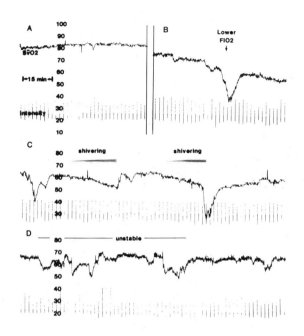

FIG 16–10.
A, a rather monotonous tracing from a cirrhotic patient with a high $S\bar{v}_{O_2}$ (see text for interpretation). A decrease in $S\bar{v}_{O_2}$ may occur due to desaturation of arterial blood, as when, in another patient with severe maldistribution of pulmonary ventilation and perfusion, inspired oxygen fraction was changed from 0.45 to 0.21 **(B).** The 25% decrease in $S\bar{v}_{O_2}$ suggests a comparable change in Sa_{O_2} (e.g., from 0.95 to 0.70) or a decrease in Pa_{O_2} from over 90 torr to less than 40 torr. Increases in oxygen consumption in patients who are unable to increase oxygen delivery may result in a decrease in $S\bar{v}_{O_2}$, as in a patient who began to shiver **(C).** Variation in multiple factors affecting oxygen consumption and delivery may be present in patients with circulatory shock. The labile nature of the $S\bar{v}_{O_2}$ emphasizes the need for a complete database before definitive therapy can be achieved **(D).**

blood ensure an adequate oxygen supply/demand balance in the myocardium. Neither does a "normal" mixed venous oxygen saturation (determined from PA blood) ensure adequate oxygen delivery to any high-oxygen-consuming organ. Fortunately, when vasoregulation is intact the total body distribution of blood flow changes in stress situations to decrease blood flow to the low-consumption organs and maintain relatively normal blood flow to the high-consumption organs so that $S\bar{v}_{O_2}$ often continues to be the best available indicator of the total body oxygen supply/demand balance.[21, 30]

Values of $S\bar{v}_{O_2}$ below 0.68 may be associated with anemia, arterial oxygen desaturation, increased oxygen consumption (due to shivering, agitation, increased activity, fever, increasing temperature), or decreases in cardiac output (Fig 16–10). Values below 0.60 or a rapidly falling $S\bar{v}_{O_2}$ may signal an impending catastrophic event.[10] Values of about 0.53 correspond to a $P\bar{v}_{O_2}$ of about 28 mm Hg (assuming a normal P50), which is often the threshold of anaerobic metabolism and lactic acidosis.[18] Unconsciousness and permanent cellular damage occur at lower levels of $S\bar{v}_{O_2}$. It should be noted that $S\bar{v}_{O_2}$ values of less than 30% have been tolerated without obvious signs of hypoxia by patients in chronic congestive heart failure.[24a] This tolerance was due in part to a right shift in the oxyhemoglobin dissociation curve, but probably also involved microvascular adaptation.

A decrease in $S\bar{v}_{O_2}$ of 0.10 is likely to be of significance regardless of the initial value. A decrease from 0.80 to 0.70 could represent a one-third drop in cardiac output, while a change from 0.60 to 0.50 represents a smaller fractional change, but it occurs when there is less reserve and a greater likelihood of tissue hypoxia. Therefore, a change in $S\bar{v}_{O_2}$ of 0.10 should trigger a more complete evaluation of the factors likely to affect the oxygen transport balance. These in-

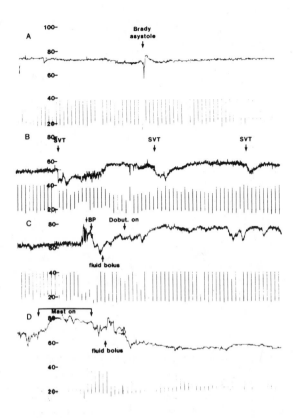

FIG 16–11.

The utility of continuously measured $S\bar{v}_{O_2}$ in improving the care of critically ill patients is demonstrated in these clinical examples. The rapidity of the response to an acute imbalance of oxygen supply/demand is shown by the immediate decrease in $S\bar{v}_{O_2}$ from 0.70 to 0.57, caused by severe bradycardia leading to 5 seconds of asystole **(A).** The period of asystole is followed by an apparent compensatory increase in $S\bar{v}_{O_2}$ and rapid return to baseline. The next patient **(B)** has a moderate to severe deficit in oxygen transport balance ($S\bar{v}_{O_2}$ = 0.52) that became acutely worse during three episodes of supraventricular tachycardia *(SVT).* The first episode caused the $S\bar{v}_{O_2}$ to decrease to 0.42. Following antiarrhythmic therapy, $S\bar{v}_{O_2}$ rose to 0.57 but later fell to 0.48 and 0.52 with recurrent bouts of arrhythmias. The patient whose $S\bar{v}_{O_2}$ tracing is shown in **C** sustained an abrupt fall in mean arterial pressure and a concomitant decrease in $S\bar{v}_{O_2}$. A fluid bolus was given, with an immediate increase in $S\bar{v}_{O_2}$ to baseline (0.64). However, because blood pressure remained labile, dobutamine was begun by continuous intravenous infusion. As blood pressure returned to normal, $S\bar{v}_{O_2}$ increased to 0.68, and after about 15 minutes increased further to about 0.77. The initial rise in $S\bar{v}_{O_2}$ is unexplained and emphasizes the need for clinical correlation with hemodynamic and oxygen transport parameters when interpreting the results of venous oximetry. In **D,** continuous venous oximetry was used in the preoperative assessment of a patient at high risk for a major abdominal procedure because of severe atherosclerotic cardiovascular disease. The initial $S\bar{v}_{O_2}$ was 0.67. When preload was augmented incrementally, first with the medical antishock trousers and then with a fluid bolus, the $S\bar{v}_{O_2}$ increased significantly. The increase in $S\bar{v}_{O_2}$ was interpreted as an improvement in oxygen transport. While the improvement was short-lived in this patient, it demonstrates the use of continuous venous oximetry in the minute-by-minute titration of therapy aimed at improving oxygen transport.

clude arterial blood gas analysis, cardiac output measurement, and the calculation of the derived cardiopulmonary parameters of arterial-venous oxygen content difference, oxygen consumption, intrapulmonary right-to-left shunt (venous admixture), and oxygen extraction (utilization) ratio. With these values in mind the clinician should be able to formulate a goal-directed therapeutic plan to correct the oxygen transport imbalance.

Continuous measurement of $S\bar{v}_{O_2}$ can be viewed as serving three major functions in critically ill patients. First, it is an indicator of the

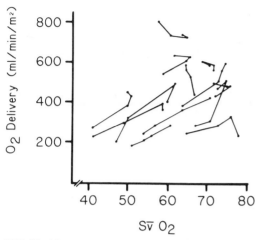

FIG 16–12.
Continuously measured $S\bar{v}_{O_2}$ may be used to improve the "efficiency" of the delivery of critical care by allowing rapid therapeutic trials to correct the cause of oxygen supply-demand imbalance. In these patients with hypoxemic respiratory failure (caused by increased venous admixture), positive end-expiratory pressure (PEEP) was applied at 5, 10, 15, and 20 cm H_2O. The effect of a therapeutic PEEP trial is demonstrated in terms of continuously measured $S\bar{v}_{O_2}$ and oxygen delivery. The authors concluded that (if oxygen consumption remains constant over the course of the PEEP trial) oxygen delivery can be optimized in a more simple and efficient manner using continuously measured $S\bar{v}_{O_2}$ rather than repeated cardiopulmonary profiles.[6] (From Fahey PJ, et al: *Chest* 1984; 86:748–752. Reproduced by permission.)

adequacy of the oxygen supply-demand balance of perfused tissues and as such may be used as an assurance of cardiopulmonary stability (see Fig 16–10,A). Second, continuously measured $S\bar{v}_{O_2}$ may function as an early warning of untoward events causing an imbalance of the oxygen supply-demand relationship (see Figs 16–10,B, C, and D).[14, 25] Third, continuously monitored $S\bar{v}_{O_2}$ may improve the efficiency of the delivery of critical care by providing immediate feedback as to the effectiveness of therapeutic interventions aimed at improving oxygen transport balance. While $S\bar{v}_{O_2}$ does not correlate well with any single determinant of oxygen transport balance in large groups of patients, a change in $S\bar{v}_{O_2}$ in an individual patient is a reliable indicator of oxygen transport imbalance, and therefore continuously measured $S\bar{v}_{O_2}$ can be used to titrate therapy to restore the balance between oxygen supply and demand without the need for frequent, serial cardiopulmonary profiles (Fig 16–11). After a clinical trial (guided by changes in $S\bar{v}_{O_2}$), a cardiopulmonary profile may be repeated to ensure that correcting one cause for oxygen transport imbalance has not created another (Fig 16–12).

While no data at this time convincingly indicate that venous oximetry per se has had any effect on outcome in critically ill patients, it remains our best continuous indicator of the oxygen supply-demand balance.

Acknowledgments

I wish to express my most sincere thanks to Joseph M. Civetta, M.D., for his careful review and suggestions regarding the manuscript for this chapter, to James V. Snyder, M.D., for his detailed editorial review, and to Hans B. Anderson, R.R.T., for his advice and assistance in the data collection done in the surgical ICU at Jackson Memorial Medical Center, Miami.

REFERENCES

1. Baele PL, McMichan JC, Marsh HM, et al: Continuous monitoring of mixed venous oxygen saturation in critically ill patients. *Anesth Analg* 1982; 61:513–517.
2. Barratt-Boyes BG, Wood EH: The oxygen saturation of blood in the venae cavae, right heart chambers, and pulmonary vessels of healthy subjects. *J Lab Clin Med* 1957; 50:93–105.
3. Christiansen I, Iverson K, Skooby AP: Benefits obtained by the introduction of a coronary care unit: A comparative study. *Acta Med Scand* 1971; 189:285.
4. Civetta JM: Critical illness: The nonsteady state. *Surg Forum* 1972; 23:153–155.
5. De La Rocha AG, Edmonds JF, Williams WG, et al: Importance of mixed venous oxygen saturation in the care of critically ill patients. *Can J Surg* 1978; 21:227–229.
6. Fahey PJ, Harris K, Vanderwarf C: Clinical experience with continuous monitoring of mixed venous oxygen saturation in respiratory failure. *Chest* 1984; 86:748–752.
7. Harken AH: The surgical significance of the oxyhemoglobin dissociation curve. *Surg Gynecol Obstet* 1977; 144:935–955.
8. Harris KW, Van der Warf CR, Fahey PJ: Continuous measurement of mixed venous O_2 saturation. *Crit Care Med* 1982; 10:216.
9. Hofvendahl S: Influence of treatment in a

CCU on prognosis in acute myocardial infarction. *Acta Med Scand Suppl* 1971; 519:1–78.

10. Jamieson WRE, Turnbull KW, Laurrieu AJ, et al: Continuous monitoring of mixed venous oxygen saturation in cardiac surgery. *Can J Surg* 1982; 25:538–543.

11. Kandel G, Aberman A: Mixed venous oxygen saturation: Its role in the assessment of the critically ill patient. *Arch Intern Med* 1983; 143:1400–1402.

12. Kazarian KK, Del Guercio LRM: The use of mixed venous blood gas determinations in traumatic shock. *Ann Emerg Med* 1980; 9:179–182.

13. Krasnitz P, Druger GL, Yorra F, et al: Mixed venous oxygen tension and hyperlactatemia: Survival in severe cardiopulmonary disease. *JAMA* 1976; 236:570–574.

14. Krauss XH, Verdouw PD, Hugenholtz PG, et al: On-line monitoring of mixed venous oxygen saturation after cardiothoracic surgery. *Thorax* 1975; 30:636–643.

15. Krouskop RW, Cabatu EE, Chelliah BP, et al: Accuracy and clinical utility of an oxygen saturation catheter. *Crit Care Med* 1983; 11:744–749.

16. Lee J, Wright F, Barber R, et al: Central venous oxygen saturation in shock: A study in man. *Anesthesiology* 1972; 36:472–478.

17. Martin WE, Cheung PW, Johnson CC, et al: Continuous monitoring of mixed venous oxygen saturation in man. *Anesth Analg* 1973; 52:784–793.

18. McMichan JC: Continuous monitoring of mixed venous oxygen saturation: Theory applied to practice, in Schweiss JF (ed): *Continuous Measurement of Blood Oxygen Saturation in the High Risk Patient.* San Diego, Beach International, Inc, 1983.

19. Mihm F, Freely TW, Rosenthal M, et al: The lack of effect of variable blood withdrawal rates on the measurement of mixed venous oxygen saturation. *Chest* 1980; 78:452–455.

20. Miller MJ: Tissue oxygenation in clinical medicine: An historical review. *Anesth Analg* 1982; 61:527–535.

21. Mitchell JH, Blomqvist G: Maximal oxygen uptake. *N Engl J Med* 1971; 284:1018–1022.

22. Nelson LD: Continuous venous oximetry in surgical patients. *Ann Surg* 1986; 203:99–103.

23. Oximetrix, Inc: *Shaw Catheter Oximetry System Instruction Manual.* Oximetrix, Inc, Mountain View, Calif, 1981.

24. Scheinman MM, Brown MA, Rapaport E: Critical assessment of the use of central venous oxygen saturation as a mirror of mixed venous oxygen in severely ill cardiac patients. *Circulation* 1969; 40:165–172.

24a. Schlichtig R, Cowden WL, Chaitman BR: Tolerance of unusually low mixed venous oxygen saturation: Adaptations in the chronic low cardiac output syndrome. *Am J Med* (in press).

25. Schmidt CR, Frank LP, Estafanous FG: Utility of continuous pulmonary artery oximetry as an early warning monitor in cardiac surgery patients. Presented at the Society of Cardiovascular Anesthesiologists Fifth Annual Meeting, San Diego, April 24–27, 1983.

26. Schweiss JF: *Continuous Measurement of Blood Oxygen Saturation in the High Risk Patient.* Beach International, Inc, San Diego, 1983.

27. Shapiro BA: *Clinical Application of Blood Gases,* ed 2. Chicago, Year Book Medical Publishers, 1977.

28. Shapiro HM, Smith G, Pribble AH, et al: Errors in sampling pulmonary artery blood with a Swan-Ganz catheter. *Anesthesiology* 1974; 40:291–295.

29. Simmons DH, Alpas AP, Tashkin DP, et al: Hyperlactatemia due to arterial hypoxemia or reduced cardiac output or both. *J Appl Physiol* 1978; 45(2):195–202.

30. Snyder JV, Carroll GC: Tissue oxygenation: A physiologic approach to a clinical problem. *Curr Probl Surg* 1982; 19:650–719.

31. Suter PM, Lindauer JM, Fairley HB, et al: Errors in data derived from pulmonary artery blood gas values. *Crit Care Med* 1975; 3:175–181.

32. Tahvanainen J, Meretoja O, Nikki P: Can central venous blood replace mixed venous blood samples? *Crit Care Med* 1982; 10:758–761.

33. Waller JL, Kaplan JA, Bauman DI, et al: Clinical evaluation of a new fiberoptic catheter oximeter during cardiac surgery. *Anesth Analg* 1982; 61:676–679.

34. Watkins GM, Rabelo A, Plzak LF, et al: The left shifted oxyhemoglobin curve in sepsis: A preventable defect. *Ann Surg* 1974; 180:213–220.

35. Watson CB: The PA catheter as an early warning system. *Anesthesiol Rev* 1983; 10:34–35.

17 The Craft of Cardiopulmonary Profile Analysis

Robert E. Fromm, Jr., M.D.

Jean-Gilles Guimond, M.D.

Joseph Darby, M.D.

James V. Snyder, M.D.

Systemic arterial and pulmonary arterial catheterization data provide us with information concerning cardiopulmonary performance that, when the data and our underlying assumptions are correct, can be invaluable in analysis and management of clinical problems. Most clinicians find it useful to manipulate these data mathematically to make the physiology more apparent. The collection of these measured and derived variables is known as the cardiopulmonary profile (CPP). In this chapter we will discuss the content of the cardiopulmonary profile, and, in a series of cases, illustrate its use in diagnosis and therapy.

In clinical medicine, the profile is always approached with a clinical picture in mind. Data from the profile and the clinical picture should be tested against each other to build a composite picture—a ''sand castle''—that incorporates all reliable findings in a rational manner. The composite is always tentative; all new information is tested against it, and when a good fit is not apparent, either the information or the constructed picture is in doubt. A review of all data (including a fresh look at the patient) is indicated in this situation.

The adequacy of oxygen transport is confirmed when the function of an organ or all organs is normal, but clinical estimates of more specific variables such as gas exchange, cardiac index, or left ventricular (LV) filling pressure are often significantly in error (see chapter 14, ''Invasive Hemodynamic Assessment Compared With Clinical Evaluation''). There are also multiple problems, both technical and in underlying assumptions, in the invasive acquisition of data (see chapter 15, ''Technical Problems in Data Acquisition''). When assessing a physiologic profile, we first look for errors by comparing the profile with previous data and with our clinical observations. Erroneous data are suspected if any values have changed markedly from a previous observation, or if clinical discrepancies are apparent. These might include oxygen consumption higher or lower than could be explained by the clinical circumstances; or low systemic vascular resistance in a patient receiving high doses of vasoconstricting drugs; or low pulmonary vascular resistance in a patient with adult respiratory distress syndrome (ARDS) and on high levels of positive end-expiratory pressure (PEEP). The physician should be familiar with the system of data acquisition. If the data collectors are not familiar with the nuances of reading resting end-expiratory pressures or the importance of simultaneous data acquisition, or if laboratory quality control is not excellent, then the CPP should not be assembled or used in the management of patient care.

Often the evidence that the CPP presents appears compatible with several pathologic conditions. Is there a variable that will discriminate between alternatives? Can the cardiopulmonary system be stressed in some way to confirm or exclude a certain disease or insult? CPP analysis is not merely a matter of selecting the diagnosis with the highest probability. It is a dynamic process that evolves as new data are obtained and therapy is instituted. Therefore, the therapeutic plan should allow for diagnoses that seem less probable, especially if the prognosis of a less likely mechanism is better with appropriate therapy than that of the initially considered disorder. A good example is case 1–1 in chapter 1, "Oxygen Transport: The Model and Reality."

CARDIOPULMONARY PARAMETERS

The variables measured in a typical profile include height, weight, cardiac output, arterial and pulmonary pressures, arterial and mixed venous blood-gas tensions, and oxygen saturations. The derived variables may include any of those listed in Table 17–1, and described below.

BSA: Body surface area is calculated from height and weight and is used to index measured and derived values to the size of the patient.

MAP: Mean arterial pressure is estimated as one-third the pulse pressure plus the diastolic pressure (DAP), or an electronically integrated value may be used.

CI: Cardiac index is calculated as cardiac output/BSA. It is the prime determinant of hemodynamic function.

SI: Stroke index is calculated as CI/heart rate and is the average volume ejected by the ventricle with each beat.

LVSWI: Left ventricular stroke work index is an approximation of the work performed by the left ventricle as it ejects its stroke volume into the aorta. It is the product of SI and (MAP − WP) and a unit correction factor of 0.0136, where WP is the occluded pulmonary artery pressure, or wedge pressure.

RVSWI: Right ventricular stroke work index is analogous to LVSWI and measures the work of the right ventricle as it ejects into the pulmonary artery. It is the product of SI and (MPAP − CVP) × 0.0136, where MPAP is mean pulmonary artery pressure and CVP is central venous pressure.

SVRI: Systemic vascular resistance index is the customary measure of resistance in the systemic circuit. It is calculated as (MAP − CVP)/CI. This may be reported as indexed torr/L/min (indexed Wood units), or multiplied by 80 to yield indexed dynes·sec/cm^5. By definition the indexed value is calculated using CI in the above formula. Thus, the indexed value is greater than the raw value when BSA is > 1.0 m^2.

$$SVRI = (MAP − CVP)/CI$$
$$= MAP − CVP/(CO/BSA)$$
$$= \frac{(MAP − CVP)}{CO} \times BSA$$

TABLE 17–1.

Derived Variables of the Cardiopulmonary Profile

VARIABLE	FORMULA	UNITS
MAP	1/3 (pulse pressure) + DAP	torr
CI	CO/BSA	L/min/m^2
SV	CO/HR × 1000	ml/beat
SI	CI/HR × 1000	ml/beat/m^2
RVSWI	(MPAP − CVP) × SI × .0136	gm · m/m^2
LVSWI	(MAP − WP) × SI × .0136	gm · m/m^2
SVRI	(MAP − CVP)/CI	torr/L/min* indexed
	(MAP − CVP)/CI × 80	dyne·sec/cm^5 indexed
PVRI	(MPAP − WP)/CI	torr/L/min* indexed
	(MPAP − WP)/CI × 80	dyne·sec/cm^5 indexed
Ca_{O_2}	(Hb × 1.36 × Sa_{O_2}) + (Pa_{O_2} × 0.003)	ml/dl
$C\bar{v}_{O_2}$	(Hb × 1.36 × $S\bar{v}_{O_2}$) + ($P\bar{v}_{O_2}$ × 0.003)	ml/dl
$C(a−\bar{v})_{O_2}$	$Ca_{O_2} − C\bar{v}_{O_2}$	ml/dl
$\dot{D}_{O_2}$ (O_2 transport)	Ca_{O_2} × CO × 10	ml/min
$\dot{V}_{O_2}$	$C(a−\bar{v})_{O_2}$ × CO × 10	ml/min
$\dot{V}_{O_2}/m^2$	$\dot{V}_{O_2}$/BSA	ml/min/m^2
$\dot{Q}va/\dot{Q}t$	$(Cc_{O_2} − Ca_{O_2})/(Cc_{O_2} − C\bar{v}_{O_2})$†	

*Also known as Wood units.
†Cc_{O_2} = (Hb × 1.36 × Sa_{O_2}) + (PA_{O_2} × 0.0031), where Sa_{O_2} = 1 when P_{O_2} > 150 torr (usually when FI_{O_2} > 0.4) and Hb ligands are absent, and PA_{O_2} = PI_{O_2} − Pac_{O_2} × FI_{O_2} + $\frac{1 − FI_{O_2}}{RQ}$, where PI_{O_2} = (BP − 47 cm H_2O) and RQ = 0.8.

PVRI: Pulmonary vascular resistance index. Analogous to SVRI, it is a measure of resistance in the pulmonary vasculature. It is calculated as (MPAP − WP)/CI and can be expressed in indexed Wood units as above or multiplied by 80 to yield dynes·sec/cm^5, indexed. Like SVRI, PVRI is a product of the nonindexed value and the BSA.

C(a − v̄)$_{O_2}$: Arteriovenous oxygen content difference is calculated as arterial oxygen content (Ca$_{O_2}$) minus venous oxygen content (Cv̄$_{O_2}$). When Ca$_{O_2}$ and V̇$_{O_2}$ are constant and all tissues are perfused, this value is inversely related to cardiac output.

V̇$_{O_2}$: Oxygen consumption is the oxygen extracted by the tissues from the arterial blood. It is calculated as C(a − v̄)$_{O_2}$ × CO × 10. It can also be indexed to BSA.

Q̇va/Q̇t (venous admixture): This number is the fraction of the cardiac output that is not oxygenated in an idealized lung. It is calculated as (Cc$_{O_2}$ − Ca$_{O_2}$)/(Cc$_{O_2}$ − Cv̄$_{O_2}$) where Cc$_{O_2}$ is the oxygen content of blood perfusing ventilated alveoli when Pa$_{O_2}$ is sufficient to fully saturate hemoglobin. This is usually assumed to be true when F$_{I_{O_2}}$ > 0.4. [The pulmonary shunt fraction (Q̇s/Q̇t) is defined as Q̇va/Q̇t at F$_{I_{O_2}}$ = 1.00.]

P50: Partial pressure of oxygen at which hemoglobin saturation is 50%. It is a measure of the affinity of hemoglobin for oxygen; a lower number indicates a leftward shift in the oxyhemoglobin dissociation curve, or increased affinity of hemoglobin for oxygen. The calculated in vivo value is more relevant clinically than when calculated for a standard temperature and P$_{CO_2}$. The in vivo P50 can be estimated from the Sv̄$_{O_2}$ and Pv̄$_{O_2}$ (corrected to body temperature) using a modification of the Hill equation (see the appendix to chapter 15, "Technical Problems in Data Acquisition").

Ḋo$_2$ (oxygen delivery or transport): This value represents the total oxygen delivered by the cardiorespiratory system. It is the product of Ca$_{O_2}$ and cardiac output, and a conversion factor of 10.

ANALYSIS BY DATA GROUPS

We find it helpful to separate the variables of the CPP into three interacting, overlapping groups: (1) the oxygen transport and demand variables, (2) the hemodynamic data, and (3) the pulmonary gas exchange variables.

Oxygen Transport and Demand Variables

These include CI, Hb, Sa$_{O_2}$, Sv̄$_{O_2}$, Pv̄$_{O_2}$, P50, and V̇$_{O_2}$. We first look at the Pv̄$_{O_2}$. If it is normal or above, then total body oxygen transport to perfused tissues is adequate, but flow may be maldistributed. Organ function is reviewed for signs of locally impaired perfusion. If the patient is otherwise without signs of circulatory failure (i.e., without end-organ dysfunction), and especially if the CI is normal or increased, it can be assumed that overall oxygen transport is acceptable. We must remain alert to the possibility of erroneous measurements. For example, a high Pv̄$_{O_2}$ and low V̇$_{O_2}$ could be due to aspiration of arterialized blood in the mixed venous sample and therefore may not truly reflect the adequacy of oxygen transport. Artifactually low Pv̄$_{O_2}$ is much less common. If the Pv̄$_{O_2}$ is decreased then oxygen transport is insufficient—because one or more of the components of oxygen delivery is compromised or because demand is high. Compromised oxygen transport may be primarily a pulmonary problem, or due to anemia or hemoglobinopathy, or due to impaired cardiac performance. The P$_{O_2}$ and saturation are assessed to evaluate the adequacy of pulmonary oxygenation. The hemoglobin and P50 are reviewed for their contribution to oxygen content. Changes in affinity of hemoglobin for oxygen occasionally play a significant role in the compromise of oxygen transport. The CI and other hemodynamic variables are then assessed (see later discussion), and increased oxygen demand is considered by reviewing the V̇$_{O_2}$. If the V̇$_{O_2}$ is increased the explanation might be hyperthermia (V̇$_{O_2}$ increases 10% for each 1° C rise in temperature), excessive muscular activity (agitation, shivering, seizures), or hyperthyroidism (see chapter 2, "Oxygen Consumption"). Metabolic rate may also be increased 10% to 100% by the stress of serious illness. The greatest elevation is seen with burns and sepsis. When the oxygen supply/demand ratio is relatively compromised, increased binding of oxygen to hemoglobin (a low P50) can make the difference between adequate oxygenation and tissue dysfunction.

Hemodynamic Data

These consist of MAP, HR, MPAP, WP, CVP, and CO, which are measured, and CI, SI, RVSWI, LVSWI, SVRI, and PVRI, which are calculated. Cardiac function is first assessed by examining cardiac index. Is it high, low, or normal? Then CI or SWI is compared with ventricular filling pressure to approximate the Frank-Starling relationship (Fig 17–1). If filling pressure is high, low CI usually indicates heart failure, which might be due to depressed contractility, excessive afterload, or both; tamponade must also be considered. SVRI is a measure of afterload and may be used to assess its contribution to decreased cardiac performance. Usually, the clearest way to evaluate ventricular performance clinically using these data is to plot LVSWI against WP, as in Figure 17–1. Similar variables are routinely calculated for the right side of the heart, but they are subject to considerable error from respiratory artifacts in pressure readings. Technical problems exist with all analyses of ventricular performance. These are explored in chapter 15, "Technical Problems in Data Acquisition."

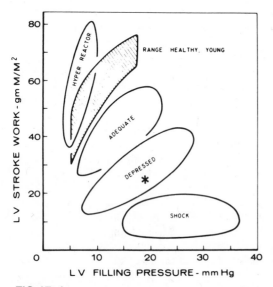

FIG 17–1.
Case 17–1. Hemodynamic consequences of myocardial infarction expressed as various levels of left ventricular (LV) function. *Hatched area* represents the range of LV function in healthy young individuals. After acute myocardial infarction, there is wide variability in the hemodynamic response. Some patients with small infarcts and increased sympathetic tone may be in the normal or hypernormal range. As the size of the infarct increases, however, function is progressively shifted down and to the right, so that all patients with cardiogenic shock fall in the lower right-hand group. (Modified from Sodeman and Sodeman,[11] by permission.)

Pulmonary Gas Exchange Variables

These include Pa_{O_2}, Sa_{O_2}, $P\bar{v}_{O_2}$, $S\bar{v}_{O_2}$, and $\dot{Q}va/\dot{Q}t$. They are closely related to the other groups. For example, a respiratory alkalosis could cause increased SVRI and $\dot{V}_{O_2}$, and decreased CI and $P\bar{v}_{O_2}$ as well.[4, 12] $\dot{Q}va/\dot{Q}t$ is many times viewed as an isolated variable reflecting lung function. Misunderstanding often arises from forgetting that $\dot{Q}va/\dot{Q}t$ is a simplistic summary of complex events. An increase in $\dot{Q}va/\dot{Q}t$ should not always be equated with deterioration in lung parenchymal structures. For example, when PEEP opens some closed alveoli, blood may be diverted to open areas with low $\dot{V}/\dot{Q}$, and thus $\dot{Q}va/\dot{Q}t$ may increase at the same time as more lung is held open. Also, calculated $\dot{Q}va/\dot{Q}t$ may be increased by intracardiac shunts without a change in pulmonary function. Similarly, Pa_{O_2} is not an isolated pulmonary value but may also be affected by hemodynamic changes. For example, changes in CI can influence Pa_{O_2}, principally by affecting $C\bar{v}_{O_2}$ or by affecting pulmonary shunting.[6] The increase in oxygen transport associated with elevated CI causes a proportional decrease in $C(a-\bar{v})_{O_2}$, or a higher $C\bar{v}_{O_2}$. The oxygen-enriched venous blood that passes through "shunt" vessels then increases Pa_{O_2}. Thus, calculated $\dot{Q}va/\dot{Q}t$ may be unchanged while Pa_{O_2} increases. Increased CI may also be associated with increased $\dot{Q}va/\dot{Q}t$, through these mechanisms: recruitment of mechanically compressed extra-alveolar vessels in "zone 4" lung,[8] relief of hypoxic pulmonary vasoconstriction,[13] pharmacologic reversal of hypoxia-constricted pulmonary vessels,[10] and decreased transit time. Note that each of these changes is due only to a change in flow pattern and does not indicate a change in the underlying pathophysiologic process. Hence, a change in Pa_{O_2} does not necessarily imply a change in "shunt," even when FI_{O_2} is constant, nor does a change in measured $\dot{Q}va/\dot{Q}t$ necessarily imply a significant change in the severity of the pulmonary injury.

The efficiency of carbon dioxide elimination, summarized in the measurement of "dead space" (Vd/Vt), is a major determinant of ventilatory requirements and therefore of airway pressure (AWP) and the potential for barotrauma and depression of CO. However, Vd/Vt is not yet commonly available in CPPs and will not be discussed further here. The importance of the concepts involved is explored further in the chapters on pulmonary physiology and the management of ventilation.

The following case summaries are presented to emphasize various aspects of CPP analysis. It might be useful for the reader to interpret each profile before reading the discussion.

CASE 17–1. *Rising Oxygen Consumption.*—A 68-year-old man with back pain and a pulsatile abdominal mass was monitored invasively during evaluation for possible dissecting aortic aneurysm (profile a). A second profile was obtained when MAP rose by 14 torr (profile b).

Discussion.—In the first profile this patient has adequate oxygen transport ($P\bar{v}_{O_2} = 34$) despite moderate anemia and depressed LV function (see Fig 17–1). In the second profile, $\dot{V}_{O_2}$ and $C(a-\bar{v})_{O_2}$ are markedly increased yet oxygen transport and hemodynamic values are not significantly different. The pronounced change in $\dot{V}_{O_2}$ with little clinical change makes a technical error likely. Because well-written computer programs are unlikely to make arithmetic errors, the problem is likely to be with a primary variable. The primary variable that has changed is $S\bar{v}_{O_2}$. Are

Cardiopulmonary Profile, Case 17–1

Measured Variables

Variable	Profile a	Profile b	Normal	Units
Ht	60	60	NA	in
Wt	75	75	NA	kg
BSA	1.72	1.72	NA	m^2
Temp	37.1	36.7	37	°C
$F_{I_{O_2}}$	0.4	0.4	NA	
PEEP	5	5	NA	cm H_2O
HR	119	104	60–100	beats/min
SAP	137	160	NA	torr
MAP	81	95	NA	torr
MPAP	31	33	9–16	torr
DPAP	27	30	8–14	torr
WP	19	21	5–10	torr
CVP	20	21	0–8	torr
CO	5.9	6.0	NA	L/min
Hb	11.2	11.1	12.5–15.5	gm/dl
pHa	7.51	7.49	7.35–7.45	
Pa_{CO_2}	40	42	35–45	torr
Pa_{O_2}	92	85	80–98	torr
Sa_{O_2}	0.96	0.96	0.95	
$P\bar{v}_{O_2}$	34	36	35–42	torr
$S\bar{v}_{O_2}$	0.61	0.42	0.68	

Derived Variables

CI	3.4	3.5	2.5–4.0	L/min/m^2
SI	29	34	35–40	ml/min/m^2
RVSWI	4.5	5.7	6–9	gm·m/m^2
LVSWI	24.4	34.0	35–47	gm·m/m^2
SVRI	17.6	21.0	27 ± 3	Wood units·m^2*
PVRI	3.6	3.5	3 ± 0.5	Wood units·m^2*
Ca_{O_2}	14.8	14.7	15–20	ml/dl
$C\bar{v}_{O_2}$	9.3	6.4	10–15	ml/dl
$C(a-\bar{v})_{O_2}$	5.5	8.2	3.5–5.0	ml/dl
$\dot{D}_{O_2}$	873	882	1,000	ml/dl
$\dot{V}_{O_2}$	326	501	NA	ml/min
$\dot{V}_{O_2}/m^2$	189	291	110–150	ml/min/m^2
P50	28.7	40.6	26–27	torr
Qva/Qt	0.15	0.10	0.05	

*Torr/L/min, indexed. The value in dyne·sec/cm^5 can be calculated by multiplying this value by 80. CO, cardiac output.

the values in the first profile artifactually high or are those in the second artifactually low? Is it a technical analysis error or a data input problem?

The mixed venous values in the first profile look valid. That is, $S\bar{v}_{O_2}$ is close to what we expect for that $P\bar{v}_{O_2}$. The patient's clinical condition is more compatible with a moderate increase than with a very severe increase in oxygen consumption, so the profile with the most deviant value (the second) is more suspect. Because only $S\bar{v}_{O_2}$ in the second profile changed, and not Sa_{O_2} or $P\bar{v}_{O_2}$, the error is probably in data input (e.g., actual $S\bar{v}_{O_2}$ was .62 rather than .42) rather than in technical analysis.

CASE 17–2. *Change in Left Ventricular Function?*—Profile a was drawn up shortly after an elderly postoperative patient arrived in the surgical ICU. It is brought to your attention as possibly representing sepsis because the cardiac output is high. You point out that the output is not high for the patient's size (CI = 3.2 L/min/m²) and in fact oxygen supply/demand is significantly compromised, as shown by $P\bar{v}_{O_2}$ of 29 torr, even though $C(a - \bar{v})_{O_2}$ is normal. The imbalance is due to moderate depression of ventricular function, anemia, and a mild increase in $\dot{V}_{O_2}$, and exists in spite of a low-normal SVRI. Allowing Pa_{CO_2} to rise will increase release of oxygen from hemoglobin, and you recommend no other therapy. Profile b is a follow-up

Cardiopulmonary Profile, Case 17–2

Measured Variables

Variable	Profile a	Profile b	Profile c	Normal	Units
Ht	74	74	74	NA	in
Wt	115	115	115	NA	kg
BSA	2.30	2.30	2.30	NA	m²
Temp	36.9	36.8	36.8	37	°C
$F_{I_{O_2}}$	0.4	0.4	0.4	NA	
PEEP	5	5	5	NA	cm H_2O
HR	99	101	101	60–100	beats/min
SAP	152	170	170	NA	torr
MAP	79	82	82	NA	torr
MPAP	28	26	26	9–16	torr
DPAP	18	20	20	8–14	torr
WP	18	16	16	5–10	torr
CVP	10	8	8	0–8	torr
CO	7.4	4.1	7.4	NA	L/min
Hb	11.4	12.6	12.6	12.5–15.5	gm/dl
pHa	7.55	7.42	7.42	7.35–7.45	
Pa_{CO_2}	32	40	40	35–45	torr
Pa_{O_2}	70	74	74	80–98	torr
Sa_{O_2}	0.96	0.96	0.96	0.95	
$P\bar{v}_{O_2}$	29	38	38	35–42	torr
$S\bar{v}_{O_2}$	0.65	0.72	0.72	0.68	

Derived Variables

CI	3.2	1.7	3.2	2.5–4.0	L/min/m²
SI	32	18	32	35–40	ml/min/m²
RVSWI	8.1	5.1	9.2	6–9	gm·m/m²
LVSWI	26.9	15.8	28.5	35–47	gm·m/m²
SVRI	21.5	41.6	23.1	27 ± 3	Wood units·m²
PVRI	3.2	7.5	4.2	3 ± 0.5	Wood units·m²
Ca_{O_2}	15.0	16.6	16.6	15–20	ml/dl
$C\bar{v}_{O_2}$	10.1	12.4	12.4	10–15	ml/dl
$C(a-\bar{v})_{O_2}$	4.9	4.2	4.2	3.5–5.0	ml/dl
D_{O_2}	1,116	683	1,233	1,000	ml/dl
$\dot{V}_{O_2}$	363	172	312	NA	ml/min
$\dot{V}_{O_2}/m^2$	157	74	135	110–150	ml/min/m²
P50	22.9	26.6	26.6	26–27	torr
Qva/Qt	0.18	0.21	0.21	0.05	

study of the patient the next day. Let us assume it has been brought to your attention by the house officer in the unit who is concerned about the drop in CI, which was reproducible and seems obviously due to a marked increase in SVR. He has also noticed a distinct drop in LVSWI at almost the same preload, and wonders if an acute myocardial infarction has occurred or some other myocardial depressant factor is involved. The house officer reports that the ECG and physical examination findings are unchanged and that the patient's urine output continues to be adequate. Should the patient be started on dopamine or dobutamine or perhaps afterload reduction?

Discussion.—On further review of the profile we see the patient's oxygen consumption has fallen from 157 to 75 ml/min/m^2, yet there has been no change in the patient's clinical appearance. $C(a - \bar{v})_{O_2}$ is almost unchanged and $P\bar{v}_{O_2}$ has actually increased, presumably because Pa_{CO_2} was allowed to rise and, hence, P50 was also higher, yielding better tissue oxygen availability. Oxygen consumption is usually relatively constant, and variations in oxygen consumption that are not clinically explainable suggest error in measurement. Because measured oxygen content is usually accurate, an error in calculated $\dot{V}_{O_2}$ is usually due to the thermodilution measurement.

A severe decrease in $\dot{V}_{O_2}$ is unlikely in the absence of an obvious underlying condition such as shock. Obviously all values derived from CO, including SVRI and LVSWI, will accordingly be artifactually distorted. Although the CO measurement should not be dismissed casually, the probability of an error in this case seems high. The cause of reproducible low CO artifacts with thermodilution technique is unclear, but may be related to the accumulation of fibrin over the thermistor.[3] The PA catheter was replaced in this patient, and profile c was obtained. The CO is identical to the first measurement, the calculated $\dot{V}_{O_2}$ is compatible with the clinical picture, and higher venous oxygen values reflect lower $\dot{V}_{O_2}$ and higher P50.

CASE 17–3. *Cardiac Crisis.*—A 61-year-old woman was transferred to the ICU with complaints of chest pain not relieved by bed rest, and shortness of breath that had become worse an hour before her arrival in the emergency department. She had a history of diabetes mellitus, hypertension, and "cardiac failure." She was tachypneic with rales at both lung bases, and an S_3 gallop could be discerned. The chest x-ray film demonstrated a large heart and prominent pulmonary vasculature. A PA catheter was placed, and profile 17–3 was obtained. Does the profile help us with the diagnosis?

Cardiopulmonary Profile, Case 17–3

Measured Variables

Variable	Profile a	Normal	Units
Ht	62	NA	in
Wt	77	NA	kg
BSA	1.78	NA	m^2
Temp	37.5	37	°C
Fi_{O_2}	0.6	NA	
PEEP	0	NA	cm H$_2$O
HR	118	60–100	beats/min
SAP	104	NA	torr
MAP	76	NA	torr
MPAP	39	9–16	torr
DPAP	25	8–14	torr
WP	14	5–10	torr
CVP	24	0–8	torr
CO	3.6	NA	L/min
Hb	13.5	12.5–15.5	gm/dl
pHa	7.36	7.35–7.45	
Pa_{CO_2}	31	35–45	torr
Pa_{O_2}	61	80–98	torr
Sa_{O_2}	0.91	0.95	
$P\bar{v}_{O_2}$	30	35–42	torr
$S\bar{v}_{O_2}$	0.55	0.68	

Cardiopulmonary Profile, Case 17–3—Continued

Derived Variables

Variable	Profile a	Normal	Units
CI	2.0	2.5–4.0	L/min/m^2
SI	17.1	35–40	ml/min/m^2
RVSWI	3.6	6–9	gm·m/m^2
LVSWI	14.5	35–47	gm·m/m^2
SVRI	25.6	27 ± 3	Wood units·m^2
PVRI	12.5	3 ± 0.5	Wood units·m^2
Ca$_{O_2}$	16.8	15–20	ml/dl
C$\bar{v}_{O_2}$	10.1	10–15	ml/dl
C(a−$\bar{v}$)$_{O_2}$	6.7	3.5–5.0	ml/dl
$\dot{D}_{O_2}$	609	1,000	ml/dl
$\dot{V}_{O_2}$	241	NA	ml/min
$\dot{V}_{O_2}$/m^2	135	110–150	ml/min/m^2
P50	27.8	26–27	torr
$\dot{Q}$va/$\dot{Q}$t	0.27	0.05	

Discussion.—CI is low with adequate filling pressure. Does this represent a myocardial infarction? It is a consideration, but let's look a little further. This patient was quite tachypneic and strained at expiration. Determining WP at resting end-expiration is difficult in these circumstances, and we suspect that WP was elevated by the increase in pleural pressure. Therefore, LV function is not as depressed as it first seemed. The pulmonary artery pressures are elevated, and PVRI is markedly increased (as suggested by the high gradient between PADP and WP). These findings are more compatible with an acute pulmonary thromboembolism, which was confirmed by pulmonary angiography. Uncritical acceptance of uncritically acquired data is hazardous.

CASE 17–4. *Cardiogenic Shock I.*—A 55-year-old man presented with complaints of anterior chest pain and a feeling of impending doom. His blood

Cardiopulmonary Profile, Case 17–4

Measured Variables

Variable	Profile a	Normal	Units
Ht	72	NA	in
Wt	96	NA	kg
BSA	2.18	NA	m^2
Temp	36.9	37	°C
F$_{I_{O_2}}$	0.5	NA	
PEEP	0	NA	cm H$_2$O
HR	121	60–100	beats/min
SAP	99	NA	torr
MAP	82	NA	torr
MPAP	25	9–16	torr
DPAP	22	8–14	torr
WP	21	5–10	torr
CVP	22	0–8	torr
CO	3.7	NA	L/min
Hb	13.8	12.5–15.5	cm/dl
pHa	7.34	7.35–7.45	
Pa$_{CO_2}$	33	35–45	torr
Pa$_{O_2}$	73	80–98	torr
Sa$_{O_2}$	0.96	0.95	
P$\bar{v}_{O_2}$	29	35–42	torr
S$\bar{v}_{O_2}$	0.52	0.68	

Cardiopulmonary Profile, Case 17–4—Continued

Derived Variables

Variable	Profile a	Normal	Units
CI	1.6	2.5–4.0	L/min/m^2
SI	14	35–40	ml/min/m^2
RVSWI	0.64	6–9	gm·m/m^2
LVSWI	11.6	35–47	gm·m/m^2
SVRI	38.1	27 ± 3	Wood units·m^2
PVRI	2.35	3 ± 0.5	Wood units·m^2
Ca$_{O_2}$	18.2	15–20	ml/dl
C$\bar{v}_{O_2}$	9.8	10–15	ml/dl
C(a $-$ $\bar{v}$)$_{O_2}$	8.4	3.5–5.0	ml/dl
D$_{O_2}$	674	1,000	ml/dl
V$_{O_2}$	311	NA	ml/min
V$_{O_2}$/m^2	142	110–150	ml/min/m^2
P50	28.1	26–27	torr
Qva/Qt	0.14	0.05	

pressure in the emergency room was 96/64 mm Hg and jugular venous distention was noted. He was oriented, anxious, mildly dyspneic, and oliguric. He was admitted to the medical ICU. The chest roentgenogram showed a large cardiac silhouette and the ECG demonstrated diffuse repolarization abnormalities. A PA catheter was inserted and the following profile was obtained.

Discussion.—The CI is profoundly depressed despite a WP of 21 torr. This is due mostly to severely depressed ventricular function.

The increase in SVRI is largely an artifact of the assumptions underlying that calculation (see chapter 15, "Technical Problems in Data Acquisition"). The low-normal pH with a low Pa$_{CO_2}$ in this setting suggests lactic acidosis. The diagnosis of cardiogenic shock is made, and a combination of inotropic support, cautious nitroprusside administration, and transfusion is contemplated. Do you agree?

Reviewing the profile we see that the DPAP pressure is 22 and CVP is 21 torr, suggesting the

Cardiopulmonary Profile, Case 17–5

Measured Variables

Variable	Profile a	Profile b	Profile c	Normal	Units
Ht	60	60	60	NA	in
Wt	70	70	70	NA	kg
BSA	1.67	1.67	1.67	NA	m^2
Temp	37.9	37.8	38.3	37	°C
FI$_{O_2}$	0.4	0.4	0.4	NA	
PEEP	0	0	0	NA	cm H$_2$O
HR	92	114	110	60–100	beats/min
SAP	96	116	86	NA	torr
MAP	69	82	60	NA	torr
MPAP	34	29	29	9–16	torr
DPAP	26	20	20	8–14	torr
WP	25	28	16	5–10	torr
CVP	18	10	12	0–8	torr
CO	2.3	2.7	3.4	NA	L/min
Hb	9.7	10.4	9.0	12.5–15.5	gm/dl
pHa	7.35	7.30	7.46	7.35–7.45	
Pa$_{CO_2}$	26	34	36	35–45	torr
Pa$_{O_2}$	100	82	85	80–98	torr
Sa$_{O_2}$	0.95	0.95	0.96	0.95	
P$\bar{v}_{O_2}$	32	34	36	35–42	torr
S$\bar{v}_{O_2}$	0.46	0.51	0.50	0.68	

Cardiopulmonary Profile, Case 17–5—Continued

Derived Variables

Variable	Profile a	Profile b	Profile c	Normal	Units
CI	1.3	1.6	2.0	2.5–4.0	L/min/m^2
SI	14.9	14.1	18.4	35–40	ml/min/m^2
RVSWI	3.2	3.7	4.3	6–9	gm·m/m^2
LVSWI	8.9	10.4	11.1	35–47	gm·m/m^2
SVRI	39.2	44.5	23.6	27 ± 3	Wood units·m^2
PVRI	7.0	6.2	6.4	3 ± 0.5	Wood units·m^2
Ca$_{O_2}$	12.9	13.7	11.9	15–20	ml/dl
C$\bar{v}_{O_2}$	6.1	7.3	6.3	10–15	ml/dl
C(a − $\bar{v}$)$_{O_2}$	6.8	6.4	5.6	3.5–5.0	ml/dl
$\dot{D}_{O_2}$	297	371	407	1,000	ml/dl
$\dot{V}_{O_2}$	156	172	192	NA	ml/min
$\dot{V}_{O_2}$/m^2	93	103	115	110–150	ml/min/m^2
P50	34.1	33.2	35.5	26–27	torr
Qva/Qt	0.09	0.11	0.11	0.05	
Dopamine	0	10	0		µg/kg/min
Dobutamine	0	0	5		µg/kg/min

possibility of cardiac tamponade. Echocardiography revealed a large pericardial effusion, and pericardiocentesis resulted in dramatic improvement in the patient's condition.

CASE 17–5. *Cardiogenic Shock II.*—A 38-year-old woman presented with pulmonary edema and atrial fibrillation. She had a history of mitral stenosis and aortic insufficiency secondary to childhood rheumatic heart disease. She had been treated with digitalis and diuretics for the previous 3 years, and her requirements for diuretics had increased gradually. Because of worsening LV function, she underwent left and right heart catheterization. On the basis of those results the patient underwent mitral and aortic valve replacement.

Discussion.—The first postoperative profile (a) shows a low P$\bar{v}_{O_2}$ despite a rightward shift in the oxyhemoglobin dissociation curve. Although P$\bar{v}_{O_2}$ of 32 torr is compatible with adequate total perfusion, the metabolic acidosis is most likely due to lactic acid production and suggests that tissue oxygen is not, or recently was not, sufficient. Oxygen transport is low primarily because of low CI and low Hb, but the possible value of raising Sa$_{O_2}$ and $\dot{D}_{O_2}$ by 5% by increasing Fi$_{O_2}$ should be kept in mind. We might conclude that vascular tone is increased reflexly to maintain blood pressure. However, an increase in SVRI with a lower CI is the result of our method of calculating SVRI, and vascular tone may not be increased at all. This problem is discussed in the section on systemic vascular resistance in chapter 15, "Technical Problems in Data Acquisition."

When informed of the results of the profile, the house officer elected to administer dopamine. The second postoperative profile (b) shows the patient's response to the dopamine administration at 10 µg/kg/min. CI and P$\bar{v}_{O_2}$ are slightly improved. SVRI is significantly increased, and myocardial oxygen need must also be increased.

The decision was made to change from dopamine to dobutamine, and the third profile shows the patient's response. We see an increase in CI accompanied by a fall in SVRI. P$\bar{v}_{O_2}$ increased, reflecting better oxygen supply/demand. LVSWI increased and WP decreased, in contrast to what we observed with the dopamine infusion.

In this case, repeated profiles permitted us to titrate our therapeutic approach to the patient. Hemodynamic monitoring is most effective when CPP measurements are repeated as the patient's condition changes and as therapeutic interventions are made.

CASE 17–6. *Cardiogenic Shock III.*—A young woman with hypercholesterolemia and subsequent chronic ischemic cardiomyopathy had required two coronary artery bypass procedures and replacement of two valves over a 10-year period. Her heart condition once again became incapacitating, and it was considered not treatable by operative intervention short of cardiac transplantation. This was undertaken, and hemodynamic performance was adequate on admission to the ICU, as evidenced by stable and adequate vascular pressures and an S$\bar{v}_{O_2}$ of 72% while dopamine, 15 µg/kg/min, and dobutamine, 20 µg/kg/min, were infused. Her cardiac condition deteriorated over the next 45 minutes, as seen in

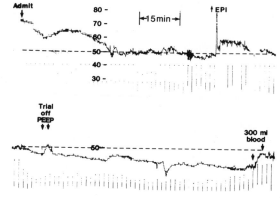

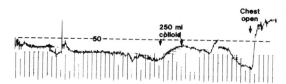

Fig 17–2.
Case 17–5. Deterioration in oxygen delivery is apparent in decline of $S\bar{v}_{O_2}$ despite initiation and then increased rate of infusion of epinephrine ($\uparrow$ EPI) to 0.18 µg/kg/min, and blood and colloid administration. The relief of focal tamponade is apparent in the vascular pressure changes as well as in the $S\bar{v}_{O_2}$.

Figure 17–2. $S\bar{v}_{O_2}$ was clearly but only transiently improved by increasing epinephrine, decreasing PEEP, and administering volume (see Fig 17–2). The severity of her illness is best reflected by the $P\bar{v}_{O_2}$ of 22 torr.

Discussion.—The oxygen imbalance is obviously due to moderately severe depression of

CI despite a WP of 12 torr and high doses of inotropic drugs. The failure is primarily of the right side of the heart, as shown by the CVP of 26 torr when MPAP was only 15 torr. This could be due to mechanical trauma to the RV during the operation and contributed to by low RV coronary perfusion pressure (MAP − RVEDP = 53 −

Cardiopulmonary Profile, Case 17–6

Measured Variables

Variable	Profile a	Normal	Units
Ht	65	NA	in
Wt	57	NA	kg
BSA	1.62	NA	m²
Temp	35.4	37	°C
FI_{O_2}	0.9	NA	
PEEP	10	NA	cm H_2O
HR	95	60–100	beats/min
SAP	90	NA	torr
MAP	53	NA	torr
MPAP	16	9–16	torr
DPAP	15	8–14	torr
WP	12	5–10	torr
CVP	26	0–8	torr
CO	3.3	NA	L/min
Hb	9.0	12.5–15.5	gm/dl
pHa	7.36	7.35–7.45	
Pa_{CO_2}	34	35–45	torr
Pa_{O_2}	66	80–98	torr
Sa_{O_2}	0.95	0.95	
$P\bar{v}_{O_2}$	22	35–42	torr
$S\bar{v}_{O_2}$	0.39	0.68	

Cardiopulmonary Profile, Case 17–6—Continued

Derived Variables

Variable	Profile a	Normal	Units
CI	2.0	2.5–4.0	L/min/m^2
SI	21.3	35–40	ml/min/m^2
RVSWI	−2.8	6–9	gm·m/m^2
LVSWI	11.9	35–47	gm·m/m^2
SVRI	13.3	27 ± 3	Wood units·m^2
PVRI	2	3 ± 0.5	Wood units·m^2
Ca_{O_2}	11.8	15–20	ml/dl
$C\bar{v}_{O_2}$	4.8	10–15	ml/dl
$C(a-\bar{v})_{O_2}$	7.0	3.5–5.0	ml/dl
$\dot{D}_{O_2}$	390	1,000	ml/dl
$\dot{V}_{O_2}$	230	NA	ml/min
$\dot{V}_{O_2}/m^2$	141	110–150	ml/min/m^2
P50	26.0	26–27	torr
$\dot{Q}va/\dot{Q}t$	0.23	0.05	

26 = 27 torr). LV preload was even lower than suggested by the WP of 12 torr; the nadir WP after abrupt removal of PEEP was only 6 torr (see chapter 15, "Technical Problems in Data Acquisition"). Additional volume administration brought only transient relief before further deterioration, despite persistently higher CVP values. It may be that RV perfusion pressure was further compromised when RVEDP was raised more than MAP.

Another possible mechanism of cardiogenic shock is focal cardiac temponade. This can occur even when the pericardium is left open postoperatively, because a clot can accumulate outside of, and compress, one or two chambers. The resulting physiology is different from that in classic tamponade because not all chambers are trapped. The diagnosis can usually be made only tentatively and often is not confirmed until drainage from a chest tube or reopening of the chest is accompanied by hemodynamic improvement. The continuous $S\bar{v}_{O_2}$ tracing reflected the effect

Cardiopulmonary Profile, Case 17–7

Measured Variables

Variable	Profile a	Profile b	Normal	Units
Ht	70	70	NA	in
Wt	76.8	46.8	NA	kg
BSA	1.94	1.57	NA	m^2
Temp	37	37	37	°C
FI_{O_2}	0.5	0.5	NA	
PEEP	5	5	NA	cm H$_2$O
HR	100	81	60–100	beats/min
SAP	104	125	NA	torr
MAP	85	102	NA	torr
MPAP	26	32	9–16	torr
DPAP	23	28	8–14	torr
WP	15	20	5–10	torr
CVP	12	8	0–8	torr
CO	7.1	7.5	NA	L/min
Hb	11.0	10.5	12.5–15.5	gm/dl
pHa	7.44	7.38	7.35–7.45	
Pa_{CO_2}	39	42	35–45	torr
Pa_{O_2}	90	122	80–98	torr
Sa_{O_2}	0.96	0.97	0.95	
$P\bar{v}_{O_2}$	52	52	35–42	torr
$S\bar{v}_{O_2}$	0.84	0.84	0.68	

Cardiopulmonary Profile, Case 17–7—Continued

Derived Variables

Variable	Profile a	Profile b	Normal	Units
CI	3.6	4.7	2.5–4.0	L/min/m^2
SI	36.5	58.7	35–40	ml/min/m^2
RVSWI	7.0	19.1	6–9	gm·m/m^2
LVSWI	34.8	65.5	35–47	gm·m/m^2
SVRI	20	19.7	27 ± 3	Wood units·m^2
PVRI	3.2	2.5	3 ± 0.5	Wood units·m^2
Ca_{O_2}	14.6	14.3	15–20	ml/dl
$C\bar{v}_{O_2}$	12.8	12.2	10–15	ml/dl
$C(a-\bar{v})_{O_2}$	1.8	2.0	3.5–5.0	ml/dl
$\dot{D}_{O_2}$	1,043	1,073	1,000	ml/dl
$\dot{V}_{O_2}$	131	153	NA	ml/min
$\dot{V}_{O_2}$/m^2	67	97	110–150	ml/min/m^2
P50	27.8	27.1	26–27	torr
$\dot{Q}$va/$\dot{Q}$t	0.38	0.28	0.05	

of each therapy in this patient, including the dramatic response to a second thoracotomy and removal of a small clot (see Fig 17–2).

CASE 17–7. *Change in BSA.*—A 17-year-old man presented with a 19-month history of chronic active hepatitis of undetermined etiology. He was known to have esophageal varices. On admission he had marked cachexia, hepatic encephalopathy, and massive ascites. The patient responded poorly to traditional medical management; hepatic function

continued to deteriorate and he received an orthotopic liver transplant.

The preoperative profile is shown as profile a. Profile b was assembled on the second postoperative day and shows a rise in CI and SWI related to an increase in LV filling.

Discussion.—Before ascribing this to a real change in cardiac performance we note that the CO, oxygen consumption, and $P\bar{v}_{O_2}$ are unchanged. The main difference in the two profiles

Cardiopulmonary Profile, Case 17–8

Measured Variables

Variable	Profile a	Normal	Units
Ht	67	NA	in
Wt	75.5	NA	kg
BSA	1.85	NA	m^2
Temp	37.5	37	°C
$F_{I_{O_2}}$	0.5	NA	
PEEP	5	NA	cm H$_2$O
HR	106	60–100	beats/min
SAP	110	NA	torr
MAP	76	NA	torr
MPAP	15	9–16	torr
DPAP	12	8–14	torr
WP	5	5–10	torr
CVP	4	0–8	torr
CO	12.2	NA	L/min
Hb	9.6	12.5–15.5	gm/dl
pHa	7.37	7.35–7.45	
Pa_{CO_2}	39	35–45	torr
Pa_{O_2}	210	80–98	torr
Sa_{O_2}	0.97	0.95	
$P\bar{v}_{O_2}$	64	35–42	torr
$S\bar{v}_{O_2}$	0.93	0.68	

Cardiopulmonary Profile, Case 17–8—Continued

Derived Variables

Variable	Profile a	Normal	Units
CI	6.5	2.5–4.0	L/min/m^2
SI	61.5	35–40	ml/min/m^2
RVSWI	9.2	6–9	gm·m/m^2
LVSWI	59	35–47	gm·m/m^2
SVRI	11.0	27 ± 3	Wood units·m^2
PVRI	1.5	3 ± 0.5	Wood units·m^2
Ca$_{O_2}$	13.2	15–20	ml/dl
C$\bar{v}_{O_2}$	12.3	10–15	ml/dl
C(a−$\bar{v}$)$_{O_2}$	0.9	3.5–5.0	ml/dl
$\dot{D}_{O_2}$	1,619	1,000	ml/dl
$\dot{V}_{O_2}$	115	NA	ml/min
$\dot{V}_{O_2}$/m^2	62	110–150	ml/min/m^2
P50	24	26–27	torr
$\dot{Q}$va/$\dot{Q}$t	0.40	0.05	

is the change in BSA due to loss of 30 kg from diuresis and intraoperative loss of ascites. The rise in CI primarily reflects the decrease in BSA, not a major change in the patient's cardiorespiratory status. On the other hand, it is possible that ventricular preload has changed more than is apparent in the CPP. Pleural pressure may be lower after a loss of 30 kg of fluid that is primarily due to ascites. Therefore, because preload is reflected by transmural end-diastolic pressure, LV preload in the first profile is more accurately thought of as a WP of 15 torr minus a pleural pressure, which is higher than normal and may be positive; LV preload in the second profile is more likely to be 20 torr minus a negative pleural pressure. Therefore, LV preload may have increased by more than the 5 torr difference in WP. For the same reasons, there may be no change or even an increase in RV preload, rather than the decrease suggested by the 4-torr reduction in CVP. Thus, this patient has the same CO despite what may be a significant increase in preload. The case reminds us of the need to remain cognizant of the assumptions inherent in our use of each variable.

CASE 17–8. *Cirrhosis.*—A 30-year-old woman with cirrhosis of the liver was admitted with acute upper GI tract bleeding and hemorrhagic shock. Blood pressure and urine output were restored with transfusion of red blood cells and volume expansion with crystalloid solution. A PA catheter was inserted to guide further therapy, and the following CPP was obtained.

Discussion.—The notable hemodynamic features of this profile are high CO and P$\bar{v}_{O_2}$ with remarkably low C(a−$\bar{v}$)$_{O_2}$ and $\dot{V}_{O_2}$, and high ve-

nous admixture. This combination suggests hyperperfusion of some beds (increased CI and P$\bar{v}_{O_2}$, low C(a−$\bar{v}$)$_{O_2}$) and inadequate perfusion of other beds (decreased $\dot{V}_{O_2}$). The adequacy of urine output and absence of other signs of organ dysfunction argue strongly against significant systemic hypoperfusion, and the possibility of artifactual measurements arises. Because $\dot{V}_{O_2}$ is calculated as the product of CO and C(a−$\bar{v}$)$_{O_2}$, error could come only from an artifactually low CO or Ca$_{O_2}$, or a high C$\bar{v}_{O_2}$. The CI is actually high and the Ca$_{O_2}$ is nearly normal, but the patient does have a markedly elevated C$\bar{v}_{O_2}$. A likely cause would be aspiration of arterialized pulmonary capillary blood resulting in a falsely high S$\bar{v}_{O_2}$ and subsequently low C(a−$\bar{v}$)$_{O_2}$ and $\dot{V}_{O_2}$. The high S$\bar{v}_{O_2}$ is also the basis of miscalculated high venous admixture.

CASE 17–9. *Shunt Calculations and the "Forgotten Variable."*—An unresponsive 50-year-old man was admitted through the emergency room after being extracted from a vehicle in an automobile accident. A PA catheter was inserted for hemodynamic monitoring. The profile (a) was unremarkable except that $\dot{Q}$va/$\dot{Q}$t was 32% despite a relatively normal chest x-ray film. The pulmonary dysfunction was ascribed to "microatelectasis" and PEEP was recommended. You compare Sa$_{O_2}$ and Pa$_{O_2}$ and recognize that the cause of the increased $\dot{Q}$va/$\dot{Q}$t is not pulmonary. You suspect that rapid improvement is likely, and do not use PEEP. The profile 8 hours later shows similar values to the first except that $\dot{Q}$va/$\dot{Q}$t is now 9%.

Discussion.—In your initial evaluation you were aware that Sa$_{O_2}$ should normally be greater

Cardiopulmonary Profile, Case 17–9

Measured Variables

Variable	Profile a	Profile b	Normal	Units
Ht	72	72	NA	in
Wt	70	70	NA	kg
BSA	1.90	1.90	NA	m^2
Temp	37	36.5	37	°C
F$_{IO_2}$	0.4	0.4	NA	
PEEP	0	5	NA	cm H$_2$O
HR	85	90	60–100	beats/min
SAP	160	160	NA	torr
MAP	113	113	NA	torr
MPAP	15	15	9–16	torr
DPAP	10	12	8–14	torr
WP	6	7	5–10	torr
CVP	10	8	0–8	torr
CO	6.2	6.9	NA	L/min
Hb	14.8	15.0	12.5–15.5	gm/dl
pHa	7.40	7.45	7.35–7.45	
Pa$_{CO_2}$	40	38	35–45	torr
Pa$_{O_2}$	110	120	80–98	torr
Sa$_{O_2}$	0.93	0.99	0.95	
P$\bar{v}_{O_2}$	32	42	35–42	torr
S$\bar{v}_{O_2}$	0.70	0.76	0.68	

Derived Variables

Variable	Profile a	Profile b	Normal	Units
CI	3.2	3.6	2.5–4.0	L/min/m^2
SI	38.2	40.1	35–40	ml/min/m^2
RVSWI	2.6	3.82	6–9	gm·m/m^2
LVSWI	55.6	58.0	35–47	gm·m/m^2
SVRI	32.2	29.0	27 ± 3	Wood units·m^2
PVRI	2.8	2.2	3 ± 0.5	Wood units·m^2
Ca$_{O_2}$	19.0	20.5	15–20	ml/dl
C$\bar{v}_{O_2}$	14.1	15.6	10–15	ml/dl
C(a$-\bar{v}$)$_{O_2}$	4.9	4.9	3.5–5.0	ml/dl
D$_{O_2}$	1,180	1,417	1,000	ml/dl
V$_{O_2}$	301	339	NA	ml/min
V$_{O_2}$/m^2	158	178	110–150	ml/min/m^2
P50	23.2	27.1	26–27	torr
Q̇va/Q̇t	0 32	0.09	0.05	

than .93 when Pa$_{O_2}$ is 110 torr. If these arterial blood measurements are valid there is either an extreme rightward shift in the oxyhemoglobin dissociation curve or abnormal hemoglobin. A significant accumulation of carboxyhemoglobin (COHb) is possible in a patient trapped in a vehicle at a busy intersection, as this patient was. Also, no rightward shift is apparent in the P50, which is calculated from values in mixed venous blood. In fact, the shift is to the left, as is expected when P50 is calculated from mixed venous values and any hemoglobin ligand is present, especially carboxyhemoglobin. Although COHb and other hemoglobin ligands are mea-

sured by most instruments used to measure oxygen saturation, they are not customarily reported unless the value is very high. Also, they are often not used to modify the calculation of Q̇va/Q̇t, and that is the basis of the artifact here. The patient's initial level of COHb was 5%. The second profile was constructed after several hours of supplemental oxygen, which rapidly reduced the patient's COHb level to 1% and normalized his Cc$_{O_2}$, thus reducing his calculated Q̇va/Q̇t to 9%. The initial Q̇va/Q̇t was overestimated (32% vs. 17%), since COHb was not accounted for in the calculation of Cc$_{O_2}$, and the real improvement in pulmonary function is not as dramatic as suggested in the

CPP. The calculations are shown at the end of the discussion.

If it is not taken into account, the presence of Hb ligands such as COHb, methemoglobin, and sulfhemoglobin can lead to large errors in the calculated $\dot{Q}va/\dot{Q}t$. These errors are most pronounced when shunt values are low.[5, 7]

Carbon monoxide (CO) has two major effects on oxyhemoglobin dissociation. First, it will lead to a shift to the left in the dissociation curve by altering the conformation of the hemoglobin molecule itself. Hemoglobin therefore binds oxygen more avidly, decreasing its availability to the tissues. The other effect is that the percent of hemoglobin binding CO is unavailable to bind and transport oxygen. This makes no difference in calculation of arterial and venous oxygen contents from Sa_{O_2} and $S\bar{v}_{O_2}$ because COHb is taken into account when those saturations are measured directly. However, pulmonary capillary oxygen content, Cc_{O_2}, is usually estimated by assuming that pulmonary capillary blood is fully saturated when alveolar P_{O_2} is greater than 150 torr (usually when $F_{I_{O_2}}$ is greater than 0.4). Thus, when COHb is significant, pulmonary capillary S_{O_2} = 1 − COHb/Hb. The different effect on the calculated Cc_{O_2} and $\dot{Q}va/\dot{Q}t$ is as follows:

Customary form: Cc_{O_2} (Eq. 17–1)
= Hb × 1.36 × 1.0 + PA_{O_2} × .003
= 14.8 × 1.36 × 1.0 + 234 × .003
= 20.8
Appropriate form: Cc_{O_2}
= Hb × 1.36 (1 − COHb/Hb) + PA_{O_2} × .003
= 14.8 × 1.36 × .95 + 234 × .003
= 19.8

Thus:
$\dot{Q}va/\dot{Q}t = (Cc_{O_2} - Ca_{O_2})/(Cc_{O_2} - C\bar{v}_{O_2})$
= (20.8 − 19.0)/(20.8 − 15.2) = .32
                (customary form)
or:
= (19.8 − 19.0)/(19.8 − 15.2) = .17
                (appropriate form)

CASE 17–10. *Intracardiac Shunts.*—You are asked to see a 69-year-old man 3 days after an anterior wall myocardial infarction is diagnosed. His condition was stable for the first 48 hours but hypotension, diaphoresis, and dyspnea developed suddenly this morning. On physical examination, you note that a loud pansystolic murmur is audible over the precordium, radiating to the axilla and posteriorly to the interscapular region.

The murmur was thought to represent either acute dysfunction of the mitral valvular apparatus or rupture of the interventricular septum.

Your patient is immediately taken to the catheterization laboratory where a PA catheter is inserted via the right subclavian vein. Venous blood is sampled and hemodynamic measurements are made in the RA, RV, and PA as the catheter is gradually advanced to wedge position, where no prominent V wave is noted.

An arterial catheter is also inserted via the right femoral artery (FA) and a ventriculography catheter is advanced to the LV.

Pressure recordings are as follows (units in torr):
FA	90/70 (mean, 76)
LV	80/5 (end-diastolic, 18)
WP	15
PA	27/20 (mean, 22)
RA	9

Apart from slightly elevated LVEDP and WP measurements, the study is unremarkable.

Oxygen saturations and contents are as follows:
	S_{O_2} (%)	O_2 content (vol%)
FA	93.8	15.2
PA	62.8	10.2
RA	40.1	6.5

There is a definite step-up in S_{O_2} from the RA to the PA, confirming the angiographically evident VSD with left-to-right shunt. One could also appreciate an early recirculation pattern on the dye dilution tracings.[1] The thermodilution cardiac output (TDCO) was 3.9 L/min.

Discussion.—The house officer is eager to enter these values directly into the computer to construct the patient's CPP, but you remind him that in the presence of a left-to-right shunt, the thermal as well as the dye-dilution cardiac output measurements are valid only for the pulmonary circuit. Because the $P\bar{v}_{O_2}$ and $S\bar{v}_{O_2}$ values represent blood taken at a site distal to the patient's intracardiac shunt, calculation of $\dot{Q}va/\dot{Q}t$ will be valid for the pulmonary circuit.

It must be noted that although pulmonary flow as determined by TDCO usually equals systemic flow, such is not the case in the presence of a left-to-right intracardiac shunt. To determine this patient's LV output it is necessary to calculate the pulmonary/systemic flow ratio, or Q_{pulm}/Q_{syst}.

This is done in the following manner: for both the pulmonary and systemic beds,

$$\dot{V}_{O_2} = CO \times C(a - \bar{v})_{O_2} \times 10 \quad \text{(Eq. 17–2)}$$

where $\bar{v}$ represents the mixed effluent from that

bed. Because oxygen uptake by the lungs is equal to systemic oxygen consumption,

$$Q_{pulm} \times C_{pulm} (a - \bar{v})_{O_2}$$
$$= Q_{syst} \times C_{syst} (a - \bar{v})_{O_2} \quad \text{(Eq. 17–3)}$$

where $C(a - \bar{v})_{O_2}$ is the oxygen content difference across the pulmonary and systemic beds, respectively.

Since, unlike the systemic circuit, the pulmonary circuit has desaturated blood entering it and saturated blood leaving it, we consider its oxygen content difference to be better equated with $C(\bar{v} - a)_{O_2}$, to avoid the negative value that would result if $C(a - \bar{v})_{O_2}$ were used. Thus, in this case, venous blood for the systemic circuit was sampled at the RA and arterial blood for the pulmonary circuit was sampled from the PA. Blood was taken from the femoral artery to sample the ve-

nous side of the pulmonary circuit and the arterial side of the systemic circuit. Rearranging this formula,

$$\frac{Q_{pulm}}{Q_{syst}} = \frac{C_{syst}(a - \bar{v})_{O_2}}{C_{pulm}(\bar{v} - a)_{O_2}} \quad \text{(Eq. 17–4)}$$

Thus, it can be seen that the ratio of pulmonary to systemic flow is equal to their reciprocal arterio-venous oxygen content differences. In this case,

$$\frac{Q_{pulm}}{Q_{syst}} = \frac{(15.2 \text{ vol}\% - 6.5 \text{ vol}\%)}{(15.2 \text{ vol}\% - 10.2 \text{ vol}\%)}$$
$$= \frac{8.7 \text{ vol}\%}{5.0 \text{ vol}\%} = 1.8/1.0$$

Since TDCO equaled 3.9 L/min, the systemic blood flow can be estimated to be 2.2 L/min.

PHYSIOLOGIC PROFILE ANALYSIS

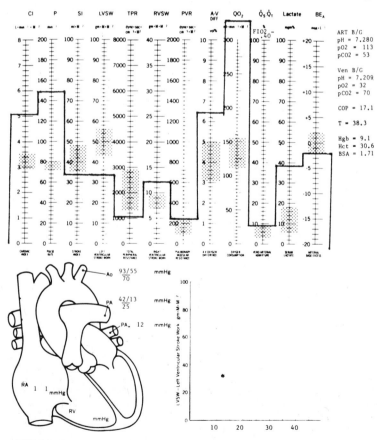

FIG 17–3.
Cardiopulmonary profile, case 17–11. (Courtesy of Kalpalatha Guntupalli, M.D.)

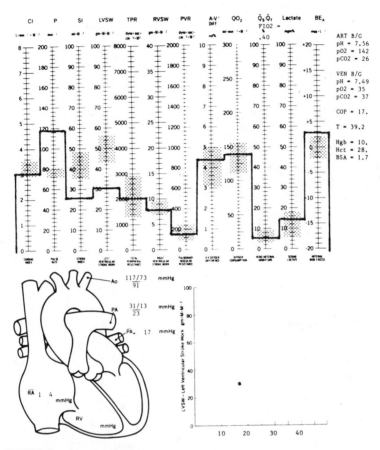

FIG 17–4.
A later cardiopulmonary profile, case 17–11. (Courtesy of Kalpalatha Guntupalli, M.D.)

Note that in the presence of an intracardiac shunt, neither thermodilution nor dye-dilution techniques reliably estimate systemic blood flow because of the inequity between pulmonary and systemic flows, and therefore calculation of derived variables is not appropriate. However, the PA catheter is useful for demonstrating the step-up in oxygen saturation in the case of a left-to-right shunt, and for estimating WP and $\dot{Q}va/\dot{Q}t$; and the pattern of the dye tracing may reveal the presence of left-to-right or right-to-left shunt.

CASE 17–11. *Rewarming.*—A 68-year-old man was admitted to the surgical ICU postoperatively after repair of an abdominal aortic aneurysm. The procedure had been prolonged by technical difficulties and the patient had a decreased core temperature. The patient was noted to be shivering as he

emerged from anesthesia; the CPP shown in Figure 17–3 was obtained. This profile is presented in a graphic form that facilitates the rapid recognition of deviation from normal values. The profile shows an elevated CI and a markedly elevated $\dot{V}o_2$. The $P\bar{v}_{O_2}$ of 32 shows that the elevated output is insufficient. (Blood gas values are listed on the right side of the form.) Serum lactate level is elevated, as is Pa_{CO_2}. Minute ventilation had to be increased 60% to return Pa_{CO_2} to normal until shivering ceased. Shortly thereafter, Pa_{CO_2} was 37 torr and pH was 7.49 (Fig 17–4). Later, when shivering had ceased, the same ventilation pattern resulted in a Pa_{CO_2} of 26 torr and pH of 7.56, and mechanical ventilation was returned to the earlier lower value.

Discussion.—The first profile (see Fig 17–3) demonstrates the large increase in oxygen consumption that may occur with the metabolic chal-

Cardiopulmonary Profile, Case 17–12

Measured Variables

Variable	Profile a	Normal	Units
Ht	67	NA	in
Wt	79	NA	kg
BSA	1.90	NA	m^2
Temp	32	37	°C
FI_{O_2}	0.9	NA	
PEEP	15	NA	cm H_2O
HR	99	60–100	beats/min
SAP	130	NA	torr
MAP	107	NA	torr
MPAP	30	9–16	torr
DPAP	22	8–14	torr
WP	12	5–10	torr
CVP	10	0–8	torr
CO	5.5	NA	L/min
Hb	13.4	12.5–15.5	gm/dl
pHa	7.32	7.35–7.45	
Pa_{CO_2}	56	35–45	torr
Pa_{O_2}	87	80–98	torr
Sa_{O_2}	0.95	0.95	
$P\bar{v}_{O_2}$	42	35–42	torr
$S\bar{v}_{O_2}$	0.74	0.68	

Derived Variables

Variable	Profile a	Normal	Units
CI	2.9	2.5–4.0	$L/min/m^2$
SI	29.3	35–40	$ml/min/m^2$
RVSWI	8.0	6–9	$gm \cdot m/m^2$
LVSWI	38	35–47	$gm \cdot m/m^2$
SVRI	33.2	27 ± 3	Wood units $\cdot$ m^2
PVRI	6.2	3 ± 0.5	Wood units $\cdot$ m^2
Ca_{O_2}	17.6	15–20	ml/dl
$C\bar{v}_{O_2}$	13.6	10–15	ml/dl
$C(a-\bar{v})_{O_2}$	4.0	3.5–5.0	ml/dl
$\dot{D}_{O_2}$	979	1,000	ml/dl
$\dot{V}_{O_2}$	221	NA	ml/min
$\dot{V}_{O_2}/m^2$	116	110–150	$ml/min/m^2$
P50	19.5	26–27	torr
$\dot{Q}va/\dot{Q}t$	0.35	0.05	

lenge of rewarming. There is a roughly proportional increase in carbon dioxide production, which commonly requires an increase in mechanically supported minute ventilation. Respiratory alkalosis may occur when the shivering stops. The graphic depiction of the CPP highlights deviations from normal in the data. Ventricular function curves can also be added to the profile analysis. However, some data are more obscure than is desirable (blood gases, $\dot{V}_{O_2}$), and following trends may be more difficult than in tabular profile forms.

CASE 17–12. *Hypothermia.*—A 58-year-old man underwent uncomplicated coronary artery by-pass surgery but returned from the operating room hypothermic, at which time a CPP was constructed. The major abnormalities in this profile are an apparent respiratory acidosis and relative hypoxemia with a high venous admixture. The blood was drawn at 32° C, variables were measured at 37° C, and the values reported were not corrected to body temperature except for the calculation of P50.

Discussion.—Using blood-gas values that are not corrected for changes in temperature is controversial in some applications and wrong in others. With hypothermia, the solubility of oxygen and carbon dioxide increases, and consequently Pa_{O_2} and Pa_{CO_2} decrease by approximately 6.0% and 4.4% per degree Celsius, respectively. In hypothermia intracellular pH rises as the pH of water rises, in order to maintain neutrality. The pH increases by approximately 0.015 units per degree Celsius. In this example, the corrected values would be pH = 7.39, Pa_{CO_2} = 45 torr, Pa_{O_2} = 61 torr, and $P\bar{v}_{O_2}$ = 29 torr. Studies in ectothermic animals and of the in vitro behavior of blood demonstrate that there is a parallel alkaline shift to maintain a constant intracellular to extracellular pH ratio. In humans the optimal in vivo pH and P_{CO_2} values at temperatures in the hypothermic range are unknown. There is, however, experimental evidence to suggest that hypothermic organs func-

tion better when perfused with blood that is alkaline.[2, 9] If we maintain pH and P_{CO_2} in the normal range when blood is at 37° C, the in vivo pH of the hypothermic patient will be to the alkaline side of normal. Therefore, it seems reasonable to use uncorrected blood gas values when managing the care of hypothermic patients.

Corrected and uncorrected P_{O_2} values will result in different calculated gas pressure gradients, such as the A-a gradient and the blood-to-tissue P_{O_2} gradient. Therefore, the P_{O_2} values should be corrected prior to calculation of A-a gradient and of in vivo P50, and when $P\bar{v}_{O_2}$ is used to assess oxygen supply/demand. Also, the calculation of P50 in hypothermia from $P\bar{v}_{O_2}$ and

Cardiopulmonary Profile, Case 17–13

Measured Variables

Variable	Profile a	Profile b	Profile c	Normal	Units
Ht	74	74	74	NA	in
Wt	120	120	120	NA	kg
BSA	2.44	2.44	2.44	NA	m^2
Temp	37	37.5	39.5	37	°C
F_{IO_2}	0.9	0.5	0.5	NA	
PEEP	20	17.5	12.5	NA	cm H_2O
HR	118	132	121	60–100	beats/min
SAP	81	142	78	NA	torr
MAP	57	94	57	NA	torr
MPAP	32	27	23	9–16	torr
DPAP	29	23	17	8–14	torr
WP	25	14	12	5–10	torr
CVP	15	9	10	0–8	torr
CO	2.12	7.97	9.58	NA	L/min
Hb	11.5	11.0	11.0	12.5–15.5	gm/dl
pHa	7.46	7.50	7.33	7.35–7.45	
Pa_{CO_2}	38	44	32	35–45	torr
Pa_{O_2}	193	85	82	80–98	torr
Sa_{O_2}	0.98	0.96	0.94	0.95	
$P\bar{v}_{O_2}$	28	35	44	35–42	torr
$S\bar{v}_{O_2}$	0.57	0.62	0.73	0.68	

Derived Variables

CI	0.87	3.27	3.93	2.5–4.0	L/min/m^2
SI	7.3	24.8	32.5	35–40	ml/min/m^2
RVSWI	1.7	6.0	5.7	6–9	gm·m/m^2
LVSWI	3.2	27	20	35–47	gm·m/m^2
SVRI	48.4	26	12	27 ± 3	Wood units·m^2
PVRI	8.07	4.0	2.8	3 ± 0.5	Wood units·m^2
Ca_{O_2}	15.8	14.6	14.3	15–20	ml/dl
$C\bar{v}_{O_2}$	9.0	9.37	11.0	10–15	ml/dl
$C(a-\bar{v})_{O_2}$	6.9	5.23	3.25	3.5–5.0	ml/dl
$\dot{D}_{O_2}$	337	1,172	1,387	1,000	ml/dl
$\dot{V}_{O_2}$	146	417	312	NA	ml/min
$\dot{V}_{O_2}m^2$	60	170	127	110–150	ml/min/m^2
P50	25.1	29	30.2	26–27	torr
Qva/Qt	0.17	0.19	0.32	0.05	

$S\bar{v}_{O_2}$ measured at 37° C will be falsely high. For example, if $P\bar{v}_{O_2}$ had not been corrected to body temperature before P50 was calculated, the calculated P50 would be 28 torr. When saturation is measured, derived values such as oxygen delivery, content, and venous admixture will usually not change significantly, but when dissolved oxygen might be a significant component of oxygen content, such as in severe anemia, or when Pa_{O_2} is very high, then the temperature-corrected value and the solubility coefficient for that temperature should be taken into account.

> CASE 17–13. *Combined Shock States.*—A 58-year-old man underwent a left hemicolectomy for carcinoma of the colon. His intraoperative course was complicated by the development of hypotension, which was treated with volume expansion and a dopamine infusion. He was still oliguric on admission to the ICU. A PA catheter was placed and CPP (a) was obtained. This demonstrated classic findings for cardiogenic shock with hypotension, low CI, and high WP. Systemic oxygen transport was marginal and the mixed venous oxygen tension was near the anaerobic threshold at 28 torr (see chapter 1, "Oxygen Transport: The Model and Reality"). An ECG confirmed the presence of an anterior wall infarction. The patient was subsequently treated with furosemide and dobutamine, and by the first postoperative day there was significant hemodynamic improvement, indicated by the rise in MAP and CI and the return of the oxygen transport variables to normal (profile b). Four days postoperatively the patient again became hypotensive and oliguric, and a third profile was constructed. CI, oxygen transport, and $P\bar{v}_{O_2}$ were all within the normal range. However, there were obvious clinical signs of inadequate tissue perfusion. The presence of fever, an elevated white blood cell count, and a low calculated SVRI supported a diagnosis of sepsis, even though there was only minimal abdominal tenderness. The patient was taken back to the operating room and a pelvic abscess was drained.

Discussion.—The CPP may reflect several hemodynamic influences at once, and each may distort the typical response to the others. This case illustrates that in patients with marginal cardiac function the classic signs of hyperdynamic septic shock may be obscured. In this example, both CI and $P\bar{v}_{O_2}$ were within the normal range. The knowledge they both had risen from the low-normal range to the high-normal range was helpful, indicating a somewhat impaired response to the septic process. CPP trend analysis is more useful than isolated observations, and the correct analysis is more often a dynamic composite than an initial classic picture.

Acknowledgment

The authors thank Henry T. Bahnson, M.D., for providing Case 13–6.

REFERENCES

1. Barry WH, Grossman W: Cardiac catheterization, in Braumwall E (ed): *Heart Disease—A Textbook of Cardiovascular Medicine*. Philadelphia, WB Saunders, 1984, vol 1, p 290.
2. Becker H, Vinten-Johansen J, Buckberg GD, et al: Myocardial damage caused by keeping pH 7.40 during systemic deep hypothermia. *J Thorac Cardiovasc Surg* 1981; 82:810–820.
3. Bjoraker DG, Ketcham TR: Catheter thrombus artifactually decreases thermodilution cardiac output measurements. *Anesth Analg* 1983; 62:1031–1034.
4. Brievik H, Grenvik A, Millen E, et al: Normalizing low arterial CO_2 tension during mechanical ventilation. *Chest* 1973; 63:525.
5. Cane RD, Shapiro BA, Harrison RA, et al: Minimizing errors in intrapulmonary shunt calculations. *Crit Care Med* 1980; 8:294.
6. Cheney FW, Colley PSL: Medical intelligence. *Anesthesiology* 1980; 52:496.
7. Cohn JD, Engler PE: Shunt effect of carboxyhemoglobin. *Crit Care Med* 1979; 7:54.
8. Hughes JMB, Glazier JB, Maloney JE, et al: Effect of lung volume on the distribution of pulmonary blood flow in man. *Respir Physiol* 1968; 4:58.
9. McConnell DH, White F, et al: Importance of alkalosis in maintenance of "ideal" blood pH during hypothermia. *Surg Forum* 1975; 26:263.
10. Prewitt RM, Wood LDH: Effect of sodium nitroprusside on cardiovascular function and pulmonary shunt in canine oleic acid pulmonary edema. *Anesthesiology* 1982; 55:537.
11. Sodeman WA Jr, Sodeman TM (eds): *Pathologic Physiology: Mechanisms of Disease*. Philadelphia, WB Saunders Co, 1974, p 287.
12. Springer RR, Clark DK, Lea AS, et al: Effects of changes in arterial carbon dioxide tension on oxygen consumption during cardiopulmonary bypass. *Chest* 1979; 75:549.
13. Suter PM, Fairley HB, Schlobohm RM: Shunt, lung volume and perfusion during short periods of ventilation with oxygen. *Anesthesiology* 1975; 43:617.

18

Functional Imaging of the Critically Ill Patient

W. Newlon Tauxe, M.D.

Howard Yonas, M.D.

David Gur, Sc.D.

B. Simon Slasky, M.D.

James V. Snyder, M.D.

Several dynamic imaging techniques have been developed recently to study disease processes. Few can be used in critically ill patients. Of those that can, some indicate oxygen transport indirectly by demonstrating tissue function, some reflect cardiac physiology, and others actually measure blood flow. The necessity of attaching or implanting iron-containing compounds in patients severely restricts the use of magnetic resonance imaging (MRI, also called nuclear magnetic resonance, or NMR) in many patients. Positron-emission tomography (PET), as of 1985, is available in only five centers in the United States. The principles on which MRI and PET studies are based are summarized in chapter 12, "Monitoring of Tissue Oxygenation." Because their usefulness in clinical practice is limited they will not be further discussed here.

Of the imaging techniques that are used in the critically ill, we will emphasize the use of nuclear medicine techniques to assess coronary blood flow and cardiac function. We will also summarize the use of nonradioactive xenon in coaxial tomography subtraction techniques to study local blood flow in the brain and other tissues.

The word *flow* must be defined carefully. In this chapter, flow per se is considered the volume of fluid moved per unit of time. Renal flow, for example, is usually represented in milliliters of plasma per minute. An *index* of flow, such as flow per unit of volume (often 100 gm), is also often expressed; these indices cannot refer to total

flow since the volume of the tissue in question is not known.

Perfusion refers to the rate of movement and distribution pattern of a substance within certain anatomical limits. It is quantified by observing the movement of a label through an organ; the volume in which it is suspended is generally not known. Sometimes perfusion refers to the end-distribution pattern of a substance fixed in an organ.

In loose clinical parlance, all of these—flow, indices of flow, and perfusion—are often referred to as flow, but a practitioner caring for a critically ill patient must recognize the differences among the three. The quantity of oxygen delivered to a tissue with "good" blood flow as measured by a labeled substance may be quite different from the quantity of oxygen delivered to a tissue in which perfusion is "good" by other criteria.

NUCLEAR MEDICINE TECHNIQUES

Only radioactive tracers and equipment that are appropriate for emergency use will be considered in this chapter. The technical details of radiotracer chemistry and of appropriate instrumentation will not be considered. All the nuclear medicine procedures described here are readily available in most large hospitals, are noninvasive, are cost-effective, and pose insignificant radiation hazard.

Functional imaging techniques related to the

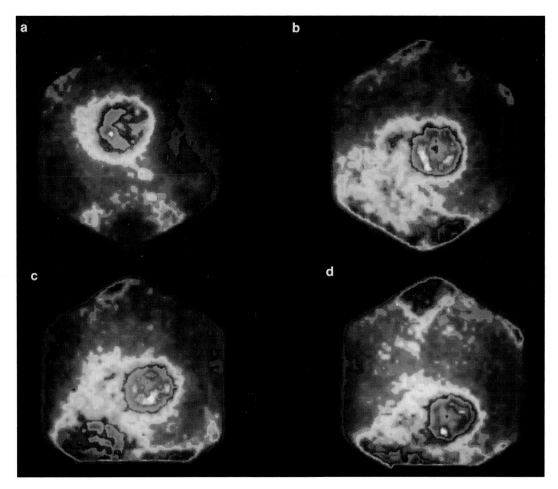

PLATE 18–1.

Scintigraphic "stress" induced after "pacing" with Dipyridamole R *(a)* and "rest" *(b)* images in LAO 45-degree projection in a patient with coronary artery disease so severe she was not able to exercise. Intensity of thallium is scaled from white (highest) through red, yellow, green, and blue. Because of high uptake, well-perfused muscle of the left ventricle is red. A dipyridamole-induced ischemic area in the posterior wall is evident on the computer-processed image *(a)*. The normal distribution, which occurred after rest, is shown by the complete white-and-red doughnut shape *(b)*. Panels *c* and *d* depict analogous stimulated and rest images and no ischemia (complete doughnuts) after surgical bypass graft. At the lower margins of some images, high uptake by liver is indicated by red.

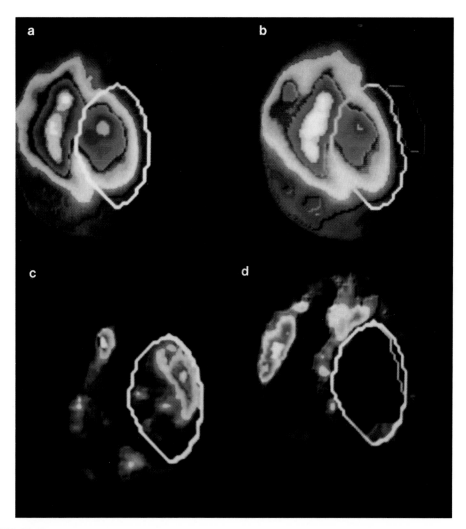

PLATE 18–2.

Computer-processed anterior projection scintigrams of a multiple-gated distribution of technetium-labeled RBCs in a patient with severe cardiomyopathy. The left ventricle is outlined in white in panel *a* and in yellow and white in panel *b*. Panel *a* depicts the end-diastolic (ED) distribution of activity and panel *b* the end-systolic (ES) distribution. Color is coded to reveal radioactivity intensity in that frame with white highest, through red, yellow, green, and blue. Distribution of activity appears quite similar in *a* and *b* because stroke volume is very low. Panels *c* and *d*, images made by subtraction. Images show regional physiology in two ways. In *c*, the image is of ED minus ES.

In this image the intensity of the *subtracted* activity is shown with the same color scale. The position of the white and red colors indicates that most of the left ventricular ejection is being accomplished by the posterolateral wall of the ventricle. In *d*, the image is ES minus ED. The minimal change in borders again indicates the small stroke volume, and that ejection is principally by the posterolateral wall. In addition, the presence of any color (in the apex, in this case) indicates an area of greater systolic than diastolic blood volume, that is, an aneurysm, for which this method is quite sensitive. Atrial contraction (atrial stroke volume) is also apparent in *c* and *d*.

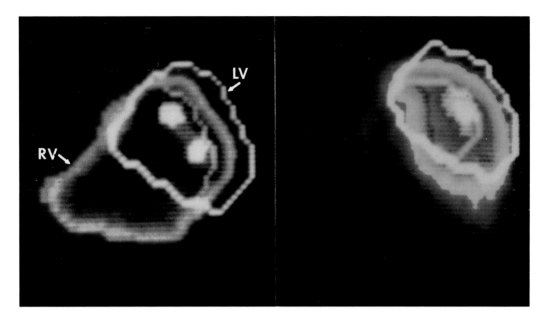

PLATE 18–3.

Scintigrams of a transplanted heart made after the injection of technetium to label patient's RBCs and subtraction of ED from ES, similar to that in Plate 18–2. Therefore, both panels reveal left ventricular "stroke volume images." The panel on the left, made three weeks after transplantation, shows both left and right ventricles, the left ventricle outlined more sharply. The image on the right was made the following day; the right ventricle is no longer evident. Clinically the right ventricle had become infarcted in the interim; it had no effective contraction, and was serving only as a conduit.

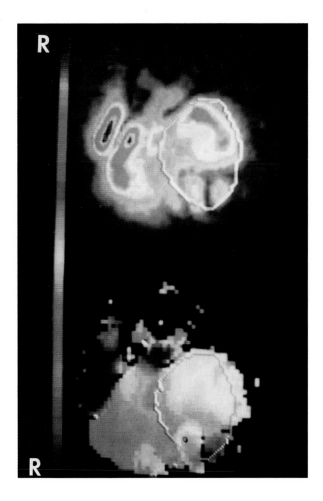

PLATE 18–4.

Computer-processed multiple-gated images (45-degree LAO) of the heart in a patient with severe cardiomyopathy. *Upper panel* shows the distribution of labeled RBCs coded to depict the intensity of the amplitude of the contraction, regardless of when the change in amplitude occurred. For the upper image, color represents intensity of contraction, with both highest and lowest shown in indigo. The greatest change in amplitude (contraction) is indicated by indigo and red colors over the right atrium and ventricle, with relatively low amplitude over the entire left ventricle. The highest contraction over the left ventricle occurs over the posterolateral wall, typical of cardiomyopathy. In the left ventricular apex there are two ellipsoidal areas of lower amplitude. In *lower panel* color is used to show time rather than intensity change. The color bar at the left now indicates time from the R wave (indigo) beginning at the lower end of the color spectrum passing through to the next R wave above (also indigo). The color of an active area is assigned according to the time at which that area reached its smallest activity (blood volume). Active areas that reach their smallest volume at the time of the R wave, such as normal atria, are indigo. Areas that reach their smallest volume midway through the R-R interval, such as normal ventricles, are green or yellow. In the image shown, most of the area representing the ventricles is green or yellow. In this case the right ventricle contracted a little before the left, as indicated by the greens. Most of the left ventricle contracted approximately midway through the R-R interval and is therefore yellow. The two ellipsoidal areas in the apex, noted above to be contracting poorly, are here contracting at times different from most of the left ventricle and from each other. The area on the left contracts slightly later than the rest of the left ventricle (tardykinesis). The area on the right contracts almost in synchrony with the atrium, shown by its blue color, indicating aneurysmal contractions or dyskinesis.

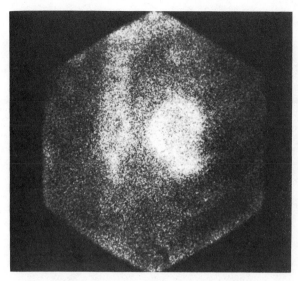

FIG 18–1.
Scintigram made 3 hours after the injection of technetium 99m–labeled pyrophosphate into a patient with a large acute anterior myocardial infarction. Uptake over the sternum is seen on the left. The uptake over the infarction is in a roughly annular form, with low uptake over the center of the infarcted area.

heart can be grouped as follows: (1) techniques that yield direct images of myocardial infarction; (2) techniques that allow assessment of coronary flow by imaging the distribution of analogues of potassium; and (3) techniques that measure cardiac movement so that defects in wall motion may be evaluated or a crude estimate of cardiac output may be made.

Myocardial Infarction Imaging

This technique was discovered quite by accident in a patient receiving technetium pyrophosphate for bone imaging. Bonte et al.[1] observed unusual uptake over the myocardium that was later correlated with an early, unsuspected myocardial infarction.

Pyrophosphate imaging is positive as early as 3½ hours after acute infarction (Fig 18–1). The maximum incidence of positivity and most intense pyrophosphate fixation occur between 1 and 3 days after infarction. Images are usually positive for 1 week, after which the incidence diminishes sharply. In a few cases images remain positive for months. We have observed this prolonged positive finding to be associated with severe disease or complications such as ventricular aneurysm.

The test may be positive before CK-MB isoenzyme levels increase. It is useful when disturbances in electrical excitation of the heart, such as bundle-branch block, interfere with the electrocardiographic (ECG) diagnosis of infarction; in right ventricular infarction; and after heart sur-

gery or chest trauma, when interpretation of changes in isoenzymes may be difficult. However, both cardioversion and chest wall trauma may introduce artifacts because of muscle injury, and studies from more than one angle may be required to discriminate them.

Myocardial Imaging With Thallium 201

Most nuclear medicine imaging studies depend on imaging some metabolic process by use of a radioactive label that is not metabolized by nearby tissues. Rates of myocardial uptake of potassium would provide an index of coronary artery blood flow. Unfortunately, no satisfactory isotopes of potassium exist for scintigraphy, so analogues that enter active muscle in a manner similar to potassium have been used. The isotope thallium 201 (^{201}Tl) is favored over isotopes of rubidium and cesium. But ^{201}Tl imaging is still unavailable in some areas and it is relatively costly. The half-life of ^{201}Tl, 3 days, is satisfactory.

Since it behaves in many ways like potassium, thallium is taken up by other tissues with which the myocardium must compete. Because of this the only satisfactory images of the left ventricle are those obtained after exercise or chemical stimulation has increased myocardial potassium uptake. Imaging must be performed immediately after injection. The patient is imaged again after a 3-hour rest. On the 45-degree left anterior oblique (LAO) view, the left ventricle appears as a ring-shaped, doughnut-like structure

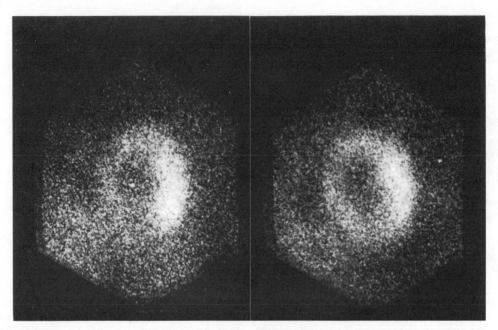

FIG 18–2.
Scintigram of thallium 201 distribution in a patient with ischemia of the ventricular septum. Relatively low uptake is seen over the septum, shown in the 45-degree left anterior oblique image *(left)*. Radioactivity increased after a 3-hour rest *(right)*. In this case reperfusion appears incomplete after 3 hours. Sometimes, more nearly complete reperfusion may be demonstrated after a longer recuperative period. This pattern is typical of an ischemic process around an infarct. Data in this case are in analogue gray scale form. They have not been processed by computer.

(Fig 18–2, right image). Ischemic areas appear as photogenic zones. Typically, zones where activity was low with exercise remain unchanged if infarction was the cause, or they may fill in if the ischemia was exercise-induced (Fig 18–2).

Unfortunately, owing to the low counting rate these changes are subtle and usually must be elucidated and quantified by computer processing. Plate 18–1 shows images of the myocardium in a patient with severe angina on minimal exertion but a negative coronary angiogram, who was stressed by an infusion of dipyridamole. Two minutes later the patient was injected with ^{201}Tl and imaged immediately. The data in analogue gray scale were not revealing, but computer processing made defective perfusion over the postero-lateral wall clearly evident (Plate 18–1, *a*). After a 3-hour rest, the scintigram was normal (Plate 18–1, *b*). On the basis of this finding, the patient underwent coronary artery bypass grafting for an estimated 90% occlusion. After surgery the process was repeated, and images were normal immediately after stressing and in repose (Plate 18–1, *c* and *d*). This study illustrates the value of stress testing by drugs when exercising is impossible.

Dynamic Studies of the Heart

Regional wall motion studies of the heart are often referred to as MUGA, or multiple-gated, studies. Briefly, these involve the labeling and reinjection of the patient's red blood cells or plasma proteins and acquiring scintigraphic data over the heart blood pool in various projections. Scintigraphy must be accompanied by an ECG signal. Scintigraphy is performed for approximately 2 minutes in each view.

The computing mechanism is programmed to recognize R waves and to examine each R-R interval. Data from each may be stored temporarily on a disk for analysis. Only intervals with a length between predetermined limits are processed. The R-R interval is divided into 16 to 24 time segments or bins. X,Y addresses from all γ-rays collected by the camera from acceptable R-R intervals are stored in the appropriate time bin. The end product is a series of 16 to 24 sequential images compiled from γ-ray X,Y addresses from many heart beats or R-R intervals, all piled into a single systole.

Each image may be smoothed or filtered or simply played back in sequence, repeating the composite R-R interval over and over. After the limits of the left ventricle are indicated to the computer (white lines surrounding images in Plate 18–2), the data can be analyzed further. Two of the frames are defined as end-diastolic (ED; Plate 18–2, *a*) and end-systolic (ES; Plate 18–2, *b*), and counting rates are determined in each of them. This permits the calculation of the left ventricular ejection fraction (EF):

$$EF = \frac{LVC_{ED} - LVC_{ES}}{LVC_{ED}} \quad (Eq.\ 18–1)$$

where LVC is the counting rate in the area designated "left ventricle" (white line) in the ED and ES frames.

A left ventricular stroke volume (LVSV) image is calculated as the difference ED − ES in the LV area (Plate 18–2, *c*). Similarly, an atrial stroke volume (ASV) can be calculated from the difference in counting rates in the atrial area in the ES and ED frames (Plate 18–2, *d*). The use of color to relate activity (see Plate 18–2, *a* and *b*) or change in activity (see Plate 18–2, *c* and *d*) emphasizes local dynamics more clearly than does gray scale. Less subtle or more diffuse processes are readily apparent in gray scale images (Plate 18–3).

Each of the images in Plates 18–3 and 18–4 is only one of the 16 to 24 images that together represent one composite contraction. Image matrices are usually assigned colors indicating various radioactivity intensity levels. Plate 18–4 shows the value of using color to indicate the amplitude of change for each area of the heart and the relative timing of that change for each area in a paired image. For example, the R-R interval may be coded so that the first segment from the R wave is assigned a single color (e.g., indigo). Then, sequential segments are color coded through the rainbow: blues, greens, yellows, reds, violets, to indigo at the next R wave. Thus, in this scheme atrial contraction may appear as indigo (since it occurs at the time of the R wave) and ventricular contraction as yellow (since it oc-

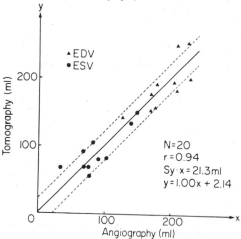

FIG 18–3.
Comparison of left ventricle volumes calculated from electrocardiographically gated SPECT images and conventional biplanar angiographic methods. Values correlate closely.

curs midway between the R waves). Areas of ventricular tardykinesis may appear as orange to red and dyskinesis as indigo or blue, indicating that there is paradoxically more blood in these areas during systole than in diastole. Thus, conduction defects and the quality and synchrony of contraction can all be made apparent in one pair of images. In Plate 18–4, all these "volumes" are based on two-dimensional matrices. True volumes can be calculated from gated, single-photon-emission computed tomographic (SPECT) images (Fig 18–3).[8] Many other variations are possible. Ejection fraction may be calculated for each segment of the left ventricle, or an entire EF matrix may be created and color-coded. The EF matrix may locate precisely where efficiency is particularly high or low. Computer processing can be carried out quite rapidly in a time frame appropriate to the emergency situation.

Cinematic images rarely add any additional information but are useful for an overall impression, especially for clinicians who are more accustomed to angiographic appearances, and for demonstrating defects to others unaccustomed to a particular processing algorithm. The computer can select premature beats or the beat following for analyses such as those described.

LOCAL BLOOD FLOW MEASUREMENT USING XENON-ENHANCED CT

Objective monitoring of local perfusion is based almost entirely on tissue function. Therefore, to monitor organ perfusion each time mentation, bowel sounds, or urine output decreases or the ST segment changes, one must question whether organ perfusion has diminished to an intolerable degree or whether the disturbance is due to another factor. Clinical impressions can be augmented by whole body or local, but still nonspecific, measurements. Thus, monitoring of toe temperature,[2] transcutaneous Po_2,[6] or tissue pH can be used to assess either generalized somatic vasoconstriction or local hypoperfusion. However, to cite a whole body variable, a normal cardiac output might represent overperfusion of some beds and none of others; and a further increase in cardiac output, such as from volume loading and inotropic therapy, might helpfully impede the coalescence of multifocal subclinical deteriorations into frank shock, or might do nothing of value.

Calculations from CT scans of various tissues during ventilation with and without nonradioactive xenon allow less invasive and more precise definition of (local) regional cerebral blood flow (CBF) and the effects of disease and therapy than has previously been possible. The technique has essentially the same restrictions as any CT technique but requires immobilization for a longer period (minutes) because it is a subtraction technique. Although the technique was developed for measuring local blood flow in the brain, it may be applicable also to the study of local blood flow in the systemic circulation. The same methodology has been used to describe local ventilation in critically ill patients.[7]

Cerebral Blood Flow*

Most methods used to map local or regional CBF involve external monitoring of the transit or clearance of inhaled or injected radioactive tracers. Although useful, these techniques estimate flow for relatively large tissue volumes of relatively superficial levels of cerebral cortex. Local

*Walter Good, M.S., played a fundamental role in developing this technology and provided the illustrations for this section.

blood flow in extremely small tissue volumes can now be derived from measurements of time-dependent concentrations of nonradioactive xenon gas.[3] This derivation is possible because xenon is a freely diffusible gas with an atomic number high enough to yield measurable increases in radiodensity even when inhaled in relatively low concentration. The derivation of local cerebral blood flow (LCBF) is based on the Fick principle. The procedure requires the acquisition of three or more images, before and during 4–6 minutes of xenon/oxygen inhalation. When venous admixture is less than 10%, end-tidal xenon levels are proportional to time-dependent xenon concentrations in arterial blood, and xenon concentrations of 35% yield satisfactory flow maps. Arterial concentration can also be assessed by quantifying the enhancement of arterial blood in vivo. These data are then used in conjunction with time-dependent xenon concentration in tissue to derive the LCBF for each tissue of interest.

CASE 18–1 (Adequacy of CBF with increased intracranial pressure, and CO_2 response).—A 19-year-old woman injured in an automobile accident was brought to the emergency room unresponsive to either verbal or painful stimulation. She was able to move her left side spontaneously and semipurposefully after resuscitation, but she remained hemiplegic on the right side. CT demonstrated a small left-sided acute subdural hematoma with two small lateral contusions of the left hemisphere. There was a minimal shift of the midline structures.

An external ventriculostomy was placed for intracranial pressure (ICP) monitoring. Initially, ICP was slightly elevated, but by the third day after admission, when hyperventilation ($Pa_{CO_2} < 30$ torr) was sustained, it remained in the normal range. When the patient was weaned from mechanical ventilation, there was a rise in Pa_{CO_2} to 35 torr and ICP rose to 15–20 torr.

Two Xe-CT blood flow studies were performed, the initial one at a Pa_{CO_2} of 23 torr and a second study 30 minutes later at a Pa_{CO_2} of 36 torr. They demonstrated relatively normal flow distribution and the expected response to Pa_{CO_2} manipulation throughout the brain, with the exception of the lateral aspect of the left hemisphere (Fig 18–4). In this area of contusion, blood flow values remained relatively hyperemic at the lower Pa_{CO_2}, demonstrating a regional loss of carbon dioxide response. However, the relatively normal flow values throughout the hemisphere at the higher Pa_{CO_2} level reassured us that weaning from the respirator was being tolerated well in spite of the mild elevation in ICP.

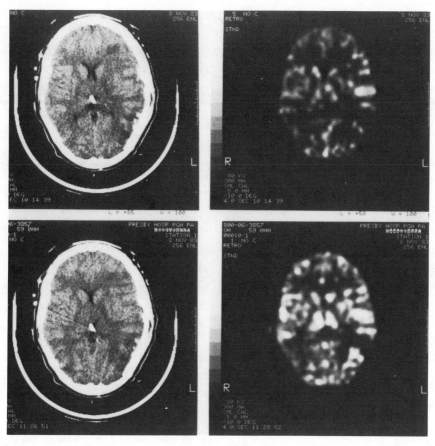

FIG 18–4.
CT images *(left)* and corresponding flow maps *(right)* of a 19-year-old patient. The scale to the left of each flow map is in ml/min/100 cc of tissue. Flow is proportional to shading, from black (zero flow) to white (80 ml/100 cc/min). The blood flow pattern shows a regional loss of autoregulation. The derived flow maps *(right)* are of the same tissue slice at Pa_{CO_2} of 23 torr *(top)* and 36 torr *(bottom),* respectively. There is relatively normal flow distribution except for the lateral aspect of the left hemisphere, where relative hyperemia persists despite the low CO_2 level. (From Yonas et al.[9] Reproduced by permission.)

The patient subsequently showed steady improvement. By the fourth week after trauma she was discharged to a rehabilitation facility with a spastic right hemiparesis and a moderate expressive aphasia.

Discussion.—Because Xe-CT blood flow mapping can be repeated at 15-minute intervals, it lends itself to the monitoring of CBF alterations caused by changes in ventilatory and drug therapy. The degree of CBF response to hyperventilation therapy can help in the decision to continue or withdraw hyperventilation. In case 18–1, the carbon dioxide response 3 days after trauma was locally impaired but flow was adequate in all areas despite an elevated ICP.

CASE 18–2 (Rapid assessment).—A 24-year-old man became unconscious without apparent cause and ceased to breathe moments later. His trachea was intubated and he was taken to the hospital. No clinical evidence of cortical or brain stem function was found. A CT scan disclosed only a small amount of subarachnoid blood over the cerebellum. The CBF examination, which added only 10 minutes to the routine CT examination, disclosed the absence of any hemispheric or brain stem blood flow (Fig 18–5). The patient met the standard clinical criteria of brain death later that day.

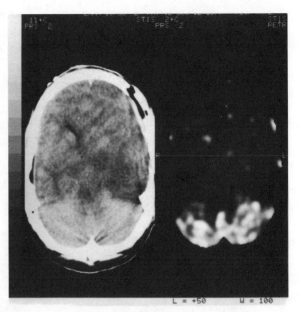

FIG 18–5.
CT scan *(left)* demonstrating compression of lateral ventricles compatible with but not diagnostic of increased ICP. The degree of impairment of flow is not apparent. The corresponding LCBF study *(right)* shows no flow in the supratentorial space but normal flows in the posterior cerebellum.

Discussion.—Xe-CT CBF examination lends itself to the frequently emergent nature of neurologic disorders. Little additional time is required to add information on flow to the anatomical data provided by the baseline CT images, and the diagnosis of a small brain stem stroke or large hemispheric infarction or death of the entire brain is made readily apparent. In this case, in spite of the lack of an etiologic mechanism adequate to explain the severe injury, the absence of brain blood flow and the implied prognosis were quickly revealed.

CASE 18–3 (Focal ischemia).—A 62-year-old woman underwent a left endarterectomy because of high-grade stenosis and recurrent neurologic events. Although the endarterectomy was performed in the standard manner without apparent intraoperative complication, in the recovery room the patient was found to be hemiplegic on her left side and aphasic. CT scanning was promptly performed, but no evidence of cerebral hemorrhage was identified on the baseline CT image (Fig 18–6,A). The CBF study, which added 10 minutes to the standard CT examination, demonstrated a near absence of flow within the entire anterior and middle cerebral artery distributions of the left hemisphere (Fig 18–6,B). This presumably was caused by an intraoperative embolism to the internal carotid that occluded both the anterior and middle cerebral arteries. The flow study also allowed a prediction of whether operative removal of the clot would be useful. If slightly higher flows (12–18 ml/100 gm/min in animal stud-

ies, as determined by other techniques) had been measured, neuronal salvage might have been significant. However, flows near zero in most of the involved area precluded meaningful recovery.

Discussion.—The absence of flow is easy to see with this methodology, and the return of flow to an ischemic region following fragmentation of an embolus has also been demonstrated. Diagnosis and therapeutic options can be quickly defined. In animals and humans, when infarction has occurred during the initial ischemic insult and then flow returns within 24–48 hours, dramatic hyperemia has been seen, accompanied by a dramatic lowering of CT values due to edema within the same region.

CASE 18–4 (Mass effect).—A 34-year-old woman was injured in an auto accident and brought to the hospital in a comatose state with a dilated left pupil and decerebrate posturing. The initial CT scan demonstrated an epidural hematoma over the left frontal lobe, which was promptly removed surgically. Although the patient initially responded favorably with a return to normal posture and normal pupillary size, her condition deteriorated 48 hours later despite ICP remaining less than 20 torr. At that time the CT scan (Fig 18–7) demonstrated the presence of bilateral intraparenchymal frontal lobe clots larger on the left side. The accompanying CBF study demonstrated not only an absence of flow in the left frontal lobe, but also severe depression of flow within the deep ganglionic regions.

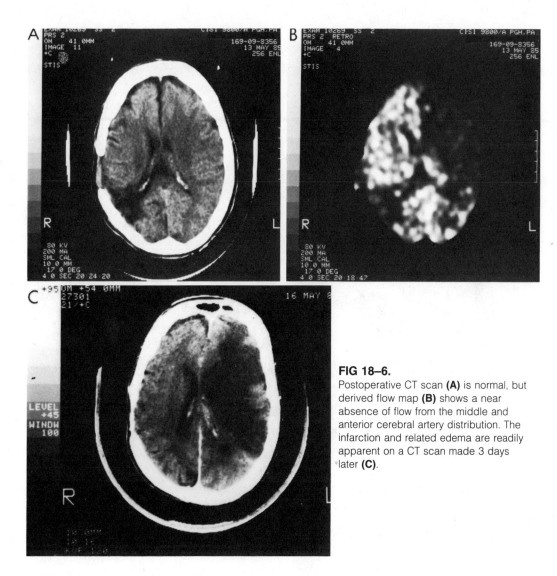

FIG 18–6.
Postoperative CT scan **(A)** is normal, but derived flow map **(B)** shows a near absence of flow from the middle and anterior cerebral artery distribution. The infarction and related edema are readily apparent on a CT scan made 3 days later **(C)**.

The patient was presumed to be undergoing central herniation, in spite of only minimal elevation of ICP, caused primarily by the left frontal lobe mass effect. The postoperative CT study demonstrated removal of the left frontal lobe mass lesion and an impressive return of more normal flow to the basal ganglia bilaterally.

Discussion.—Local CBF information coupled with CT scanning provides an understanding of how mass lesions distribute forces within the immediately surrounding parenchyma as well as on distant tissues, sometimes despite minimal elevation of ventricular fluid pressure. The effect of mass in each dural compartment is readily apparent and thus provides a further understanding

of how intracranial mass lesions can affect blood flow to the brain. Measurement of ventricular fluid pressure is not a valid monitor of the external pressure on capillaries, which has solid as well as fluid components.

Xenon-Enhanced CT Evaluation of Blood Flow in Other Tissues

The Xe-CT technique of evaluating tissue perfusion has potential for clinical use in abdominal and retroperitoneal disorders. Preliminary nonhuman primate studies have confirmed the feasibility of this noninvasive method to quantitate blood flow and tissue perfusion in the liver and kidneys.[4] Clinically, multilevel studies of the abdo-

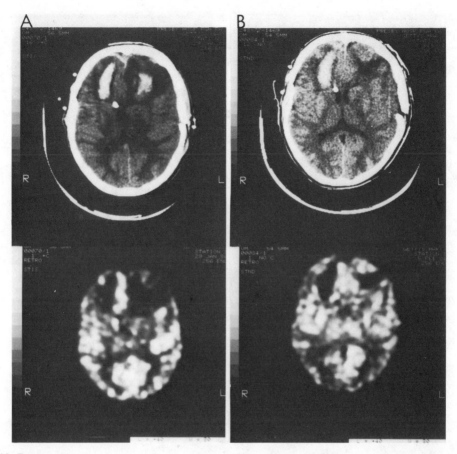

FIG 18–7.
CT scan 48 hours after head injury *(top left)* shows bilateral frontal lobe hemorrhages with minimal shift, and the presence of a catheter in the right ventricle. The corresponding blood flow study *(bottom left)* shows severe depression of flow in all of the left frontal lobe and in the deep ganglionic tissues, suggesting compression of the basal ganglia (central hernia- tion) due to mass effect, primarily from the left frontal lobe. Flow in the medial right frontal lobe is preserved despite an adjacent intraparenchymal blood clot and the pressure effects in the left frontal area. The post- operative scan *(top right)* shows absence of the left frontal lobe, and brain stem flow is improved in the flow map.

men have been successful. The technique has not been verified as carefully in these tissues as in the brain, but derived blood flow maps of the liver and kidney have given values that are in the range of those expected from other techniques. Diminished perfusion of the liver has been demonstrated by this method in hepatic artery thrombosis, sclerosing cholangitis, chronic active hepatitis, and primary biliary cirrhosis.[5]

The future use of xenon-enhanced CT for measurement of blood flow in the abdomen and retroperitoneal space is, at this stage, purely speculative. Disturbance in blood flow and tissue perfusion is at the core of much pathology in those spaces. Hence, a noninvasive, accurate, and reliable technique of quantitating flow could significantly improve diagnosis, understanding of flow-related disorders, and the clinical titration of vasoactive drug therapy.

We expect that after further evaluation the method described will provide more precise information on changes in distribution of blood flow in patients in shock and other vasoderegulated states or visceral disorders. It may be possible to show the local influence of general resuscitative and specific vasoactive drug therapy on each of several tissues at once. Use of the technique at the level of the lumbar vertebrae might allow quantitation of local flow simultaneously in any tissue that maintains a constant position, such as in liver, spleen, kidneys, pancreas, muscle, and bone.

At its present stage, there are two caveats to the use of Xe-CT mapping methods in the liver and kidney. First, the dual blood supply to the liver calls into question the validity of using the end-tidal xenon concentration measurement from the portal circulation as input information. This may bias the derived blood flow values for the liver toward the underestimation of flow. The problem must be addressed before absolute values of blood flow to the liver can be accurately derived. At this stage, the flow maps appear to be more useful for evaluating flow ratios and relative flow rates to liver and spleen than for quantitating absolute flow. Abnormal liver/spleen flow ratios with dominant splenic perfusion have been observed in patients with cirrhosis and other causes of portal hypertension prior to liver transplantation. Hepatic perfusion is monitored in these patients following transplantation.

The second caveat is that the flow of blood through the renal cortex is relatively rapid and the speed of available scanners is technically limited. This calls into question the validity of assuming that instantaneous equilibration of xenon concentrations in tissues and blood can be reached. Again, the net result is a bias toward underestimation of flow through the renal cortex.

Case 18–5. A CT scan and blood flow study of the brain were performed in an elderly woman because of persistent coma 2 weeks after head injury. At the same time a flow study of the kidneys was performed to assess renal failure (Fig 18–8).

Discussion.—Renal perfusion appears sufficient, so renal cortical necrosis is unlikely and renal function is likely to return.

SUMMARY

Techniques for frequent or continuous monitoring of oxygen supply and demand have improved to

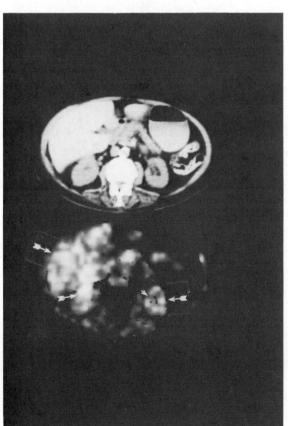

FIG 18–8.
CT scan at the level of the upper abdomen *(top)* with corresponding derived blood flow map *(bottom)*. Good tissue perfusion is indicated by the bright areas *(arrows)* in the hepatic and renal parenchyma. Variation in brightness in the area of renal parenchyma suggests irregular tissue perfusion bilaterally, but cortical necrosis is unlikely, and recovery of renal function appears likely. The dark areas *(arrow)* in the center of the kidney indicate low flow to the renal pelves. As expected, low flow is seen in the paraspinal musculature.

allow routine clinical application. However, having identified a deficiency in overall oxygen supply/demand (low venous oxygen) or possible maldistribution of oxygen supply (tissue dysfunction with normal venous oxygen), we must analyze cardiac dynamics and distribution of systemic blood flow more precisely and routinely. The nuclear medicine and xenon-enhanced CT techniques are potentially widely available techniques that seem to satisfy these needs and therefore to be practical tools for research investigation and perhaps routine clinical application in the critically ill patient.

Acknowledgment

The authors thank John B. Cone, M.D., for his editing of this manuscript.

REFERENCES

1. Bonte FJ, Parkey RW, Graham KD, et al: A new method for radionuclide imaging of myocardial infarction. *Radiology* 1974; 110:473–474.
2. Douglas ME, Downs JB: Applied physiology and respiratory care, in Shoemaker WC (ed): *The Society of Critical Care Medicine: State of the Art*. Fullerton, Calif, Society of Critical Care Medicine, 1982, vol 3, E:1.
3. Gur D, Wolfson SK, Yonas H, et al: Progress in cerebrovascular disease: Local cerebral blood flow by xenon enhanced CT. *Stroke* 1982; 13:750–758.
4. Gur D, Yonas H, Wolfson SK, et al: Xenon/CT Blood Flow Mapping of the Kidney and Liver. *J Comput Assist Tomogr* 1984; 8(6):1124–1127.
5. Gur D, Good WF, Herbert DL, et al: Blood flow mapping in the human liver by the xenon/CT method. *J Comput Assist Tomogr* 1985; 9(3):447–450.
6. Leith DE: Barotrauma in human research. *Crit Care Med* 1976; 4:159.
7. Snyder JV, Pennock B, Herbert D, et al: Local lung ventilation in critically ill patients using nonradioactive xenon-enhanced transmission computed tomography. *Crit Care Med* 1984; 12:46–51.
8. Tauxe WN, Soussaline F, Todd-Pokropek A, et al: Determination of organ volume by single photon emission tomography. *J Nucl Med* 1982; 23:984–987.
9. Yonas H, Snyder JV, Gur D, et al: Local cerebral blood flow alterations (Xe-CT method) in an accident victim. *J Comput Assist Tomogr* 1984; 8:990–991.

PART 5

Ventilatory Support: Physiology and Technique

19

The Development of Supported Ventilation: A Critical Summary

James V. Snyder, M.D.

In this chapter, various approaches to ventilatory support are presented as though they were developed independently of each other, so that the advantages and disadvantages of each may be defined. Limited space precludes adequate recognition of many individuals for their contributions.

THE HIGH VT APPROACH

Development

The introduction of positive-pressure ventilation during the polio epidemics of 1958–1959 changed respiratory care and remarkably improved outcome from respiratory failure. External negative-pressure (Cuirass) ventilators were preferred as late as 1963 because of complications associated with intubation and positive-pressure ventilation.[32] Subsequent changes were spearheaded by physicians at the Massachusetts General Hospital and reported in their excellent publications.[7, 36, 58]

After seeing increased arterial-alveolar oxygen gradients [$\dot{D}(A-a)_{O_2}$] and decreased compliance during controlled ventilation with normal tidal volume (Vt),[24, 48] a number of investigators suggested that high volume ventilation would be beneficial. They emphasized the prevention or early reversal of atelectasis, noting that the longer atelectasis has been allowed to persist, the higher are the pressures needed for reinflation of alveoli. They saw that patients under general anesthesia who had the largest fall in arterial carbon dioxide tension (Pa_{CO_2}) had the least fall in arterial oxygen tension (Pa_{O_2}).[35] In dogs, compliance was increased by sustained passive inflation and by using high Vt.[35, 48] Dogs ventilated with a Vt of less than 25 ml/kg of body weight invariably showed an increase in $\dot{D}(A-a)_{O_2}$ and physiologic

shunting. Oxygenation was best with Vt values of 62.7 and 87.5 ml/kg. The pulmonary shunt (Qs/Qt) decreased with increases in Vt of up to 25 ml/kg, as did $\dot{D}(A-a)_{O_2}$ with Vt up to 50 ml/kg.[35] In closed-chested dogs, surface activity decreased with very high Vt, but did not when Vt was less than 50 ml/kg.[36(p 15)] In humans, however, a Vt of 27 ml/kg often caused barotrauma. A Vt of 10–15 ml/kg became widely recommended.[7] Periodic "sighing" was believed useful by some[7, 68] but eventually given up by most.[36] When high minute and tidal volumes became routine, large deadspace volumes (Vd) and ratios of deadspace to tidal volume (Vd/Vt) of over 80% were observed; deadspace in nonemphysematous patients averaged 2.84 times normal.[36] The approach recommended then was consistent with the concepts promoted in this text: the correct way to lower Pa_{CO_2} in such cases is not just to increase Vt more, but to improve the distribution of pulmonary ventilation relative to perfusion.[7] To do so, the individual patient's regional pulmonary physiology must be analyzed to guide a systematic search for the ventilator settings that will result in the best possible distribution of ventilation and perfusion in that patient. This entails a process of repeated trial and evaluation, as well as ongoing evaluation to manage pathophysiologic changes over time. Because practitioners do not appreciate that there are distinct alternatives, increasing ventilation is still the most common approach to lowering Pa_{CO_2}. Thus, a Vt of 25–50 ml/kg, shown to improve function experimentally, was incorporated into clinical practice in some institutions. However, a high incidence of barotrauma, especially when positive end-expiratory pressure (PEEP) was introduced, encouraged a more conservative and physiologic approach.[9]

Although respiration could be supported just as effectively by a constantly attended pressure-limited ventilator, volume-limited ventilation became the preferred mode because compliance changes do not influence tidal or minute ventilation. Adding security straps to secure airway connections increased the safety of volume-limited ventilators by preventing leaks in the connecting tubing. Assisted ventilation allowed the patient to set the ventilator rate so the patient required less sedation. Furthermore, paralysis, with its physiologic disadvantage,[25] psychological discomfort, and disasters from accidental disconnections, could then usually be avoided.

The regional aspects of pulmonary pathophysiology were well described in the early 1970s.[72, 80] Two conditions were recognized as invariably present in acute respiratory failure (ARF). The first is an abnormal pattern of gas distribution, with closure of alveoli or airways, or both. The second is an increase in pulmonary extravascular water, with interstitial edema caused by pulmonary vascular congestion or by loss of integrity of the pulmonary capillary endothelium.[58] As noted by Pontoppidan et al.,[58(p 6)]

> Both conditions tend to become manifest on a regional basis dictated by the effect of gravity on the distribution of ventilation, blood flow, and extravascular water. They result in a reduction of functional residual capacity, a decrease in pulmonary compliance and mismatching of ventilation an1 blood flow. These are the hallmarks of ARF.

The importance of the relation between lung volume at end-inspiration and lung volume at which appreciable airway closure begins (closing volume, also called closing capacity) was stressed. In these observations, "the greater the closing volume in relation to inspiratory lung volume, the more pronounced the effect on gas exchange." The analysis by Pontoppidan et al. continued,[58(p 12)]

> If airways remain closed throughout inspiration, gas trapped in air spaces distal to the point of closure is absorbed by the blood more or less rapidly, according to gas composition and solubility. The end result is atelectasis unless airways are periodically opened by an active or passive deep inspiration. If perfusion continues, venous admixture (shunting) will also occur. Re-expansion of gas exchanging airspaces may be delayed or refractory because high distending pressures are needed to expand collapsed alveoli.

Nonpulmonary factors such as obesity and abdominal distention, immobilization, paralysis, narcotic drugs, and pain were thought to contribute to the reduction of functional residual capacity (FRC). Pulmonary factors such as increased surface tension, interstitial edema, and pulmonary inflammation were recognized to promote alveolar and airway closure.[58(p 13)]

PEEP was shown to increase arterial oxygenation in anesthetized, mechanically ventilated patients,[26] then in patients with severe ARF.[3, 45, 47] The increase in Pa_{O_2} with end-expiratory pressure was shown to be related to the resulting increase in lung volume,[23] and a linear relation was found between change in FRC and end-expiratory pressure. FRC increased by 400 ml or more for each 5 cm H_2O of added end-expiratory pressure.[36(p 18)] In normal lungs that had been degassed, the pulmonary shunt (Qs/Qt) decreased linearly with increases in lung volume up to 70% of total lung capacity.[2] The critical influence of the relation between closing capacity (CC) and inspiratory lung volume on venous admixture was observed, as was the change in the relation with age.[50] In this study, when FRC exceeded CC, $\dot{D}(A-a)_{O_2}$ did not change with anesthesia and was not affected by Vt. When CC exceeded inspiratory lung volume $\dot{D}(A-a)_{O_2}$ increased significantly with anesthesia. During anesthesia, changing from a small Vt to a large Vt decreased $\dot{D}(A-a)_{O_2}$ when it increased inspiratory lung volume from below to above CC.[78]

The Current Approach: High Vt

The "current" approach described here (Table 19–1) represents our perception of what has become wide practice across the United States, although practices vary between and within institutions.[1, 8, 11, 16, 36, 58, 66, 68] Recent trends such as

TABLE 19–1.

Conventional (High Vt) Support of Ventilation

1. Use assisted volume-limited ventilation, Vt = 10–15 ml/kg.
2. Use PEEP to lower $F_{I_{O_2}}$ to .7 (or .5), with no decrease in cardiac output.
3. Wean from PEEP first, then from mechanical support, then extubate.

Corollaries:
Venous admixture is a problem of FRC relative to closing volume.
PEEP causes low cardiac output and barotrauma.
CO_2 elimination is not a problem.
Mechanical ventilation provides security.

using a lower Vt, a lower fraction of inspired oxygen (F_{IO_2}), and intermittent mandatory ventilation (IMV) are ignored for the purposes of this characterization. Treatment of ARF includes increasing F_{IO_2} until toxic levels (.5 to .7) are needed to keep Pa_{O_2} adequate (60–90 torr) during spontaneous breathing. Intubation and assisted mechanical ventilation of the patient is mandated by carbon dioxide retention or hypoxemia despite toxic F_{IO_2}. Large tidal volumes (10–15 ml/kg) are used to diminish or prevent progressive lung collapse.[6, 24, 35, 77] The resulting increase in lung expansion with these techniques sometimes allows a decrease in F_{IO_2}. PEEP may permit an additional decrease but, because of the danger of reducing cardiac output and of barotrauma, PEEP is administered only to keep F_{IO_2} at less than toxic levels and may be limited to 10–15 cm H_2O.[70] Venous admixture decreases markedly when FRC or end-expiratory lung volume exceeds CC.

Problems and Modifications of the High Vt Approach

The approach described uses high Vt because the volume and function of the lung depend on its pressure-volume history. High Vt, however, may contribute to morbidity, especially when respiratory failure is severe, by several mechanisms. First, when PEEP is required, high Vt is a principal cause of high peak airway pressure (AWP) and probably of barotrauma. Second, as the disadvantages of long-term muscle paralysis and controlled ventilation became appreciated and the mode of assisted ventilation was developed, the use of a high mechanical Vt with an increased (patient-triggered) breathing rate caused respiratory alkalosis.[80] The lower Pa_{CO_2} caused significant hemodynamic sequelae[12] and, surprisingly, mild increases in oxygen consumption.[15, 41] When Vt was set at 10 ml/kg, the lower limit of the recommended high Vt range, respiratory alkalosis still occurred to a dangerous degree in one of ten patients. High Vt was still considered essential to prevent hypoxemia, so respiratory alkalosis was countered by increasing deadspace[74] and increasing F_{ICO_2}.[54] Third, when the high Vt approach is applied to a lung with underlying pathology, the cyclic stretching can induce further structural damage, as will be described in chapter 24, "Respirator Lung."

Several important influences are not adequately addressed in the currently accepted application of ventilatory support. (1) The more subtle benefits of a lower F_{IO_2} are not considered. (2) Whereas high Vt is used to keep the lung open and PEEP is withheld to avoid barotrauma, using PEEP may result in lower peak AWP from both lower Vt and improved compliance, and therefore reduce the risk of barotrauma. (3) The contribution of inefficient carbon dioxide elimination (high Vd/Vt) to increases in required minute ventilation and therefore to increases in mean and peak AWP (and the complications of high AWP) is not commonly considered. Until the disease process is advanced, the principal concern with carbon dioxide elimination is respiratory alkalosis rather than inefficiency. (4) The therapeutic benefit of PEEP has been related to normalization of overall FRC, whereas it is actually the changes in regional volumes and airway closure that are important. (5) PEEP has been regarded only as a tool to improve oxygenation; its potential importance in diminishing the ill effects of mechanical ventilation merits consideration.

INTERMITTENT MANDATORY VENTILATION

The term intermittent mandatory ventilation (IMV) refers to two significantly different mechanical ventilation systems, each of which allows the patient to inhale spontaneously at the same F_{IO_2} as in the mechanical breaths.[19, 20] Thus, mean AWP is lower, and the hypocarbia that may be associated with assisted or controlled ventilation is avoided. As initially described,[19] IMV delivered mechanical Vt of 12–15 ml/kg as needed to prevent respiratory distress; PEEP was not an essential component but was added as desired. The ventilator systems initially used for IMV have characteristics that minimize the work of breathing. In these systems mechanical breaths are initiated independently of the patient's spontaneous efforts; hence uncoordinated ventilation can occur.

With both the original and the subsequent commercial systems, IMV provided a method of keeping the lung splinted open with PEEP while using high peak AWP less frequently. Thus IMV lowered the mean AWP for a given level of PEEP and perhaps reduced the risk of barotrauma. With IMV, respiratory muscles can be exercised through the entire period of ventilatory support. However, the Vt, the work done by the patient, and the coordination of spontaneous breaths vary with the system used (see Table 22–1 in chapter 22, "Technical and Semantic Aspects of Ventilator Support").

Problems and Modifications

Commercial ventilators have been developed or modified (Bourns Bear I, Bennett MA 2, Siemens) to deliver IMV. "Advantage" is taken of the patient trigger (assist) mechanism built into most ventilators to provide IMV. With the synchronized IMV systems, mechanical breaths are synchronized with the patient's effort (SIMV), and peak and mean AWP are lower.[34] But with most commercial systems spontaneous breaths require more effort by the patient because he must trigger a demand valve, and there is a delay between the patient's effort and the delivery of the gas. Most patients readily tolerate the delay and increased work inherent in these demand valve systems, but some patients with minimal ventilatory reserve struggle as the ventilator rate is decreased, and some breathe easier via a T tube than when assisted by a demand valve IMV system. Therefore, weaning with assisted ventilation and periods of spontaneous breathing through an open T tube have been recommended.[54, 56] Others find this controversy is unnecessarily polarized.[21, 55] The distinct differences and advantages of continuous flow versus demand valve (IMV vs. SIMV) systems, and the important influence of particular features in each, are still not widely appreciated. These are elaborated in chapter 22, "Technical and Semantic Aspects of Ventilator Support."

POSITIVE END-EXPIRATORY PRESSURE

Early Observations

Positive pressure for spontaneously breathing patients in pulmonary edema was recommended by Bullow in 1937[14] and Barach et al. in 1938,[4] and reevaluated by Greenbaum et al. in 1975.[30] Frumin and his associates demonstrated an increase in arterial oxygenation with PEEP in anesthetized, mechanically ventilated patients in 1959.[26] Safar in 1959 recommended that "continuous positive pressure ventilation . . . be reserved for special indications, such as pulmonary edema."[67] PEEP became widely accepted when oxygenation was improved in patients with severe ARF.[3, 45, 47] The degree of increase in Pa_{O_2} with PEEP was related to the resulting increase in lung volume.[23, 47] For example, 5 cm H_2O of PEEP produced a mean increase in Pa_{O_2} of 68 torr and in FRC of 0.35 L.[47] However, Downs et al. showed that the relation between PEEP and Pa_{O_2} is unpredictable, and that PEEP could sometimes increase shunting.[18]

The remarkable influence of continuous positive airway pressure (CPAP) on the course of infant respiratory distress syndrome (IRDS) was reported by Gregory et al. in 1971.[31] The success of CPAP given by mask[30, 62] and endotracheal tube encouraged the conceptual separation of the components of respiratory support. That is, one can choose to use independent expiratory pressure to improve oxygenation, intubation for airway protection, and inspiratory pressure to improve carbon dioxide elimination.

The value and cost of PEEP continue to be debated. The few studies reported are of unclear value even when physiologic criteria for application of PEEP are used, because the physiologic response to PEEP and therefore its appropriate application may be different from that which was presumed in those studies.[53, 69, 79]

In summary, simplistic conclusions about the effect of PEEP on outcome are inadequate. There is ample evidence showing that PEEP per se does not inherently heal or harm. In appropriate circumstances, PEEP can contribute to cardiopulmonary deterioration or to stabilization and improved function. Principles of application of PEEP are presented in chapter 22, "Technical and Semantic Aspects of Ventilator Support," and chapter 25, "The Open Lung Approach: Concept and Application." The role that PEEP and other aspects of ventilatory support might play in modifying pulmonary pathophysiology is discussed in chapter 24, "Respirator Lung."

Physiologic Criteria for Application of PEEP

The optimal level of PEEP for each patient depends entirely on which therapeutic goals are considered primary. Different goals and the physiologic criteria and *implied* premises of approaches to treatment are summarized in Table 19–2. These approaches concur in that none allows compromise of systemic oxygenation to the point of tissue dysfunction.

TABLE 19–2.

Principal Characteristics of Different Approaches to PEEP Application*

TERM	APPROACH	IMPLIED PREMISE
Best PEEP	PEEP to maximum $\dot{D}o_2$; inotrope as needed	Systemic oxygenation is the primary goal of PEEP, and any possible benefit to the lungs of further increases in FRC is not warranted if $\dot{D}o_2$ will be diminished.
High PEEP	Qs/Qt less than 12%; increase intravascular volume and inotrope as needed	There is sufficient value in maintaining the lung open that some reduction in $\dot{D}o_2$ may be acceptable but not so much as to cause tissue dysfunction
Least wedge (least PEEP)	Vasodilate, inotrope to minimize WP with adequate $\dot{D}o_2$ (PEEP only to improve Sa_{O_2})	Goal should be to minimize water in lung; neither maintenance of function (e.g., $\dot{Q}va/\dot{Q}t$) nor maintenance of structure (e.g., FRC) warrants application of PEEP if systemic oxygenation is adequate
Open lung, minimal airway pressure	Directed recruiting to open lung, splint with PEEP as needed to improve efficiency of ventilation	Lung closure has pathophysiologic consequences to lung remaining open, especially when gas exchange is inefficient; pathophysiologic cycles are broken and gas exchange is more efficient when lung is kept open

*From Snyder JV, et al.[71] Reproduced by permission.

Suter's "Best PEEP"

Suter and associates[73] administered PEEP in 3 cm H_2O increments to 15 patients with radiologically homogeneous lung dysfunction. They then correlated data with the level of PEEP at which oxygen transport was maximal, and found that the mean static compliance was highest and mean deadspace was lowest when mean oxygen transport was highest (Fig 19–1).

The study by Suter et al. was a landmark because it provided a database to document the response of the relatively homogeneously insulted lung to PEEP, and confirmed that applying PEEP could decrease alveolar deadspace and improve the efficiency of ventilation. As they subsequently explained, as PEEP is increased, alveolar overdistention eventually predominates over recruitment, with a resulting decrease in compliance, and this effect is related to a decrease in cardiac output and an increase in alveolar deadspace. They agreed that the coincidence of compliance, hemodynamic, and gas exchange zeniths depends on many variables, especially blood volume and peripheral vascular responsiveness, but they also pointed out that "such simple generalizations often have wide application in the hands of astute clinicians."[22] Their observations were difficult to reconcile with Riley's simplified approach to the mismatch of ventilation and perfusion, and therefore encouraged deeper inquiry.

Problems and Modifications. The concept that there is a level of PEEP at which oxygen transport and pulmonary static compliance are maximal and alveolar deadspace is minimal is philosophically appealing because that level would interfere least with cardiopulmonary function. The assumption that underlies the concept is that the primary goal of treatment is to improve systemic oxygen transport, without consideration of any potential benefit to the lung. We differ with this view. The findings of Suter and col-

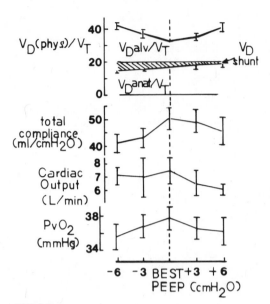

FIG 19–1.
"Best PEEP" of Suter et al. The observed correspondence of minimal alveolar deadspace *(V_Dalv/V_T)* and minimal depression of cardiac output with maximal static compliance in this group of patients gave some insight into the physiology involved. The change in direction for each factor is related to a change in the proportion of lung that is newly recruited compared with the proportion of lung that is stretched to a volume of less compliance and increased pulmonary vascular resistance. In contrast, anatomical deadspace *(V_Danat/V_T)* is shown to progressively increase, and the effect of shunting venous CO_2 to arterial blood (deadspace effect of shunt, V_D shunt) is shown to decrease as PEEP is increased. (Modified from Suter et al.[73] Reproduced by permission)

leagues are not easily applied to individual patients. As could be predicted from the wide standard deviation in the correlation between highest oxygen transport and maximal static compliance, these physiologic zeniths and nadirs may not be simultaneous in individual patients. Thus, although the PEEP at which static compliance was highest correlated with the PEEP at which oxygen transport was maximal for the entire group in Suter's study, this correlation is not reliable in individual patients. Futhermore, arterial oxygen content and therefore the level of PEEP that is optimal by Suter's definition can usually be augmented ("best" PEEP can be shifted to the right in Fig 19–1) by volume loading and inotropic support.

"High PEEP"

The application of PEEP at levels higher than that associated with maximal oxygen transport[18, 27, 42, 43] reflects a belief that PEEP per se may be beneficial to the lung. Its most obvious potential benefit would be to allow a decrease in FI_{O_2} to less toxic levels. (The toxicity of FI_{O_2} as low as 0.4 is reviewed in chapter 26, "Cellular Mechanisms in Adult Respiratory Distress Syndrome." Other possible beneficial effects of high PEEP are discussed in chapter 25, "The Open Lung Approach: Concept and Application.") The clinical evidence cited to support using high levels of PEEP is impressive, but the reported comparisons are uncontrolled,[10] and the available data are not conclusive.

Problems and Modifications. It has become apparent that when intravascular volume is adequate, the hemodynamic and pulmonary effects of increased AWP are more tolerable. The lung in ARF can tolerate higher pressures than a normal lung can. The concern regarding a high incidence of barotrauma has diminished, and chest tubes usually are not inserted prophylactically when high levels of PEEP are used. Proponents of high PEEP claimed that the lung benefited from being held open, and their approaches sought to enhance both lung function and systemic oxygenation, rather than systemic oxygenation only. The common use of IMV with higher levels of PEEP not only diminishes peak and mean AWP directly, by diminishing the number of mechanical breaths, but also may improve the efficiency of ventilation. Nonetheless the use of PEEP to expand closed lung may be more hazardous than more directed techniques. Once the lung is adequately expanded and splinted open, high PEEP may then be more safely accompanied by normal rather than high Vt.

"Least PEEP" (Least Wedge)

The approach suggested by Prewitt and Wood[33, 60, 61, 81] assumes that reductions of pulmonary edema and of FI_{O_2} levels are primary goals of ventilatory support. Changes in oxygenation and mechanical support of the lung architecture are significant only as they influence lung water content and FI_{O_2}. Prewitt and Wood attempt to minimize wedge pressure (WP) in order to decrease lung water content. Therefore, they suggest that the goals of cardiovascular management in acute hypoxemic respiratory failure should be (1) to use the lowest WP that will keep cardiac output adequate and (2) to use the least PEEP that will maintain adequate oxygen saturation of hemoglobin with a nontoxic inspired oxygen concentration. They suggest using inotropic and systemic vasodilating drugs to achieve these ends.[81]

Despite the appeal of the logic, the underlying premise that the lung water content is of primary importance in relation to function or outcome is unproved.[63, 64] The sensitivity of lung water to hydrostatic pressure in "nonhydrostatic" pulmonary edema is important to emphasize, and the use of inotropic drugs and reducing afterload to keep cardiac output adequate with minimal pulmonary capillary pressure may be beneficial in some cases. However, the variable effects of vasodilator therapy on pulmonary function,[81] the possible maldistribution of cardiac output, and a lack of data showing a change in outcome prevent acceptance of these principles as fundamental guidelines.

Effect of PEEP on Venous Admixture and on Lung Water

Because in arguments about its proper use PEEP has been stated to increase and to decrease both $\dot{Q}va/\dot{Q}t$ and lung water, those relations will be summarized. The effect of PEEP on venous admixture depends significantly on the degree of inhomogeneity of disease. Regardless of any beneficial effect PEEP might have on local V/Q, the influence of the same level of PEEP in other lung regions might cause deterioration of $\dot{Q}va/\dot{Q}t$, which is an assessment of the whole lung. For example, after acid aspiration, if much of the lung is still normal, the increased AWP associated with increased PEEP can increase pulmonary vascular resistance in the normal lung and cause increased blood flow and increased transmural capillary pressure to the insulted lung. Venous admixture is then increased while the severity of the insult is unchanged. A higher level of PEEP, a change in posture, or an effective recruiting maneuver followed by sufficient PEEP to sustain recruitment may then dramatically decrease $\dot{Q}va/\dot{Q}t$. Thus there is no reliable relation between venous admixture and either PEEP or FRC. An increase in lung water can contribute to venous admixture, but it does so indirectly and the

correlation between $\dot{Q}va/\dot{Q}t$ and lung water is also poor.[13, 68]

Even in the normal lung, lung water content is not influenced by PEEP in any single direct way. Interstitial water increases as the lung expands.[64] This may be why the application of PEEP to normal sheep lung causes a transient decrease in lymph flow, which then returns to baseline.[75] PEEP has not been shown to decrease the accumulation of fluid in the lung[17, 40, 46, 49, 51, 52, 64, 76] unless the PEEP lowered (transmural) pulmonary arterial hydrostatic pressure.[66] The latter is an important exception: PEEP does appear to diminish lung water in conditions of fluid overload.

The Influence of PEEP on Outcome: Observations in Humans

Infant Respiratory Distress Syndrome

CPAP appeared to reduce the mortality rate of IRDS from more than 75% to 25% in 20 patients, and then to zero in 16 patients.[31] Tidal volume and minute volume decreased significantly with increases in CPAP to 4, 8, and 12 torr, with no consistent change in Pa_{CO_2}. In a more recent study, administration of continuous CPAP (mean airway pressure, 6 cm H_2O) to infants with IRDS slowed the progression and then reversed the course of the syndrome, whether applied early (as soon as F_{IO_2} of 0.3 was required to maintain Pa_{O_2} at 50 torr) or late (when F_{IO_2} of 0.5 was required to maintain Pa_{O_2} at 50 torr) (Fig 19–2).[37] In addition, the early application of CPAP dramatically reduced the severity and duration of the disease, compared with later treatment (see Fig 19–2). *It may be that IRDS, once established, is a self-enhancing process; when the positive feedback is interrupted, as by CPAP, the progressive decline in function (oxygenation) is reversed and returns toward normal.*

IRDS has been ascribed to delayed maturation of alveolar epithelial cells and a consequent decrease in the production of surfactant. IRDS is usually not present at birth but develops over a few hours postnatally. Hence, whereas surfactant deficiency (or dysfunction) exists from birth, the physiologic, radiologic, and clinical changes of IRDS, which progress over hours, must be due to some additional factor that might be common to infant and adult mechanical breaths. Progressive lung closure when loss of surfactant function ex-

FIG 19–2.

Response of respiratory index $[P(A-a)_{O_2}/Pa_{O_2}]$ to early and late application of CPAP (*dashed line,* prior to CPAP; *solid line,* during CPAP). Equal progression of dysfunction in the two groups is apparent in the equal slopes prior to institution of CPAP. Improvement in function with application of CPAP is only temporary, but rate of progression of dysfunction was diminished by early and late CPAP. Ultimate severity was more limited by early CPAP. The respiratory index indicates the severity of the IRDS.[37] (From Hegyi and Hiatt.[38] Reproduced by permission.)

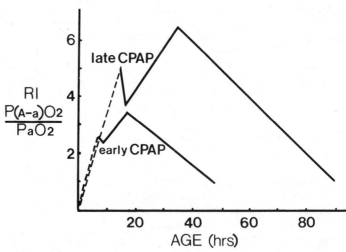

ceeds surfactant production capacity is described in chapter 24, "Respirator Lung."

Adult Respiratory Distress Syndrome

Schmidt and co-authors gave CPAP to every other adult patient in a series of 112 at risk for ARF after upper abdominal surgery.[69] All patients were mechanically ventilated in the same manner except that 8 cm H_2O PEEP was added to the treated group during mechanical ventilation. In control patients the tracheas were extubated when spontaneous ventilation was judged adequate, whereas the "treated" group received CPAP via endotracheal tubes for an additional 24 hours. The groups were well matched in all other major respects. Although the effects of bias in management cannot be ruled out, the results suggest that maintaining increased end-expiratory pressure, as summarized in Table 19–3, has some prophylactic value in prevention of both ARDS and other pulmonary complications. It would be more convincing to see benefit from such therapy if it were applied according to specific physiologic criteria rather than uniformly to all patients.

Weigelt and co-authors[79] randomly assigned 135 patients at risk for ARDS to one of two treatment groups: applicaton of PEEP, or PEEP only to treat hypoxemia. Of the 79 patients retained in the study, the 45 who received early PEEP had a lower incidence of respiratory failure, lower pulmonary-related mortality, and lower overall mortality, compared with the 34 to whom PEEP was administered only for hypoxemia. However, the

appropriateness of the criteria used in the study has been questioned.[53]

Pepe and associates gave 8 cm H_2O PEEP "early" (at the time mechanical ventilation was initiated) to 44 of 92 patients well defined to be at risk for ARDS and withheld PEEP from a similar group of 38 patients. Although there was a trend toward earlier extubation of patients who received PEEP, the difference was not statistically significant, and the incidence of ARDS was similar in the two groups.[53]

TABLE 19–3.

Effect of Prophylactic PEEP and CPAP on Respiratory Variables and Complications in 56 Treated Patients and 56 Controls*

VARIABLE	CPAP	CONTROL	P
$F_{I_{O_2}}$ at 24 hr	.34	.40	= .01
Pa_{O_2} at 24 hr (torr)	106	97	
ARDS†	1‡	10§	<.01
Other respiratory complications:			
Pneumonia	5	12	
Lobar atelectasis	1	6	
Pleural effusion	3	4	
Platelike atelectasis	1	3	
Asthma	1	0	
Total	11	25	= .01

*Data taken from Schmidt et al.[69]
†Pa_{O_2} less than 60 torr with $F_{I_{O_2}} = .6$, or decreasing Pa_{O_2} on increasing $F_{I_{O_2}}$; respiratory frequency greater than 36/minute; typical fluffy infiltrates on roentgenogram.
‡Ascribed to fluid overload and congestive failure; reversed with diuresis.
§Three died in respiratory failure.

Thus, the influence of end-expiratory pressure on outcome seems dramatic in IRDS but continues to be debated in ARDS. It is possible that other aspects of ventilator support are relevant to outcome, and that the differing conclusions of studies to date are due to failure to view the interaction between lung pathophysiology and ventilatory support on a sufficiently broad scale. Such a broad overview is presented in chapter 24, "Respirator Lung," and a related therapeutic approach is discussed in chapter 25, "The Open Lung Approach: Concept and Application."

EXTRACORPOREAL RESPIRATORY SUPPORT

Extracorporeal Membrane Oxygenation

Early observations of extracorporeal membrane oxygenation (ECMO) showed that patients could be supported for prolonged periods, but the rate of survival was low.[5, 39] Continued perfusion of the injured lung was considered to be an important mechanism of further injury, and therefore the inclusion of venoarterial bypass and the use of near-total support were emphasized.[5] Efforts to maintain the lung open prior to or during ECMO were not emphasized. Of 25 patients treated at one center, pulmonary function improved in 13 sufficiently that the patients could be removed from ECMO to conventional ventilatory support. These included 4 of 5 patients with shock lung following trauma and 4 of 4 with fat emboli; 4 of these 8 who were returned to conventional support survived. Only 4 of 12 patients with pneumonia could be removed from ECMO, and none survived. Signs considered unfavorable included a long initial illness, a persistent "severe fixed shunt," pulmonary fibrosis, increasing hypercapnia, and uncontrollable disseminated intravascular coagulation.

A prospective randomized study to evaluate prolonged ECMO concluded that it did not increase the probability of long-term survival in patients with severe ARF.[82] Again, maintenance of the lungs in an open state was not emphasized; ventilator frequency and Vt were decreased in most patients, and compliance was noted to be lower on ECMO. It is possible that lung that had been kept open with mechanical ventilation was allowed to collapse on ECMO. The mode of bypass was venoarterial, with a decrease in arterial blood flow from 3.5 to 2.4 L/m^2/min.

Extracorporeal Removal of Carbon Dioxide

Other observations made during experimental use of extracorporeal membrane perfusion to support patients in severe respiratory failure support the concept that some of the progressive lung injury may be due to mechanical ventilation. Developed and applied clinically by Kolobow and Gattinoni and their colleagues,[28, 29, 44] this approach consists of low-rate IMV with a peak AWP of 45 cm H_2O, PEEP of 15–20 cm H_2O, and venovenous bypass of 25% of cardiac output to remove most carbon dioxide. Patients are paralyzed initially, then allowed to breathe spontaneously. Weaning from bypass is started when improvement in lung compliance allows spontaneous breathing with CPAP. The approach is called low frequency positive-pressure ventilation–extracorporeal CO_2 removal (LFPPV-ECCO$_2$R). Patients were considered as candidates for the system when they (1) met the controlled ECMO study gas exchange entry criteria,[82] and (2) had a total static lung compliance lower than 30 ml/cm H_2O at 8–10 ml/kg inflation. In 17 patients for whom data are reported, the average Pa$_{O_2}$ was 50 torr when the average F$_{I_{O_2}}$ was 0.81, and Pa$_{CO_2}$ was 46 torr when minute ventilation was almost three times normal. In spite of this severity of dysfunction, 10 of the 17 recovered fully from ARF. The time on extracorporeal support was 1 to 13 days (average, 6.5). Improvement in lung function, compliance, and radiologic image occurred in these 10 patients and in 4 others who died of nonrespiratory causes. Improvement was sometimes dramatic in less than 24 hours.[28] The authors contrast this result with 90% mortality in the ECMO study, for which similar gas exchange criteria were used. It is not clear that this comparison is appropriate because the duration of illness is an important prognostic factor and is not discussed in this study. Regardless, the described changes are dramatic. This improvement could hardly have been a benefit of the extracorporeal process, and because a venovenous system was used there was no decrease in pulmonary artery blood flow or pressure. As the authors imply, the benefit may have been a result of obviating the ill effects of conventional ventilation.

HIGH-FREQUENCY VENTILATION

High-frequency ventilation (HFV) refers to a variety of ventilatory support techniques in which higher than standard respiratory rates are used. Reports of effective gas exchange with peak pressures as low as 4 torr, rates of 100 to 1,500 per minute, and tidal volumes as low as ½–2 ml/kg have excited interest in the possibility of significant modifications of ventilation patterns and have stimulated new interest in the physics and physiology of gas transport and exchange. The demonstration that gas exchange could be effectively supported using "tidal volumes" less than anatomical deadspace was startling in several respects. Simple concepts of deadspace required revision. The maintenance of oxygenation at equal levels of PEEP and lower mean AWP demonstrated that increased Vt was not necessary to keep the lung open if adequate PEEP was used and if the lung was intermittently recruited. Insight into the physiology of ventilatory support has been enhanced by observations using HFV, and conventional approaches are being modified accordingly. The optimal design and utilization of HFV remain to be developed and are discussed further in chapter 23, "High-Frequency Ventilation."

REFERENCES

1. Al-Jurf AS: Positive end-expiratory pressure (editorial). *Surg Gynecol Obstet* 1981; 152:653.

2. Anthosisen NR: Effect of volume and volume history of the lungs on pulmonary shunt flow. *Am J Physiol* 1964; 207:235.

3. Ashbaugh DG, Petty TL, Bigelow DB, et al: Continuous positive-pressure breathing (CPPB) in adult respiratory distress syndrome. *J Thorac Cardiovasc Surg* 1969; 57:31.

4. Barach AL, Martin J, Eckman M: Positive pressure respiration and its application to the treatment of acute pulmonary edema. *Ann Intern Med* 1938; 12:754.

5. Bartlett RH, Gazzaniga AB, Fong SW, et al: Prolonged extracorporeal cardiopulmonary support in man. *J Thorac Cardiovasc Surg* 1974; 68:918.

6. Bendixen HH, Hedley-Whyte J, Chir B, et al: Impaired oxygenation in surgical patients during general anesthesia with controlled ventilation. *N Engl J Med* 1963; 269:991.

7. Bendixen HH, Egbert LD, Hedley-Whyte J, et al (eds): *Respiratory Care.* Saint Louis, CV Mosby Co, 1965, p 145.

8. Blaisdell FW, Lewis FR Jr (eds): *Respiratory Distress Syndrome of Shock and Trauma: Post-Traumatic Respiratory Failure.* Philadel-

phia, WB Saunders Co, 1977, pp 151–177.

9. Bone RC, Francis PB, Pierce AK: Pulmonary barotrauma complicating positive end-expiratory pressure. *Am Rev Respir Dis* 1975; 111:921.

10. Bone RC: Treatment of adult respiratory distress syndrome with diuretics, dialysis, and positive end-expiratory pressure. *Crit Care Med* 1978; 6:136.

11. Bone RC: Treatment of severe hypoxemia due to the adult respiratory distress syndrome. *Arch Intern Med* 1980; 140:85.

12. Brievik H, Grenvik A, Millen E, et al: Normalizing low arterial CO_2 tension during mechanical ventilation. *Chest* 1973; 63:525.

13. Brigham KL, Kariman K, Harris TR, et al: Correlation of oxygenation with vascular permeability surface area but not with lung water in humans with acute respiratory failure and pulmonary edema. *J Clin Invest* 1983; 72:339.

14. Bullow JGM (ed): *The Management of the Pneumonias for Physicians and Medical Students.* New York, Oxford Medical Publications, Oxford University, 1939, p 241.

15. Cain SM: Increased oxygen uptake with passive hyperventilation of dogs. *J Appl Physiol* 1970; 28(1):4.

16. Connors AF, McCaffree DR, Rogers RM: Lung injury associated with abnormal coagulation (the microembolism syndrome). *Disease-A-Month* 27:39, 1981.

17. Demling RH, Staub NC, Edmundo LH Jr: Effect of end-expiratory airway pressure on accumulation of extravascular lung water. *J Appl Physiol* 1975; 38:907.

18. Downs JB, Klein EF, Modell JH: The effect of incremental PEEP on Pa_{O_2} in patients with respiratory failure. *Anesth Analg* 1973; 52:210.

19. Downs JB, Klein EF, Desautels D, et al: Intermittent mandatory ventilation: A new approach to weaning patients from mechanical ventilators. *Chest* 1973; 64:331.

20. Downs JB, Douglas ME: Applied physiology and respiratory care, in Shoemaker WC (ed): *The Society of Critical Care Medicine: State of the Art.* Fullerton, Calif, Society of Critical Care Medicine, 1982, vol 3, pp E:1–35.

21. Downs JB, Douglas ME: Intermittent mandatory ventilation: Why the controversy? *Crit Care Med* 1981; 9:622.

22. Fairley HB, Isenberg MD, Suter PM: Reply to: End-expiratory pressure and oxygen transport (letter). *N Engl J Med* 1975; 292:1131.

23. Falke KJ, Pontoppidan H, Kumar A, et al: Ventilation with end-expiratory pressure in acute lung disease. *J Clin Invest* 1972; 51:2315.

24. Ferris BG, Pollard DS: Effect of deep and quiet breathing on pulmonary compliance in man. *J Clin Invest* 1960; 39:143.

25. Froise AB, Bryan AC: Effects of anesthesia and paralysis on diaphragmatic mechanics in man. *Anesthesiology* 1974; 41:242.

26. Frumin MJ, Bergman NA, Holaday DA, et al: Alveolar-arterial O_2 differences during artificial respiration in man. *J Appl Physiol* 1959; 14:694.

27. Gallagher TJ, Civetta JM: Goal-directed therapy of acute respiratory failure. *Anesth Analg* 1980; 59:831.

28. Gattinoni L, Pesenti A, Rossi GP, et al: Treatment of acute respiratory failure with low-frequency positive-pressure ventilation and extracorporeal removal of CO_2. *Lancet* 1980; 8:292.

29. Gattinoni L, Pesenti A, Pellizola A, et al: Extracorporeal carbon dioxide removal in acute respiratory failure. *Ann Chir Gynaecol* 1982; 71(S196):77.

30. Greenbaum DM, Millen JE, Eross B, et al: Continuous positive airway pressure without tracheal intubation in spontaneously breathing patients. *Chest* 1976; 69:615.

31. Gregory GA, Kitterman JA, Phibbs RH, et al: Treatment of the idiopathic respiratory-distress syndrome with continuous positive airway pressure. *N Engl J Med* 1971; 284:1333.

32. Hamilton WK: Workshop on intensive care units. *Anesthesiology* 1964; 25(2):192.

33. Harrison WD, Raizen M, Ghignone M, et al: Treatment of canine low pressure pulmonary edema. *Am Rev Respir Dis* 1983; 128:857.

34. Heenan TJ, Downs JB, Douglas ME, et al: Intermittent mandatory ventilation: Is synchronization important? *Chest* 1980; 77:598.

35. Hedley-Whyte J, Laver MB, Bendixen HH: Effect of changes in tidal ventilation on physiologic shunting. *Am J Physiol* 1964; 206:891.

36. Hedley-Whyte J, Burgess GE, Feeley TW, et al (eds): *Applied Physiology of Respiratory Care,* ed 1. Boston, Little Brown & Co, 1976.

37. Hegyi T, Hiatt I: Respiratory index: A simple evaluation of severity of idiopathic respiratory distress syndrome. *Crit Care Med* 1979; 7:500.

38. Hegyi T, Hiatt I: The effect of continuous positive airway pressure on the course of respiratory distress syndrome: The benefits of early initiation. *Crit Care Med* 1981; 9:38.

39. Hill JD, Ratliff JL, Fallat RJ, et al: Prognostic factors in the treatment of acute respiratory insufficiency with long-term extracorporeal oxygenation. *J Thorac Cardiovasc Surg* 1974; 68:905.

40. Hopewell PC: Failure of positive end-expiratory pressure to decrease lung water content in alloxan-induced pulmonary edema. *Am Rev Respir Dis* 1979; 120:813.

41. Karetzky MS, Cain SM: Effect of carbon dioxide on oxygen uptake during hyperventilation in normal man. *J Appl Physiol* 1970; 28:8.

42. Kirby R, Perry J, Calderwood H, et al: Cardiorespiratory effects of high positive end-expiratory pressures. *Anesthesiology* 1975; 43:533.

43. Kirby RR, Downs JB, Civetta JM, et al: High level positive end expiratory pressure (PEEP) in acute respiratory insufficiency. *Chest* 1975; 67:156.

44. Kolobow T, Gattinoni L, Tomlinson T: An alternative to breathing. *J Thorac Cardiovasc Surg* 1978; 75:261.

45. Kumar A, Falke KJ, Geffin B, et al: Continuous positive-pressure ventilation in acute respiratory failure: Effects on hemodynamics and lung function. *N Engl J Med* 1970; 283:1430.

46. Luce JM, Robertson HT, Huang J, et al: Does positive end-expiratory pressure affect the resolution of oleic acid-induced injury in dogs? (abstract). *Am Rev Respir Dis* 1981; 123:S68.

47. McIntyre RW, Laws AK, Ramachandran PR: Positive expiratory pressure plateau: Improved gas exchange during mechanical ventilation. *Can Anaesth Soc J* 1969; 16:477.

48. Mead J, Collier C: Relation of volume history of lungs to respiratory mechanics in anesthetized dogs. *J Appl Physiol* 1959; 14(5):669.

49. Miller W, Rice D, Ugder K, et al: Effect of PEEP on lung water content in experimental noncardiogenic pulmonary edema. *Crit Care Med* 1981; 9:7.

50. Nunn JF, Bergman NA, Coleman AJ: Factors influencing the arterial oxygen tension during anaesthesia with artificial ventilation. *Br J Anaesth* 1965; 37:898.

51. Pare PD, Warrimer B, Baile EM, et al: Redistribution of pulmonary extravascular water with positive end-expiratory pressure in canine pulmonary edema. *Am Rev Respir Dis* 1983; 127:590.

52. Peitzman A, Corbett W, Shires T, et al: The

effect of increasing end-expiratory pressure on extravascular lung water. *Surgery* 1981; 90:439.

53. Pepe PE, Hudson LD, Carrico JC: Early application of positive end-expiratory pressure in patients at risk for the adult respiratory-distress syndrome. *N Engl J Med* 1984; 311:281.

54. Petty TL: IMV vs. IMC (letter). *Chest* 1975; 67:6.

55. Petty TL: In defense of IMV (letter). *Respir Care* 1976; 21:121.

56. Petty TL: Intermittent mandatory ventilation: Why the controversy? *Crit Care Med* 1981; 9:620.

57. Pontoppidan H, Geffin B, Lowenstein E: Medical progress: Acute respiratory failure in the adult. *N Engl J Med* 1972; 287:690.

58. Pontoppidan H, Geffin B, Lowenstein E: *Acute Respiratory Failure in the Adult.* Boston, Little, Brown & Co, 1973.

59. Poulton EP, Oxon DM: Left-sided heart failure with pulmonary edema: Its treatment with the pulmonary plus-pressure machine. *Lancet* 1936; 231:981.

60. Prewitt R, Wood L: Effect of sodium nitroprusside on cardiovascular function and pulmonary shunt in canine oleic acid pulmonary edema. *Anesthesiology* 1981; 55:537.

61. Prewitt R, McCarthy J, Wood L: Treatment of acute low pressure pulmonary edema in dogs, relative effects of hydrostatic and oncotic pressure, nitroprusside, and positive end-expiratory pressure. *J Clin Invest* 1981; 67:409.

62. Rasanen J, Heikkila J, Nikki P: Continuous positive airway pressure by face-mask in acute cardiogenic pulmonary edema: A randomized study (abstract). *Crit Care Med* 1984; 12(3):325.

63. Rinaldo JE: PEEP therapeutic or simply supportive for heart failure and the adult respiratory distress syndrome? (letter) *Am J Med* 1983; 75(3):448.

64. Rizk NW, Murray JF: PEEP and pulmonary edema. *Am J Med* 1982; 72:381.

65. Rogers RM (ed): *Respiratory Intensive Care.* Springfield, Ill, Charles C Thomas, Publisher, 1977.

66. Russell JA, Hoeffel J, Murray JF: Effect of different levels of positive end-expiratory pressure on lung water content. *J Appl Physiol* 1982; 53:9.

67. Safar P (ed): *Respiratory Therapy.* Philadelphia, FA Davis Co, 1965, p 123.

68. Said SI, Longacher JW, Davis RK, et al: Pulmonary gas exchange during induction of pulmonary edema in anesthetized dogs. *J Appl Physiol* 1964; 19:403.

69. Schmidt G, O'Neill W, Kotb K, et al: Continuous positive airway pressure in the prophylaxis of the adult respiratory distress syndrome. *Surg Gynecol Obstet* 1976; 143:613.

70. Shelhamer JH, Natason C, Parrillo JE: Positive end expiratory pressure in adults. *JAMA* 1984; 251:2692.

71. Snyder JV, Schuster DP, Culpepper J, et al: *Mechanical Ventilation: Physiology and Application. Curr Probl Surg* 1984, vol 21.

72. Staub NC: The pathophysiology of pulmonary edema. *Hum Pathol* 1970; 1:419.

73. Suter PM, Fairley HB, Isenberg MD: Optimum end-expiratory airway pressure in patients with acute pulmonary failure. *N Engl J Med* 1975; 292:284.

74. Suwa K, Geffin B, Pontoppidan H, et al: A nonogram for deadspace requirement during prolonged artificial ventilation. *Anesthesiology* 1968; 29:1206.

75. Taylor AE: Personal communication, 1982.

76. Toung T, Saharia P, Permutt S, et al: Aspiration pneumonia: Beneficial and harmful effects of positive end-expiratory pressure. *Surgery* 1977; 82:279.

77. Vissick WW, Fairley HB, Hickey RF: The effects of tidal volume and end-expiratory pressure on pulmonary gas exchange during anesthesia. *Anesthesiology* 1973; 39:285.

78. Weenig CS, Peitak S, Hickey RF, et al: Relationship of preoperative closing volume to functional residual capacity and alveolar-arterial oxygen deficiency during anesthesia with controlled ventilation. *Anesthesiology* 1974; 11:3.

79. Weigelt JA, Mitchell RA, Snyder WH: Early positive end-expiratory pressure in the adult respiratory distress syndrome. *Arch Surg* 1979; 114:497.

80. West JB (ed): *Ventilation/Blood Flow and Gas Exchange,* ed 2. Philadelphia, FA Davis Co, 1970.

81. Wood L, Prewitt RM: Cardiovascular management in acute hypoxemic respiratory failure. *Am J Cardiol* 1981; 47:963.

82. Zapol WM, Snider MT, Hill JD, et al: Extracorporeal membrane oxygenation in severe acute respiratory failure. *JAMA* 1979; 242:2193.

20   Pulmonary Physiology

James V. Snyder, M.D.

MECHANICS OF VENTILATION AND PERFUSION

Lung function depends on the matching of ventilation and perfusion at the local level. Local compliance and resistance to blood and gas flow in diseased lungs can vary widely in adjacent regions. Hence, both normal and abnormal physiology must be understood so that the approach to ventilatory support can incorporate principles appropriate to disparate conditions.

Determinants of Lung Volume

Observations in Normal and Insulted Lungs

Reports of changes in lung volume, such as those due to atelectasis, and the effects of efforts to prevent or reverse them usually concern lungs that are either normal or rather uniformly insulted. Review of both is reasonable preparation for planning therapy when both conditions exist in the same lung. Normal human and dog lungs undergo a decrease in compliance over 0.5 to 2 hours when ventilated spontaneously or mechanically at a normal tidal volume (Vt) in the absence of positive end-expiratory pressure (PEEP) or sighs.[31, 66] Compliance can be restored to control by raising airway pressure (AWP) to 40 cm H_2O for 10–15 sec. Bendixen et al. described a decrease in compliance of about 20% over an average of 75 minutes in anesthetized patients being mechanically ventilated with a pressure of 15–20 cm H_2O at a rate of 20–25/min.[6] Maximal compliance was restored with sustained inflation of 30 cm H_2O for 15 sec. Oxygenation but not compliance was further improved by AWP of 40 cm for 15 sec. Apparently the lower pressure left sufficient lung unrecruited that oxygenation was impaired by a small degree of venous admixture, but overall compliance was normalized. Ben-

dixen et al. also observed that atelectasis could occur and be grossly visible in the isolated lung, yet inapparent on radiographic examination.[6] Nunn et al. observed an effect of age: in anesthetized individuals under the age of 43 who did not have cardiorespiratory disease, venous admixture did not change during 1 hour of ventilation with Vt of about 10 ml/kg, but it did increase in older patients. Venous admixture could be reduced by hyperinflation of the lungs when 40 cm H_2O was maintained for 40 sec. Lower pressures and the use of 5 cm H_2O PEEP were not effective in reducing venous admixture.[73] Visick et al. observed maximal compliance and gas exchange in normal supine adults under anesthesia when Vt was 15 ml/kg, compared with 5 ml/kg or with 5 ml/kg with 10 cm H_2O PEEP.[96] Thus, normal lungs progressively decrease in volume and compliance when Vt is maintained at resting levels without sighs or PEEP. Alveolar and airway collapse can occur and is more likely in older individuals even without identified pulmonary disease (Fig 20–1). From these and other observations it seems clear that larger than normal Vt may be adequate to prevent lung closure and may not be harmful in patients with normal lungs. PEEP may be useful if closing capacity is increased owing to subtle chronic effects, but it may be unnecessary. The use of an erect position may increase functional residual capacity (FRC) above closing capacity.[19] However, once lung collapse has occurred, a sustained increase in AWP to 40 cm H_2O may be required to open normal lungs.

The response of injured lung is somewhat different. Suter et al.[93] observed that compliance, venous admixture, and the deadspace-to-Vt ratio all improved as PEEP was increased in 15 patients with diffuse acute pulmonary disease (see Fig 19–2 in chapter 19, "The Development of Supported Ventilation: A Critical Summary"). Observations in two lung models by Kolton and

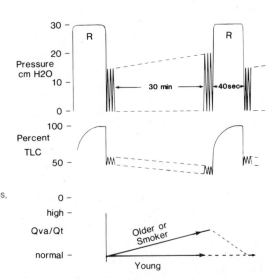

FIG 20–1.

Effect of low Vt on compliance and function in normal lungs. Sustained low (normal) Vt allows a progressive decrease in compliance. If the lung volume at which a significant number of airways close is above normal, venous admixture ($\dot{Q}va/\dot{Q}t$) can increase promptly. R denotes a sustained increase in pressure to recruit closed lung. *TLC* is total lung capacity. (Drawn from data in multiple sources, as referenced in the text.)

associates added further insightful contrasts to the findings in normal humans.[50] After rabbit lungs were surfactant-depleted by lung lavage, recruitment pressures of 30 cm H_2O were ineffectual when applied during conventional mechanical ventilation with moderate PEEP (Fig 20–2). However, when Vt was kept low (2–3 ml/kg) by

high-frequency ventilation, higher PEEP levels could be achieved using the same mean AWP as during conventional mechanical ventilation (CMV). This prevented abrupt collapse of alveoli and airways during expiration, keeping the lungs open and functioning well despite peak AWP levels that were lower than those used during CMV.

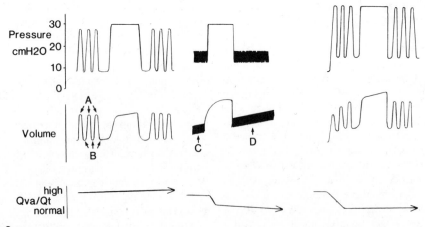

FIG 20–2.

Approximate pressure and volume changes when a surfactant-depleted lung model is ventilated with three ventilator patterns. In A no benefit is seen in either lung volume or oxygenation when recruitment pressures of 30 cm H_2O are applied for 15 seconds during CMV with Vt values of 10–15 ml/kg and 9 cm H_2O PEEP. C and D correspond to Figures 20–3, **C** and **D**. When Vt of 2–3 ml/kg is applied at 15 Hz (high-frequency oscillatory ventilation), higher PEEP is maintained for the same mean AWP, resulting in larger lung volumes and some decrease in venous admixture. A recruitment pressure of 30 cm H_2O dur-

ing HFO ventilation causes a further abrupt increase in lung volume and a decrease in $\dot{Q}va/\dot{Q}t$ that is sustained for long periods. Further gradual increases in lung volume may also occur at fixed pressure settings during HFO ventilation. A and B correspond to Figures 20–3, **A** and **B**. In C, CMV PEEP is adjusted upward to achieve mean lung volumes equal to B. These settings decrease $\dot{Q}va/\dot{Q}t$ comparably but at the cost of high peak and mean airway pressures. (Figures and related text produced in consultation with Alison B. Froese, M.D.)

Even greater gains in oxygenation and lung volume could be achieved during small-volume, high-frequency ventilation when a brief recruitment maneuver to 30 cm H_2O AWP was utilized.[49] Lung volume and oxygenation continued to improve gradually with delivery of small Vt, presumably owing in some cases to additional recruitment of closed lung. These relations are diagramed in Figure 20–2(B). In these models, the limiting factor in sustaining good oxygenation appeared to lie in the expiratory rather than the inspiratory phase of the ventilator pattern. Alveoli and airways could be opened satisfactorily by recruitment maneuvers during either CMV or high-frequency oscillation (HFO), but they could be kept open only if the minimal AWP during expiration was above the critical closing pressures of the injured lung. It is important to appreciate the rapidity with which injured lung can close after recruitment. In lung lavage and oleic acid models, and probably in injured lungs, collapse is immediate (Fig 20–3).

Thus, observations in normal individuals cannot reliably be applied to patients with pulmonary disease, and unfortunately the range of pulmonary insult that must be dealt with clinically is much more varied in severity and homogeneity than that in animal models. Understanding patients often requires integration of physiologic observations from healthy and diseased lungs, because the patient often has components of both.

Airway and Alveolar Dynamics

Analysis of lung volume dynamics must include consideration of the number of alveoli open, their compliance, effective transpulmonary pressure, airway resistance, and time. Airways in dependent lung tend to close as the normal lung is decreased in volume from FRC. Supportive tissue in the lung helps to hold airways open, but this function deteriorates after age 18. As a result, in middle-aged supine men a significant portion of the lung is closed at FRC. The number of alveoli open depends on lung volume as well as on pulmonary parenchymal factors. Lower FRC, such as occurs with pleural effusion or obesity, is likely to close additional lung in such patients. Muscle paralysis not only allows FRC to decrease, but also increases the gradient of relative alveolar volume (larger at the top, smaller at the bottom). At residual volume, about one half of the normal lung may be "closed" from the trachea.[68]

Alveolar and airway collapse depends on the mechanical properties of the walls, the surface tension–reducing properties of the film lining the walls, and the extra-alveolar forces acting to hold the walls apart.[57, 68] Figure 20–4 shows the estimated compliance curve of alveoli in normal and acutely diseased lungs. Once open, alveoli in the same state of health probably have the same compliance curve. Because of the weight of the lung, alveoli in dependent areas experience lower static transpulmonary pressure than those in nondependent areas, and are therefore smaller. The abrupt "all-or-none" opening shown in the alveolar compliance curves in Figure 20–4 differs from the progressively rising curve that characterizes inflation from residual volume of the whole lung in Figure 20–5.[91] The lower compliance of the lung at low volumes actually reflects normal compliance of fewer alveoli. The progressive rise in the curve probably reflects opening of airways and alveoli.[68] Once open, alveoli behave elastically. In normal lungs, the pressure-volume relation at lung volume greater than 50% of total lung capacity is due primarily to this elastic character, but recruitment/derecruitment is more important at lung volumes less than 40% of total lung capacity.[70]

Acute diffuse parenchymal disease decreases the number of functional lung units at any given distending pressure. The functional loss may include collapse of some airways and alveoli, and a decrease in distensibility of others. The depressed and right-shifted whole lung compliance curves seen in acute respiratory failure (ARF) (see Fig 20–5)[67, 81, 91] reflect both the changes in individual alveolar compliance and the loss of alveoli to airway obstruction and flooding. At the other extreme, any alveolus that can be expanded at all can be stretched to its elastic limit (the horizontal part of the compliance curve), at which point large increases in pressure may minimally increase volume. Overexpansion causes compression of pulmonary microvasculature and increases the probability of alveolar rupture. Because of these changes, when PEEP is added the distribution of both ventilation and perfusion to uppermost lung is likely to decrease.[43] However, the net effect on lung function is dependent on other factors, such as whether other areas of the lung are opened, the relative resistance to blood flow in dependent lung, and the influence on venous return. Standard pressure-volume curves (see Fig 20–5) show that the normal lung is fully distended by an AWP of about 30 cm H_2O. How-

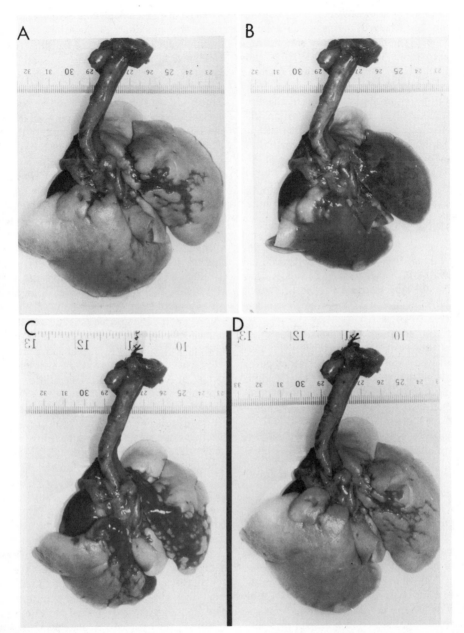

FIG 20–3.
The need for PEEP to sustain lung volume after lung injury. **A,** after injury by lavage, the lung is fairly well expanded with each mechanical ventilation of 10–15 ml/kg body weight. However, gross atelectasis recurs virtually instantaneously with every exhalation despite PEEP of 9 cm H_2O (**B**), and recruitment must be repeated with every breath. These photographs correspond to inflation and deflation (*A* and *B*) in Figure 20–2. **C,** PEEP is increased but Vt is reduced to keep AWP the same as during the ventilation in **A** and **B.** Lung volume is intermediate between **A** and **B,** and atelectasis (and recurrent recruitment) is not as severe. **D,** mean AWP is again the same as in the **A-B** pattern; the difference from **C** is only an additional recruiting maneuver, which provided the pressure required to open more alveoli, after which the higher PEEP keeps them open. **C** and **D** correspond to *C* and *D* in Figure 20–2. (From Kolton et al.[50] Reproduced by permission.)

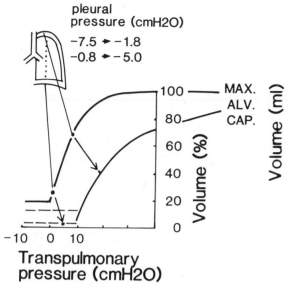

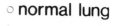

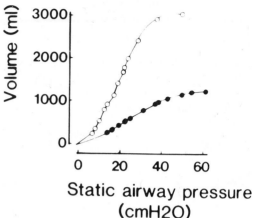

FIG 20–4.
Compliance curves of normal (*upper*) and diseased (*lower*) alveoli, in contrast to whole lung. The effect of the vertical gradient of pleural surface pressure on static distribution of gas within the normal lung and within the lung with acute parenchymal alveolar disease is apparent, as is the characteristic "all-or-none" opening. It is assumed (for simplification) that intrinsic static mechanical properties of the lungs are uniform, which is unlikely in disease. Values of pleural surface pressure at the apex and base for normal lung were computed assuming that the gradient does not change with lung volume. Pleural pressures for the diseased lung are estimates. At full inspiration all normal lung regions are expanded virtually uniformly, despite the pleural surface pressure differences down the lung, but at lower lung volumes the pleural surface pressure gradient causes the upper regions to be expanded more than the lower zones. In diseased lung, maximum alveolar capacity requires higher distending pressure, and the alveolus may have a smaller than normal volume, or may collapse completely, at end-exhalation (*dashed line*). *Max. alv. cap.*, maximum alveolar capacity. (Modified from Milic-Emili.[68] Reproduced by permission.)

FIG 20–5.
Static pressure-volume curves from two patients, one with neurogenic respiratory failure and no apparent parenchymal disease and the other with severe bilateral parenchymal disease. (From Suter et al.[91] Reproduced by permission.)

ever, individual alveolar compliance might be different, with some alveoli more compliant and some less compliant than the lung as a whole. Experimentally, when alveoli are kept from expanding, and thus stopped from restraining their neighbors (see Fig 24–2 in chapter 24, "Respirator Lung"),[27] their neighbors demonstrate improved compliance. Also, although we will usually refer to transpulmonary pressure as the distending force for the lung, alveolar expansion is a result of the *transepithelial* pressure gradient between alveolar and interstitial pressure. Because strongly negative interstitial pressures can be generated, alveolar distending forces may be considerably greater than suggested by the AWP. We shall term this pressure gradient "effective transpulmonary pressure."

Because their compliance curve is depressed and shifted to the right, diseased alveoli or airways may require a higher than normal transpulmonary pressure to open, and a greater increase in pressure for any comparable increase in volume. Thus, diseased alveoli and airways might be collapsed at FRC and not only at residual volume, and might require 30 cm H_2O or more AWP just to open. Disease factors affecting local compliance include increased elastic forces in ARF due to increased alveolar surface tension, interstitial edema, or alveoli filled with water or pus. Loss of elasticity in chronic obstructive pulmonary disease (COPD) causes increased compliance.

Effective Transpulmonary Pressure

Effective transpulmonary pressure is the distending pressure of the alveolus, that is, AWP minus local interstitial pressure. In normal lungs at FRC interstitial pressure approximates pleural pressure. Diaphragmatic contraction may generate a greater distending pressure for basilar alveoli and may be important in maintaining basilar lung volume at higher levels than have been observed in static studies.[33] Contraction of inspiratory muscles during exhalation can contribute to lower pleural pressure and increase FRC; active narrowing of the larynx during exhalation can have the same effect.[13, 17]

In nonuniformly distended lungs the local distending pressure increases in collapsed areas (Fig 20–6). This *interdependence of air space distention* supports uniform expansion of air spaces. To demonstrate this concept, Mead et al.[67] glued a number of thin-walled latex balloons to each other to simulate distal air spaces, and inflated all with the same distending pressure. A central balloon was then opened to atmospheric pressure, simulating resorption atelectasis or decreased surfactant. The resulting forces were manifest in the distortion of the balloons. Figure 20–6 shows that the open peripheral balloons open even wider. More significant for this discussion, the same forces are pulling to open the collapsing ''lung.'' Further expansion of the peripheral lung increases these forces, which are transmitted through the interstitium (glue) to pull open the part of the lung that is tending to collapse.

Implications of the Pressure-Volume Curve

Measurement of the lung and chest wall pressure-volume relationship has been suggested as having clinical application.[44, 62, 63] A widely applicable technique for measuring dynamic and static relations between pressure and volume has been described by Bone.[11] Total (lung + thorax) compliance is improved as new units (airways and alveoli) are opened and add their compliance. In normal lungs, airway closure seems to be evenly distributed in the horizontal level,[9] and the inflection point (Fig 20–7) of a pressure-volume curve may represent the point at which all airways have opened.[68] Whenever a large number of airways open at the same time in the course of lung inflation, improved compliance may be seen, with an abrupt decrease in venous admixture ($\dot{Q}va/\dot{Q}t$).[62, 64] Matamis et al. compared the inspiratory and expiratory compliance curves with blind interpretation of roentgenograms and with duration of adult respiratory distress syndrome (ARDS) in 19 patients with bilateral diffuse opacities on the chest x-ray film.[64] They saw

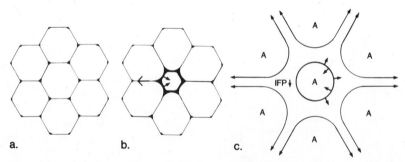

FIG 20–6.

The mechanical stabilization of adjacent air spaces (interdependence) was demonstrated in a model of thin-walled latex balloons, representing alveoli (A), glued together and inflated to equal pressure (normal, a). Any tendency of the central space to collapse, for example, owing to loss of surfactant or resorption atelectasis, tends to be countered by increased outward forces resisting the collapse (arrows, b). Similar forces are generated when the outer balloons are inflated more than the central balloon. The influence of these forces of interdependence on interstitial fluid pressure (*IFP*) is suggested in the enlargement (c): the forces tending to cause collapse, for example, an increase in surface tension (*arrows directed centrally*), stretch adjacent normal tissue and thus increase outward-acting radial stress (*large arrows along alveolar septa*). This radial stress is transmitted to the collapsed tissue hydraulically (*small outward arrows*) as well as through solid elements. Thus, local IFP becomes more subatmospheric, and transudation from enclosed vessels increases out of proportion to the change in pleural pressure. (Illustrations *a* and *b* modified from Mead et al.,[67] by permission.)

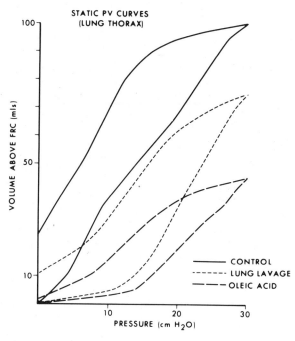

FIG 20-7.
Typical in vivo pressure-volume curves of respiratory system in control, lung lavage, and oleic acid lesions. Volumes reported are those greater than functional residual capacity (*FRC*). (From Kolton et al.[50] Reproduced by permission.)

a remarkable correlation between the alveolar patterns on the radiographs of patients with ARDS and breaks in the ascending pressure-volume curves of the patients. Similar changes in shape were seen in the ascending pressure-volume curves of rabbit lungs after lung lavage and after oleic acid infusion (see Fig 20–7).[50]

A changing slope on the ascending pressure-volume curve probably indicates that a significant number of airways close and must be reopened with every breath and that an increase in PEEP sufficient to prevent this should be considered. The pressure at which airways close, or the critical closing pressure, is lower than the critical opening pressure. Therefore, PEEP lower than the inflection point pressure might prevent collapse. While use of PEEP in this range has been associated with improvement in venous admixture in a lung lavage model,[50] diversion of blood to closed areas of the lung might counter this effect or even increase venous admixture, especially when the lung disease is nonhomogeneous.

Unfortunately, using the pressure-volume curve to find the level of PEEP at which all lung units are open does not work as well in most patients as it does in models. That is because regional lung physiology is commonly nonhomogeneous in patients. PEEP therapy improves compliance by opening collapsed air spaces (in-creased FRC), thereby placing the end-expiratory point on a steeper part of the pressure-volume curve.[91] FRC is also increased by distention of units already open, but this does not improve function or compliance. Recall that as individual lung units expand to the upper, horizontal part of the compliance curve, whole lung compliance decreases. The change in whole lung compliance is the sum of compliance changes in each part, and generalizations must be applied with caution in individual cases. Even normal lungs inflate unevenly from completely collapsed states.[1] Thus, in nonhomogeneous lung disease, even if compliance improves and venous admixture decreases with the addition of PEEP, indicating opening of a number of lung units at a particular opening pressure, a significant proportion of the lung may still be closed and stay closed until much higher airway pressures are reached. If the open lung has already reached the horizontal part of the compliance curve at the same time that the closed lung is finally opened, there may be no break in the compliance curve of the whole lung.[72] Similarly, if increasing levels of PEEP open closed lung units (tending to improve venous admixture), but at the same time overdistend open units and divert blood flow to closed parts of the lung, there may be little net effect on venous admixture until the last lung units are opened, and arterial oxygenation improves abruptly. This seems a likely explanation for the fact that changes in shunting are sometimes minimal until high levels of PEEP are applied.[47, 48, 50]

Kolton et al. compared HFO with CMV at various mean AWP levels; their findings are insightful.[50] HFO provided equal oxygenation as CMV at equal mean AWP when mean AWP was less than opening pressure. Opening pressure was defined as the upward inflection of the compliance inflation limb of the curve. However, when mean AWP was higher then opening pressure, oxygenation with HFO was better than with CMV. When lung was recruited by increasing AWP to 30 cm H_2O for 15 sec, the higher lung volume and improved oxygenation was sustained with the original HFO settings, but with the original CMV settings the lung immediately collapsed to its prerecruitment volume and level of oxygenation. In one model (lavage), oxygenation was superior with HFO at all mean AWP values greater than opening pressure, but in an oleic acid model, oxygenation was not better with HFO until mean AWP was 5–10 cm H_2O higher than opening pressure. This suggests that two mechanisms are operative in changes in venous admixture following recruitment. In the lavage model, in which oxygenation was improved with HFO at all mean AWP values greater than opening pressure, the principal influence on oxygenation is the recruitment and splinting open of closed airways and alveoli. This mechanism is also the cause of the improvement in compliance. However, failure of oxygenation to improve until mean AWP was 5–10 cm H_2O higher than opening pressure

suggests the interplay of several factors in the oleic acid model.

In the latter case, at the same time that new units were being recruited, presumably more blood was diverted to closed lung, initially causing a compensatory increase in venous admixture. A similar sequence seems to occur with stepwise addition of PEEP during CMV, as shown in Figure 20–8.

Measurement of total ''static'' compliance (Cst) is preferable to measurement of ''dynamic'' or ''effective'' compliance for the assessment of pulmonary parenchymal changes, because total Cst depends only on the elastic properties of the respiratory system, whereas dynamic compliance additionally reflects inspiratory flow and resistance of airways. In the presence of pulmonary parenchymal disease, total Cst predominantly reflects alterations in pulmonary compliance because chest wall compliance is approximately constant between FRC and total lung capacity in normal humans.[91] If Cst is observed while either Vt or PEEP is progressively increased, Cst often increases at first, then decreases again.[91] The decrease in Cst has been used as an index of the excessiveness of pulmonary overdistention relative to recruitment.[12, 28, 91, 93] Just as PEEP alters Cst by moving the end-expiratory point on the pressure-volume curve, changes in Vt alter Cst by moving the end-inspiratory point of tidal ventilation on the pressure-volume curve. With large values for Vt and at high end-expiratory pressures, ventilation reaches the upper, flatter part of the pressure-volume curve, particularly in patients with a reduced inspiratory capacity. This

FIG 20–8.
Projected effects of acid aspiration to dependent lung, and application of low and high levels of PEEP. In c, FRC is restored to normal by overdistention of lung units already open rather than by recruitment of closed lung units, and blood flow is diverted to collapsed lung. In d, a further increase in AWP has finally opened the injured alveolus and improved lung function. N, normal; ↑ indicates increase. (From Snyder et al.[87] Reproduced by permission.)

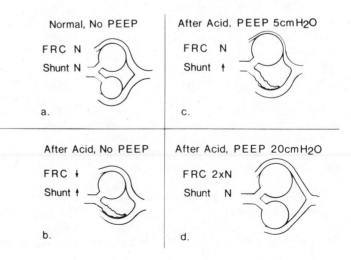

Normal, No PEEP
FRC N
Shunt N
a.

After Acid, PEEP 5cm H2O
FRC N
Shunt ↑
c.

After Acid, No PEEP
FRC ↑
Shunt ↑
b.

After Acid, PEEP 20cm H2O
FRC 2xN
Shunt N
d.

decrease in compliance is important because it warns one of overdistension of lung that is open. The possible consequences of an increase in local pulmonary vascular resistance (PVR) and of pulmonary rupture at this point should be apparent, and it should also be kept in mind that when disparate conditions coexist in an individual subject, local overdistension probably occurs at lower pressures.

Lung Volume and Time

The influence of time on lung volume and recruitment must also be considered, although it is not easy to quantify or incorporate into compliance diagrams. Its influence is clear when, after a sustained inflation, the return to a "normal" Vt causes progressive decrease in compliance and FRC and an increase in $\dot{Q}va/\dot{Q}t$ over minutes to hours (see Fig 20–1).[31, 66] In this circumstance, the lung appears to have undergone *stress relaxation* in addition to opening of closed alveoli. The term "stress relaxation" refers to a change in the elasticity of the lung according to the volume at which it is held. For example, when the lung is distended to a given volume and kept there, the tissues adapt so that elastic recoil and distending pressure actually decrease with time.[99] Prostaglandins partly mediate this change.[8] The adaptation is reversed when the lung is not fully expanded for a period of time; the lung then "creeps," or adjusts elastically, so that it contains a lower volume for a given distending pressure. Periodic "stretching" is therefore required to maintain lung compliance even when lung closure does not occur.

Another subtle influence of time is the effect of gas trapping when the expiratory time constant is long with respect to the time allowed for exhalation. This is familiar as a cause of lung overexpansion in obstructive lung disease, but it can also occur when airway resistance is normal, such as when expiratory time is diminished by increasing ventilator rates, especially during high-frequency ventilation.[2, 15, 81]

The Role of PEEP

Functional lung volume is the composite result of body posture, inspiratory muscle tone, expiratory time relative to expiratory time constant, alveolar stability, the recent pressure-volume history of the lung, and the adequate control of secretions. Each of these factors merits consideration when PEEP is used. PEEP may be required to minimize alveolar and airway closure with each exhalation. If PEEP is insufficient, some lung units opened by recruiting efforts will close during exhalation. When PEEP is sufficient to keep alveoli above their closing pressures, periodic recruiting maneuvers are usually still needed to recoup the progressive loss of tissue compliance that occurs secondary to creep, and also to reopen lung units that close as a result. A further increase in PEEP might preclude any need for recruiting and reversal of creep, but it also increases the risk of excessive peak AWP and barotrauma, especially when volume ventilators are used. A reduction in Vt simultaneous with the use of PEEP diminishes those risks.

The results of high-frequency ventilation in two lung models mentioned above support these tenets (see Figs 20–2 and 20–3). On the basis of these observations, we recommend not necessarily high-frequency ventilation but a modified approach to CMV. It is likely that a better combination of improved gas exchange and lower AWP can be obtained with CMV if every effort is made to reduce peak AWP when PEEP is increased. Reducing mechanical deadspace and Vt and increasing respiratory frequency, if necessary, are examples of techniques for reducing AWP.

Sighs Alone Versus Recruiting and PEEP to Maintain Lung Open. A Vt of 15 ml/kg can maintain better compliance and gas exchange in normal lungs than can a low Vt, even with PEEP.[96] However, abnormal surface lining may require a high distending pressure to *maintain* as well as to create distention.[50] Therefore, we should not be surprised that in experimental respiratory failure, sighing with normal Vt has not consistently improved compliance[4] or oxygenation. Sighs may not recruit collapsed lung, or the lung may recollapse rapidly.[2, 50] Airways require a higher pressure to open than is needed when they collapse. Therefore, airways need a higher pressure to be ventilated when they are allowed to collapse between sighs than when PEEP keeps them from collapsing. These factors favor the use of PEEP to sustain volume in injured lung rather than the use of high Vt or of repeated sighing to regain lost volume.

Sequential Increase in PEEP Versus Directed Recruiting to Open Closed Lung. A sustained elevation in pressure recruits collapsed lung more effectively than does a brief elevation to higher levels. Since effective recruiting is often followed by the clearing of mucus from the trachea, it may be that lung areas distal to occluding plugs are gradually expanded with gas, either directly via the enlarged bronchus, or via adjacent open lung areas through collateral pathways of ventilation such as the pores of Kohn, interbronchiolar channels of Martin, and alveolar-bronchiolar channels of Lambert.[94] Viscous and elastic forces must also be overcome, as during stress-relaxation. Finally, prostaglandin physiology seems to have an important influence on FRC, and it is altered by PEEP.[8]

In spite of these theoretical justifications, PEEP may be as unimpressive at first as sighing was in the studies mentioned above.[71] After acid aspiration in swine lungs, FRC was increased to normal with 5 cm H_2O PEEP, but oxygenation remained depressed. PEEP of 20 cm H_2O restored arterial P_{O_2} to normal levels, at a point where FRC was by then twice normal.[79] What aspect of physiology explains areas of lung collapse (manifested by depressed oxygenation) when lung volume is greater than normal? This is a common coincidence when lung units of widely different health and compliance exist in the same subject. We imagine that the increase in FRC with 5 cm H_2O PEEP in the study mentioned above was due to overdistention of the normal lung areas, with little effect on the insulted lung. In this case the focal lung injury is only exaggerating the preferential inflation of nondependent lung that occurs when tracheal pressure is increased to lungs with diffuse disease. The collapsed areas were not opened until the peak and PEEP pressures were further increased. The sequence is diagramed in Figure 20–8. Thus, incremental increases in PEEP can effectively open closed lung areas,[26, 34] but lower cardiac output and sustained overinflation of relatively normal lung, with increased risk of barotrauma and diversion of lung blood flow, may be a cost of this approach. It is possible to use body posture changes to direct the forces of recruiting to relatively specific areas. The principles of directed recruiting are described with that technique in chapter 21. Directed recruiting, combined with a lower level of PEEP than is required when PEEP alone is used for recruitment, is likely to be effective, with less risk of barotrauma or prolonged hypoperfusion. Directed recruiting should be tried in other models of alveolar injury that have not responded to conventionally applied PEEP.[5]

To summarize, when Vt is maintained at resting levels the normal lung at end-exhalation gradually shrinks, and lungs that otherwise function normally can undergo progressive alveolar and/or distal airway closure. Both increased Vt and PEEP tend to prevent loss of volume. Acute pulmonary disease, head injury, and other extra-pulmonary events decrease stability of the lung, and PEEP is required to prevent collapse. While PEEP is effective in stabilizing open lung areas, the use of increasing levels of PEEP to recruit closed parts of the lung may subject the patient to unnecessary risks, compared with the use of the combined principles of directed recruitment of closed lung plus a level of PEEP adequate to splint open the lung once it has been recruited.

Barotrauma

A major concern in the application of high AWP to open lung or to maintain lung volume is the risk of epithelial disruption. Barotrauma is related to the transepithelial pressure gradient (between alveolar and interstitial pressures) and to the degree of alveolar distention.[14, 46, 60] As hypothesized by Macklin and Macklin, the pressure differential is created by lower interstitial pressure, due to increased alveolar size (see Fig 20–6) and to decreased distending pressure in extra-alveolar vessels, and by increased alveolar pressure.[60] Air ruptures into the perivascular space and dissects proximally up vascular sheaths to the mediastinum and then can variably extend to cause subcutaneous emphysema, pneumothorax, or pneumoperitoneum. Alveolar pressure is determined largely by AWP. Interstitial pressure is altered by many factors, most of which cause it to become more subatmospheric as the lung is inflated. Interstitial pressure is also lower when the blood vessels that are passing through are not distended,[14, 54] such as those downstream from capillaries closed by distended alveoli. The site of tissue disruption is usually not noted; we would expect it to occur predominantly in superior and anterior lung. Gravity influences the pleural pressure to be lowest over this region in the semierect position, and pulmonary vessels are the least filled there. Thus, body position is likely to be a determinant of the site of barotrauma for the same reasons it can be exploited in recruiting closed lung.

While there is no firm proof, the risk of barotrauma is probably strongly influenced by any inhomogeneity of the response to each mechanical breath and to any recruiting maneuver. When lung segments are inflated to 40 cm H_2O experimentally and neighboring lung regions are prevented from inflating, the inflated segments may be distended to three to four times their normal maximum volume, which causes increased microvascular permeability[27] and increased risk of barotrauma. From observations on the pulmonary edema that occurs after expansion of atelectatic lung it appears that interstitial pressure in freshly recruited lung is considerably more negative than normal (see discussion of effects of lung expansion on interstitial fluid pressure, in chapter 24, ''Respirator Lung''). We would expect this greater increase in transepithelial pressure to further increase the risk of barotrauma. Therefore, open lung, especially when freshly recruited, may be particularly susceptible to barotrauma when adjacent areas have not responded.

The relationship between alveolar and interstitial pressure when alveolar volume is held constant is different from the pressure gradient during lung expansion. If lung volume changes insignificantly when peak AWP is increased, as during a Valsalva maneuver or cough or because of poor compliance, then interstitial pressure increases as much as alveolar pressure, the gradient is unchanged, and barotrauma is unlikely.[14] Thus, barotrauma is less likely at a given AWP in poorly compliant and homogeneously insulted lungs. Barotrauma may still occur with coughing if discrepancies in airway obstruction allow much more rapid evacuation of some areas than of others, establishing a pressure gradient sufficient to disrupt the tissue.

Several investigators have studied specific risk factors for barotrauma. (1) Increased alveolar size (without increased alveolar pressure) was investigated by Griffin, who induced barotrauma in experimental animals with alveolar expansion in a negative-pressure chamber. (2) Lenaghan et al. studied the effect of intravascular volume and showed in a closed-chested dog model that in normovolemic dogs, lung rupture occurs at 48.3 torr intratracheal pressure.[54] In dogs bled to a systolic arterial pressure of 40 torr, lung rupture occurred at 25 torr intratracheal pressure. Caldwell et al.,[14] in animal studies, found no correlation between barotrauma and the alveolar-arterial pressure gradient, but they did not measure perivascular pressure. There have been no clinical studies on the effect of intravascular volume status on barotrauma risk. (3) How much AWP

is dangerous has been the subject of many studies. Nennhaus reviewed the literature on inflation pressure and barotrauma and concluded that pressures less than 25 cm H_2O are safe, those greater than 80 cm H_2O are unsafe, and those between 25 and 80 cm H_2O are variably risky. Parker and associates demonstrated that microvascular permeability in dog lungs increased in all lungs when AWP exceeded 42 cm H_2O, but in only one experiment at a lower AWP.[74]

Most of us would agree that patients on positive-pressure ventilation are at higher risk for barotrauma if they are exposed to higher pressures. Some argue that PEEP increases the risk of barotrauma. Many series demonstrate that pneumothorax occurs more often in patients on PEEP. It is our opinion that the risk of barotrauma is indeed increased with PEEP as it is commonly applied. However, we hypothesize that this results primarily from increased peak pressure rather than from PEEP per se. Recognizing the effect of low intravascular volume on interstitial pressure, we also suspect that the use of PEEP in a relatively hypovolemic patient may be likely to potentiate barotrauma through depression of venous return. In 171 patients treated for respiratory failure with mechanical ventilation, the incidence of barotrauma was 43% when peak pressure was greater than 70 cm H_2O, 8% when peak pressure was 50–70 cm H_2O, and did not occur at pressures less than 50 cm H_2O.[75] Other studies that conclude that PEEP is the risk factor do not give data on peak pressure. In a study by Kumar et al.,[51] PEEP did not correlate with barotrauma (range of PEEP, 0–14 cm H_2O), but peak pressures greater than 36 cm H_2O did. A study of 200 patients by Cullen and Caldera[20] included only one with a pneumothorax that was related to mechanical ventilation; this patient had a peak pressure greater than 70 cm H_2O and was on 12–15 cm H_2O PEEP. (4) Other factors that may increase the risk of barotrauma in mechanically ventilated patients include aspiration pneumonia,[24] COPD,[51, 89] inflation time,[23] and poor chest compliance.[28] Additional factors that may have an effect, such as lung infarction and infection, have not been well studied. The duration of treatment with mechanical ventilation has been suggested as a risk factor but not clearly demonstrated, and the evidence is contradictory.[20, 76] Steier, de Latorre, and others have suggested that ventilation with volume-limited machines is more risky than with pressure-cycle ventilators; however, they do not provide data regarding their patients' peak pressures. In the study by Kumar et al.,[51] the type of ventilator used did not correlate with risk. It has been suggested by Kirby and others that IMV (as opposed to assist/command or command mode) may decrease the risk of barotrauma, but this possibility has not been studied. Elliott et al. reported poor compliance in patients who subsequently experienced barotrauma compared with those who did not; they decreased the incidence of barotrauma in their patients by using compliance curves to regulate Vt in patients on PEEP, but the number of patients in the study was too small for firm conclusions to be drawn.[28]

Role of Diaphragmatic Inhibition

Ford and Guenter provided a useful perspective in a recent editorial.[32] They found parallels in gas exchange and low FRC and vital capacity between patients recovering from upper abdominal surgery, obese supine patients, and those with muscle weakness or diaphragm failure, and observed that these dysfunctions did not occur following lower abdominal surgery. They recounted experimental examples of diaphragmatic inhibition after stimulation of splanchnic nerves or viscera. Patients and animals shifted from abdominal to rib cage breathing for 24–48 hours after upper abdominal surgery, and the animals demonstrated increased use of expiratory muscles, which caused lung volume to cycle below the previous FRC and passive movement of the diaphragm despite its lack of contraction. Ford and Guenter pointed out that failure of the diaphragm to contract, combined with increased expiratory effort, may be responsible for the changes in gas exchange and lung volume, as well as for failure of analgesia and standard respiratory therapy maneuvers to abolish postoperative respiratory complications. They suggested that the reflex inhibition of the diaphragm might be overridden voluntarily and might be effectively compensated for by continuous positive airway pressure (CPAP).[32]

Distribution of Ventilation

The determinants of local ventilation are local compliance, local airway resistance, and the local change in transepithelial pressure. Local alveolar compliance in normal lung depends on relative alveolar volume, which in turn depends on the gravity-oriented position of the alveolus in the lung and on total lung volume, as indicated in

Figure 20–4.[68] With spontaneous ventilation at normal FRC, ventilation of the lung base is greater than ventilation of the apex. However, at low lung volumes the proportion of gas delivered to upper lung units is greater than that delivered to dependent units, because the lower units are closed.[68]

Airway resistance varies with airway edema, interstitial elasticity, bronchoconstriction, and physical obstruction from collapse or mucus. Airway caliber increases with local alveolar expansion and is diminished in atelectatic lung;[71] these influences might be partly mediated by prostaglandins.[8]

Transpulmonary pressure may be altered more at the lung base than in the higher lung by diaphragmatic contraction at the lung base (Fig 20–9).[33] The resulting distribution of ventilation to dependent lung is an important aspect of the efficiency of spontaneous ventilation.[3, 41, 78, 84]

Distribution of Perfusion

The distribution of regional perfusion in normal erect lung at normal FRC is diagramed in Figure 20–10.[100 (p 42)] Determinants of regional perfusion are gravity, lung volume, local changes in interstitial pressure, vasomotor tone, and vascular change due to disease processes such as fibrosis and hepatic cirrhosis. Gravity causes a decrease in pulmonary arterial (PA) pressure up the lung and an increase in PA pressure and venous distention (which decreases venous resistance) down the lung. Gravity also influences the degree of lung expansion, with secondary effects on perfusion. Interstitial pressure is higher (less subatmospheric) in dependent lung; this elevation of interstitial pressure is likely to be the basis of the decrease in blood flow seen in the most dependent lung, as shown in Figure 20–10.

The effects of lung volume on vessel lumina and therefore on vascular resistance differ for vessels exposed directly to alveolar pressure (alveolar vessels) and for those not subject to direct pressure from the alveolus (extra-alveolar vessels).[45] The cumulative effect of lung volume on these separable beds is shown in Figure 20–11. PVR is least at normal end-expiratory lung volume; lung collapse increases resistance to flow through extra-alveolar vessels, and lung expansion causes flow resistance by compression of alveolar vessels. These effects of lung volume on vascular resistance occur with regional lung volume changes as well. Thus, as open lung areas

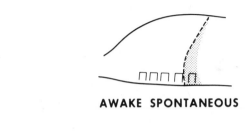

AWAKE SPONTANEOUS

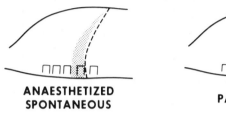

**ANAESTHETIZED
SPONTANEOUS**

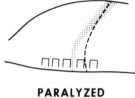

PARALYZED

FIG 20–9.
Diaphragm position and placement during tidal breathing in supine subjects. *Dashed line* denotes control functional residual capacity (FRC) position of the diaphragm. *Shaded area* represents diaphragmatic excursion during tidal breathing. FRC is lower with anesthesia and paralysis. Ventilation is directed posteriorly when spontaneous, and anteriorly when mechanical. (From Froese et al.[33] Reproduced by permission.)

become more distended by increased PEEP, more flow may be diverted to less distended regions, resulting in an increase in high V/Q regions.[77] In fact, PEEP-induced improvement in Pa_{O_2} in many patients may be wholly explained on the basis of changes in distribution of blood flow.[77] Patients who have a sufficient intravascular volume may not show this.[63]

In addition to the effect of lung volume, pulmonary vascular resistance may increase with hypoxia, acidemia, and increased sympathetic stim-

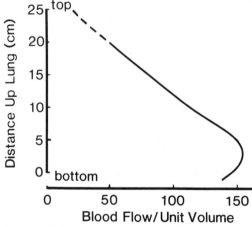

FIG 20–10.
Distribution of blood flow according to vertical level in the lung. Flow is diminished in nondependent lung by gravity and by compression of alveolar vessels if Paw is increased. Flow may be diminished in the less expanded dependent lung by increased interstitial pressure and by hypoxic vasoconstriction. (From West.[100] Reproduced by permission.)

ulation. The influence of hypoxia is immediate, whereas reduction of flow due to atelectasis may occur over an hour.[25] Because flow to unventilated lung is diminished, hypoxic pulmonary vasoconstriction (HPV) tends to improve overall gas exchange.[38, 95]

The increased PVR seen in ARF may be due to alveolar compression of capillaries in inflated lung, HPV, and increased interstitial pressure in collapsed lung; microembolism and macroembolism, and in situ thrombosis;[40] and to arterial wall thickening and disruption or disappearance of the pulmonary vascular bed.[86] On the other hand, PVR has been calculated to be closer to normal in respiratory insufficiency with high levels of PEEP when intravascular volume and cardiac output are maintained.[35] HPV has been shown experimentally to increase pulmonary edema if flow is constant;[70] other causes of increased vascular resistance probably have the same effect. The degree of vasoconstriction varies in different individuals.[69]

HPV is diminished by increased cardiac output,[85] increased $P\bar{v}_{O_2}$,[92] sepsis, and multiple drugs,[55, 97] including the prostaglandin inhibitor indomethacin,[39] and in proportion to left atrial pressure (LAP).[7] Inhibition of pulmonary vasomotor tone can alter the response to PEEP by allowing easier diversion of blood flow from overdistended to still closed lung.[95] Inhibition of HPV also can occur as a side effect of the inflammatory response to pneumonia or systemic sepsis.[56] This might explain why $\dot{Q}va/\dot{Q}t$ in septic patients seems poorly responsive to PEEP, in that blood flow is more easily diverted from normal lung to

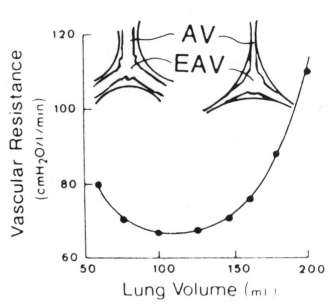

FIG 20–11.
Effect of lung volume on pulmonary vascular resistance when the transmural pressure of the capillaries is held constant. At low lung volumes, resistance is high because the extra-alveolar vessels (*EAV*) become narrow. At high volumes, the alveolar vessels (*AV*) are stretched and their caliber is reduced (data from a dog lobe preparation). (Modified from West.[100] Reproduced by permission.)

poorly ventilated lung when the vessels of the latter remain unconstricted.[18] On the other hand, agents that enhance HPV might improve V/Q distribution and in particular might diminish the diversion of blood flow from open to closed lung when AWP is increased.[80]

Increased collateral circulation is a possible explanation for large gradients between the obstructed PA pressure (wedge pressure, WP) and LAP reported in five septic patients[53] and with nitroprusside therapy following cardiac surgery.[61] Thus, WP may be 5–10 torr higher than LAP in patients receiving vasodilators[61] and has been reported to be up to 25 torr higher than LAP in sepsis.[53] These observations need to be verified. The clinical implication is that such individuals may have inadequate intravascular volume despite an elevated WP.

Gas Transport and Exchange

Riley Analysis Versus V/Q Distribution

Riley and Cournand[79] suggested that the lung can usually be thought of as consisting of three kinds of alveoli: those that are ventilated and perfused "normally" (V/Q = 1), those perfused but not ventilated (shunt unit, V/Q = 0), and those ventilated but not perfused (deadspace). We can calculate from arterial and mixed venous blood gases and $F_{I_{O_2}}$ the degree to which the lung behaves as though it were shunting venous blood past nonventilated alveoli:

$$\dot{Q}va/\dot{Q}t = (Cc_{O_2} - Ca_{O_2})/(Cc_{O_2} - C\bar{v}_{O_2})$$

where Cc_{O_2} is calculated pulmonary end-capillary oxygen content, and Ca_{O_2} and $C\bar{v}_{O_2}$ are measured arterial and mixed venous oxygen contents.

With a few other assumptions, the deadspace is calculated:

$$Vd/Vt = (Pa_{CO_2} - P\bar{E}_{CO_2})/Pa_{CO_2}$$

where Vd/Vt is the fraction of Vt that is "wasted" and $P\bar{E}_{CO_2}$ is mixed expired P_{CO_2}.

Although these simplifications by Riley and Cournand are useful, one must not forget that alveoli vary in function through a continuum. The problem with the Riley approach is the tendency to ignore regional inhomogeneities.[63, 77] For example, many physicians have come to think of alveolar P_{CO_2} as equal to arterial P_{CO_2}. Alveolar P_{CO_2} actually varies according to local V/Q, from low values in high V/Q areas to values at least as high as mixed venous blood in low V/Q areas. The term alveolar P_{CO_2} (PA_{CO_2}) refers to a conceptual average value. We usually think of improvement in Vd/Vt as due to less ventilation or more perfusion of high V/Q areas; however, improved ventilation of low V/Q areas can have a dramatic effect on carbon dioxide elimination, as shown in the decline in deadspace when PEEP was initially increased in patients with diffuse pulmonary insults (see Fig 19–2 in chapter 19, "The Development of Supported Ventilation: A Critical Summary").[65, 93] To summarize this contrast, we can note that ventilation of dependent lung is usually more efficient than ventilation of nondependent lung; but reference to the recruitment and ventilation of closed lung as a decrease in Vd/Vt does little to explain the mechanism. The term *efficiency of gas exchange* is more suggestive of the physiology involved than this concept of deadspace. It was because of similar problems with simplistic interpretations of the term "pulmonary shunt" ($\dot{Q}s/\dot{Q}t$) that the term "venous admixture" ($\dot{Q}va/\dot{Q}t$) was introduced. The terms "shunt effect" or "equivalent shunt" and "deadspace effect" or "effective deadspace" are also useful efforts to emphasize the distinction.

Riley was justified in his simplistic summary of gas exchange. As summarized by Farhi,[29] many of us, "understandably perturbed at being asked to look simultaneously at oxygen uptake, carbon dioxide output, ventilation, perfusion, gas exchange ratio, and partial pressures of O_2 and CO_2 in the inspired gas, in the alveoli, and in the mixed venous blood, have given up the seemingly hopeless struggle."[29] We were therefore well served and escaped considerable hardship by the gift of these idealized concepts of shunt and deadspace. Thirty-five years later we seem able to manipulate therapy with sufficient focus that some reexploration of the underlying physiology is required. As a practical matter for those practicing and developing intensive care medicine, the relations need to be restated only to the level of complexity that is useful to current therapy. Hence, the terms venous admixture and efficiency of ventilation are compromises encouraging deeper inquiry into the underlying assumptions. For those "hardy souls willing to make one more attempt to unravel these relationships and probe their implications," Farhi's exposition is an excellent source.[29]

A number of circumstances relate to the efficiency of carbon dioxide elimination. Mixed venous carbon dioxide content ($C\bar{v}_{CO_2}$) increases with an increased metabolic rate, an increased respiratory quotient, or a decreased cardiac output. In these circumstances an inefficient system, such as occurs when there is ventilation predominantly of high V/Q areas, will be less able to compensate for the elevated $C\bar{v}_{CO_2}$, and arterial P_{CO_2} will also rise. Another variable relating to efficiency of carbon dioxide elimination is F_{IO_2}. Transfer of carbon dioxide from the capillaries to the alveoli, in low V/Q areas where incomplete

arterial oxygen saturation is obtained, can be improved by increasing F_{IO_2}. This phenomenon is due to the fact that the binding of oxygen by hemoglobin causes release of chemically bound carbon dioxide, with subsequent elevation of first capillary and then alveolar P_{CO_2}. This is a consequence of the Haldane effect, which has been credited with about half of the total carbon dioxide elimination.[49] Prolonging the inspiratory phase of mechanical ventilation by adding a pressure-maintained plateau increases the time for alveolar-capillary equilibration in the expanded state. PEEP is another variable in carbon dioxide elimination efficiency. There are two mechanisms (at least) by which PEEP might decrease "deadspace" that do not involve "ventilated but unperfused alveoli." First, the addition of PEEP recruits and splints open alveoli that were closed. These are converted from true shunt alveoli to units with low V/Q. Alveoli with low V/Q have a high alveolar P_{CO_2}. Any portion of Vt that is now distributed to these carbon dioxide–rich alveoli was previously distributed to alveoli with a higher V/Q and lower carbon dioxide concentration. Therefore, more carbon dioxide molecules are eliminated with the same Vt. Second, it is interesting to conjecture that one of the causes of increased Vd/Vt in ARDS may be related to limitation of diffusion of carbon dioxide into the alveolus. That is, injured lung units may not open until near the end of inspiration and may close immediately after exhalation begins; the time spent open can be quite short. In addition, the change in volume can be relatively quite large, especially since the starting volume might be nil. Capnograms in ARDS patients commonly demonstrate that airway carbon dioxide is lower than normal throughout the early part of exhalation. This suggests that the alveolar gas exhaled first is from high V/Q (low carbon dioxide) regions. Yet we would expect the least compliant and therefore rapidly emptying alveoli to be in the lung base where perfusion is high, V/Q should be low, and PA_{CO_2} should be high. This observation could be explained by the relatively large but very brief expansion of these dependent alveoli, proposed above. If equilibration cannot occur during the brief period of expansion of the basilar alveoli at high AWP, the carbon dioxide from these early emptying alveoli will be low despite their low V/Q ratios. The time for carbon dioxide equilibration would be enhanced either by the addition of sufficient PEEP to prevent lung closure or by the incorporation of an inspiratory plateau. Since carbon dioxide equilibration occurs very quickly, it is no surprise that washout of an inert gas was not improved by incorporating an inspiratory hold during ventilation of animals,[22] but such studies look only at ventilation and do not adequately account for local perfusion or V/Q. Therefore such findings are not necessarily relevant to carbon dioxide elimination or exchange of more soluble gases. Thus, efficiency of dependent lung carbon dioxide elimination may improve without change in local minute ventilation or perfusion.

The clinical implications of the physiology discussed above are apparent when a patient in respiratory failure due to a diffuse pulmonary insult finally requires endotracheal intubation and mechanical support.

CASE 20–1.—Thirty minutes prior to intubation, an exhausted but previously healthy patient with viral pneumonitis sat at 60 degrees, breathing spontaneously with tidal volumes of 400 ml at a rate of 35/min. Exhaled minute volume was 14 L/min. After intubation it was discovered that Vt settings of 1,000 ml at a frequency of 20/min (minute volume of 20 L/min) were required to achieve the same level of Pa$_{CO_2}$, at which the patient's ventilation was controlled. Although mean AWP increased from -2 cm H$_2$O to $+15$ cm H$_2$O, intrapulmonary shunt was increased. (The data in this case are comparable to observations in many patients, simplified to present changes clearly.)

Comment.—The principal reasons gas exchange became so inefficient—that is, "deadspace" and "shunt" increased so much—are the following. (1) Anatomical deadspace increases with inflation pressure. (2) Nondependent lung should be most compliant in acute parenchymal lung disease and therefore should receive the first and perhaps most of the Vt, yet it is least efficient at gas transport (high ventilation to perfusion ratio). (3) If higher inspiratory flow is used to deliver higher Vt, distribution to nondependent lung is favored because the latter is less resistant to flow.[3] The result is even more wasted ventilation. (4) The greater distention of alveoli due to increased transpulmonary pressure in nondependent lung is likely to compress adjacent pulmonary capillaries, causing redistribution of blood flow to "shunt" vessels in closed, dependent lung[10] and making both oxygenation and carbon dioxide elimination less efficient. (5) Loss of regional mechanics: the diaphragm is no longer directly pulling open the dependent, low V/Q lung, which

is the most efficient region in terms of carbon dioxide elimination. Local V/Q decreases further, resulting in increased venous admixture.[84]

If the addition of PEEP improves the efficiency of carbon dioxide elimination, it may be possible to decrease minute ventilation, as by decreasing Vt to minimize the increase in peak inspiratory pressure, without increasing Pa$_{CO_2}$. However, increases in PEEP that do not significantly recruit closed lung are likely to decrease efficiency of ventilation.[10, 93] Therefore, as lung is recruited and splinted open with PEEP, it might be possible to simultaneously decrease venous admixture, F$_{IO_2}$, and peak inspiratory pressure with no increase in carbon dioxide or mean AWP and no decrease in cardiac output. The changes actually seen in each application vary, however, in part because lung disease is rarely homogeneous. Improved ventilation of low V/Q areas should be a primary goal in manipulation of therapy for the patient.

Quantitation of Alveolar Efficiency

In spite of our conceptual objections, the efficiency of carbon dioxide elimination is reasonably summarized in the measurement of Vd/Vt. Because efficiency of carbon dioxide elimination is an important determinant of minute ventilation and therefore of peak and mean AWP, it may be more useful to monitor this variable than is suggested by current practice. Simple methods for doing so are summarized in chapter 31, "Ventilatory Support of the Failing Circulation." Vd/Vt is weighted toward the ventilation component of "deadspace"; quantitation of the blood flow components of gas exchange efficiency is improved by more accurate calculation of *pulmonary end-capillary carbon dioxide concentration* (Cc$_{CO_2}$), similar to the calculation of average Pa$_{CO_2}$. Cc$_{CO_2}$ is derived as follows.[52] Ca$_{CO_2}$ is the sum of the products of C$\bar{v}_{O_2}$ times the fraction of the cardiac output that is not involved in gas exchange, and Cc$_{CO_2}$ times the fraction of cardiac output that perfuses ventilated alveoli:

$$Ca_{CO_2} = C\bar{v}_{CO_2} \times \dot{Q}s/\dot{Q}t + Cc_{CO_2}\,(1 - \dot{Q}s/\dot{Q}t) \quad \text{(Eq. 20–1)}$$

Solving equation 20–1 for Cc$_{CO_2}$:

$$Cc_{CO_2} = \frac{Ca_{CO_2} - C\bar{v}_{CO_2} \times \dot{Q}s/\dot{Q}t}{1 - \dot{Q}s/\dot{Q}t}$$

$$\text{(Eq. 20–2)}$$

The end-capillary carbon dioxide content of capillaries perfusing ventilated alveoli (Cc_{CO_2}) is dependent on (1) the carbon dioxide load presented to the alveoli, that is, $C\bar{v}_{CO_2}$ multiplied by the rate of blood flow past ventilated alveoli; (2) the efficiency of transfer of carbon dioxide from blood to these alveoli; and (3) the volume and timing of ventilation of these alveoli.

WORK OF BREATHING AND RESPIRATORY MUSCLE FUNCTION

The mechanical work done on the lungs to move air is called work of breathing. Work of breathing can be expressed as $W = P(dV)$, where W denotes work, P denotes change in pressure, and dV denotes the sum of volume changes.

The respiratory muscles must overcome elastic, flow-resistive, and inertial forces in order to move this volume of gas for ventilation. The lung compliance curve graphing measured AWP against inhaled and exhaled volume changes can be used to diagram work done on the lung. Transmural pressures are used to assess elastic and flow-resistive work; or pleural pressure can be used to include externally imposed work (Fig 20–12).

If the patient's curve is abnormally shifted down and to the right, as in ARDS, more pressure will be required to move the same volume, and elastic work will therefore be increased. Similarly, the position on the compliance curve (for example, the FRC) will affect work: at the extremes of low and high FRC, more pressure is needed to move volume. In addition, any increase in Vd/Vt increases work as more total minute ventilation is required to eliminate carbon dioxide. An increase in carbon dioxide production, as from higher oxygen consumption or respiratory quotient, increases work by the same mechanism. Consider the effect of CPAP on the work of breathing. Normal lungs may be distended to the less compliant part of the compliance curve and undergo an increase in Vd/Vt, and inspiratory muscles may be shortened to a less efficient length and position.[30, 59] All these factors can increase the work of breathing.[36] However, CPAP could expand a diffusely injured lung to a more compliant condition and diminish airway resistance, requiring less work to move the same volume, and also improve efficiency of carbon dioxide elimination, thus requiring lower minute ventilation to eliminate the same carbon dioxide load; because of these reductions in work, oxygen consumption and the carbon dioxide load would decrease further.

Flow-resistive work is seen in this diagram as the further pressure required to overcome such factors as turbulence and friction (see Fig 20–12).

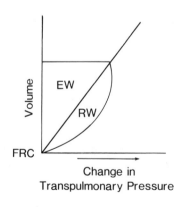
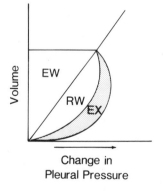

FIG 20–12.
Pressure and lung volume changes during inspiration. When the transpulmonary pressure is used to calculate the work of inspiration (*left*) the result is the sum of the work of overcoming elastic (*EW*) and resistive (*RN*) forces in the lung. The external work load related to an inspiratory drop in AWP is literally subtracted out of the work estimate. The external work load is included when pleural pressure is used to calculate work (*right*). To maintain the same inspiratory flow and volume when inspiratory AWP is allowed to drop, the additional drop in pleural pressure must equal the change in AWP. Therefore, the external work load can be calculated as the product of the change in AWP and the sum of volume changes. More simply, the external work load is proportional to the decrease in AWP over time.

Determining work by measuring pressures and volumes, as discussed above, cannot evaluate the amount of inertial work done or antagonistic work done by muscles working paradoxically against those moving air. Another approach to measuring work of breathing is to assess changes in oxygen consumption with incremental changes in level of ventilation. If all other variables are constant, the change in oxygen consumption must be due to the change in ventilatory work done. This technique has inherent difficulties, as the method of causing increasing ventilation (e.g., carbon dioxide inhalation vs. voluntary hyperventilation) may itself affect oxygen consumption.

When the muscle demand for energy needed to accomplish the work of breathing exceeds the energy supplied to it, muscle fatigue and then failure occurs.[58, 82] Factors increasing the demand of muscles for energy include more work to be done (e.g., tachypnea, stiff lungs), poor muscle efficiency (hyperinflation), and increased carbon dioxide production (shivering, fever, or working hard to breathe). Factors affecting the energy supply to muscles include low cardiac output or hemoglobin, poor nutritional status, and impaired muscle perfusion. The maximally contracting diaphragm may even impair its own perfusion.

Thus, an imbalance of energy supply and demand leads to muscle fatigue. Fatigue is manifested progressively by tachypnea, the recruiting of accessory muscles, an alternating pattern of muscle use, paradoxical muscle motion, discoordination, and finally ventilatory failure. In this way muscle failure may provide a final common pathway for respiratory failure due to many different precipitating causes. That this phenomenon is clinically relevant has been shown by several authors,[16, 37] who have demonstrated that abnormal muscle function correlates with respiratory deterioration and difficulty in weaning from mechanical ventilation.

Treatment of fatigued muscles includes treatment of the underlying conditions, adequate oxygenation, improving regional V/Q to reduce deadspace (which is wasted ventilation and therefore wasted work), improving lung compliance to reduce the work of breathing, and resting the fatigued muscles (mechanical ventilation). In addition, theophylline can be administered to increase diaphragmatic contractility. Rest is most important if muscle fatigue is already established. Mechanical ventilation for up to 48 hours may be required for relief of muscle fatigue. In some pa-

tients with chronic muscle dysfunction, respiratory muscle training may be useful. Resistive endurance training may enhance exercise endurance and the ability to tolerate the activities of daily living in COPD patients.[88] Similarly, muscle training has improved respiratory muscle endurance and strength and prevented fatigue in quadriplegic patients.[42]

The implications of respiratory muscle physiology for the management of mechanical ventilators have not yet been clarified. The basic principles that the muscles should be properly rested before they are put to work and that muscles should not be allowed to atrophy seem straightforward. The best way to achieve these goals is currently being debated.[98] Intermittent mandatory ventilation (IMV) is advocated by some as permitting ongoing muscle exercise to prevent atrophy, but giving enough machine support to avoid fatigue. Because the external work load imposed by various IMV circuits varies widely, statements about the value and role of IMV should be made and interpreted cautiously. On the other hand, other writers have advocated the use of assisted ventilation to provide complete rest for fatigued muscles, followed by T tube weaning to provide progressive muscle training, adequately resting the muscles with assisted ventilation between T tube trials. Some clinicians advocate decreasing the sensitivity of the assist sensor on the mechanical ventilator used in the assist mode, which thereby requires the patient to work harder to initiate mechanical breaths, as an exercise for respiratory muscles. Good clinical studies of the effect of mechanical ventilation and weaning mode on respiratory muscle function have not been done.

THE SPECTRUM OF SPONTANEOUS TO CONTROLLED VENTILATION

The Effect of Spontaneous Ventilation on Systemic Perfusion

The effect of spontaneous ventilation is to enhance venous return to the right side of the heart, and simultaneously to inhibit left ventricular systole. Ventilation by positive AWP has the opposite effects. Both effects occur through the influence of ventilation on pleural pressure. The effect on venous return is more pronounced in hypovolemia; the effect on left ventricular systole is more pronounced when contractility is compromised and ample venous return is ensured. Both spontaneous and mechanical inspiration to high alveolar volumes can increase right ventricular afterload.[101] Thus, an intravascular volume status that is appropriate for spontaneous ventilation without PEEP commonly proves inadequate when AWP is increased, and an intravascular volume status appropriate for high pressure ventilation is excessive at lower AWP. Also, the function of a poorly contracting left ventricle may be significantly impaired by negative pleural pressure (spontaneous ventilation) and augmented by positive pleural pressure. These relations are explored more completely in chapter 21, "Hemodynamic Effects of Artificial Ventilation," and chapter 32, "Ventilatory Support of the Failing Circulation."

Spontaneous Versus Assisted Versus Controlled Ventilation

Currently available mechanical ventilators provide a continuous spectrum of ventilation patterns, from spontaneous ventilation to complete mechanical support.

The distribution of V and Q and the resulting efficiency of gas exchange for both carbon dioxide and oxygen are generally best with spontaneous ventilation. The diaphragm most effectively inflates dependent alveoli and dependent vessels are better perfused because of gravity. However, several additional factors must be considered. These are patient exhaustion, cardiac output, and venous pressure. It is obviously more work for a patient to breathe spontaneously than to be ventilated by a machine. This is true regardless of how inefficient gas exchange with mechanical ventilation might be, or how much AWP or pleural pressure might increase, or how cardiac output and venous pressure might be affected. When the patient is unable to ventilate spontaneously, for example, because of paralysis or exhaustion, the costs of controlled ventilation must be borne. The principal advantages of mechanical ventilation are relief for the patient from the work of breathing and the recruiting effect of increased transpulmonary pressure. Also, the left ventricular afterload and preload reduction by positive pressure ventilation may benefit some patients. The differences in the spectrum from spontaneous to controlled ventilation are diagramed in Figure 20–13. Review of these multiple simultaneous effects emphasizes that the op-

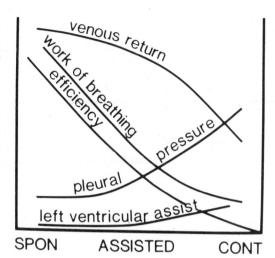

Ventilation Pattern

FIG 20–13.
Spectrum of spontaneous (*Spon*) to controlled (*Cont*) ventilation. Pleural pressure and venous return are inversely related, as are efficiency and transpulmonary inflation pressure. The exact relations will vary widely; those shown are arbitrary. Significant left ventricular assistance usually requires special apparatus. (From Elliott and Snyder.[27a] Reproduced by permission.)

timal ventilation pattern for a given patient depends on the current physiology of that patient.

A consideration sometimes raised against assisted ventilation is that of respiratory alkalemia, which some authors feel occurs less frequently with IMV. Severe respiratory alkalemia can usually be avoided during assisted ventilation if Vt is limited to 10 ml/kg.[21]

IMV Versus Assisted Ventilation/T Tube Program for Weaning

The more rapidly support is withdrawn and the more unstable the patient's condition, the more closely the patient must be observed. Because IMV allows weaning in minute steps, less frequent observations may suffice for most of a prolonged weaning phase. Likewise, assisted ventilation permits less frequent observation than does low IMV ventilation. We have occasionally observed weaning to proceed more slowly than necessary when either IMV or T tube weaning is used by formula or habit rather than by consideration of the patient's capacity and needs. The patient should usually be allowed to resume spontaneous ventilation as soon as he or she is capable, with extubation as soon as it is safe. Use of a demand valve system for spontaneous breaths is acceptable when the patient can easily initiate ventilation, and may be preferable when lack of coordination with the ventilator results in "bucking." When the patient's ventilatory reserve is borderline, however, the use of a continuous flow system with a low-resistance circuit PEEP valve is important to minimize the work of spontaneous breathing. How the components of the circuit influence the work of breathing is described in chapter 21, "Hemodynamic Effects of Artificial Ventilation."

Patients may be taken abruptly from assisted ventilation to a T tube, but they must be closely observed during the transition, especially if they are weaned from PEEP at the same time. When mechanical ventilation is removed, maintenance of CPAP diminishes the threat of lung closure and excessive increase in venous return.

Acknowledgment

The author thanks Judith A. Culpepper, M.D., for her insightful review of these concepts.

REFERENCES

1. Anthonisen NR: Effect of volume and volume history of the lungs on pulmonary shunt flow. *Am J Physiol* 1964; 207:235.

2. Askanazi J, Wax SD, Neville JF, et al: Prevention of pulmonary insufficiency through prophylactic use of PEEP and rapid respiratory rates. *J Thorac Cardiovasc Surg* 1978; 75:267.

3. Bake B, Wood L, Murphy B, et al: Effect of inspiratory flow rate on regional distribution of inspired gas. *J Appl Physiol* 1974; 37:8.

4. Balsys AJ, Jones RL, Man SFP, et al: Effects of sighs and different tidal volumes on compliance, functional residual capacity and arterial oxygen tension in normal and hypoxemic dogs. *Crit Care Med* 1980; 8:641.

5. Barrett CR, Bell AL, Ryan SF: Effect of positive end-expiratory pressure on lung compliance in dogs after acute alveolar injury. *Am Rev Respir Dis* 1981; 124:705.

6. Bendixen HH, Hedley-Whyte J, Chir B, et al: Impaired oxygenation in surgical patients during general anesthesia with controlled ventilation. *N Engl J Med* 1963; 269:991.

7. Benumof JL, Wahrenbrock EA: Blunted hypoxic pulmonary vasoconstriction by increased vascular pressures. *J Appl Physiol* 1975; 38:846.

8. Berend N, Christopher KL, Boekel NF: The effect of PEEP on functional residual capacity of prostaglandin production. *Am Rev Respir Dis* 1982; 126:646.

9. Bindslev L, Hedenstierna G, Santesson J, et al: Airway closure during anaesthesia, and its prevention by positive and expiratory pressure. *Acta Anaesthesiol Scand* 1980; 24:199.

10. Bindslev L, Hedenstierna G, Santesson J, et al: Ventilation-perfusion distribution during inhalation anaesthesia. *Acta Anaesthesiol Scand* 1981; 25:360.

11. Bone RC: Diagnosis of causes for acute respiratory distress by pressure-volume curves. *Chest* 1976; 70:740.

12. Bone RC, Francis PB, Pierce AK: Pulmonary barotrauma complicating positive end-expiratory pressure. *Am Rev Respir Dis* 1975; 111:921.

13. Bryan AC: Maintenance of an elevated FRC in the newborn. *Am Rev Respir Dis* 1984; 129:209.

14. Caldwell EJ, Powell RD, Mulooly JP: Interstitial emphysema: A study of physiologic factors involved in experimental induction of the lesion. *Am Rev Respir Dis* 1970; 102:516.

15. Cartwright DW, Willis MM, Gregory GA: Functional residual capacity and lung mechanics at different levels of mechanical ventilation. *Crit Care Med* 1984; 12:422.

16. Cohen CA, Zagellaum G, Gross D, et al: Clinical manifestations of inspiratory muscle fatigue. *Am J Med* 1982; 73:308.

17. Collett PW, Brancatisano T, Engel LA: Changes in the glottic aperture during bronchial asthma. *Am Rev Respir Dis* 1983; 128:719.

18. Cotev S, Perel A, Kalzenelsen R, et al: The effect of PEEP on oxygenating capacity in acute respiratory failure with sepsis. *Crit Care Med* 1976; 4:186.

19. Craig DB, Wahba WM, Don HF, et al: "Closing volume" and its relationship to gas exchange in seated and supine positions. *J Appl Physiol* 1971; 31:717.

20. Cullen DJ, Caldera DL: The incidence of ventilator-induced pulmonary barotrauma in critically ill patients. *Anesthesiology* 1979; 50:185–190.

21. Culpepper J, Rinaldo J, Grenvik A, et al: Effect of ventilator mode on tendency to respiratory alkalosis (abstract). *Am Rev Respir Dis* 1983; 127:104.

22. Dammann JF, McAslan C, Maffeo CJ: Optimal flow pattern of mechanical ventilation of the lungs. *Crit Care Med* 1978; 6:293.

23. Day R, Goodfellow AM, Apgar V, et al: Pressure-time relations in the safe correction of atelectasis in animal lungs. *Pediatrics* 1952; 10:593.

24. de Latorre FJ, Tomasa A, Klamburg J, et al: Incidence of pneumothorax and pneumomediastinum in patients with aspiration pneumonia requiring ventilatory support. *Chest* 1977; 72:141.

25. Domino KB, Chen L, Alexander CM, et al: Time course and responses of sustained hypoxic pulmonary vasoconstriction in the dog. *Anesthesiology* 1984; 60:562.

26. Downs JB, Klein EF, Desautels D, et al: Intermittent mandatory ventilation: A new approach to weaning patients from mechanical ventilators. *Chest* 1973; 64:331.

27. Egan EA: Lung inflation, lung solute permeability, and alveolar edema. *J Appl Physiol* 1982; 53:121.

27a. Elliott JL, Snyder JV: Non-relation between alveolar ventilation and Pa_{CO_2}. *Crit Care Med* 1979; 7:134.

28. Elliott CG, Morris AH, Cengiz M, et al: Ventilatory mechanisms and pneumothorax in the adult respiratory distress syndrome (ARDS) (abstract). *Am Rev Respir Dis* 1978; 117(S):111.

29. Farhi LE: Ventilation-perfusion relationship and its role in alveolar gas exchange, in Caro CG (ed): *Advances in Respiratory Physiology*. Baltimore, Williams & Wilkins Co, 1966, p 149.

30. Farkas GA, Roussos CH: Acute diaphragmatic shortening: In vitro mechanics and fatigue. *Am Rev Respir Dis* 1984; 130:434.

31. Ferris BG, Pollard DS: Effect of deep and quiet breathing on pulmonary compliance in man. *J Clin Invest* 1960; 39:143.

32. Ford GT, Guenter CA: Toward prevention of postoperative pulmonary complications. *Am Rev Respir Dis* 1984; 130:4–5.

33. Froese AB, Bryan AC: Effects of anesthesia and paralysis on diaphragmatic mechanics in man. *Anesthesiology* 1974; 41:242.

34. Gallagher TJ, Civetta JM: Goal-directed therapy of acute respiratory failure. *Anesth Analg* 1980; 59:831.

35. Gallagher T, Civetta J: Normal pulmonary vascular resistance during acute respiratory insufficiency. *Crit Care Med* 1981; 9:647.

36. Gherini S, Peters RM, Virgilio RW: Mechanical work of the lungs and work of breathing with positive end-expiratory pressure and continuous positive airway pressure. *Chest* 1979; 76:251.

37. Gilbert R, Ashutosk K, Auchincloss JH: Clinical value and observations of chest and abdominal motion in patients with pulmonary emphysema. *Am Rev Respir Dis* 1977; 119:155.

38. Glasser SA, Domino KB, Lindgren L, et al: Pulmonary blood pressure and flow during atelectasis in the dog. *Anesthesiology* 1983; 58:225.

39. Gordon JB, Wetzel RC, Gioia FR, Sylvester JT: Indomethacin blocks the attenuation of the hypoxic pulmonary vascular response seen with high frequency ventilation (abstract). *Crit Care Med* 1984; 12:322.

40. Greene R, Zapol W, Snider M, et al: Early bedside detection of pulmonary vascular occlusion during acute respiratory failure. *Am Rev Respir Dis* 1981; 124:593.

41. Grimby G, Hedenstierna G, Lofstrom B: Chest wall mechanics during artificial ventilation. *J Appl Physiol* 1975; 38:576.

42. Gross D, Ladd HW, Riley EJ, et al: The effect of training on strength and endurance of the diaphragm in quadriplegia. *Am J Med* 1980; 68:27.

43. Hammon JW, Wolfe WG, Moran JF, et al: The effect of positive end-expiratory pressure on regional ventilation and perfusion in the normal and injured primate lung. *J Thorac Cardiovasc Surg* 1976; 72:680.

44. Holzapfel L, Robert D, Perrin F, et al: Static pressure-volume curves and effect of positive end-expiratory pressure on gas exchange in adult respiratory distress syndrome. *Crit Care Med* 1983; 11:591.

45. Howell JBL, Permutt S, Proctor DF, et al: Effect of inflation of the lung on different parts of pulmonary vascular bed. *J Appl Physiol* 1961; 16:71.

46. Kao DK, Tierney DF: Air embolism with positive pressure ventilation of rats. *J Appl Physiol* 1977; 42:368.

47. Kirby R, Perry J, Calderwood H, et al: Cardiorespiratory effects of high positive end-expiratory pressures. *Anesthesiology* 1975; 43:533.

48. Kirby RR, Downs JB, Civetta JM, et al:

High level positive end expiratory pressure (PEEP) in acute respiratory insufficiency. *Chest* 1975; 67:156.

49. Klocke RA: Mechanism and kinetics of the Haldane effect in human erythrocytes. *J Appl Physiol* 1973; 35:673.

50. Kolton M, Cattran CV, Kent G, et al: Oxygenation during high frequency ventilation compared with conventional mechanical ventilation in two models of lung injury. *Anesth Analg* 1982; 61:323.

51. Kumar A, Pontoppidan H, Falke KJ, et al: Pulmonary barotrauma during mechanical ventilation. *Crit Care Med* 1973; 1:181.

52. Kuwabara S, Duncalf D: Effect of anatomic shunt of physiologic deadspace to tidal volume ratio: A new equation. *Anesthesiology* 1969; 31:575.

53. Lefcoe MS, Sibbald WJ, Holliday RL: Wedged ballon catheter angiography in the critical care unit. *Crit Care Med* 1979; 7:449.

54. Lenaghan R, Silva YJ, Walt AJ: Hemodynamic alterations associated with expansion rupture of the lung. *Arch Surg* 1969; 99:339.

55. Leventhal JP, Parsons GH, Hansen MM, et al: Effect of sodium nitroprusside on hypoxic pulmonary vasoconstriction (abstract). *Am Rev Respir Dis* 1979; 119(S):329.

56. Light RB, Mink S, Wood LDH: The pathophysiology of gas exchange and pulmonary perfusion in pneumococcal lobar pneumonia dogs. *J Appl Physiol* 1981; 50:524.

57. Macklem PT, Murphy B: The forces applied to the lung in health and disease. *Am J Med* 1974; 57:371.

58. Macklem PT: Respiratory muscles: The vital pump. *Chest* 1980; 78:753.

59. Macklem PT: Hyperinflation (editorial). *Am Rev Respir Dis* 1984; 129:1.

60. Macklin MT, Macklin CC: Malignant interstitial emphysema of the lungs and mediastinum as an important occult complication in many respiratory diseases and other conditions: An interpretation of the clinical literature in the light of laboratory experiment. *Medicine* 1944; 23:281.

61. Mammana RB, Hiro S, Levitsky S, et al: Inaccuracy of pulmonary capillary wedge pressure when compared to left atrial pressure in the early postsurgical period. *J Thorac Cardiovasc Surg* 1982; 84:420.

62. Mankikian B, Lemaire F, Benito S, et al: A new device for measurement of pulmonary pressure-volume curves in patients on mechanical ventilation. *Crit Care Med* 1983; 11:897.

63. Matamis D, Lemaire F, Harf A, et al: Redistribution of pulmonary blood flow induced by positive end-expiratory pressure and dopamine infusion in acute respiratory failure. *Am Rev Respir Dis* 1984; 129:39.

64. Matamis D, Lemaire F, Harf A, et al: Total respiratory pressure-volume curves in the adult respiratory distress syndrome. *Chest* 1984; 86:58.

65. McIntyre RW, Laws AK, Ramachandran PR, et al: Positive expiratory pressure plateau: Improved gas exchange during mechanical ventilation. *Can Anaesth Soc J* 1969; 16:477.

66. Mead J, Collier C: Relation of volume history of lungs to respiratory mechanics in anesthesized dogs. *J Appl Physiol* 1959; 14:669.

67. Mead J, Takishima T, Leith D: Stress distribution in lungs: A model of pulmonary elasticity. *J Appl Physiol* 1970; 28:596.

68. Milic-Emili J: Pulmonary statics, in Widdicombe JG (ed): *MTP International Review of Sciences: Respiratory Physiology*. Physiology series, vol 2. Baltimore, University Park Press, 1974, p 127.

69. Miller MA, Hales CA: Stability of alveolar hypoxic vasoconstriction with intermittent hypoxia. *J Appl Physiol* 1980; 49:846.

70. Mitzner W, Sylvester JT: Hypoxic vasoconstriction and fluid filtration in pig lungs. *J Appl Physiol* 1981; 51:1965.

71. Murtagh PS, Proctor DF, Permutt S, et al: Bronchial mechanics in excised dog lobes. *J Appl Physiol* 1971; 31:403.

72. Nielson D, Olsen DB: The role of alveolar recruitment and derecruitment in pressure and volume hysteresis in lungs. *Respir Physiol* 1978; 32:63.

73. Nunn JF, Bergman NA, Coleman AJ: Factors influencing the arterial oxygen tension during anaesthesia with artificial ventilation. *Br J Anaesth* 1965; 37:898.

74. Parker JC, Townsley MI, Rippe B, et al: Increased microvascular permeability in dog lungs due to high peak airway pressures. *J Appl Physiol* 1984; 57:809.

75. Peterson GW, Baier H: Incidence of pulmonary barotrauma in a medical ICU. *Crit Care Med* 1983; 11:67.

76. Pollack MM, Fields AI, Holbrook PR: Pneu-

mothorax and pneumomediastinum during pediatric mechanical ventilation. *Crit Care Med* 1979; 7:536.

77. Ralph DD, Robertson T, Weaver J, et al: Distribution of ventilation and perfusion during positive end-expiratory pressure in the adult respiratory distress syndrome. *Am Rev Respir Dis* 1985; 131:54.

78. Rehder K, Sessler D, Rodarte JR: Regional intrapulmonary gas distribution in awake and anesthetized-paralyzed man. *J Appl Physiol* 1977; 42:391.

79. Riley RL, Cournand A: Ideal alveolar air and the analysis of ventilation-perfusion relationships in the lungs. *Alveolar Air Relations* 1979; 1:825.

80. Romaldini H, Rodriquez-Roisin R, Wagner PD, et al: Enhancement of hypoxic pulmonary vasoconstriction by Almitrine in the dog. *Am Rev Respir Dis* 1983; 128:288–293.

81. Rose D, Downs J, Heenan T: Temporal responses of functional residual capacity and oxygen tension to changes in positive end-expiratory pressure. *Crit Care Med* 1981; 9:79.

82. Roussos C, Macklem PT: The respiratory muscles. *N Engl J Med* 1982; 307:786.

83. Saari AF, Rossing TH, Solway J, et al: Lung inflation during high-frequency ventilation. *Am Rev Respir Dis* 1984; 129:333–336.

84. Schmid E, Rehder K: General anesthesia and the chest wall. *Anesthesiology* 1981; 55:668.

85. Schumacker PT, Newell JC, Saba TM, et al: Ventilation-perfusion relationships with high cardiac output in lobar atelectasis. *J Appl Physiol* 1981; 50:341.

86. Snow RL, Davies P, Pontoppidan H, et al: Pulmonary vascular remodeling in adult respiratory distress syndrome. *Am Rev Respir Dis* 1982; 126:887.

87. Snyder JV, Carroll GC, Schuster DP, et al: *Mechanical Ventilation: Physiology and Application. Curr Probl Surg* 1984, vol 21.

88. Sonne LJ, Davis JA: Increased exercise performance in patients with severe COPD following inspiratory resistive training. *Chest* 1982; 81:436.

89. Steier M, Ching N, Roberts EB, et al: Pneumothorax complicating continuous ventilatory support. *J Thorac Cardiovasc Surg* 1974; 67:17.

90. Summer WR, Permutt S, Sagawa K, et al: Effects of spontaneous respiration on canine left ventricular function. *Circ Res* 1979; 45:719.

91. Suter PM, Fairley HB, Isenberg MD: Effect of tidal volume and positive end-expiratory pressure on compliance during mechanical ventilation. *Chest* 1978; 73:158.

92. Suter PM, Fairley HB, Schlobohm RM: Shunt, lung volume, and perfusion during short periods of ventilation with O_2. *Anesthesiology* 1975; 43:617.

93. Suter PM, Fairley HB, Isenberg MD: Optimum end-expiratory airway pressure in patients with acute pulmonary failure. *N Engl J Med* 1975; 292:284.

94. Terry PB, Traystman RJ, Newball HH, et al: Collateral ventilation in man. *N Engl J Med* 1978; 298:10.

95. Thomas HM, Garrett RC: Strength of hypoxic vasoconstriction determines shunt fraction in dogs with atelectasis. *J Appl Physiol* 1982; 53:44.

96. Visick WD, Fairley HB, Hickey RF: The effects of tidal volume and end-expiratory pressure on pulmonary gas exchange during anesthesia. *Anesthesiology* 1973; 39:285.

97. Weir EK: Hypoxic pulmonary vasoconstriction (editorial). *Chest* 1982; 82:519.

98. Weisman IM, Rinaldo JE, Rogers RM, et al: Intermittent mandatory ventilation. *Am Rev Respir Dis* 1983; 127:641–47.

99. West JB: *Regional Differences in the Lung.* New York, Academic Press, 1977.

100. West JB: *Respiratory Physiology: The Essentials,* ed 2. Baltimore, Williams & Wilkins Co, 1979.

101. Whittenberger J, McGregor M, Berglund E, et al: Influence of state of inflation of the lung on pulmonary vascular resistance. *J Appl Physiol* 1960; 15:878.

21

The Hemodynamic Effects of Artificial Ventilation

Michael R. Pinsky, M.D.

The widespread use of positive pressure ventilation in critically ill patients has shown that the resulting complex cardiopulmonary interactions can significantly affect cardiovascular homeostasis. Since oxygen transport to the tissues is a function both of arterial oxygen content and of cardiac output, it is important to understand how positive pressure ventilation affects the circulation. The goal of this chapter is to differentiate between the hemodynamic effects of artificial ventilation and those of spontaneous ventilation. These effects are due to mechanical[15, 20] and neurohumoral reflex mechanisms.

The heart, existing within the thorax, is a pressure chamber within a pressure chamber. Thus, changes in intrathoracic pressure (ITP) will affect the pressure gradient for blood returning to the chest (venous return)[21] and leaving the chest (left ventricular output).[9] Similarly, as lung volumes change, pulmonary vascular resistance[69] and capacitance[43] vary, and at high lung volumes, mechanical heart-lung interactions may occur.[68] All of these changes can affect cardiac performance. Since ITP rises during positive pressure inspiration and falls during spontaneous inspiration, the effects of positive pressure ventilation on cardiovascular performance may not be the same as those of spontaneous ventilation even though lung volumes may increase to a similar extent with both modes of breathing. To better understand these dynamics we will evaluate the effects of fixed changes in airway pressure (AWP), ITP, and lung volume on right ventricular (RV) and left ventricular (LV) performance. An analysis of the dynamic effects of spontaneous (negative pressure) and positive pressure ventilatory cycles on cardiac performance will follow. The chapter ends with a discussion of the different artificial ventilatory modes available.

RIGHT VENTRICULAR PERFORMANCE

Preload

At any level of cardiac contractility and heart rate, RV systolic performance is determined by diastolic (preload) and systolic (afterload) components. The force of ventricular contraction is directly related to end-diastolic myocardial fiber length.[42] For the RV this fiber length may be proportional to end-diastolic volume, as it is for the LV.[61] This comparison has not been made because it is difficult to measure RV volume. The irregular and varying shape of the RV makes contrast angiography inaccurate.[21] First-pass radionuclide angiocardiography can measure RV ejection fraction[32] and by inference can estimate RV volume. Equilibrium-gated blood pool imaging has also been used, but it is difficult to separate RV volumes from overlying vascular structures. Sibbald et al.,[59] however, have found that equilibrium-gated blood pool imaging yielded reproducible results. They demonstrated that RV end-diastolic volume (RVEDV) correlates with RV stroke volume. Changes in RVEDV (preload), in turn, are determined by the diastolic compliance of the ventricle and its filling pressure. RV diastolic compliance may decrease in response to acute chamber dilation, ischemia, neurohumoral stimulation, or overdistention of the LV (reverse interdependence).[63] RV distending pressure is the intracavitary pressure minus extracavitary (pericardial) pressure. Extracavitary pressure rarely equals atmospheric pressure, and during respiration may fluctuate widely. Therefore, to accurately estimate RV distending pressure, this extracavitary pressure may be measured. In practice, it is extremely difficult to measure pericardial pressure. If the pericardium does not limit diastolic filling, the pleural pressure can be used to approximate pericardial pressure.

Pleural Pressure

Pleural pressure is the pressure in the pleural space between the inner surface of the chest wall and the outer surface of the lung. Pleural pressure throughout most of the thorax at end-expiration is negative relative to atmospheric pressure, because the lungs and chest wall are above and below their resting volumes, respectively. Measuring pleural pressure is problematic, primarily because gaining access to the pleural space is difficult and methods of estimating the pressure are inaccurate. Since pleural pressure at end-expiration is negative, if the pleural space is exposed to atmospheric pressure air will passively enter the pleural space. Thus, placing a measuring catheter in the pleural space may result in a pneumothorax by the inadvertent entry of air. The measured pressure may not represent pleural pressure over other areas of the lung or when the air is evacuated. To circumvent this problem, esophageal pressure can be measured as an estimate of pleural pressure.[34] Although esophageal pressure swings follow negative swings in pleural pressure during spontaneous inspiration in upright humans, esophageal pressure may underestimate positive swings in pleural pressure, because of the stinting effect of the mediastinum or the esophagus on intraluminal esophageal pressure. When pleural pressure is measured directly, it is important to remember that pleural surface pressure may not be the same as pleural fluid pressure. When the chest wall and lung are separated by fluid, pleural surface and fluid pressures are equal. However, when the two surfaces oppose each other, as they do normally, local deformational pressures are produced that decrease pleural fluid pressure but do not change pleural surface pressure.[1] Under most conditions, it is the pleural surface pressure that is physiologically important. Thus, for measuring pleural surface pressure, the measuring device should be small and flat enough not to deform the pleural space. Although pleural pressure has been measured with chest tubes, fluid-filled catheters, and collapsible soft plastic

catheters, it is most accurately quantitated with air-filled, thin-walled balloon catheters, of which various types are available.[33]

Intrathoracic Pressure and the Concept of Transmural Pressure

Since measurements of pleural pressure are used to estimate pericardial pressure, pleural pressure should be measured near the pericardium—the juxtacardiac pleural pressure. Not all measurements of pleural pressure reflect juxtacardiac pleural pressure because ITP is not uniform throughout the thoracic cavity.[68] As lung volume increases, juxtacardiac pleural pressure increases relative to lateral chest wall pleural pressure, as the heart is compressed between the two expanding lungs. Many studies use lateral chest wall pleural pressure to calculate transmural cardiac pressures, and thus may underestimate increases in juxtacardiac pleural pressure induced by increasing lung volumes. However, small changes in juxtacardiac pleural pressure can usually be inferred from changes in either lateral chest wall pleural pressure or esophageal pressure since the degree of error is small. To simplify the discussion in this review, we will assume ITP to be a common pressure throughout the pleural and pericardial space. Since the RV receives its blood from the right atrium, which is easily deformed by ITP, RV distending pressure can be approximated as right atrial pressure (RAP) minus ITP, or transmural RAP. The driving pressure for venous return from the body to the heart, however, is determined by the pressure gradient between the small systemic veins and RAP, both measured relative to atmospheric pressure.[21] Since the right atrium is an intrathoracic structure, changes in ITP will directly affect RAP. During spontaneous inspiration, for example, as ITP becomes more negative RAP will also decrease. Thus, the pressure gradient between the systemic veins and the right atrium increases, accelerating venous blood flow.[5] Spontaneous inspiration is usually associated with an increase in venous return, which manifests itself as an increase in both transmural RAP and RVEDV (preload), augmenting RV stroke volume. By increasing ITP, positive pressure inspiration increases RAP, thus decreasing the pressure gradient for venous return and decelerating venous blood flow.[36] This decrease in venous return decreases transmural RAP and RVEDV, which in turn decrease RV stroke volume and, ultimately, cardiac output. The reciprocal change in RAP and transmural RAP (RV filling pressure) during both spontaneous (intermittent negative-pressure) breathing and intermittent positive-pressure breathing (IPPB) is shown in Figure 21–1. Note that RAP tends to follow pleural pressure. The resulting reciprocal change in venous blood flow into the RV induces a parallel change in transmural RAP. These fluctuations in RAP during ventilation should not be confused with the steady-state effect of intravascular volume loading on RAP and transmural RAP. With volume loading, both mean RAP and transmural RAP increase, although their phasic reciprocal relation persists.

Venous Return and ITP

Since the pressure gradient for venous blood flow can be defined as RAP minus the hydrostatic pressure in the small venules,[21] the driving pressure can decrease from an increase in RAP, a decrease in peripheral venous pressure, or both. Thus the decrease in the pressure gradient for venous return during positive pressure breathing is exacerbated by any condition that decreases venous pressure in the periphery, such as hypovolemia or decreased vasomotor tone. The decrease can be minimized by decreasing mean ITP (decreasing mechanical inspiratory time or increasing inspiratory flow rate for a fixed tidal volume, Vt) to decrease RAP,[4] or by infusing volume or using vasotonic agents to increase systemic venous pressure.[27] Remember, however, that when pulmonary parenchymal compliance is low, AWP increases do not increase ITP as much as when lung compliance is normal.[18] Thus, in patients with stiff lungs, artificial ventilation may have less of an effect on venous return and overall cardiovascular homeostasis than would be expected if the lungs were normal.

Right Ventricular Afterload

RV afterload can be defined as RV systolic wall stress, which is a function of end-diastolic volume and systolic RV pressure.[31, 61] Since the RV and the pulmonary circulation are surrounded by an ITP that may not equal atmospheric pressure, functional systolic RV pressure is more accurately defined as pulmonary artery pressure (PAP) relative to ITP, that is, transmural PAP. Increases in transmural PAP impede RV ejection. If the RV does not eject as completely, RV end-systolic volume will increase and stroke volume will initially decrease, causing an increase in RVEDV. For cardiac output to remain unchanged, RV filling pressures must be further increased to compensate for the increased afterload. This increase in transmural RAP causes a parallel increase in absolute RAP. Although chronically increased sympathetic tone and fluid retention increase the upstream pressure and return the pressure gradient for venous return toward normal, so that cardiac output is normal despite elevated transmural PAP,[19] acute elevations of transmural PAP may profoundly compromise hemodynamic function. Transmural PAP may increase either from a passive backup of pressure from the LV or from increased pulmonary vascular resistance (PVR).

Most increases in transmural PAP seen during artificial ventilation are caused by increased PVR. As lung volume increases above functional

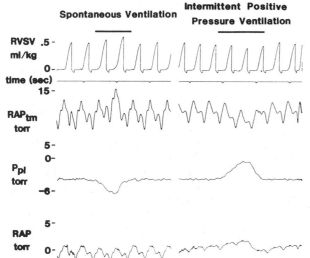

FIG 21–1.
Trend recordings of, from bottom to top, right atrial pressure (*RAP*), juxtacardiac pleural pressure (*P_pl*), RAP measured relative to pleural pressure, called transmural RAP (*RAP_tm*), and right ventricular stroke volume (*RVSV*) during spontaneous (*left*) and positive pressure (*right*) breathing in intact anesthetized dogs. Inspiration is depicted as solid bars. Note that RAP and P_pl follow each other, but that RAP_tm (right ventricular filling pressure) moves in the opposite direction. As RAP_tm varies so does RVSV on the subsequent beat. See text for discussion.

residual capacity (FRC), PVR increases as alveolar vessels are compressed.[43] Overdistention of the lungs, as occurs with obstructive airway disease, large Vt ventilation, or the application of excessively high positive end-expiratory pressure (PEEP), will increase PVR. Normal resting Vt is about 5–10 ml/kg,[64] which increases PVR at end-inspiration in a normal lung by no more than 12%.[58] Accordingly, Piene and Sund[44] have noted that RV systolic performance changes minimally during normal ventilation. Therefore, changes in lung volume occurring during normal ventilation in patients without pulmonary hypertension do not affect RV performance through increases in PVR. Artificial ventilation may actually decrease PVR in certain conditions. In acute respiratory failure, resting lung volumes are often below FRC and alveolar hypoxia may be present.[48] When lung volume falls below FRC, PVR also rises from compression of extra-alveolar vessels. In addition, hypoxia can increase PVR by inducing vasoconstriction.[2] If artificial ventilation increases the concentration of oxygen in the alveoli or returns lung volume to its normal end-expiratory level, then PVR may decrease. Canada et al.[12] have recently demonstrated that in a dog model with normal lungs, increasing end-expiratory volumes by the use of 10 cm H_2O PEEP increases PVR. After the induction of acute respiratory failure by oleic acid the same amount of PEEP decreases PVR. Thus, the effects of positive pressure ventilation on RV performance depend on the degree to which venous return is compromised and PVR is affected. In most patients, however, positive pressure ventilation increases RAP, either by passive transmission of ITP to intrathoracic venous structures or by RV dilation secondary to increases in PVR. Increasing RAP decreases the pressure gradient for venous return[21, 46] and decelerates venous blood flow, and thus cardiac output is lower during IPPB than during spontaneous breathing.[16] *The most common and important hemodynamic effect of artificial ventilation is to decrease cardiac output by decreasing the pressure gradient for venous return.*

LEFT VENTRICULAR PERFORMANCE

LV performance, like RV performance, is determined by its preload (LV end-diastolic volume, LVEDV), contractility, afterload (systolic wall stress), and heart rate (HR).[54] When LV contractility is not reduced, LV stroke volume is regulated by the Frank-Starling mechanism and depends primarily on LVEDV. Small changes in HR or LV afterload, as may occur during positive pressure ventilation, do not significantly change stroke volume.[42]

LV Preload and Ventricular Interdependence

Artificial ventilation can significantly alter LVEDV in several ways. First, as described in the previous section on RV performance, if RAP increases due to an increase in either ITP or RV afterload, venous return will decrease. This must eventually decrease pulmonary venous blood flow and LVEDV. Second, since LVEDV is determined by LV diastolic compliance and distending pressure, changes in either will change end-diastolic volume. If the RV dilates during artificial ventilation (because lung inflation increases the RV systolic pressure), LV diastolic volume may be compromised in two ways: leftward shift of the interventricular septum[7] may decrease LV diastolic compliance (ventricular interdependence), or the semirigid pericardium may limit absolute biventricular end-diastolic volume.[8, 23] If septal shift is responsible for a decrease in LVEDV, then LV diastolic compliance should decrease, whereas if the pericardium limits LV diastolic filling, then LV compliance will not change but pericardial pressure will rise and LV distending pressure will fall. Marini and associates[28] directly measured pericardial pressure in dogs and found that increasing positive airway pressure decreased LV distending pressure but did not decrease diastolic compliance. When LV distending pressure was returned to control levels LV performance returned to normal. Similarly Rankin and colleagues[53] studied the deformational characteristics of the LV in dogs with normal lungs using ultrasonic crystals to measure the anterior-to-posterior axis and the septal-to-free-wall minor axis. They found a decrease in LV chamber size that was slightly more pronounced in the septal-to-free-wall minor axis, and a transient decrease in RV chamber size in response to a sudden 15 cm H_2O increase in AWP. This finding suggests that in a normal heart, increasing lung volume and ITP causes a minimal though measurable septal shift. These investigators also found that steady-state decreases in stroke volume correlate with an overall decrease in LVEDV.[38] Sudden increases in AWP may dilate the RV by increasing PVR,[24] but also immediately decrease venous return, thus decreasing RVEDV. Therefore, ventricular interdependence is probably not a significant factor in depressing steady-state LV performance during positive pressure ventilation unless marked cardiomegaly or large increases in transmural PAP occur.

Independent of ventricular interaction, as lung volume increases the expanding lungs compress the cardiac fossa (the space within the thorax where the heart rests).[10] Wallis et al.[68] have demonstrated that this mechanical heart-lung interaction decreases LVEDV by increasing juxtacardiac pleural pressure and that this effect becomes more important as lung volume or heart size increases beyond normal limits. Since the compliance of the LV measured relative to juxtacardiac pleural pressure does not change,[28] increasing LV filling pressure by volume infusion usually overcomes the decrease in LVEDV and restores cardiac output to normal.[49]

Although septal shift, pericardial limitation of volume, and mechanical heart-lung interaction are different mechanisms, functionally they all maintain adequate LVEDP (measured relative to atmosphere) but reduce LVEDV. Thus, all three mechanisms decrease the "effective" LV diastolic compliance, and all three respond to intravascular volume challenge. Therefore, positive pressure ventilation may decrease LV preload either by decreasing venous return to the RV or by decreasing effective LV diastolic compliance.

LV Afterload and the Concept of Systolic Pressure Load

Since the LV ejects its stroke into an aorta that has free extrathoracic drainage, changes in ITP may affect the ejecting LV independent of aortic pressure measured relative to atmosphere. Buda et al.[9] have shown that in conditions in which ITP varies widely, the LV systolic pressure load is more accurately represented by LV pressure relative to ITP than by LV pressure alone. For a given aortic pressure, positive swings in ITP will decrease the transmural LV pressure and decrease LV afterload, whereas negative swings in ITP will increase LV afterload (Fig 21–2). Vigorous spontaneous inspiratory efforts as in upper airway obstruction,[25] bronchospasm,[60] or decreased lung compliance[35] significantly decrease ITP and thereby increase LV afterload by increasing the

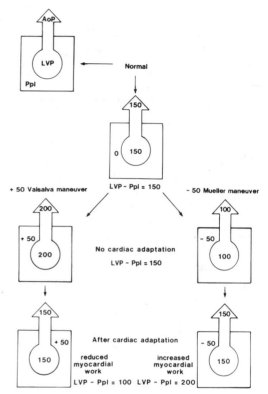

FIG 21–2.
Diagram depicts the effects of changes in pleural pressure (P_{pl}) on the amount of work the heart must perform to maintain a constant aortic pressure (*AoP*). Top, representation of left ventricle surrounded by thorax ejecting blood into an extrathoracic aorta with $P_{pl} = 0$. A left ventricular pressure (*LVP*) of 150 torr will generate an AoP of 150 torr. The pressure across the wall of the left ventricle (*LVP* – P_{pl}) will be 150 torr. If a 50-torr Valsalva maneuver is performed with no myocardial adaptation, then *LVP* – P_{pl} and myocardial work will be constant and AoP will reflect the change in P_{pl} of 50 torr. To maintain a 150-torr AoP the myocardium does not have to generate as great a transmural pressure, and *LVP* – P_{pl} will decrease to 100 torr. For a minus-50-torr Mueller maneuver, the opposite is true: to maintain an AoP of 150 torr, *LVP* – P_{pl} must be increased to 200 torr and the myocardium must perform more work.

transmural LV pressure. In such patients positive pressure ventilation may improve LV performance by abolishing the negative swings in ITP seen during spontaneous inspiration as well as by adding positive ITP during the positive pressure breaths. Recently, Calvin and associates[11] studied patients with severe LV dysfunction who were dependent on changes in LV afterload for changes in LV performance and relatively less responsive to changes in preload. They found that increasing ITP by adding PEEP did not depress LV function, and in some patients improved LV performance. Mathru and associates[30] demonstrated that in patients with elevated LV filling pressures (≥ 15 torr) and presumably decreased myocardial performance, increasing ITP by applying 10 cm H_2O PEEP improved cardiac output, whereas in patients with low LV filling pressure (<15 torr) the same amount of PEEP decreased cardiac output. Artificial ventilation then may improve LV performance for a given LV preload by eliminating the negative swings in ITP seen during spontaneous ventilation as well as by decreasing LV afterload. Thus, increases in ITP will affect LV performance by decreasing LV end-diastolic compliance and decreasing LV afterload. To the extent that cardiac performance depends on venous return and LVEDV, positive pressure ventilation can decrease blood flow. If LVEDV can be maintained, increases in ITP would not be expected to depress LV performance, and may improve LV performance when contractility is depressed by decreasing LV afterload.

Neural and Humoral Effects of Positive Pressure Ventilation

Neuroreflex mechanisms and humoral cardiac depressant substances have been shown to influence the cardiovascular response to positive pressure ventilation.[15, 20, 57, 70] Lung hyperinflation induces a reflex vasodilation, bradycardia, and negative inotropic response. This vasodepressor response is directly proportional to Vt.[65] The receptors for this response, whose nerve fibers travel in the *vagus* nerve, *tonically* inhibit the vasomotor center.[19, 40] Cassidy and associates[14] demonstrated that unilateral hyperinflation of an unperfused lung in dogs decreased blood pressure and stroke volume. Vagotomy abolished this response. This depressor reflex appears to be related primarily to the degree of lung stretch.[56] Lung inflation may also produce humoral substances that may depress myocardial performance,[41] alter the distribution of peripheral blood flow,[26] and stimulate fluid retention.[72] Priebe and colleagues[50] demonstrated that PEEP resulted in a redistribution of renal blood flow with fluid retention due primarily to the fall in cardiac output. When cardiac output is maintained during IPPB

with or without PEEP, blood flow distribution and renal function are preserved. This appears to be directly related to stretch receptors in the right atrium, which stimulate secretion of antidiuretic hormone if atrial volume decreases.[6]

Cardiac Performance During the Ventilatory Cycle

Throughout the ventilatory cycle, phasic and continual changes occur in lung volume, transpulmonary pressure, and ITP that instantaneously affect blood flow. The degree to which blood flow is affected depends on the state of the heart, lungs, and vasculature, so the effect of any mode of ventilation on cardiovascular performance will not be uniform for all clinical conditions. However, under normal conditions with Vt ventilation in the range of 5–15 ml/kg, the hemodynamic effects of either spontaneous or positive pressure ventilation are reasonably predictable. They are summarized in Table 21–1. Since the cardiovascular system is never in a circulatory steady state, measurements averaged throughout the respiratory cycle may not accurately represent the hemodynamic interactions present during specific phases of the respiratory cycle. Analyzing the moment-to-moment changes in ITP and blood flow increases an understanding of the overall hemodynamic effects of artificial ventilation. The instantaneous changes in intrathoracic vascular pressures and ventricular output during spontaneous and positive pressure ventilation in a dog model are illustrated in Figures 21–3 and 21–4, respectively.

Spontaneous ventilation decreases RAP (see Fig 21–3) by decreasing ITP. This increases the pressure gradient for venous return, which in turn increases RV filling pressure (transmural RAP), resulting in an increase in RV stroke volume and

TABLE 21–1.

Factors Determining Heart-Lung Interactions

Changes in intrathoracic pressure
  Altered pressure gradient for venous
    return
  Altered pressure gradient for LV ejection
Changes in lung volume
  Changes in pulmonary vascular
    resistance
  Ventricular interdependence*

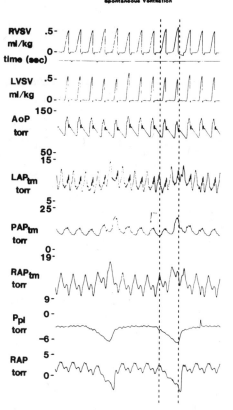

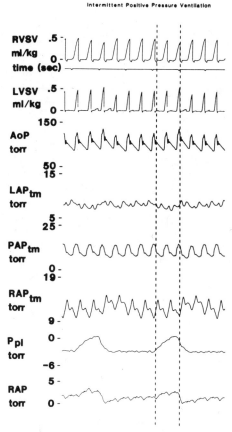

FIG 21–3.

Recordings of various hemodynamic variables during spontaneous ventilation in an intact anesthetized dog. RV stroke volume (*RVSV*) and LV stroke volume (*LVSV*) are derived by integrating the flow signals from flow probes placed on the main pulmonary artery (*PA*) and aorta, respectively. Also displayed are the corresponding instantaneous pressures for the aorta (*AoP*), airway (*Paw*), pleural space (*P_{pl}*) and right atrium (*RAP*), as well as the transmural (relative to P_{pl}) left atrial (*LAP_{tm}*), pulmonary arterial (*PAP_{tm}*), and right atrial (RAP_{tm}) pressures. RAP_{tm} and LAP_{tm} approximate the filling pressures of the RV and LV, respectively. The *vertical dotted lines* serve as reference points for the start and end-inspiration for the second of the two breaths displayed. Note the inverse relationship between P_{p1} and RV filling pressure, and that RVSV changes in a similar fashion to RAP_{tm} and not RAP. See text for discussion.

FIG 21–4.

Recordings of the same hemodynamic variables as shown in Figure 21–3 during intermittent positive pressure ventilation at approximately the same tidal volume and frequency. Abbreviations and symbols are as in Figure 21–3. Note both the inverse relationship between P_{pl} and RPA_{tm} and the oppositive effect of inspiration on RVSV in this Figure, as compared to spontaneous inspiration in Figure 21–3. See text for discussion.

transmural PAP on the following systole. Intrathoracic blood volume increases, and within two to three cardiac cycles, as the increased blood flow reaches the LV, transmural LAP and LV stroke volume increase as well. This phasic lag in the outputs of the two ventricles in response to respiration-induced changes in venous return to the RV can be such that the peak output of each ventricle is 180 degrees out of phase with the other. This can complicate assessment of the effects of ventilation on LV performance.[55] In general, the phasic variations in RV stroke volume during the ventilatory cycle are greater than those in the LV because the capacitance of the pulmonary circulation is greater than the capacitance of the systemic venous system. Spontaneous inspiration, however, concomitantly increases transmural LAP, which does not represent a transfer of the increased venous return to the left side of the heart. Transmural LAP may increase by any of four mechanisms: direct transmission of the pressure pulse from the pulmonary artery (no change in preload),[27] acceleration of pulmonary venous blood flow during inspiration, which squeezes alveolar vessels (increase in preload),[36] interdependent decrease in LV diastolic compliance from the suddenly dilated RV (decrease in preload),[23, 63] or decrease in LV ejection when negative ITP increases the LV systolic pressure load (increase in afterload).[9] Ventilation-associated changes in aortic pressure and flow are usually less than those in the pulmonary circulation since systemic venous return is greatly affected by small changes in RAP and the pulmonary vascular capacitance can absorb a large variation in venous blood flow,[43] whereas during quiet breathing similar changes in transmural aortic pressure do not affect LV systolic performance.[9, 61] However, to the extent that spontaneous respiratory efforts change ITP and lung volume, affecting venous return and LV diastolic compliance, LV output may also be affected. In the example illustrated in Figure 21–3, spontaneous inspiratory efforts decrease LV stroke volume and aortic pressure despite a rise in transmural LAP (LV filling pressure). If this form of pulsus paradoxus were due to the transmission of the negative ITP to the arterial tree, systolic aortic pressure would decrease without changing the aortic pulse pressure, transmural aortic pressure, or LV stroke volume.[51, 71] Since LV stroke volume, aortic pulse pressure, and calculated transmural aortic pressure also decrease, LV performance is diminished. This may occur from a decrease in LV preload due to decreasing LV diastolic compliance by ventricular interdependence or from an increase in LV afterload created by the decrease in ITP. For LV afterload to increase, however, LVEDV must increase, such that LV systolic wall stress increases despite a decrease in transmural aortic pressure. Without knowledge of relative changes in LV volumes during inspiration, it is impossible to ascertain the extent that either mechanism is operative. In the setting of decreased lung compliance or increased resistance to inspiration, spontaneous inspiratory efforts may be associated with profound negative swings in ITP that will increase venous return and reduce LV output, tending to pool blood in the chest, promoting pulmonary edema, and further decreasing lung compliance. This negative feedback process has been postulated to be a

cause of pulmonary edema in asthma[60] and upper airway obstruction,[25] and may be important in the progression of pulmonary edema associated with acute myocardial infarction. Placing such deteriorating patients on artificial ventilation, by alleviating these exaggerated negative swings in ITP, will decrease intrathoracic blood volume and can decrease afterload, and may allow for a more rapid resolution of the pulmonary edema process than would have otherwise occurred. Similarly, spontaneous expiratory grunting by increasing ITP may relieve pulmonary vascular congestion in pulmonary edema states.[22, 47]

POSITIVE PRESSURE VENTILATION

The Oxygen Cost of Breathing

The work of breathing under normal resting conditions is minimal, accounting for approximately 5% of the total oxygen consumption. However, with increasing elastic loads (pulmonary edema or fibrosis) or resistive loads (bronchospasm or airway collapse) the respiratory muscles may use more than 50% of the total oxygen delivery.[52] This stress can overtax a failing cardiovascular system even if the oxygen-carrying capacity and blood volume are acceptable for resting conditions. As the work of breathing increases, blood flow to the respiratory muscles also will increase, which may compromise flow to other organs. For example, if cardiac output is limited, this increased consumption of oxygen by respiratory muscles may limit the capacity for exercise. If ventilation-perfusion imbalance exists, the decreasing mixed venous oxygen content associated with increased oxygen consumption may cause arterial oxygen content and oxygen delivery to fall, as deoxygenated blood flows through intrapulmonary shunts. Artificial ventilation, by eliminating the work cost of breathing, will decrease oxygen consumption and may increase mixed venous oxygen content and therefore arterial oxygen content without primarily affecting either gas exchange or cardiac output.

Intermittent Positive Pressure Ventilation

Positive pressure inspiration (see Fig 21–4) increases AWP and distends the lungs, causing ITP to increase. Increased ITP increases RAP and in turn decreases venous return, RV filling pressure, and RV stroke volume. Since the pulmonary circulation is intrathoracic and has a relatively high capacitance relative to the right side of the heart, transmural LAP (LV filling pressure) and LV stroke volume will not vary as much as transmural RAP and RV stroke volume during ventilation despite similar changes in venous return and pulmonary arterial blood flow.[45] The decrease in LV stroke volume seen with positive pressure ventilation in Figure 21–4 is delayed by two or three beats from that of the RV and represents the decrease in venous return to the left side of the heart. Such decreases in LV stroke volume will be accentuated when there is functional hypovolemia, decreased vasomotor tone, large Vt breathing, or prolonged inspiratory time.[55] The former two factors decrease the upstream pressure for venous return and the latter two increase the backpressure to venous return.[10, 26–28] Inspiratory increases in LV stroke volume (reverse pulsus paradoxus) may also occur during positive pressure ventilation in heart failure; they are manifested by an increase in aortic pulse pressure over end-expiratory levels.[29] Such matching of inspiration to pulse pressure changes usually does not indicate relative hypovolemia, but rather decreased LV contractility and/or volume overload. Although pulsus paradoxus suggests cardiac or pulmonary pathology, it is not enough to ascertain that the aortic pulse pressure and systolic aortic pressure vary with artificial ventilation. The timing of such changes and their direction relative to the cycle are also important. For example, in hypovolemia the relation of the pulse variation to the phase of the respiratory cycle varies depending on ventilatory frequency, since this pulsus is generated by changes in venous return reaching the LV. In asthma and in severe LV failure with volume overload, however, changes in ITP directly change mean arterial pressure and aortic pulse pressure.

Continuous Positive Airway Pressure

End-expiratory airway pressure relative to atmospheric pressure may be zero or positive, independent of the mode that generates tidal breaths. When positive expiratory (and inspiratory) AWP is applied during spontaneous ventilation it is referred to as continuous positive airway pressure (CPAP), and when applied during pressure breathing it is referred to as positive end-expiratory pressure (PEEP). Both CPAP and PEEP are used in respiratory failure to improve gas exchange. Acute respiratory failure is often associ-

ated with a decrease in FRC, owing partly to lung collapse.[2, 34] By increasing end-expiratory AWP, collapsed or closed lung areas may expand, allowing FRC to increase. To the extent that closed lung is opened by CPAP or PEEP, PVR will tend to decrease. If collapsed alveoli reexpand, hypoxic pulmonary vasoconstriction may be reversed, further lowering PVR. If pulmonary parenchymal compliance is nonuniform owing to nonhomogeneous lung disease, however, then end-expiratory AWP may overexpand compliant areas, leaving diseased regions collapsed. This would increase resistance to blood flow in the "healthy" lung, thereby shunting RV output to collapsed lung areas. Thus, the effects of CPAP or PEEP on PVR and gas exchange are variable and dependent on the degree to which each local lung volume is normalized and hypoxia relieved. As PVR decreases, RV volume and filling pressure will decrease, improving both venous return and LV filling without increasing intrathoracic blood volume. If positive AWP returns the lungs to a more compliant state, reducing the elastic load on the respiratory muscles, the work cost of breathing will be reduced. Venus et al.[66] were able to use CPAP without mechanical ventilation to successfully treat previously healthy young adults with the adult respiratory distress syndrome, without causing carbon dioxide retention. CPAP and PEEP have similar hemodynamic effects for the same mean ITP,[17, 67] but since CPAP is associated with spontaneous ventilation, for a given level of end-expiratory AWP, mean ITP will be higher with PEEP.

Intermittent Mandatory Ventilation

Intermittent mandatory ventilation (IMV), by interspersing a fixed number of mechanically delivered positive pressure breaths during spontaneous ventilation, mitigates the detrimental hemodynamic effects of positive pressure breathing by minimizing the increase in ITP. Cardiac output and oxygen delivery may improve more than with assisted or controlled mechanical breathing if the primary limiting factor to blood flow is venous return. By decreasing ITP and the pressure gradient for venous return during spontaneous breaths, IMV will improve venous return during those breaths. However, in patients with normal ventricular function and normal intravascular volume, there is no evidence that steady-state cardiac output is different between IMV and positive pressure breathing matched for ventilatory characteristics.[30] In the patient with borderline oxygen transport not due to hypovolemia, IMV may be less useful, since its use may be associated with the increased oxygen consumption from increased work of breathing and with increased pulmonary edema from increased intrathoracic blood volume. Thus, in the unstable patient with limited oxygen transport, and especially with severe congestive heart failure, IMV offers no cardiovascular advantages over positive pressure breathing and may be deleterious. In hemodynamically stable patients the two modes of ventilation appear to have similar cardiovascular effects. It is possible that IMV at low rates diminishes barotrauma and improves the distribution of V/Q. Also, the exercise of respiratory muscles is presumed useful if oxygen transport is sufficient.

High-Frequency Ventilation

Recently, a new mode of ventilation using respiratory frequencies up to 900 breaths per minute and tidal volumes sometimes less than anatomical deadspace has been shown to provide adequate alveolar ventilation. A major problem in assessing the hemodynamic effects of high-frequency ventilation (HFV) as commonly used is the inaccuracy inherent in measuring AWP and lung volume with this mode of ventilation. However, changes in ITP and lung volume are small during the short respiratory cycles of HFV, and thus a characteristic effect of HFV is a relative steady state hemodynamically. Indeed, Oberg and Sjostrand originally used HFV to eliminate the "respiratory artifact" on the cardiac pressure tracings.[37] This equilibrium approximates that seen with apneic CPAP and has a similar effect on cardiac output as other forms of positive pressure ventilation that create the same mean ITP and lung volume.[62] High-frequency jet ventilation (HFJV) is a type of HFV that delivers pulses of gas at high velocity. Delivery of these pulses in a fixed timing relative to cardiac activity can have significant effects on cardiac performance (see chapter 31, "Ventilatory Support of the Failing Circulation: Phasic High Intrathoracic Pressure Support and Cardiac Cycle–Specific Ventilation").

CLINICAL APPLICATIONS

The overall effect of artificial ventilation on cardiovascular performance has not been precisely defined, primarily because phasic and steady-state characteristics that determine cardiac performance are inherently difficult to assess. On the basis of the studies reviewed herein, however, certain statements can be made regarding the hemodynamic effects of artificial ventilation. If ventilatory maneuvers are divided into those that generate negative swings in ITP (e.g., spontaneous ventilation with or without CPAP, and spontaneous breaths during IMV) and those that cause positive swings (e.g., positive pressure ventilation), the effects of these maneuvers can be separated into factors that alter venous return to the RV, ventricular interdependence, and LV afterload.

When cardiac function is normal, venous return is the primary determinant of cardiac output. Increases in RAP induced by positive pressure ventilation will decrease cardiac output by increasing the backpressure to venous blood flow. This decrease in venous return will be especially pronounced in hypovolemic states (hemorrhage or dehydration) and when vasomotor tone is decreased in sepsis, spinal shock, or autonomic blockage. In these clinical settings, increases in ITP by any means, whether induced by positive breathing, by CPAP, or by hyperinflation in patients with airflow obstruction, will be associated with a decrease in cardiac output. A decrease in venous return induced by positive pressure breathing may be responsible for the often observed cardiovascular collapse seen in some patients immediately after endotracheal intubation and "bagging" for acute respiratory failure. Since the reduction in blood pressure and cardiac output is due to decreased venous blood flow, appropriate treatment should restore the normal pressure gradient for venous return. This can be accomplished by administering fluids, elevating the legs, applying a pressure suit (MAST), and minimizing the increase in ITP by decreasing inspiratory time, decreasing Vt, or using the minimal amount of PEEP necessary to keep the lung open. IMV, by interspersing spontaneous breaths with mechanically delivered ones, also minimizes the increase in ITP. However, IMV may confound the management of fatigued or hypervolemic patients, or those in whom oxygen transport is borderline. If patients requiring fluid resuscitation are at significant risk of developing pulmonary edema, then LV filling pressures and cardiac output should be measured by pulmonary artery catheterization as a guide to fluid and vasopressor management. It is important to remember in the hemodynamic evaluation of such patients that pulmonary artery occlusion pressure (wedge pressure, WP) may not accurately reflect LV filling when hyperinflation or high levels of PEEP (> 12 cm H_2O) are present.[39] In such settings other parameters of blood flow such as cardiac output, mixed venous oxygen saturation, arterial-venous oxygen differences, and urine output can be monitored. Low LV filling pressure in spite of elevated WP due to PEEP can be detected in dogs and perhaps in man by observing the mode of the WP tracing immediately after removing PEEP (see chapter 15, "Technical Problems in Data Acquisition"). If fluid resuscitation and ventilator manipulation fail to sustain mean arterial pressure adequately for perfusion of vital organs, vasopressors may be indicated.

When PAP rises acutely, RV systolic performance can be compromised. Hyperinflation, excessive use of PEEP, pulmonary thromboembolism, and hypoxic pulmonary vasoconstriction can induce acute cor pulmonale. As RAP increases, venous blood flow decreases. The dilated RV impinges on the LV, decreasing LV diastolic compliance and filling, which further decreases cardiac output. Minimizing hyperinflation by bronchodilator therapy, minimum inspiratory time ratio, and minimum necessary levels of PEEP will decrease PVR. Opening closed lung areas and using supplemental oxygen may reverse hypoxic vasoconstriction. However, increasing RV filling pressure by volume infusion will result in improved cardiac output in all but the most advanced forms of cor pulmonale[44, 59] and may allow time for other selective forms of therapy to become effective.

When the LV fails, intrathoracic blood volume increases, and spontaneous inspiration only increases it further. If pulmonary venous pressure is elevated either from volume overload or from severe LV failure, pulmonary edema may develop, decreasing pulmonary compliance and alveolar gas exchange and increasing the work of breathing. If attempts to reverse these processes with peripheral vasodilators, inotropic agents, or diuretics, for example, are not successful, or when severe hypoxemia associated with pulmonary edema necessitates endotracheal intubation, positive pressure breathing (including CPAP) will decrease intrathoracic blood volume by decreasing venous return and may improve cardiac performance by increasing ITP. This should manifest itself as either an improvement or no change in cardiac output, associated with a decreasing

LV filling pressure. To the extent that extra work of breathing had impeded oxygen delivery and that positive pressure ventilation improves alveolar gas exchange, oxygen delivery to the tissues will also improve.

Acknowledgment

Work was supported in part by the Veterans Administration. Dr. Pinsky was the recipient of a Veterans Administration Career Development Award.

REFERENCES

1. Agostoni E: Mechanics of the pleural space. *Physiol Rev* 1972; 52:57–128.
2. Ahmed T, Oliver W Jr: Does slow-reacting substance of anaphylaxis mediate hypoxic pulmonary vasoconstriction? *Am Rev Respir Dis* 1983; 127:566–571.
3. Berend N, Christopher KL, Voelkel NF: Effect of positive end-expiratory pressure on functional residual capacity: Role of prostaglandin production. *Am Rev Respir Dis* 1982; 126:641–647.
4. Braunwald E, Binion JT, Morgan WL, et al: Alterations in central blood volume and cardiac output induced by positive pressure breathing and counteracted by metraminol (Aramine). *Circ Res* 1957; 5:670–675.
5. Brecher GA, Hubay CA: Pulmonary blood flow and venous return during spontaneous respiration. *Circ Res* 1955; 3:210–214.
6. Brennan CA Jr, Malvin RL, Joachmin KE, et al: Influence of right and left atrial receptors on plasma concentrations of ADH and renin. *Am J Physiol* 1971; 221:273–278.
7. Brinker JA, Weiss I, Lappe DL, et al: Leftward septal displacement during right ventricular loading in man. *Circulation* 1980; 61:626–633.
8. Brookhart JM, Boyd TE: Local differences in intrathoracic pressure and their relationship to cardiac filling pressure in the dog. *Am J Physiol* 1947; 148:434–444.
9. Buda AJ, Pinsky MR, Ingels NB, et al: Effect of intrathoracic pressure on left ventricular performance. *N Engl J Med* 1979; 301:453–459.
10. Butler J: The heart is in good hands. *Circulation* 1983; 67:1163–1168.
11. Calvin JE, Driedger AA, Sibbald WJ: Positive end-expiratory pressure (PEEP) does not depress left ventricular function in patients with

pulmonary edema. *Am Rev Respir Dis* 1981; 124:121–128.

12. Canada E, Benumof JL, Tousdale FR: Pulmonary vascular resistance correlated in intact normal and abnormal canine lungs. *Crit Care Med* 1982; 10:719–723.

13. Carter RS, Snyder JV, Pinsky MR: Filling pressure during PEEP as measured by nadir wedge pressure after airway disconnection. *Am J Physiol* 1985; 249:H770–H776.

14. Cassidy SS, Eschembacher WL, Johnson RJ Jr: Reflex cardiovascular depression during unilateral lung hyperinflation in the dog. *J Clin Invest* 1979; 64:620–629.

15. Conway CM: Haemodynamic effects of pulmonary ventilation. *Br J Anaesth* 1975; 47:761–766.

16. Cournand A, Motley HL, Werko L, et al: Physiologic studies of the effect of intermittent positive pressure breathing on cardiac output in man. *Am J Physiol* 1948; 152:162–174.

17. Dorinsky PM, Whitcomb ME: The effect of PEEP on cardiac output. *Chest* 1983; 84:210–216.

18. Ellman H, Denbin H: Lack of a diverse hemodynamic effect of PEEP in patients with acute respiratory failure. *Crit Care Med* 1982; 10:706–711.

19. Glick G, Wechsler AS, Epstein SE: Reflex cardiovascular depression produced by stimulation of pulmonary stretch receptors in the dog. *J Clin Invest* 1969; 48:467–472.

20. Grenvik A: Respiratory, circulatory and metabolic effects of respiratory treatment. *Acta Anaesthesiol Scand Suppl* 19, 1966.

21. Guyton AC, Lindsey AW, Abernathy B, et al: Venous return at various right atrial pressures and the normal venous return curve. *Am J Physiol* 1957; 189:690–715.

22. Harrison VC, Heese H deV, Klein M: The significance of grunting in hyaline membrane disease. *Pediatrics* 1968; 41:549–559.

23. Janicki JS, Weber KT: The pericardium and ventricular interaction distensibility, and function. *Am J Physiol* 1980; 238:H494–H503.

24. Jardin FF, Fercot J-C, Gueret P, et al: Echocardiographic evaluation of ventricles during continuous positive pressure breathing. *J Appl Physiol* 1984; 56:619–627.

25. Lee KWT, Downes JJ: Pulmonary edema secondary to laryngospasm in children. *Anesthesiology* 1983; 59:347–349.

26. Lenfant C, Howell BJ: Cardiovascular adjustments in dogs during continuous pressure breathing. *J Appl Physiol* 1960; 15:425–428.

27. Maloney JE, Bergel DH, Blazier JB, et al: Transmission of pulsatile blood pressure and flow through the isolated lung. *Circ Res* 1968; 23:11–24.

28. Marini JJ, Culver BN, Butler J: Mechanical effect of lung distension with positive pressure in cardiac function. *Am Rev Respir Dis* 1981; 124:382–386.

29. Massumi RA, Mason DT, Vera Z, et al: Reversed pulsus paradoxus. *N Engl J Med* 1973; 289; 1272–1275.

30. Mathru M, Roa TLK, El-Etr AA, et al: Hemodynamic response to changes in ventilatory patterns in patients with normal and poor left ventricular reserve. *Crit Care Med* 1982; 10:423–426.

31. Matthay RA, Berger HJ: Non-invasive assessment of right and left ventricular function in acute and chronic respiratory failure. *Crit Care Med* 1983; 11:329–338.

32. Matthay RA, Berger HJ, Davies RA, et al: Right and left ventricular exercise performance in chronic obstructive pulmonary disease: Radionuclide assessment. *Ann Intern Med* 1980; 93:234–239.

33. McMahon SM, Permutt S, Proctor DF: A model to evaluate pleural surface pressure measuring devices. *J Appl Physiol* 1969; 27:886–871.

34. Milic-Emili J, Mean J, Turner JM, et al: Improved technique for estimating pleural pressure from esophageal balloons. *J Appl Physiol* 1964; 19:207–211.

35. Milic-Emili J, Ruff F: Effects of pulmonary congestion and edema on the small airways. *Bull Physiol Pathol Respir* 1977; 7:1181–1196.

36. Morgan BC, Abel FL, Mullins GL, et al: Flow-patterns in cavae, pulmonary artery, pulmonary vein, and aorta in intact dogs. *Am J Physiol* 1966; 210:903–909.

37. Oberg PA, Sjostrand U: Studies on blood-pressure regulation: III. Dynamics of arterial blood pressure on carotid-sinus nerve stimulation. *Acta Physiol Scand* 1971; 81:96–105.

38. Olsen CO, Tyson GS, Maier GW, et al: Dynamic ventricular interaction in the conscious dog. *Circ Res* 1983; 52:85–104.

39. O'Quin R, Marini JJ: Pulmonary artery occlusion pressure: Clinical physiology, measure-

ment, and interpretation. *Am Rev Respir Dis* 1983; 128:318–326.

40. Painal AS: Vagal sensory receptors and their reflex effects. *Physiol Rev* 1973; 53:59–88.

41. Patten MT, Liebman PR, Hechtman HG: Humorally mediated decreases in cardiac output associated with positive end-expiratory pressure. *Microvasc Res* 1977; 13:137–144.

42. Patterson SW, Piper H, Starling EH: The regulation of the heart beat. *J Physiol* 1914; 48:465–513.

43. Permutt S, Howell JBL, Proctor DF, et al: Effect of lung inflation on static pressure-volume characteristics of pulmonary vessels. *J Appl Physiol* 1961; 16:64–70.

44. Piene H, Sund T: Does normal pulmonary impedance constitute the optimal load for the right ventricle? *Am J Physiol* 1982; 242:H154–H160.

45. Pinsky MR: Determinants of pulmonary arterial blood flow variation during respiration. *J Appl Physiol* 1984; 56:1237–1243.

46. Pinsky MR: Instantaneous venous return curves in an intact canine preparation. *J Appl Physiol* 1984;56:756–771.

47. Pinsky MR, Matuschak GM, Itzkoff JM: Respiratory augmentation of left ventricular function during spontaneous ventilation in severe left ventricular failure by grunting: An auto-EPAP effect. *Chest* 1984; 86:267–269.

48. Pontoppidan H, Green B, Lowenstein E: Acute respiratory failure in the adult. *N Engl J Med* 1972; 87(part 1):690–698.

49. Prewitt RM, Wood LDH: Effect of positive end-expiratory pressure on ventricular function in dogs. *Am J Physiol* 1979; 236:H534–H544.

50. Priebe HJ, Heimann JC, Hedley-Whyte J: Mechanisms of renal dysfunction during positive end-expiratory pressure ventilation. *J Appl Physiol* 1981; 50:643–649.

51. Robotham JL, Rabson J, Permutt S, et al: Left ventricular hemodynamics during respiration. *J Appl Physiol* 1979; 47:1295–1303.

52. Roussos C, Macklem PT: The respiratory muscles. *N Engl J Med* 1982; 307:786–797.

53. Rankin JS, Olsen CO, Arentzen, CE, et al: The effects of airway pressure on cardiac function in intact dogs and man. *Circulation* 1982; 66:108–120.

54. Sarnoff SJ: Myocardial contractility as described by the ventricular function curves: Observations on Starling's law of the heart. *Physiol Rev* 1955; 35:107–122.

55. Scharf SM, Brown R, Saunders N, et al: Hemodynamic effects of positive pressure inflation. *J Appl Physiol* 1980; 49:124–131.

56. Schrender JJ, Jansen JRC, Versprill A: Contribution of lung stretch depressor reflex to non-linear fall in cardiac output during PEEP. *J Appl Physiol* 1984; 56:1578–1582.

57. Shepherd JT: The lungs as receptor sites for cardiovascular regulation. *Circulation* 1981; 63:1–10.

58. Shuler RH, Ensor C, Gunning RE, et al: The differential effects of respiration on the left and right ventricles. *Am J Physiol* 1942; 137:620–627.

59. Sibbald WD, Driedger AA, Myers ML, et al: Biventricular function in the adult respiratory distress syndrome: Hemodynamic and radionuclide assessment with special emphasis on right ventricular function. *Chest* 1983; 84:126–134.

60. Stalcup SA, Mellins RB: Mechanical forces producing pulmonary edema in acute asthma. *N Engl J Med* 1977; 297:592–596.

61. Suga H, Sagawa K: Instantaneous pressure-volume relationships and their ratio in the excised, supported canine left ventricle. *Circ Res* 1974; 35:117–126.

62. Szele C, Shahvari MBG: Comparison of cardiovascular effects of high frequency ventilation and intermittent positive pressure ventilation in hemorrhagic shock (abstract). *Crit Care Med* 1981; 9:161.

63. Taylor RR, Corell JW, Sonnenblick EH, et al: Dependence of ventricular distensibility on filling of the opposite ventricle. *Am J Physiol* 1967; 213:711–718.

64. Tobin MJ, Chadha TS, Jenouri G, et al: Breathing patterns: I. Normal subjects. *Chest* 1983; 84:202–205.

65. Vatner SF, Rutherford JD: Control of the myocardial contractile state by carotid chemo- and baroreceptors and pulmonary inflation reflexes in conscious dogs. *J Clin Invest* 1978; 63:1593–1601.

66. Venus B, Jacobs HK, Lim L: Treatment of the adult respiratory distress syndrome with continuous positive airway pressure. *Chest* 1979; 76:257–261.

67. Vuori A, Jalonen J, Laaksonen V: Continuous positive airway pressure during mechanical ventilation and spontaneous ventilation: Effects on central hemodynamics and oxygen trans-

port. *Acta Anaesthesiol Scand* 1979; 23:459–462.

68. Wallis TW, Robotham JL, Compean R, et al: Mechanical heart-lung interaction with positive end-expiratory pressure. *J Appl Physiol* 1983; 54:1039–1047.

69. Whittenberger JL, McGregor M, Berglund E, et al: Influence of state of inflation of the lung on pulmonary vascular resistance. *J Appl Physiol* 1960; 15:878–882.

70. Widdicombe JG: Respiratory reflexes, in *Handbook of Physiology*. Section 3: *Respiration*. Fenn WD, Rabin H (eds). Washington, DC, American Physiological Society, 1964; pp 585–630.

71. Wise RA, Robotham JL, Summer WR: Effects of spontaneous ventilation on the circulation. *Lung* 1981; 159:175–192.

72. Zehr JE, Hasbarger JA, Risz KD: Reflex suppression of renin secretion during distention of cardiopulmonary receptors in dogs. *Circ Res* 1976; 38:232–239.

22 _____ Technical and Semantic Aspects of Ventilator Support

James V. Snyder, M.D.

Judy Culpepper, M.D.

Currently available mechanical ventilators provide a continuous spectrum of ventilation patterns, from spontaneous ventilation to complete mechanical support. Most of the technical aspects of mechanical ventilation have been well described.[15] In this chapter we limit our discussion to the wide spectrum of patient needs, and the failure of current semantic distinctions to match those needs. We will also review several technical aspects that we think deserve emphasis, especially the mechanical support of spontaneous ventilation.

TERMINOLOGY

It is important that the clinician be aware of the limitations of currently used respiratory therapy terminology. We will consider several illustrative examples (Fig 22–1).

The term continuous positive airway pressure (CPAP) means that airway pressure remains positive during the respiratory cycle, but it does not say whether the pressure varies or is constant. Therefore, it encompasses extremes ranging from inspiratory pressure equaling expiratory pressure to inspiratory pressure less than expiratory pressure and only slightly higher than atmospheric. The higher inspiratory pressure is more likely to impair venous return, whereas allowing inspiratory pressure to drop to atmospheric (called expiratory positive airway pressure, EPAP) is associated with increased work of breathing, higher venous admixture, and lower functional residual capacity (FRC).[18] Thus, the same term may be applied to patterns that have very different physiologic effects.

The terms that refer to ventilator mode settings are also ambiguous. A patient with a spontaneous respiratory rate of 16/min who is then mechanically ventilated by a machine set in the intermittent mandatory ventilation (IMV) mode with a rate of 25/min (suppressing the patient's spontaneous drive) is, in effect, receiving controlled ventilation. Similarly, when the synchronized IMV rate is set close to the patient's spontaneous breathing rate, the pressure tracing and the resulting physiology may be identical to those seen in assisted ventilation. Finally, in the *pressure assist mode* available, for example, on the Siemens 900 C, Bennett 7200, and Engstrom Erica models, the ventilator's inspiratory flow can be regulated to merely compensate for airway pressure (AWP) loss occurring with the patient's inhalation, in which case it resembles a CPAP circuit with little work of breathing; or the system can generate more assistance to inspiration and resemble intermittent positive pressure breathing (IPPB). Because terminology can be misleading, it is useful to consider how much positive or negative airway and pleural pressure is generated each time a patient and system are evaluated in order to understand the physiologic implications.

SUPPORT OF SPONTANEOUS VENTILATION

Demand Valve Versus Continuous Flow

When equipment is arranged to support the spontaneously breathing patient (with or without IMV), either a demand valve or a continuous flow system supplies the gas from which the patient takes his spontaneous breaths (Table 22–1). Demand valve systems can increase the patient's work of breathing[10, 13] if the response of the valve is slow or if delivered flow is inadequate. This may cause intolerable stress during sponta-

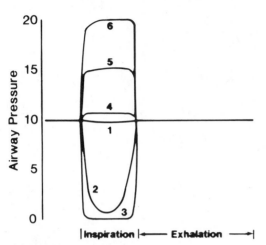

FIG 22–1.

Terminology overlap: Inspiratory pressure can vary widely in a given ventilation pattern, and the pressure changes that occur with one system may overlap those in another system. For example, the CPAP system that allows inspiratory pressure to approach atmospheric (2) has a similar effect as EPAP (3), whereas when inspiratory pressure in a CPAP system does not drop (1), CPAP may approximate low positive-pressure ventilation (4) in effect. The pressure assist mode may be set to provide a minimal pressure over PEEP, and then simulate CPAP, (4) or it can be set higher (5,6) and simulate conventional IPPB in effect.

neous breaths for a weak patient. Figure 22–2 shows the pressure and flow response of a commercially available demand valve system to mechanical simulation of a patient with a weak inspiratory effort. With the demand valve there is a time delay between the beginning of the patient's inspiratory effort (decrease in AWP) and the beginning of gas flow from the ventilator. Thus, there is an inherent lack of coordination between

the patient's effort and the mechanical response, which results in greater work of breathing with this system. Other factors that affect the work of breathing of a patient on a demand valve system include the level of the demand valve threshold, the volume of the chamber containing the pressure sensor, and the level of gas flow from the demand valve. A weak patient may breathe more confortably and effectively from a well-designed continuous flow system than from a demand valve system. If a weak patient requires mechanical ventilation and a well-designed continuous flow circuit is not available, weaning may be possible only by alternating assisted ventilation and T tube weaning.

On the other hand, the demand valve system permits synchronization of machine breaths with the patient's respiratory efforts (synchronized IMV, or SIMV). SIMV may be much more comfortable than unsynchronized breaths for a vigorous, reactive patient who fights or ''bucks'' the ventilator. It must be emphasized that one can usually alleviate discoordination between the patient and the ventilator when nonsynchronized IMV is used by sensitive manipulation of ventilatory settings, combined, if necessary, with judicious sedation. However, SIMV is particularly useful when respiratory muscle strength is not a concern and when sedation is contraindicated, for example, after head trauma.

The demand valve system allows convenient measurement of the patient's minute ventilation and exhaled tidal volumes (Vt), which facilitates continuous monitoring with appropriate alarms. These measurements are difficult to make with a continuous flow system; even when a double exhalation valve system is used to separate a patient's exhaled gas volume from the continuous source flow gas, when PEEP is used it is difficult

TABLE 22–1.

Comparison of Demand Valve System and Continuous Flow System For Spontaneous Ventilation*

SYSTEM	PRO	CON
Demand valve	Synchronous with patient effort Volumes can be monitored	Short inspiratory effect and delayed electronic sensing result in late delivery of gas flow, low Vt, and more work
Continuous flow	Minimal work of breathing	Asynchronous Volume monitoring is difficult

*From Snyder et al.[20] Reproduced by permission.

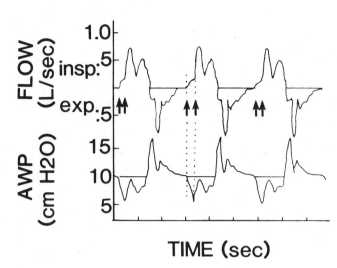

FIG 22–2.
Response of a commercial demand valve system (Bournes Bear I[R]) set to deliver CPAP with maximal sensitivity to a "weakened" mechanical patient simulator (the "patient" has a Vt of 500 ml, respiration rate of 20/min, and inspiratory flow of .75 L/sec (45 L/min). The delay from initiation of patient effort to response of the demand valve (space between arrows) is insignificant in patients with normal ventilatory mechanics but becomes larger as the patient's inspiratory flow diminishes and as the mechanical (tubing) volume that must be evacuated to trigger the system is increased. Note the oscillatory nature of both flow and pressure with this system. (Modified from Snyder JV et al:[20] Reproduced by permission.)

to balance the system so that both accurate volume measurements and minimal work of breathing are obtained.[23] Alternative approaches to monitoring, such as capnography,[19] inductive plethysmography,[21] and pneumotachography, are not rendered inaccurate by continuous flow systems.

Modifications of Demand Valve Systems

It seems theoretically possible to decrease the response time of the demand valve (without increasing the frequency of premature ventilator response) and thus to reduce the work of breathing. We suspect that manufacturers could adapt their systems by diminishing the volume containing the sensor, by using an airway carbon dioxide or gas-flow sensor rather than pressure to trigger the demand valve, and by increasing the flow from the demand valve. However, some of these changes are likely to worsen the choppy flow now delivered by some demand systems. Also, the sluggish response of the demand valve can be compensated for in some available systems by programming the ventilator to maintain a slightly more positive pressure during inspiration*.[11]

Continuous Flow Systems: Plumbing is Critical

Greenbaum et al.[12] and Venus et al.[22] have shown that oxygenation can be improved independently of mechanical breaths by the use of CPAP. Using such a CPAP system, the patient can obtain the benefits of spontaneous breathing

*Pressure assist mode, discussed earlier.

discussed in chapter 20, "Pulmonary Physiology." However, a poorly constructed system can add to the patient's work of breathing, making it difficult or impossible for him to tolerate using it. The following principles characterizing continuous flow CPAP systems have been elaborated primarily by Douglas and Downs[7] and technical details have been reviewed recently by Kakmarek et al.[14] A mechanical simulation of a spontaneously breathing patient, diagramed in Figure 22–3, is valuable for demonstrating and comparing such systems.

In CPAP, AWP is continuously positive during spontaneous ventilation. Inspiratory pressure (IPAP) is therefore always positive, but it may be less than the pressure during exhalation (EPAP). The drop in IPAP below EPAP depends on the mechanical characteristics of the CPAP system, the flow of gas to the patient, and the patient's inspiratory flow. The work of breathing increases with a drop in pressure during inhalation, as diagramed in Figure 22–1. This increase in patient work is similar to the effect that suction applied to the system during inspiration would create. For the purposes of discussion, it is convenient to divide the CPAP system into its expiratory and inspiratory limbs (Fig 22–4).

Expiratory Limb

The resistance of the expiratory limb has significant influence on the drop in AWP with inspiration, and therefore on the work of breathing. The ideal PEEP valve is a threshold valve, that is, the desired pressure is reached with minimal

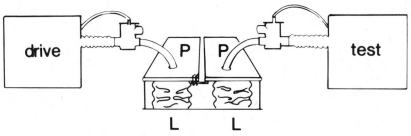

44

FIG 22–3.

Mechanical simulation of a spontaneously breathing patient. A bar is secured to the top plate (*P*) of the driven lung (*L*) in a Dixie Lung Model[R] (Michigan Instruments, Inc., Grand Rapids, Mich.) to lift the top plate of the other lung, which thus simulates a patient. Controlled ventilation of one lung at various rates, flows, and volumes by the drive ventilator establishes a similar and reproducible ventilatory "effort" by the other lung. The arrangement is useful for comparing systems designed for spontaneous or assisted ventilation. Modification was suggested by the manufacturer. (From Snyder JV et al.[20] Reproduced by permission.)

flow and then stays constant despite increasing flow. However, the pressures maintained by some commercially available PEEP valves vary significantly with flow; we refer to these as resistance-type valves in contrast to threshold-type valves (Fig 22–5).[4] As the patient inhales source flow, less is available to the valve. Thus, when a resistance PEEP valve is used, pressure drops with decreasing flow through the valve during inspiration, and the patient must work harder to overcome this external work load. Unfortunately the same problem occurs during every spontaneous breath whenever mechanical ventilators are modified to provide continuous flow, because the exhalation valves, especially those of mushroom design, have significant resistance.[6] When changing from IMV with PEEP to CPAP, it is convenient simply to stop the mechanical breaths on a system adapted for continuous flow; however, replacement of the ventilator circuit by an appropriately designed, separate CPAP circuit is likely to result in less work of breathing for the patient because of less resistance in the expiratory limb.

With either the IMV or the CPAP circuit, the drop in IPAP may be due to an inadequate source flow relative to the patient's inspiratory flow. When a threshold system is used it is appropriate simply to increase the source flow. However, if there is expiratory limb resistance and the source flow rate is turned up in an effort to compensate, the higher flow passing through the same circuit results in further elevation of PEEP, but the dif-

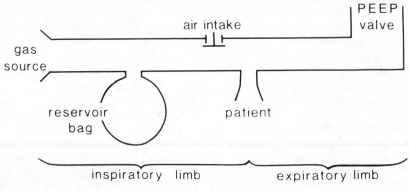

FIG 22–4.

Continuous flow CPAP system. Work of breathing is least when the resistance of the expiratory limb is low and source flow is higher than peak inspiratory flow. Elastic loading of a reservoir bag is also helpful. (From Snyder JV et al.[20] Reproduced by permission.)

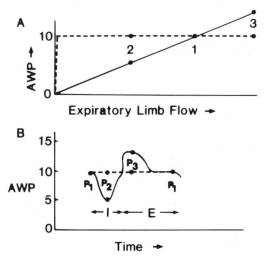

FIG 22–5.
Flow-pressure characteristics of a CPAP expiratory limb with resistance but no threshold characteristics (*solid line*) and of a limb with a 10 cm H_2O threshold but no additional resistance (*dashed line*). If the patient's peak inspiratory flow is sufficient to lower the flow through the expiratory limb from flow 1 to flow 2, inspiratory AWP will drop to point 2 (in both **A** and **B**) when the resistance system is used, but not at all with the threshold system.

ference between inspiratory and expiratory AWP (and therefore the work of inspiration) is unchanged. Resistance in the expiratory limb is also increased by the accumulation of water in the tubing between the patient and the PEEP valve and, in some systems, by unnecessary one-way valves or other high-resistance components.[6]

Patient-exhaled gas added to the bias flow may transiently increase AWP. This increased expiratory work is usually accomplished passively by the elastic recoil in the expanded lungs, but it may also be accomplished actively, in which case it is manifested as expiratory muscle tension.

Inspiratory Limb

When the source flow of gas is greater than the patient's inspiratory flow, the characteristics of the inspiratory limb are minimally important and no reservoir bag is necessary. However, when patient inspiratory flow exceeds source flow the properties of the inspiratory limb can cause a significant decrease in IPAP. A reservoir bag is commonly included in the inspiratory limb to provide the additional volume of gas demanded by the patient in this situation.

The ideal reservoir bag would have elastic properties such that AWP would not change significantly with bag volume changes during patient inhalation. A reservoir bag that does not maintain pressure when volume is removed is useful as a volume source, but its use will be associated with a drop in IPAP and therefore an increase in the work of breathing. This is true of some commercially available bags.[6] Reservoir bag pressure is better sustained if the bag is elastic-loaded,[10] or briefly stretched to several feet in diameter before it is added to the circuit.[5] Even with an optimal reservoir bag, any resistance in the system between bag and patient decreases IPAP and increases work of breathing. This effect can be minimized by using large-diameter connector tubing and eliminating one-way valves in the inspiratory limb. Eliminating the one-way valve between the bag and the patient requires that source flow be sufficient (at least twice minute volume) to prevent rebreathing of expired gas. However, increasing source flow (this time to minimize rebreathing in the inspiratory limb) will again increase PEEP when a PEEP device with substantial resistance is used. Thus, *the decrease in IPAP (and its resulting increase in work of breathing) is least when a threshold-type PEEP valve is used and there is minimal resistance in the expiratory limb, and either source flow is greater than patient inspiratory flow or the reservoir maintains pressure.*

The inspiratory limb should include an emergency intake valve. During normal operation of the system, the positive pressure keeps this one-way valve closed and prevents entrainment of room air. If source flow is inadvertently shut off the patient can inhale room air through the valve. A system pressure alarm will alert personnel to this and other mechanical failures.

TECHNICAL ASPECTS OF MECHANICAL VENTILATION

Monitoring Efficiency of Ventilation

The efficiency of carbon dioxide elimination is an important variable in determining the required mechanical minute volume, as discussed in chapters 19, "The Development of Supported Ventilation: A Critical Summary," and 20, "Pulmonary Physiology." It is therefore a potentially

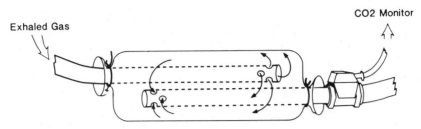

FIG 22–6.
Mixing bag for monitoring mixed expired PCO_2 ($P\overline{E}CO_2$). Variation in the $P\overline{E}CO_2$ reading indicates inadequate mixing. The tubes should be repositioned within the bag, or a larger bag may be required. Extra holes are cut near the ends of the tubes to prevent obstruction and resulting increase in PEEP.

important determinant of peak and mean AWP, and of the probability of barotrauma and depression of venous return. There are conceptual objections to using the term "deadspace," but measurement of the deadspace to tidal volume ratio (Vd/Vt) remains the most efficient means of quantifying the efficiency of carbon dioxide elimination. Because changes in ventilatory support can significantly alter Vd/Vt just as they may alter venous admixture ($\dot{Q}va/\dot{Q}t$), measurement of Vd/Vt can be a comparably important variable to monitor in mechanically ventilated patients. Such monitoring is uncommon, in part because the potential usefulness is not widely appreciated, but also because monitoring as it is usually done is a particularly ungainly process. Convenient means to monitor Vd/Vt more frequently are therefore desirable and are described here.

Monitoring of Vd/Vt is based on the Enghoff modification of the Bohr equation:

$$Vd/Vt = (Pa_{CO_2} - P\overline{E}_{CO_2})/Pa_{CO_2}$$

where $P\overline{E}_{CO_2}$ is mixed expired PCO_2. Inspired PCO_2 is assumed to be insignificant. Obviously, Pa_{CO_2} is included in every arterial blood gas analysis. In addition, Pa_{CO_2} is closely and continuously approximated by transcutaneous PCO_2 monitoring.[17] The mixed expired PCO_2 is easily monitored in the effluent of a low-resistance mixing bag through which all exhaled gas is passed. An inexpensive mixing system that uses a plastic trash bag and a capnograph instrument is diagramed in Figure 22–6. The adequacy of gas mixing is assured by the absence of detectable fluctuations in the continuous capnograph reading. Vd/Vt can be calculated after observing the $P\overline{E}_{CO_2}$ each time arterial blood is aspirated for PCO_2 measurement, or more frequently if a trans-cutaneous carbon dioxide monitor is used, or continuously if the readings by the two devices are appropriately integrated in a simple computer device.

Intermittent Mandatory Ventilation

The CPAP systems described earlier are, of course, similar to the circuits used to provide continuous flow of gas for spontaneous breaths by the patient on IMV. The principal difference is the presence of the exhalation valve in the IMV system, which adds significantly to expiratory limb resistance and therefore to the work of breathing. The machine superimposes volume-limited positive pressure mechanical breaths. With demand valve SIMV systems, these machine breaths can be initiated by a spontaneous breath and therefore do not disrupt the patient's breathing pattern, as discussed earlier.

Assisted Ventilation

Assisted ventilation systems provide mechanical breaths triggered by every spontaneous patient breath, usually with a "backup" control rate that will provide mechanical breaths in the absence of patient triggering. Altering the control rate has no direct influence on the rate of ventilation unless it is set higher than the patient's spontaneous rate. The sensitivity of the trigger is an important variable: if it is too sensitive it will trigger prematurely, controlling ventilation at a higher rate than is needed rather than assisting. If it is not sensitive enough the work of breathing is increased, and discoordination of machine and patient effort may occur.

Controlled Ventilation

The controlled ventilation mode does not permit the patient to take spontaneous breaths, which may be psychologically as well as physiologically disturbing for the patient,[9] and it is virtually never preferable to either assisted or IMV mode. When a patient is receiving assisted ventilation and there is concern regarding the function of the respiratory center or occasional inability to trigger the demand valve, then setting a high control rate just below the rate at which the patient is generating assisted breaths is an appropriate security measure but should not be confused with controlled ventilation. Similarly, in the IMV mode with a high machine breath rate almost all the work can be done for the patient without preventing his making efforts on his own. Even when controlled ventilation is required, the assisted or IMV modes are preferred, because they provide a system that responds when the patient's demands become greater than the control settings.

PEEP Valves

PEEP can be provided through separately attachable PEEP valves (as discussed), or it can be achieved by pressurizing the in-line exhalation valve. These tend to be resistance valves, which increase the work of breathing during any spontaneous breaths if a continuous flow circuit is used.

Inspiratory-Expiratory Ratio

The ratio of inspiratory to expiratory time (I:E ratio) has been considered important since Cournand et al. described its prominent influence on cardiac output in dogs.[3] It is important for other effects as well. The I:E ratio can be adjusted by changing ventilator rate, inspiratory flow rate, inspiratory time, or Vt. Longer, slower inspiration may improve ventilation of areas with long time constants.[1] However, it remains unclear whether this has clinical benefit. For example, Conners and co-workers[2] showed that patients with chronic obstructive pulmonary disease had improved oxygenation and Vd/Vt ratio with higher machine inspiratory flow rates and shorter I:E ratios, presumably because exhalation time was prolonged. On the other hand, high inspiratory

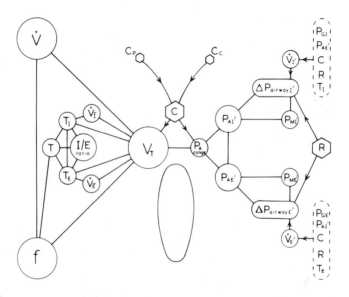

FIG 22–7.

Relationship among many of variables used in mechanical ventilation. (From Mushin et al.[16] Reproduced by permission.) Abbreviations: C, total compliance; C_C, chest wall compliance; C_P, pulmonary compliance; f, respiratory frequency; P_{AI}', alveolar pressure at end of inspiratory phase; P_{MI}', machine pressure, usually similar to mouth pressure, at end of inspiratory phase; Δ P' airway I', pressure drop across airway (from machine to alveoli) at end of inspiratory phase; P_{AE}' P_{ME}' and ΔPairway E' corresponding pressures at end of expiratory phase; P_A range, $P_{AI} - P_{AE}$; P_{GI}, inspiratory generated pressure (if any); P_{GE}, expiratory generated pressure (if any); R, resistance (from machine to alveoli); T, respiratory period; T_I, inspiratory time; T_E, expiratory time; V_T, tidal volume; V, total minute-volume ventilation; $\dot{V}_I$, mean inspiratory flow rate; $\dot{V}_E$, mean expiratory flow rate; $\dot{V}_I'$, flow rate at end of inspiratory phase; $\dot{V}_E'$, flow rate at end of expiratory phase.

flows can increase peak AWP, which may predispose the patient to barotrauma. Higher I:E ratios may be associated with higher FRC and less airway closure, serving then as a dynamic substitute for PEEP. However, as Cournand et al. noted, pleural pressure may be higher and venous return impaired. Finally, if the inspiratory time is too long and flow too slow for the patient, she may struggle to get gas faster than the machine supplies it; this causes discoordination and increases the work of breathing.

Interrelation of Variables

Tidal volume, PEEP, inspiratory flow, and inspiratory time all affect peak inspiratory pressure, as do the patient variables compliance and resistance. Respiratory rate, Vt, and exhalation time all affect PEEP. Flow cannot be changed without altering the I:E ratio or the inspiratory plateau. Inspiratory flow, expiratory retard, and PEEP all influence mean and peak AWP. The differences between pressures at the ventilator, in the proximal airway, in the distal airway, and in the pleural space are important. In short, as discussed in detail by Mushin et al.[16] and illustrated in Figure 22–7, all the variables on the ventilator have interlocking effects. Studying this diagram of interrelations diagramed is a time-consuming but worthwhile exercise.

REFERENCES

1. Bake B, Wood L, Murphy B, et al: Effect of inspiratory flow rate on regional distribution of inspired gas. *J Appl Physiol* 1974; 37:8.

2. Conners AE, McCaffree R, Gray BA: Effect of inspiratory flow rate on gas exchange during mechanical ventilation. *Am Rev Respir Dis* 1981; 124:537.

3. Cournand A, Motley HL, Werko L, et al: Physiological studies of the effects of intermittent positive pressure breathing on cardiac output in man. *Appl J Physiol* 1948; 152:162.

4. Culpepper J, Snyder J, Pennock B, et al: Effect of PEEP value resistance on airway pressure and inspiratory work (abstract). *Crit Care Med* 1983; 11:220.

5. Culpepper J, Snyder J, Pinsky M, et al: Resistance in the inspiratory limb of continuous positive airway pressure systems (abstract). *Crit Care Med* 1983; 11:220.

6. Culpepper J: Unpublished data.

7. Douglas ME, Downs JB: Applied physiology and respiratory care, in Shoemaker WC (ed):
The Society of Critical Care Medicine: State of the Art. Fullerton, Calif, Society of Critical Care Medicine, 1982, vol 3, pp E:1–35.

8. Downs JB, Klein EF, Desautels D, et al: Intermittent mandatory ventilation: A new approach to weaning patients from mechanical ventilators. *Chest* 1973; 64:331.

9. Earl J: Controlled ventilation: A horror story (or Take me off the ventilator so I can breathe). *Respir Care* 1979; 24:193.

10. Gibney RTN, Wilson RS, Pontoppidan H: Comparison of work of breathing on high gas flow and demand valve continuous positive airway pressure systems. *Chest* 1982; 82:692.

11. Gjerde GE, Katz JA, Kraemer RW: Inspiratory work and airway pressure with continuous positive airway pressure delivery systems. *Crit Care Med* 1984; 12:272.

12. Greenbaum DM, Snyder JV, Grenvik A: Continuous positive airway pressure without tracheal intubation in spontaneously breathing patients. *Chest* 1976; 69:615.

13. Henry W, West G, Wilson R: A comparison of oxygen uptake between a high continuous flow constant positive airway pressure (CPAP) system and a demand breath CPAP system by use of the Beckman metabolic measurement. *Respir Care* 1983; 28:1273.

14. Kakmarek RM, Dimas S, Reynolds J, et al: Technical aspects of positive end-expiratory pressure (PEEP): I. Physics of PEEP devices. II. PEEP with positive pressure ventilation. III. PEEP with spontaneous ventilation. *Respir Care* 1982; 27:1478.

15. Kirby RR, Smith RA, Desautels DA (eds): *Mechanical Ventilation*. New York, Churchill Livingstone, 1985.

16. Mushin WW, Rendell-Baker L, Thompson PW, et al: *Automatic Ventilation of the Lungs*. Philadelphia, FA Davis Co, 1969.

17. Severinghaus JW: Transcutaneous monitoring of arterial Pco_2, in Spence AA (eds): *Respiratory Monitoring in Intensive Care*. New York, Churchill Livingstone, 1982, pp 85–91.

18. Schlobohm R, Falltrick R, Quan S, et al: Lung volumes, mechanics, and oxygenation during spontaneous positive-pressure ventilation: The advantage of CPAP over EPAP. *Anesthesiology* 1981; 55:416.

19. Snyder JV, Elliott FL, Grenvik A: Capnography, in Spence AA (ed): *Respiratory Monitoring in Intensive Care*. New York, Churchill Livingstone, 1982, p 100.

20. Snyder JV, Carroll GC, Schuster DP, et al: *Mechanical Ventilation: Physiology and Application. Curr Probl Surg* 1984, vol 21.

21. Tobin MJ, Jenouri G, Lind B, et al: Validation of the respiratory inductive plethysmograph in patients with pulmonary disease. *Chest* 1983; 83:615.

22. Venus B, Jacob HK, Lim L: Treatment of the adult respiratory distress syndrome with continuous positive airway pressure. *Chest* 1979; 76:257.

23. Weled B, Winfrey D, Downs J: Measuring exhaled volume with continuous positive airway pressures and intermittent mandatory ventilation: Techniques and rationale. *Chest* 1979; 76:166.

23 _____ High-Frequency Ventilation

Alison Froese, M.D.

The goal of this chapter is not to duplicate the extensive reviews already published,[16, 24, 38, 41, 43, 62, 67, 75] but to delineate both the strengths and weaknesses of the current information base so that we can develop some appreciation of both the promise and the conundrums presented by high-frequency ventilation (HFV) today.

It is now fact that effective gas transport can be sustained indefinitely by ventilation at higher than normal frequencies, even when the tidal volume (Vt) is only a fraction of the volume of the conducting airways. Gas transport can be achieved over a wide range of frequencies with a variety of devices and in many different pathologic states. In the midst of the plethora of data reported, it is important to stand back and ask critically whether or not this new modality in fact improves management of ventilation. Is HFV any better than the conventional approach? Answers to this question are contradictory, ranging from uncritical optimism through cautious interest to reactionary negativism.

SOURCES OF CONFUSION

Multiplicity of Devices

There are many reasons for the current confusion in the field of HFV. First, an incredible variety of systems has been reported in one study or another. Many are designed "in house," and rarely are two units exactly the same (even two originating in the same institution) until the device reaches commercial production. Even then, modifications can be made by the user, especially of the patient circuit, that may appear minor but substantially affect the function of that particular device. Therefore, even "experts" in the field may read an article and be unable to discern the exact functional characteristics of the system

being reported. Recently, increasing awareness of this problem[2, 46] has stimulated authors to provide much more complete descriptions of the particular system they used, but more vigilance is still needed in this area.

Uncontrolled and Unidentified Variables

A second problem that contributes to uncertainty in the field is investigators' failure to identify and monitor all important variables. Such failure represents not deliberate omission, but rather honest ignorance of the importance of certain variables and/or of the existence of physiologically significant artifacts that, we can see in retrospect, flawed many studies performed during the evolution of HFV. For example, in many early studies of HFV (both jet and oscillatory forms) mean airway pressure (AWP) was not even a measured, let alone a controlled, variable. We now recognize that without knowledge of that variable, many observations cannot be interpreted adequately. As research continues, undoubtedly other significant variables will be identified that are not now routinely defined. For example, recent experience suggests that characterization of the pressure-time profile produced in the trachea by an HFV device may be important, since the occurrence of asymmetric waveforms during the use of an oscillator-type device appears to be associated with increased risk of lung hyperinflation.[68]

Inadequacies of Experimental Design

Much confusion in the field of HFV has arisen from lack of carefully structured hypotheses in some studies. Limitations in the technology available for measuring certain variables, such as delivered stroke volume when the frequency is 5–30 Hz, have also seriously hampered protocol design. At times, investigators have been so intrigued with a new technique that they have jumped to the conclusion that because an HFV device works well in a particular situation, it is better than other techniques. Reports on the use of high-frequency jet ventilation (HFJV) for bronchoscopy or tracheal reconstruction are an example.[8, 27] HFJV has not been adequately compared to low-frequency jet or conventional ventilation for the same procedure.[4, 30]

Erroneous Presumptions

No scientific experiment is free of underlying assumptions. However, if these assumptions are not clearly defined and submitted to objective testing, they are better termed presumptions. A recurring presumption in much of the HFV literature is that the goal in using HFV devices is to ventilate at the lowest possible peak and mean AWP. Current experience indicates that this presumption may lead to suboptimal use of HFV devices. The basic presumption was and remains true when high-frequency devices are used primarily to "rescue" patients with large air leaks in whom conventional ventilation fails to support gas exchange. However, when the pathophysiologic problem is one of diffuse alveolar instability with extensive atelectasis, the aim is no longer necessarily to achieve mean AWPs lower than those generated by conventional ventilation. A rationale that is appropriate for a relatively rare condition, tracheobronchial cutaneous fistula, cannot automatically be extrapolated to a much more common problem, diffuse atelectasis. The presumed value of lowering AWP arises from the unproved assumption that absolute pressure is the villain. However, it is equally valid to speculate that it is not peak or mean AWP per se, but rather a large change in pressure applied to a collapsed parenchyma that damages lung tissue. There are two very different assumptions that lead to very different experimental designs. They may both prove to be correct under certain carefully defined circumstances. One thing is sure: when such fundamental assumptions aren't clearly delineated, confusion fills the void.

CLASSIFICATION OF HFV DEVICES

The physical characteristics of many HFV systems are summarized in several recent reviews. This section focuses on their functional characteristics.

In the early years of HFV, classifications were based primarily on the historical sequence of development. The term high-frequency positive pressure ventilation (HFPPV) was used for the modality introduced by Sjöstrand and his colleagues in Sweden in 1967 in which tidal volumes of 3–4 ml/kg were delivered at 60–100 breaths per minute.[75] The modality used a pneumatically controlled system with minimal compressible volume and no gas entrainment and achieved gas exchange at lower peak AWPs. HFJV became the more common approach in North America as Klain and Smith,[51] Carlon et al.,[16] and others combined the concept of higher ventilating rates with the equipment used for jet ventilation at ordinary frequencies. Operating frequencies of 100–200/min have since become customary for HFJV. High-frequency flow interruptors (HIFI) are closely related to jet ventilators. No fundamental difference between HIFI and HFJV has been documented, although their pattern of usage has differed, with HIFI generally used in combination with a basal level of conventional mechanical ventilation (CMV).

In the early 1970s researchers in Germany who were studying myocardial response to pressure pulses[55] and researchers in Canada who were trying to enhance intrapulmonary gas mixing[7] discovered that, rather surprisingly, adequate carbon dioxide elimination and oxygen uptake could be sustained indefinitely simply by small-volume, sinusoidal flow oscillations at the airway at rather high frequencies of 10–40 Hz (600–2,400 min). Because the waveform used was sinusoidal, the term high-frequency oscillatory ventilation, or high-frequency oscillation (HFO), was coined.

In the past 10 years, as research on HFPPV, HFJV, and HFO has progressed, considerable confusion has arisen over the nonuniform terminology in the literature. In several instances, exactly the same ventilator has appeared in two different articles under completely different names, as authors have sought to comply with what seemed to be the consensus of the moment.[32, 55]

It has been suggested that to improve communications we establish a system of nomenclature based on an important functional property of these systems, namely, the nature of the expiratory phase (active versus passive).[38] The operating frequency was once thought to be a useful distinction, since HFJV tended to be used at a frequency of 1–3 Hz and HFO at a frequency of 10–40 Hz. As research has progressed, however, jet ventilators have been used at higher and higher frequencies while HFO has come down to the 3–5 Hz range in some studies, so that their operational frequency ranges overlap. Nevertheless there do appear to be significant differences in the performance of "jet ventilators" and "oscillators." It is not yet clear which may be "better," or under what circumstances, or why, but there is no question that they are different when it comes to the frequency at which obligatory increases in lung volume (also known as auto-PEEP, inadvertent PEEP, or gas trapping) tend to occur.

Although there are a number of minor differences between jet ventilators and oscillators, such as inspiratory waveform and customary inspiratory-expiratory (I:E) ratio, the most distinctive difference lies in the expiratory phase. Jet ventilators and flow interrupters (such as the Emerson V-2) all actively inject a pulse of gas into the lungs but have a passive exhalation phase during which gas is driven out of the lungs solely by passive recoil of the lung and chest wall. To date, HFO devices have all used some type of reciprocating pump—a bellows, piston, or loudspeaker—that actively pushes gas into the lungs and then actively draws an equal volume of gas out of the system. In recent bench tests of a number of current HFV devices, all assessed at a constant reference frequency of 15 Hz, several models with active expiratory phases appeared to be functionally equivalent, while models with passive exhalation formed a distinctly different functional grouping.[37]

Therefore, I wish to strongly reiterate an earlier plea[38] that all reports of HFV clearly characterize the system used as either a high-frequency ventilator with active expiration (HFV-A) or as one with a passive expiratory phase (HFV-P), considering both the flow generator and the circuit in the categorization. Such an approach is essential to avoid further confusion as new hybrids appear that add active expiration to HFJV devices, and as circuit modifications introduce passive expiratory phases to devices that are otherwise classic oscillators. Perhaps HFV-P and HFV-A could be adopted as generic terms to be used when referring to these broad categories of HFV devices. When a specific ventilator is referred to, its customary acronym could be used, along with the appropriate designation "-P" or "-A" so the reader was immediately informed of this functional parameter. For example, one would then use HFJV-P to denote the customary jet ventilator but specify HFJV-A if the device had been modified to make expiration active. Similarly, the classic oscillator would be labeled HFO-A unless its expiratory phase were made passive, in which case the designation would be HFO-P.

In this text, the old terminology is used in reference to existing literature; we recognize that HFO always implies HFV-A, while HFJV and HFPPV always imply HFV-P.

ARE HFV DEVICES BETTER?

HFV devices are effective. Whether or not they are "better" than existing conventional devices is a much more complex question. The continued search for new ventilators is based on the tacit assumption that current ventilatory support is not yet perfect. It may even be that some of the problems that ensue over the course of treatment may be partly the result, not just the cause, of the ventilator therapy (see chapter 24, "Respirator Lung").

Any attempt to improve ventilatory support must seek to transport oxygen and carbon dioxide more effectively while decreasing lung injury (both acute and chronic), and do all this without impairing cardiac output. These goals are laudatory, but some may be mutually exclusive. Measures that minimize acute barotrauma may be detrimental to oxygenation. As indicated earlier, this intrinsic conflict has led to a great deal of uncertainty about whether we should pursue high pressures or low pressures during HFV. Undoubtedly some trade-off will have to be made in our efforts to minimize risk and maximize benefit. The biggest barrier to progress in this area currently is the lack of an accurate rank-ordering of all the various mechanisms that have been implicated as playing some role in lung injury (e.g., F_{IO_2}, peak pressure, magnitude of pressure or volume cycles, lung distention). Also, the possible mitigating influence of cofactors, such as the development of protein leak into the alveoli, is not known.[48]

Is HFV Better for Special Procedures?

High-frequency systems have been used extensively for special procedures such as bronchoscopy and laryngoscopy[8, 30] or tracheal surgery.[26, 27] In all of these procedures there is competition for access to the airway, and it is convenient to use a system that can deliver the necessary Vt through a small cannula. However, there is no clear evidence that the operating frequency matters in this application. The same procedures can be handled successfully with low-frequency ventilation through a cannula.[4, 30] A physical characteristic of the delivery system, not the operating frequency, appears to be the critical feature in this application. Laser resection of tracheobronchial tissue appears to be one situation in which decreased motion of the surgical field does confer a definite advantage to the endoscopist.[84]

It has been postulated that high-frequency systems would facilitate operative procedures by reducing movement of the diaphragm and upper abdominal organs that can interfere with visualization of or access to certain operative sites. However, no clear-cut benefit has emerged in evaluations to date.[21, 72] Some surgeons like it; others prefer to have fewer large displacements every minute, and a motionless field in between. Possible applications during microneurosurgery are still under investigation.

The anticipated ability of HFV to minimize intracranial pressure (ICP) in patients with elevated ICP has also proved to be of limited applicability. The use of lower mean AWP achieved some lowering of ICP during HFJV in one animal model with normal lungs and elevated ICP,[81] but not in a different model of elevated ICP.[73] In the presence of concurrent pulmonary dysfunction, if mean AWPs were increased during HFJV as well as during CMV to achieve adequate gas exchange, differences in ICP and cerebral perfusion pressure with the two ventilatory modalities were negligible.[73]

Is HFV Better With Established Barotrauma?

In the past 5 years numerous clinical reports have affirmed that HFV ventilators—both with passive and with active expiratory phases—can be life-saving in patients with massive air leaks under circumstances in which conventional ventilators fail to move adequate gas volumes to the alveoli to eliminate carbon dioxide.[10, 12, 16, 20, 33, 60, 83] Since all the original clinical experience was obtained using jet ventilators, in which entrainment of additional gas is characteristic, it was proposed that entrainment may be an important mechanism in the therapeutic efficacy of HFJV in major air

leaks.[83] However, it seems likely that the reduction of Vt in HFJV simply decreases the driving pressure across the air leak and permits adequate gas volumes to reach the gas-exchanging alveolar surface. Air leaks with or without pulmonary interstitial air have also been successfully treated using HFO devices, without air entrainment.[10, 12, 20] Characteristically resolution during both HFO and HFJV has occurred while carbon dioxide elimination has been improved at lower mean and peak AWPs than during CMV. Further experimental work is needed to delineate precisely which features of HFV account for its therapeutic efficacy in this particular clinical situation.

Is HFV Better at Carbon Dioxide Elimination?

Yes. As experience accumulates with both HFV-A and HFV-P devices it is increasingly clear that HFV ventilators are extremely effective in terms of AWP at transporting carbon dioxide in both normal and abnormal lung, except possibly in the presence of diffuse bronchospasm.[21] Repeatedly, patients who retained carbon dioxide despite numerous adjustments of pressures and rate during CMV have had Pa_{CO_2} normalized by HFV at the same or lower peak and mean AWPs.[10, 12, 16, 20, 33, 60, 83] This feature may prove useful when respiratory alkalosis at low transrespiratory pressures is desired, as in the treatment of persistent fetal circulation.[39]

HFV is not, however, particularly efficient in terms of minute volume. During CMV, approximately 60% of the minute volume generally participates in alveolar gas exchange. During HFV this figure can be as low as 5% at frequencies of 10–20 Hz.[64] Therefore HFV can be viewed as a pressure effective, though not a volumetrically efficient, means of transporting carbon dioxide.

The high-frequency modalities are not all equally effective at carbon dioxide transport, however. Typically, HFV-A devices can achieve carbon dioxide elimination over a wide frequency range (1–50 Hz). With HFV-P devices carbon dioxide elimination is frequency dependent.[3] Normocapnia is attainable in both normal and abnormal lung at frequencies of less than 200–300/min. At higher rates normocapnia can sometimes be achieved by increasing driving pressure and shortening the percent inspiratory time, but eventually carbon dioxide retention, usually in association with lung hyperinflation, will limit the usable frequency.

Is HFV Better at Oxygenation?

This question must be addressed in terms of the major clinical causes of hypoxemia: inadequate alveolar ventilation, extensive ventilation/perfusion mismatch with large areas of low but non-zero $\dot{V}/\dot{Q}$ ratio, and increased intrapulmonary shunting (diffuse atelectasis).

Hypoxia Secondary to Alveolar Hypoventilation

When patients are hypoxic from inadequate alveolar ventilation, as occurs with massive air leaks, HFV generally improves oxygenation as it corrects carbon dioxide retention.[10, 12, 16, 20, 33, 60, 83]

Hypoxia Secondary to Low $\dot{V}/\dot{Q}$ Regions

Starting with the earliest reports of many of the high-frequency modalities, numerous anecdotes have accumulated in which oxygenation with HFV appeared to be much better than oxygenation with CMV in a variety of circumstances. Speculation evolved that enhanced interregional and intraregional gas mixing during HFV would make ventilation/perfusion ratios more homogeneous throughout the lung. In a few human subjects with chronic obstructive lung disease (and $\dot{V}/\dot{Q}$ mismatch presumed on that basis), rather striking decreases in calculated venous admixture were observed during HFO, compared with CMV.[13] In both animal and human studies, rapid intrapulmonary mixing has been observed both within[58] and between[69] lung regions. However, no larger trials have been performed to test whether or not HFV ventilators can improve oxygenation significantly through the postulated impact on regions with low (but nonzero) $\dot{V}/\dot{Q}$ ratios. Although animal modeling has been attempted, results have been inconclusive primarily because of difficulties in developing a stable, relevant model of extensive $\dot{V}/\dot{Q}$ mismatch. However, one can legitimately question whether this is a very important issue to pursue, since in patients with extensive $\dot{V}/\dot{Q}$ mismatch but little intrapulmonary shunting, oxygenation is not really a therapeutic problem. Their hypoxia responds readily to small increases in F_{IO_2}. Their problems lie in weaning, not oxygenation.

Hypoxia Due to Intrapulmonary Shunting

In the presence of diffuse atelectasis, HFV ventilators, like conventional ventilators, improve oxygenation only when used with appropriate distending pressures to maintain alveolar volume. The principle established by Boros[9] for conventional ventilators was confirmed first by Marchak et al.[56] and Thompson et al.[80] for HFO and later by Schuster et al.[70, 71] and Rouby et al.[66] for HFJV. In the presence of diffuse atelectasis, oxygenation is tightly linked to maintenance of an adequate alveolar gas-exchanging volume and therefore, to a first approximation, oxygenation is proportional to the mean AWP applied across the respiratory system to splint alveoli open (Fig 23–1).

The relationship between mean AWP and oxygenation has seemed to be the single concept that best unifies the broad database of oxygenation during HFV. However, this concept ignores the established pressure-volume behavior of the lung, which exhibits considerable hysteresis. That is, for any given lung and any given trans-respiratory pressure, there exists a variety of possible lung volumes ranging from the relatively low volume (and greater hypoxia) of the inflation limb to the higher volume (and lesser hypoxia) of the deflation limb. Therefore, conceptually, mean AWP and oxygenation cannot be uniquely interrelated. This variable relation was demonstrated in studies performed using HFO in which oxygenation was significantly better with HFO than with CMV, under circumstances in which HFO maintained a larger mean lung volume than CMV even though both ventilators were operated at the same mean AWP.[53] Kolton et al. then demonstrated in two animals models of diffuse lung injury that one could increase mean lung volume and improve oxygenation by using a brief volume recruitment maneuver.[53] Conceptually, one can think of this as an attempt to move the operating position of the injured lung from the "inflation limb" to the "deflation limb" of its pressure-volume relationship. Such maneuvers are more effective during HFV than CMV primarily because the small cyclic pressure swings of HFV make the minimum (or PEEP) pressure of a ventilatory cycle higher during HFV than during CMV operating at the same mean AWP, thereby reducing alveolar derecruitment during expiration. When lung injury has occurred, alveolar collapse may occur during the first exhalation after recruitment.

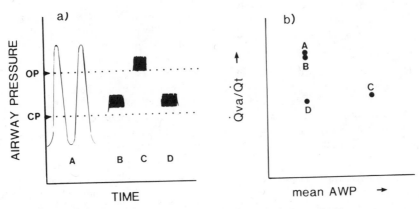

FIG 23–1.
a) *A*-CMV at moderate mean AWP. *B*-HFV at equal mean AWP, higher PEEP, and lower peak AWP. Gas exchange is no better than at *A* because peak pressures are also below opening pressures (*OP*) of some alveoli. *C*-HFV at higher mean AWP but still with lower peak AWP than at *A*. Both opening and closing pressures (*CP*) are exceeded and oxygenation improves. *D*-HFV at mean AWP equal to *A* and *B* after a brief sustained inflation is used to exceed OP and recruit alveolar volume, and then PEEP is reduced to a level that keeps alveoli above CP. **b)** venous admixture (Qva/Qt) corresponding to ventilatory pattern in **(a)**.

Therefore, after a recruiting maneuver it may be important to allow exhalation only to the maintenance AWP (Fig 23–2). This concept has yet to be systematically explored and applied to the various forms of HFV in use today, although the principle undoubtedly provides the rationale for why many protocols with periodic "sighs" or background levels of intermittent mandatory ventilation (IMV) have come into use on a pragmatic basis over the past few years.[6, 10]

Analysis of the many early reports of HFJV reveals that much of the success in terms of oxygenation was probably secondary to the use of rather high mean AWP, although this must be deduced by extrapolation from later studies, since accurate intratracheal pressures are not reported in much of the early literature. Rouby's reports clearly document a link between oxygenation and mean AWP[66] and demonstrate as well that increases in mean AWP will eventually exact a price in cardiac output,[40] although this price can be moderated to some extent by synchronizing the jet with the cardiac cycle (see chapter 31, "Ventilatory Support of the Failing Circulation"). Schuster and colleagues did much to clarify the role of mean AWP in oxygenation during HFJV in carefully controlled animal and human studies.[70, 71] Again, they demonstrated that with

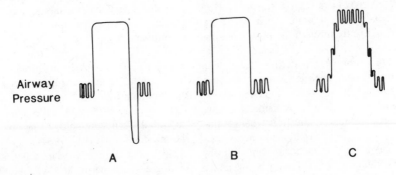

FIG 23–2.
Example of a volume recruiting maneuver (*A*) that is followed by a dip in AWP during which derecruitment may occur. *B, C*, examples of two types of recruiting maneuvers during which AWP is never allowed to dip below the minimum maintenance AWP.

diffuse lung injury (oleic acid in dogs, ARDS in humans) oxygenation was improved beyond that achieved by CMV only if the HFV device was operated at a higher mean AWP. Note that volume recruitment maneuvers were not used in any of this early work.

Therapeutically, we tend to recoil from using higher mean AWP levels because we expect an inevitable link between the associated high peak inspiratory pressures and acute barotrauma. Kirby and associates[50] tried to break this link by coupling super-PEEP with the maximum possible contribution from spontaneous breaths to decrease the lung's exposure to high peak pressures while still using high distending pressures. Directed recruiting has also been used to reduce the need for, and damage from, high peak AWP. When recruiting efforts open closed lung and sufficient PEEP is used to prevent lung closure, high Vt is no longer needed and Vt need only be sufficient to eliminate carbon dioxide. Although to a degree this may be achieved simply by reducing Vt from CMV ventilators, HFV ventilators provide us with a more effective tool to achieve the goal of an open lung with minimal AWP. Because smaller pressure and volume swings can be used during HFV, one can use a higher *mean* AWP and still keep the *peak* AWP lower than during CMV (see Fig 23–1, *A* vs. *C*). As in conventional ventilation, lung volume can be further enhanced by specific volume recruitment maneuvers during HFO (see Fig 23–1, point *D*). One can think of HFV as a potential means of delivering high PEEP with built-in carbon dioxide removal (see chapter 25, "The Open Lung Approach: Concept and Application"). One can speculate that for maintenance of lung volume the best combination of ventilator stroke volume and frequency would be the one that produced the smallest possible fluctuations in lung volume around the desired mean value, while sustaining gas transport. (Note that this issue is theoretical at present.) In this context, we need to determine whether, for these purposes, HFV is any better at one or the other end of the frequency spectrum.

To date, clinical data on the role of lung volume in the efficacy of HFV are still limited because so many reports antedate accurate monitoring of intratracheal pressure and/or lung volume. However, this concept is a key to the future evaluation of HFV's ability to correct defects in oxygenation caused by diffuse atelectasis. It is important to recognize that in the only large comparative trial of CMV and HFJV reported to date, in which no significant difference in outcome could be detected between the two modalities, no specific volume recruitment maneuvers were used during HFJV.[15] It is possible that if HFJV were to be used with a deliberate volume recruitment strategy, differences might emerge.

Does HFV Cause Less Lung Injury?

Only tentative conclusions can be drawn about the extent of lung injury with HFV. It is tempting to conclude that a device that permits resolution of an injury that occurred with a different ventilator (e.g., bronchopleural cutaneous fistula or pulmonary interstitial air developing on CMV) must itself be "less injurious" to lung tissue. However, HFV ventilators have also produced injury. Disastrous, sometimes fatal, barotrauma has occurred in a number of instances in which "jetting devices," both high frequency and manually operated, have continued to force gas into the lungs while gas exit was in some way impeded.[25] At high driving pressures, such complications can evolve extremely rapidly. Also, a number of centers have seen an unusual incidence of necrotizing tracheitis in infants treated with HFJV.[59, 60] This incidence has tended to decrease but not disappear with improved humidification techniques, which suggests there may be an aspect of direct trauma from the high-velocity jet pulses. This concern requires further study. In a few clinical studies prohibitive bronchospasm has occurred during trials of HFV.[21, 83]

The impact of several hours of ventilation on lung morphology has been examined in normal animals in which both active expiratory (HFO)[32, 34] and passive expiratory (HFJV)[49] techniques have been compared with CMV. No differences have been seen morphologically or in the amount or composition of lung phospholipids.[34, 82] Although a small amount of transudate accumulated in the pleural space of dogs undergoing 32 hours of HFO,[63] lymph flow studies have not shown any impairment of lung fluid clearance during HFO in either normal or abnormal lungs.[29, 47] The impact of HFV on mucociliary clearance remains controversial.[31, 42, 57]

Whether HFV ventilators can support gas exchange in IRDS or ARDS with less structural injury than is caused by CMV is still unclear, but experimental observations are promising. Hamilton et al. found better oxygenation and less structural damage (i.e., less epithelial necrosis and hyaline membrane formation) in rabbits made surfactant deficient by repeated saline lavage who were ventilated by HFO rather than CMV for 5–20 hours.[44] In that study a deliberate volume recruitment maneuver was performed at the beginning of the treatment period, and both ventilators were operated at the same mean AWP. In that particular protocol, the HFO study group was exposed to different ventilator characteristics and also was maintained at a different operating lung volume, since alveolar recruitment proved very effective in the HFO-treated rabbits only.

HFJV has not been shown to produce comparable results, but the difference may relate to experimental design. In one protocol no volume recruitment was attempted and rather low mean AWP was used.[54] In another, a volume recruitment maneuver was used in only half the animals and HFJV was delivered at considerably lower mean AWP levels than CMV.[61]

Further clarification of this issue should emerge from the comparative studies of two forms of HFV and conventional ventilation in baboons with hyaline membrane disease.[6, 19] In short-term studies, HFV appeared to cause earlier saccular recruitment, while in studies of longer duration less structural injury was observed after HFO-A than after either CMV or HFV using a flow interrupter with passive expiration (HIFI-P).[19] In a preliminary comparative study of HFO-A and CMV in human neonates and using a protocol aimed at early recruitment of lung volume, we found that we could lower the F_{IO_2} requirement faster using HFO-A than using CMV, without any apparent increase in acute or chronic lung injury.[39] Following this protocol, similar mean AWP levels were used in both HFO-A- and CMV-treated infants, but these mean AWP levels were deliberately used early in the HFO-A-treated infants to reverse atelectasis, whereas in the CMV-treated infants comparable mean AWP levels were not reached until the second day of treatment, when they became necessary to support carbon dioxide elimination.

SPECIAL TACTICAL ISSUES IN HFV

Gas Trapping

A number of studies now document the phenomenon of intrapulmonary gas trapping, "auto-PEEP," or "inadvertent PEEP";[3, 5, 18, 68, 74]

these are synonyms for the occurrence of potentially deleterious, unwanted hyperinflation of the lungs. This problem has been described most commonly during HFV-P (HFJV or HIFI), the devices being dependent on passive exhalation of gas that was driven in by a high pressure source. The hyperinflation generally increases with increasing frequency and driving pressure.[3, 5, 18] For any given frequency it can be reduced by lengthening the fraction of the cycle spent in expiration. The hazard is intensified by any factor that increases resistance to exhalation, especially when a high minute volume is being used. The presence of mucus or a bend in the endotracheal tube will have negligible effect during CMV but can markedly increase mean AWP during HFJV. Similarly, although using HFJV to maintain ventilation during tracheal suctioning can be advantageous, the practice can be hazardous if pulmonary dysfunction is severe and high mean AWP and high minute volume are required. In the latter case, if the expiratory path is narrowed by the presence of the suction catheter while minute volume is maintained and suction is not applied, serious barotrauma can ensue.

Responses to the problem of hyperinflation have varied. Some have suggested that one could simply accept the gas trapping and thenceforth select the operating frequency on the basis of what distending pressure was desired. That is, one could increase the rate to increase lung distention therapeutically and decrease the rate to avoid overdistention. Although such an approach is feasible (if pulmonary distending pressures and mechanics are well characterized), it limits the range of usable ventilator frequencies. If there were some compelling reason to ventilate at a high rate (for example, to minimize cycle volume), one might be unable to do so safely. Alternatively, one could apply continuous suction to the circuit behind the jet to assist the expiratory phase during HFJV and extend the usable range of frequency and driving pressure.[77] With this approach appropriate, automatic safeguards must be in place to prevent excessive negative pressures from being applied accidentally to the lungs.

More rarely, lung hyperinflation has been described in some HFO systems.[68, 74, 78] Predictably, the degree of hyperinflation is proportional to the lung compliance. Despite our deliberate efforts to detect it, hyperinflation has not been observed in any of the extensive animal and human studies performed either by this author[39] or by

Bryan et al.[12] when using an oscillator system at 15 Hz with an unvalved circuit that incorporates a bias flow of 8–10 L/min. With this system we obtain a symmetric sinusoidal pressure waveform at the top of the endotracheal tube. However, if certain changes are made in the circuit, such as dropping the bias flow rate, one can produce asymmetric pressure profiles of the type demonstrated by Saari et al. (see Figure 5 in their paper).[68] It is likely that all high-frequency systems are potentially vulnerable to the development of lung hyperinflation, but for different reasons. HFV devices with passive expiration appear to engender gas trapping at rates of 300–400 breaths per minute because of problems regarding the time constant: the expiratory period simply becomes less than the passive time constant of the lung. This phenomenon seems to appear consistently throughout the HFJV database, despite the use of a variety of ventilators and circuits. This mechanism is simply inherent in the fundamental design of HFV devices with passive expiration and can be overcome only by assisting expiratory flow in some way, such as by adding suction during the expiratory phase. When HFV devices with active expiration are used, the phenomenon occurs less frequently and appears to be influenced strongly by the design of the system. Gas trapping during HFV-A may represent a state in which gas is sucked out of the lung faster than the critical wave speed of the small airways, at which point expiratory flow limitation (a "choke" point) develops with a corresponding intrapulmonary pressure gradient across it.[22] Since the maximum flow that can pass through a tube at critical wave speed increases with the radius and the elastance of the tube wall, one would predict that flow limitation would be least likely to occur in stiff lungs (high elastance) ventilated at a high mean AWP (increased airway dimensions), as in the treatment of IRDS or ARDS. Conversely, flow limitation and hyperinflation would be most probable during ventilation of very compliant lungs with small airways obstruction (e.g., COPD) at low transrespiratory pressures. One would also predict that flow limitation would be more likely when using a closed HFO-A system, with high impedance connections to the fresh gas source and expiratory pathway, since in this case the high expiratory flow rates demanded by the ventilator can be provided only by flow out of the lungs. Conversely, open systems, with no valves or restrictions on inlet and exit gas flow pathways, may be less prone to development of intrapulmonary flow limitation and hyperinflation since gas aspirated during exhalation can come partially from the circuit rather than the lungs. These characteristics of flow limitation may explain why hyperinflation has been described several times with high impedance circuits, but not with the "open" bias flow design.

The above argument implies that systems with active expiration may have a greater usable range of operating frequency than HFV-P devices, without inducing potential deleterious hyperinflation. However, as so many factors potentially influence the occurrence of hyperinflation, it is mandatory that any HFV user take appropriate action to control hyperinflation.

Pressure Monitoring

Inaccurate or inappropriate pressure monitoring has plagued the study of HFV. One problem has been related to the use of transducer/catheter systems with unknown or inadequate frequency response. Such systems make any statements about dynamic pressure profiles highly suspect, although mean pressures may be reflected accurately. A more serious problem has been the site of pressure measurement. Most major discrepancies in pressure assessment can be traced to errors in the site. Some early users of HFJV even sampled their monitoring pressures external to the jet itself (somewhere in the ancillary circuit proximal to the jet tip), rather than distal to the point of jet entry. Such sampling produces values that systematically underestimate true intrapulmonary pressure.[45, 85] Such inaccuracy not only limits one's understanding of the performance of the HFV device, but is also hazardous to patient safety.

The low-pressure zone that most often leads to erroneous estimates of intrapulmonary pressure (both peak and mean values) is the zone upstream of the jet injector tip itself.[45, 85] This of course is the low-pressure region responsible for entrainment. If the jet injector is located at the top of the endotracheal tube so that flow patterns can spread out through the tube before reaching the tip, the endotracheal tube itself may behave as a jet cannula as the high-velocity gas pulses pass out of the smaller tube (the "injector") into the larger trachea (the "diffusor"). Therefore, a second low-pressure zone can occur just below the tip of the endotracheal tube, even with high jet placement, and introduce a further discrepancy of

2–3 cm H_2O.[1] Third, pressure differentials can occur within the airways, such that alveolar pressures exceed central AWP, in association with the hyperinflation phenomenon discussed earlier.[1, 79] Faced with such a plethora of possible artifacts, we strongly recommend the approach of Rouby et al.[66] They validated AWP measurements, sampled at a site 10 cm below the injector nozzle, by comparing them with relaxation pressures measured during periods of brief occlusion of all tubing connected to the patient. This isolated the lungs from the ventilator and provided an estimate of the operative mean transrespiratory distending pressure free from potential flow-related artifacts. In view of the importance of accurate pressure monitoring for patient safety, we recommend that only tracheal monitoring sites situated approximately 10 cm below the jet tip be used, that the accuracy of a monitoring technique be established in animal trials before it is used in humans, and that relaxation pressures be used to further confirm a monitoring system's performance.

Safety Devices

Because of the high rates and high pressures used during HFV, safety systems must be designed very carefully. Alarms alone are not enough. *There must be* automatic *shut-off mechanisms that can instantaneously prevent any further gas delivery into the lungs, or any further suction out of the lungs in systems that incorporate a negative pressure source.* Such devices must be tailored for each specific HFV-P or HFV-A device. The monitor that triggers a safety device must be fed an accurate, appropriate signal. In the case of HFJV devices, this means a tracheally sampled pressure, as discussed above. In the case of HFV-A (oscillator) devices, we have used circuit pressures to run our safety devices after validating the system using relaxation pressure measurements.

Volume Recruitment

Volume recruitment strategies during HFV are still very poorly defined. There are enough data from animal and human studies to substantiate that a recruitment maneuver should be incorporated into HFV to exceed the opening pressures of collapsed alveoli. But what? And how? A variety of combined modes have appeared, with the ''low''-frequency mode operating at anything from 1–100 min, but there is little factual basis upon which to select among them.[10, 28] Kolton et al. introduced the alternative concept of using

brief periods of a deliberate increase in inflation pressure (an SI, or sustained inflation).[53] These are isolated events, used only when needed, and occur at rather long intervals.

We are left with a wide range of options: from perhaps two to ten ordinary CMV breaths per minute with superimposed HFV, to pure HFV with a sustained inflation once every 1 to 12 hours! The former is obviously the simpler approach, since it can be preset and automatic. The latter requires ongoing assessment and response by a primary care individual (nurse, respiratory therapist, or physician). The former automated system provides alveolar recruitment periods of a second or less (in infants), whereas the manual approach uses 10- to 15-second periods of raised pressure, which may be long enough to call interdependence forces into play to aid in alveolar recruitment. Until we have a clearer idea of both the time dependence of alveolar recruitment and the causes of lung injury, rational selection among these options will remain impossible. In this context it is important to recognize the totally arbitrary nature of many of the clinical protocols that have been described to date.

A number of questions need to be answered. First, how does one know the volume recruitment maneuvers are working? If one uses periodic CMV breaths all the time, how does one know they are contributing anything more than the HFV alone? How does one select frequency and peak pressure? If one uses intermittent SI maneuvers, it is easier to assess efficacy, because one can look for a step-change in oxygenation monitored by some on-line technique. In infants it has been our policy that if no benefit is seen, no further SI maneuvers are attempted, since there is no point in exposing the lung to potential risk without demonstrable benefit. If there is a clear response, then the maneuver is used whenever needed. Again, we need to question how vigorously we should pursue volume recruitment. Byford et al. found a dose-response relationship between magnitude of improvement in oxygenation and the amount of pressure used for the SI.[14] Eventually a plateau was reached at which further increases in SI pressure yielded no further benefit. However, as the SI pressure increases the risk of barotrauma will also increase, so some sort of trade-off—still poorly defined—appears inevitable.

I strongly doubt that rote prescription of volume recruitment maneuvers during HFV will ever be optimal, given the wide variability of opening pressures and time dependence required for alveolar recruitment in lungs injured by different processes to variable degrees. Instead, we must focus on developing procedures for ongoing evaluation and titration of therapy using on-line estimates of "shunt," such as pulse oximetry or transcutaneous Po_2 monitoring.

One thing is clear, however. Observations in both animals and humans demonstrate that volume recruitment can be evanescent. Therefore, whatever the approach, one must be careful that during the expiratory phase immediately *after* the CMV breath or sustained inflation, AWP is not allowed to fall *below* maintenance levels, or any benefit gained may be lost. This requires careful attention to circuit design (see Fig 23–2).

Choice of Ventilator Settings

This issue remains embarrassingly vague after years of HFV experience. The problem is that there is no "optimal" setting for carbon dioxide elimination. A whole host of Vt and frequency combinations will do the job. "Jetters" seem to work at rates of 150–200/min and "oscillators" at 10–20 Hz, but these frequencies are used more by habit than by reason. We lack a solid rational basis for selection. Such a basis will probably emerge from studies of mechanisms of lung injury, not of gas transport per se. For example, it has been suggested that the frequency that produced the smallest alveolar pressure swings per unit of volume flow might be optimal. Up to resonant frequency, a decrease in alveolar pressure swings should be accompanied by a decrease in pressure swings at the airway opening.[35] Dorkin et al.[23] found that in infants with RDS the resonant frequency is much higher (>40 Hz) than in the normal infant (3–7 Hz).[86] If minimization of alveolar and airway pressure amplitudes can be shown to aid resolution of the pathologic process, even higher frequencies than have been used clinically to date may prove valuable. More data are needed to clarify such decisions about ventilator settings.

One practical issue relevant to operating frequency should be noted. As frequencies during HFV become higher and higher (e.g., ~30 Hz), eventually a point is reached where oscillations of the chest wall are not seen. Gas exchange is attained without visible motion, and visual cues can no longer be used to diagnose problems such as a blocked endotracheal tube or ventilator disconnection. Under these circumstances, appropriately designed pressure monitors and on-line indicators of oxygenation are essential.

GAS TRANSPORT AND HFV

We lack space to discuss this issue fully. However, Chang has provided an excellent recent review.[17] During HFV, the secondary mixing mechanisms that we usually ignore as insignificant when analyzing classic bulk flow transport are of major importance. With Vt much smaller than deadspace no single ventilatory cycle can physically transport gas molecules from alveolus to airway. However, if each cycle follows asymmetric flow profiles so that the pattern of flow in does not exactly match the pattern of flow out, and there are additional mixing processes as from turbulent eddies, then with each stroke there will be some net transport of gas molecules. That is, some molecules pushed in will not be pulled out again. Although each cycle is too small to do the job, with hundreds of cycles per minute carbon dioxide and oxygen transport can readily be achieved, with net movement down their respective concentration gradients. Considering the high flows of HFV, rapid cycling frequencies, abrupt flow reversals, and many airway branch points in the lung, one can easily see how asymmetric velocity profiles and secondary mixing processes can occur during HFV.

This process of gas transport is variously referred to as "augmented diffusion," "augmented dispersion," or an "effective diffusivity."[36] These terms have engendered considerable confusion. It is important to realize that these terms, in and of themselves, say nothing fundamental about the actual mechanisms of transport in HFV. They simply provide one with a shorthand way of talking about it. This approach pursues a tradition in fluid mechanics, whereby phenomena are modeled as a problem of *apparent* or *virtual* diffusion. That is, one says transport is occurring *as if* the fluid were moving with a certain diffusivity, and one then performs experiments to find out empirically which variables influence the extent of the transport.

These principles have emerged from studies to date:

1. Although we talk a great deal about apparent diffusivity in HFV, *molecular* diffusivity

(D_{mol}) is of minimal importance. Only about 5% of total transport is influenced by D_{mol}.[52]

2. Gas transport by HFV is not particularly efficient, with effective alveolar ventilation approaching only 5%–10% of minute volume at high frequencies.[64]

3. Intrapulmonary gas mixing is enhanced by HFV, compared with CMV. The extent of mixing is proportional to $Vt^{\sim 1.5} \times f$.[58]

4. Carbon dioxide transport out of the lung increases with increases in both stroke volume and rate, but Vt has the stronger influence such that $\dot{V}_{CO_2} \propto f \times Vt^{-2}$.[11, 76]

5. Eucapnia can be achieved with lower products of $Vt \times f$ if the fresh gas front is moved to the tip rather than the top of the endotracheal tube, to reduce transport distances.[65] (This option may not always be practical, as in small infants, and can influence the accuracy of pressure measurements.)

One must emphasize that all the detailed transport analyses to date have been done using sinusoidal flow oscillations (i.e., HFO), because sinusoidal flow is easier to analyze and model. Comments about transport during HFJV inevitably must be made by analogy to the sine wave flow profile of HFO, with its active expiratory phase. These extrapolations may not be totally accurate. More actual comparisons among different high-frequency modalities are needed to clarify issues such as whether or not the use of an active versus passive expiratory phase influences gas transport efficiency.

FUTURE DIRECTIONS

Despite the frustrations, confusion, arguments, and artifacts that have plagued the development of HFV, a core of excitement remains among investigators who have sufficient successes to realize that there is potential here—if we can only have enough insight to pick our way through the maze. HFV devices are not magic machines that will solve all the problems of ventilation. Nevertheless they are intrinsically different from our conventional ventilators, and these differences offer some distinctly new therapeutic options, particularly in the area of lung volume recruitment and maintenance, and in the treatment of air leaks.

Further research is needed that will systematically clear up the areas of confusion referred to in this chapter. This research must include a balance of carefully designed trials in the laboratory and in humans. A very important step will be the up-coming randomized multicenter trial of HFO and CMV in infants with RDS, which will provide us with a large body of data on the use of these two ventilatory modalities in a relatively homogeneous disease state. If HFV works under those fairly "pure" conditions, we will then ask whether the same approach could be of benefit in the more disparate pathologic states encountered in the adult.

In the long term, success will be mixed until enough evidence accumulates to show whether or not the early use of HFV is valid, since prevention of lung injury is more promising than cure. Above all we must think systematically, not only about which ventilator we use to treat a given patient, but about how we use it, and why we select that particular therapeutic strategy. In all this we must recognize that the therapeutic goal in mechanical ventilation of the lungs can no longer be stated just in terms of F_{IO_2}, Pa_{O_2}, Pa_{CO_2}, and pH, or even oxygen delivery. The impact of our therapies on the underlying pathophysiologic processes is now also up for scrutiny and must become an integral part of our therapeutic rationale.

REFERENCES

1. Armengol J: *Studies of hemodynamics, gas exchange and lung mechanics with metal bellows oscillatory ventilation in dogs,* thesis. Edmonton, Alberta, University of Alberta, 1985.
2. ATS, ACCP, DLD-NHLBI: High Frequency Ventilation Workshop. New Orleans, Dec 5–7, 1982. *Chest* (in press).
3. Banner MJ, Gallagher TJ, Banner TC: Frequency and percent inspiratory time for high-frequency jet ventilation. *Crit Care Med* 1985; 13:395–398.
4. Baraka A, Muallem M, Noueihid R, et al: Oxygen jet ventilation of patients with tracheal T-tube. *Anesth Analg* 1982; 61:622–623.
5. Beamer WC, Prough DS, Royster RL, et al: High-frequency jet ventilation produces auto-PEEP. *Crit Care Med* 1984; 12:734–737.
6. Bell RE, Kuehl TJ, Coalson JJ, et al: High-frequency ventilation compared to conventional positive-pressure ventilation in the treatment of hyaline membrane disease in primates. *Crit Care Med* 1984; 12:764–768.
7. Bohn DJ, Miyasaka K, Marchak BE, et al:

Ventilation by high frequency oscillation. *J Appl Physiol* 1980; 48:710–716.

8. Borg U, Eriksson I, Sjöstrand U: High-frequency positive pressure ventilation (HFPPV): A review based upon its use during bronchoscopy and for laryngoscopy and microlaryngeal surgery under general anesthesia. *Anesth Analg* 1980; 59:594–603.

9. Boros SJ: Variation in inspiratory-expiratory ratio and airway pressure waveform during mechanical ventilation: The significance of mean airway pressure. *J Pediatr* 1979; 94:114–117.

10. Boynton BR, Mannino FL, Davis RF, et al: Combined high-frequency oscillatory ventilation and intermittent mandatory ventilation in critically ill neonates. *J Pediatr* 1984; 105:297–302.

11. Brusasco V, Knopp TJ, Rehder K: Gas transport during high frequency ventilation. *J Appl Physiol* 1983; 55:472–478.

12. Bryan AC: Unpublished data.

13. Butler WJ, Bohn DJ, Bryan AC, et al: Ventilation by high-frequency oscillation in humans. *Anesth Analg* 1980; 59:577–784.

14. Byford LJ, Finkler JH, Froese AB: Lung volume recruitment during high frequency ventilation in surfactant deficient rabbits. *Fed Proc* 1985; 44:1557.

15. Carlon GC, Howland WS, Ray C, et al: High-frequency jet ventilation: A prospective randomized evaluation. *Chest* 1983; 84:551–559.

16. Carlon GC, Kahn RC, Howland WS, et al: Clinical experience with high frequency jet ventilation. *Crit Care Med* 1981; 9:1–6.

17. Chang HK: Mechanisms of gas transport during ventilation by high-frequency oscillation. *J Appl Physiol* 1984; 56:553–563.

18. Chiaranda M, Rubini A, Fiore G, et al: Hemodynamic effects of continuous positive-pressure ventilation and high-frequency jet ventilation with positive end-expiratory pressure in normal dogs. *Crit Care Med* 1984; 12:750–754.

19. Coalson J, Kuehl T, Ackerman N, et al: Ventilator-associated lung injury in the premature baboon with hyaline membrane disease (abstract). *Am Rev Respir Dis* 1985; 131(suppl):A251.

20. Cornish D, Ackerman N, Yoder B, et al: High frequency oscillation in the management of infants with pulmonary interstitial emphysema (abstract). *Am Rev Respir Dis* 1985; 131(suppl):A250.

21. Crawford M, Rehder K: High-frequency small-volume ventilation in anesthetized humans. *Anesthesiology* 1985; 62:298–304.

22. Dawson SV, Elliott EA: Wave-speed limitation on expiratory flow: A unifying concept. *J Appl Physiol* 1977; 43:498–515.

23. Dorkin HL, Stark AR, Werthammer JW, et al: Respiratory system impedance from 4 to 40 Hz in paralyzed intubated infants with respiratory disease. *J Clin Invest* 1983; 72:903–910.

24. Drazen JM, Kamm RD, Slutsky AS: High-frequency ventilation. *Physiol Rev* 1984; 64:505–543.

25. Egol A, Culpepper J, Snyder J: Barotrauma and hypotension resulting from jet ventilation in critically ill patients. *Chest* 1985; 88:98–102.

26. El Baz N, El-Ganzouri A, Gottschalk W, et al: One-lung high-frequency positive pressure ventilation for sleeve pneumonectomy: An alternative technique. *Anesth Analg* 1981; 60:683–686.

27. El Baz N, Holinger L, El-Ganzouri A, et al: High-frequency positive-pressure ventilation for tracheal reconstruction supported by tracheal T-tube. *Anesth Analg* 1982; 61:796–800.

28. El Baz N, Faber LP, Doolas A: Combined high-frequency ventilation for management of terminal respiratory failure: A new technique. *Anesth Analg* 1983; 62:39–49.

29. Enderson BL, Rice CL, Beaver CW, et al: High frequency ventilation and the accumulation of extravascular lung water. *J Surg Res* 1984; 36:433–437.

30. Flatau E, Lewinsohn G, Konichezky S, et al: Mechanical ventilation in fiberoptic-bronchoscopy: Comparison between high frequency positive pressure ventilation and normal frequency positive pressure ventilation. *Crit Care Med* 1982; 10:733–735.

31. Forrest JB, Chambers C: High-frequency ventilation does not depress respiratory cilia function. *Can Anaesth Soc J* 1983; 30:S77.

32. Frank I, Noack W, Lunkenheimer PP, et al: Light- and electron-microscopic investigations of pulmonary tissue after high-frequency positive-pressure ventilation (HFPPV). *Anaesthesist* 1975; 24:171–176.

33. Frantz ID III, Werthammer J, Stark AR: High-frequency ventilation in premature infants with lung disease: Adequate gas exchange at low tracheal pressure. *Pediatrics* 1983; 71:483–488.

34. Frantz ID III, Stark AR, Davis JM, et al: High frequency ventilation does not affect pulmo-

nary surfactant, liquid, or morphologic features in normal cats. *Am Rev Respir Dis* 1982; 126:909–913.

35. Fredberg JJ, Keefe DH, Glass GM, et al: Alveolar pressure nonhomogeneity during small-amplitude high-frequency oscillation. *J Appl Physiol* 1984; 57:788–800.

36. Fredberg JJ: Augmented diffusion in the airways can support pulmonary gas exchange. *J Appl Physiol* 1980; 49:232–238.

37. Fredberg JJ: Personal communication.

38. Froese AB: High-frequency ventilation: A critical assessment, in Shoemaker WC (ed): *Critical Care: State of the Art*. Fullerton, Calif, Society of Critical Care Medicine, 1984, vol 5.

39. Froese AB: Unpublished data.

40. Fusciardi J, Rouby JJ, Benhamou D, et al: Hemodynamic consequences of increasing mean airway pressure during high-frequency jet ventilation. *Chest* 1984; 86:30–34.

41. Gallagher TJ, Klain M, Carlon GC: Present status of high frequency ventilation. *Crit Care Med* 1982; 10:613–617.

42. George RJ, Moore-Gillon V, Geddes DM: High frequency oscillations improve nasal mucociliary transport. *Lancet* 1984; 2:10–12.

43. Gillespie DJ: High-frequency ventilation: A new concept in mechanical ventilation. *Mayo Clin Proc* 1983; 58:187–196.

44. Hamilton PP, Onayemi A, Smyth JA, et al: Comparison of conventional and high-frequency ventilation: Oxygenation and lung pathology. *J Appl Physiol* 1983; 55:131–138.

45. Heard SO, Banner MJ, Jaeger MJ: Airway pressure measurement during high frequency jet ventilation (abstract). *Crit Care Med* 1984; 12:262.

46. James LS, Hudson WA (chairmen): High-frequency ventilation for immature infants: Report of a conference, March 2–4, 1982. *Pediatrics* 1983; 71:280–287.

47. Jefferies AL, Hamilton P, O'Brodovich HM: Effect of high-frequency oscillation on lung lymph flow. *J Appl Physiol* 1983; 55:1373–1378.

48. Jobe A, Ikegami M, Jacobs H, et al: Permeability of premature lamb lungs to protein and the effect of surfactant on that permeability. *J Appl Physiol* 1983; 55:169–176.

49. Keszler M, Klein R, McClellan L, et al: Effects of conventional and high frequency jet ventilation on lung parenchyma. *Crit Care Med* 1982; 10:514–516.

50. Kirby RR, Downs JB, Civetta JM, et al: High level positive end expiratory pressure (PEEP) in acute respiratory insufficiency. *Chest* 1975; 67:156–163.

51. Klain M, Smith RB: High frequency percutaneous transtracheal jet ventilation. *Crit Care Med* 1977; 5:280–287.

52. Knopp TJ, Kaethner T, Meyer M, et al: Gas mixing in the airways of dog lungs during high-frequency ventilation. *J Appl Physiol* 1983; 55:1141–1146.

53. Kolton M, Cattran CB, Kent G, et al: Oxygenation during high-frequency ventilation compared with conventional mechanical ventilation in two models of lung injury. *Anesth Analg* 1982; 61:323–332.

54. Kumar BS, Beney K, Jastremski M, et al: High-frequency jet ventilation versus conventional ventilation after surfactant displacement in dogs. *Crit Care Med* 1984; 12:738–741.

55. Lunkenheimer PP, Frank I, Ising H, et al: Intrapulmonaler Gaswechsel unter simulierter Apnoe durch transtrachealen, periodischen intrathorakalen Druckwechsel. *Anaesthesist* 1972; 22:232–237.

56. Marchak BE, Thompson WK, Duffty P, et al: Treatment of RDS by high frequency oscillatory ventilation: A preliminary report. *J Pediatr* 1981; 99:287–292.

57. McEvoy RD, Davies NJ, Hedenstierna G, et al: Lung mucociliary transport during high frequency ventilation. *Am Rev Respir Dis* 1982; 126:452–456.

58. Moffatt SL, Byford LJ, Forkert L: Intrapulmonary gas mixing during high frequency oscillation in humans (abstract). *Fed Proc* 1984; 43:322.

59. Ophoven JP, Mammel MC, Gordon MJ, et al: Tracheobronchial histopathology associated with high-frequency jet ventilation. *Crit Care Med* 1984; 12:829–832.

60. Pokora T, Bing D, Mammel M, et al: Neonatal high-frequency jet ventilation. *Pediatrics* 1983; 72:27–32.

61. Quan SF, Militzer HW, Calkins JM, et al: Comparison of high-frequency jet ventilation with conventional mechanical ventilation in saline-lavaged rabbits. *Crit Care Med* 1984; 9:759–763.

62. Quan SF, Otto CW, Calkins JC, et al: High-frequency ventilation: A promising new method of ventilation. *Heart Lung* 1983; 12:152–155.

63. Rehder K, Schmid ER, Knopp TJ: Long-term

high-frequency ventilation in dogs. *Am Rev Respir Dis* 1983; 128:476–480.

64. Rieke H, Hook C, Meyer M: Pulmonary gas exchange during high-frequency ventilation in dogs. *Respir Physiol* 1983; 54:1–17.

65. Rossing TH, Solway J, Saari AF, et al: Influence of the endotracheal tube on CO_2 transport during high-frequency ventilation. *Am Rev Respir Dis* 1984; 129:54–57.

66. Rouby JJ, Fusciardi J, Bourgain JL, et al: High-frequency jet ventilation in postoperative respiratory failure: Determinants of oxygenation. *Anesthesiology* 1983; 59:281–287.

67. Saari AF, Rossing TH, Drazen JM: Physiological bases for new approaches to mechanical ventilation. *Annu Rev Med* 1984; 35:165–174.

68. Saari AF, Rossing TH, Solway J, et al: Lung inflation during high-frequency ventilation. *Am Rev Respir Dis* 1984; 129:333–336.

69. Schmid ER, Knopp TJ, Rehder K: Intrapulmonary gas transport and perfusion during high-frequency oscillation. *J Appl Physiol* 1981; 51:1507–1514.

70. Schuster DP, Snyder JV, Klain M: Comparison of venous admixture during high-frequency ventilation and conventional ventilation in oleic acid-induced pulmonary edema in dogs. *Anesth Analg* 1982; 61:735–740.

71. Schuster DP, Klain M, Snyder JV: Comparison of high frequency jet ventilation to conventional ventilation during severe acute respiratory failure in humans. *Crit Care Med* 1982; 10:625–630.

72. Seki S, Fukushima Y, Goto K, et al: Facilitation of intrathoracic operations by means of high-frequency ventilation. *J Thorac Cardiovasc Surg* 1983; 86:388–392.

73. Shuptrine JR, Auffant RA, Gal TJ: Cerebral and cardiopulmonary responses to high-frequency jet ventilation and conventional mechanical ventilation in a model of brain and lung injury. *Anesth Analg* 1984; 63:1065–1070.

74. Simon B, Weinmann G, Mitzner W: Mean airway pressure and alveolar pressure during high-frequency ventilation. *J Appl Physiol* 1984; 57:1069–1078.

75. Sjöstrand U: High-frequency positive-pressure ventilation (HFPPV): A review. *Crit Care Med* 1980; 8:345–364.

76. Slutsky AS, Kamm RD, Rossing TH, et al: Effects of frequency, tidal volume, and lung volume on CO_2 elimination in dogs by high frequency (2–30 Hz) low tidal volume ventilation. *J Clin Invest* 1981; 68:1475–1484.

77. Snyder JV: Unpublished data.

78. Solway J, Rossing TH, Drazen JM: Expiratory flow limitation causes dynamic hyperinflation during high frequency ventilation. *Fed Proc* 1985; 44:1557.

79. Sutton JE Jr, Glass DD: Airway pressure gradient during high-frequency ventilation. *Crit Care Med* 1984; 12:774–776.

80. Thompson WK, Marchak BE, Froese AB, et al: High-frequency oscillation compared with standard ventilation in pulmonary injury model. *J Appl Physiol* 1982; 52:543–548.

81. Todd MM, Toutant SM, Shapiro HM: The effects of high-frequency positive-pressure ventilation on intracranial pressure and brain surface movement in cats. *Anesthesiology* 1981; 54:496–504.

82. Truog WE, Standaert TA, Murphy J, et al: Effect of high-frequency oscillation on gas exchange and pulmonary phospholipids in experimental hyaline membrane disease. *Am Rev Respir Dis* 1983; 127:585–589.

83. Turnbull AD, Carlon G, Howland WS, et al: High-frequency jet ventilation in major airway or pulmonary disruption. *Ann Thorac Surg* 1981; 32:468–474.

84. Vourc'h G, Fischler M, Michon F, et al: Manual jet ventilation v. high frequency jet ventilation during laser resection of tracheo-bronchial stenosis. *Br J Anaesth* 1983; 55:973–975.

85. Waterson CK, Militzer HW, Quan SF, et al: Airway pressure as a measure of gas exchange during high-frequency jet ventilation. *Crit Care Med* 1984; 12:742–746.

86. Wohl MEB, Stigol LC, Mead J: Resistance of the total respiratory system in healthy infants and infants with bronchiolitis. *Pediatrics* 1969; 43:495–509.

24 _____ Respirator Lung

James V. Snyder, M.D.

Alison Froese, M.D.

Some forms of artificial ventilatory support can be deleterious to the lung. The idea that conventional mechanical ventilation may potentiate pulmonary damage is not new, but it remains unproved. This chapter provides a pathophysiologic basis to explain the ill effects of some ventilation patterns and the benefit of others. Very similar pathophysiologic mechanisms may explain the spontaneous deterioration in lung function seen in the infant respiratory distress syndrome (IRDS) and the reversal of that course by positive pressure ventilation.

This discussion represents a paradigm shift—a change in the scheme normally used to understand and explore observations;[29] it is a deliberate attempt to restructure the conceptual framework with which we approach therapeutic dilemmas in critical care. In this sense it is an attempt to take the scattered pieces of the jigsaw puzzle provided by each existing published investigation and see whether they fit with better congruity if we omit one basic assumption—that ventilators do not contribute to lung injury—and start instead with a different one: that the method used to support gas exchange in the injured lung can have a major influence on the evolution of the pathophysiologic process.

Initial outcome studies of mechanical ventilation demonstrated progression of lung injury. Subsequent studies, however, showed that oxygen in high concentrations, not mechanical ventilation per se, was the major factor precipitating this progressive dysfunction. Thus, mechanical ventilation was exonerated as a major contributor to the nonspecific morphological changes in acute respiratory failure (ARF).[2, 7, 22, 23, 48] Two conditions are invariably present in ARF: an "abnormal pattern of gas distribution, with closure of alveoli or airways, and an increase in pulmonary extravascular water, with interstitial edema caused by . . . loss of integrity of capillary endothelium, with exudation of plasma into the interstitium."[48 (p 5)] Recently, numerous physiologic mechanisms have been identified by which high volume ventilation might contribute to precisely this type of pathophysiologic picture. If such mechanisms can be shown to accelerate or prolong ARF significantly, then reinstatement of the term "respirator lung" would seem appropriate.

The extension of multifocal, early ARF[8] to more diffuse terminal fibrosis[24, 49] could be due to oxygen toxicity, progression of the primary process, or superimposition of a new process such as sepsis. However, a growing body of evidence suggests that cyclic stretching of a lung with underlying pathology can, of itself, induce further structural damage. Much of the evidence comes from premature, surfactant-deficient lungs, which are structurally fragile as well as prone to alveolar collapse.[11, 33, 39] One could argue that these data are unduly influenced by tissue fragility, but a very similar picture can be seen in adult lungs made surfactant-deficient and therefore atelectasis-prone.[18] The improvement in pulmonary function associated with diminished ventilatory support combined with extracorporeal carbon dioxide removal ($ECCO_2$) of patients in severe ARF is compatible with the hypothesis[15] that the pulmonary problem is not due merely to primary pulmonary parenchymal fragility. In addition, allowing some lung regions to stay collapsed may have functional effects on these units and eventually structural effects on the lung remaining open. Does the form of mechanical ventilatory support in ARF cause detrimental effects on lung structure and function and eventually on outcome? Similarly, could altering the mode of support modify the course of ARF? The mode of ventilation is less likely to be a prominent influence on ARF if the primary cause is unabated. In the following sections, we present several pathophysiologic mechanisms of lung injury and show how they can produce secondary pulmonary dysfunction that can be exaggerated (a form of "respirator lung") or ameliorated by the ventilatory support provided.

INFLUENCE OF VENTILATORY PATTERN ON PATHOPHYSIOLOGY: MECHANISMS

In the lungs of patients with ARF, the alveoli may be open, closed, or opening and closing cyclically with each breath. Several factors may influence alveolar integrity, including cyclic opening and closing of lung already injured and overdistention (of both injured and uninjured lung tissue). Alveolar volume changes also affect surfactant activity. Changes in alveolar volume and surface tension activity can affect microvascular permeability and interstitial fluid accumulation.

Cyclic Opening of Closed Lung

The lung tissue that appears most sensitive to "respirator-induced" changes in function is that fraction of bronchioles and alveolar ducts that open and close with each breath. McAdams et al. ventilated premature rhesus monkeys and found that even 5 minutes of conventional mechanical ventilation (CMV) induced hyaline membrane formation with epithelial necrosis in the terminal airways.[33] Nilsson et al. studied immature rabbit pups and observed terminal airway injury after brief periods of CMV in animals that were surfactant-deficient. The pathologic picture revealed collapsed air spaces in conjunction with cystic overdistention of terminal bronchioles and alveolar ducts.[39] A strikingly similar pattern has recently been reported in the lungs of three adults who died of ARDS.[5]

Enhorning and Robertson reasoned that in surfactant deficiency the air-fluid interface during lung expansion must lie in the cylindrical terminal airway, rather than in the alveolar space itself.[10] The surface tension forces generated across a cylinder are only half those generated across the spherical interface at the mouth of an alveolus (by the Laplace relation). Therefore, to

inflate alveoli one must apply a force twice as large as that which can be counterbalanced by conducting airway surface forces. If tissue tensile strength is inadequate, overdistention of conductive airways will occur prior to alveolar reexpansion. If persistent, this inhomogeneity of tensile forces may lead to permanent cystic changes in the terminal airways. However, if alveoli are open, the surface forces across their walls are less than the airway wall (alveolar radius is now large) and the terminal bronchioles act as an air conduit rather than as a target for overdistention. Following this line of reasoning, one could argue that maintaining an adequate residual *alveolar* volume is essential to decompressing terminal airways, besides being good for gas exchange. From this argument it follows that (1) in open lung (normal lung), if cyclic volume changes occur no respirator-induced structural injury will result; (2) in atelectatic lung (surfactant-deficient, as in prematurity), if cyclic volume changes do not occur no structural injury will occur (e.g., in utero, and perhaps in the patient on ECCO$_2$ removal; (3) in diffuse air space collapse (IRDS or ARDS), cyclic volume changes in repeatedly collapsing lung cause epithelial necrosis in terminal airways, hyaline membranes, and chronic structural damage. This hypothesis, that repeated opening and closing of lung results in structural lung damage, is at present unproved.

In our experience this three-part synthesis is consistent with clinical observations by us and others. Dependably, cyclic ventilation of the normal lung is innocuous. Inevitably, ARDS and IRDS lead to diffuse alveolar damage or bronchopulmonary dysplasia.[5, 6] Gattinoni and colleagues reported similar observations, in which putting the lung to rest (avoiding cyclic mechanical stretching) was an important contribution to resolution of the lesions.[15] A fourth option, however, is presented by extension from the work of Hamilton and associates and will be supported in the remainder of this chapter. They studied the effect of CMV and high-frequency oscillatory ventilation (HFO) in surfactant-deficient rabbits. They found that surfactant-deficient lung ventilated conventionally showed evidence of structural damage (hyaline membranes and early epithelial necrosis) after as little as 5 hours of therapy. When compared with the earlier observations of Kolton et al.[28] (which were described in chapter 20, "Pulmonary Physiology"), it appears that CMV at the settings used by Hamilton et al. resulted in the surfactant-deficient lung cycling between extremes of extensive atelectasis (despite PEEP of about 6 cm H_2O) to full inflation (at peak inspiration) with each conventional mechanical breath. However, the lungs ventilated by HFO were ventilated in such a way that atelectatic alveoli were recruited early and then splinted open mechanically by a higher level of PEEP. The HFO-ventilated lungs showed minimal structural damage.

These data suggest to us a fourth option: With diffuse air space injury (IRDS or ARDS), sustained reexpansion with superimposed small volume excursions minimizes structural injury induced by mechanical ventilation. It is currently thought that in the alveolar epithelium, type I cells are the pulmonary parenchymal cells most susceptible to injury. Injury of type I cells is followed by (1) proliferation of type II cells, (2) migration of the type II cells along the surface of the alveolar epithelial basement membrane, and (3) differentiation of some type II cells into type I cells. Successful repair of the alveolus depends critically on an intact epithelial basement membrane. By preserving the architecture of the epithelial surface, the basement membrane defines the topography of epithelial cellular replacement.[52]

If increased airway pressure (AWP) disrupts the epithelial basement membrane, both epithelialization and patterns of fibrosis are likely to be altered. PEEP has been considered a potential cause of such disruption. A case report of PEEP-induced overdistention of air spaces as a complication of paraquat lung injury has been used to support the idea that high AWP may be detrimental to the lung, even if it is immediately life-saving.[30] Because lesions such as those seen in that reported case are not typical of paraquat lung when AWP is not increased,[55] concern about the effects of high AWP seems justified. Whereas CPAP seems to have caused air space overdistention in this reported case, it is likely that mechanical ventilation, even without PEEP, would cause greater pressure gradients and disruption of the fragile membranes remaining after a paraquat insult. When the insult causes destruction of the basement membrane, as with this poisoning, no mode of ventilatory support will be satisfactory. PEEP has also been held to correlate significantly with bronchiolectasis in patients with severe ARDS, but the data presented were insufficient to exclude other factors, such as oxygen or high peak AWP, as causative.[57]

Causes of Overexpansion

Overexpansion of open areas of the lung is another primary process by which mechanical ventilation might cause pulmonary deterioration. When a tidal volume (Vt) up to 50 ml/kg has been used experimentally without significant ill effect (see chapter 20, "Pulmonary Physiology"), why would Vt of only 10–15 ml/kg be detrimental? It is not the Vt delivered to the whole lung that is important but the regional differences in lung expansion due to local differences in parenchymal compliance, airway resistance, and pleural pressure. These differences can cause regional inflation to vary widely despite a common upper airway pressure. Delivery of 15 ml/kg, which is about one seventh of total lung capacity, can cause some regions of the lung to overinflate if the remainder of the lung is less distensible. The following related mechanisms can contribute to local overexpansion (Table 24–1).

1. Tidal volume that is three times normal, as is commonly ordered, obviously increases lung expansion threefold.

2. Any airway resistance, as might be caused by mucosal edema, for example, directs ventilation to areas with open airways. Functional loss of one third of the lung would result in a 50% increase in ventilation of the lung remaining open. A Vt of 15 ml/kg would then cause the same excursion in the lung remaining open as would a Vt of 22.5 ml/kg.

3. The elastic recoil of the distal lung units can vary widely, and volume excursion will be inversely proportional to it. If one-half the lung

TABLE 24–1.

Contributions to Local Overexpansion

Increased delivered Vt

Airway resistance or closure, directing volume to open lung

Wide variation in local compliance

Inactive diaphragm → loss of base-directed ventilation

Overexpansion → increased deadspace, increased minute ventilation

Overexpansion → increased shunting → increased hypoxic drive

Obstruction of adjacent airways, increasing local compliance

Higher CO_2 production, requiring increased minute ventilation remaining open has a compliance one fifth of normal while the rest of the lung is unchanged, the expansion of the uninjured lung will almost double.

4. The contraction of the diaphragm normally directs ventilation to the lung base, but the distribution of ventilation during mechanical breaths is toward more open, nondependent lung regions; again, lung units that are already open become more distended.

5. Overexpansion of the open lung by each of the mechanisms just described can compress alveolar vessels, thereby increasing the resistance to blood flow, which diverts the flow to more closed areas of the lung. Ventilation is then less efficient (deadspace is increased), and a higher minute ventilation is needed to keep carbon dioxide elimination constant. An increase in Vd/Vt from 0.3 to 0.6 necessitates doubling of minute ventilation to maintain Pa_{CO_2}. An increase in Vd/Vt from .4 to .5 makes a 20% increase in minute ventilation necessary to maintain a consistent Pa_{CO_2}. The required increase in minute ventilation may again cause additional microvascular overdistention and inefficiency, and establish a deleterious cycle (Fig 24–1). This diversion of blood flow from open lung may explain why patients with radiologic evidence of extensive pulmonary disease have a high Vd/Vt of 0.65, compared with patients who have essentially normal

lungs on x-ray studies.[46] An inadequate intravascular volume can also contribute to a cycle of increased deadspace and increased minute ventilation. The common observation of increased Vd/Vt in ARF is difficult to explain except by these alterations in V/Q ratios, because anatomical pulmonary vascular obstruction is not a uniform component of ARF.[14]

6. Similarly, the diversion of blood from open to closed lung regions can increase venous admixture and stimulate an increase in hypoxic respiratory drive. If ventilation is increased as a result, the same cycle of more overdistention and inefficiency is established (see Fig 24–1). In each of these cases, not only will the higher volume be delivered to the open lung, but, with a volume-limited ventilator, it will be delivered at a higher pressure.

7. The radiologic finding of "compensatory" distention of an open lung region adjacent to a collapsed lobe or lung is familiar. Experimental observations suggest that the expansive forces involved are more potent than might be apparent. In rabbits, when AWP was increased to 40 cm H_2O, a small area of lung increased twofold to threefold in volume when all of the lung was allowed to inflate, and sixfold to twelvefold when the adjacent lung area was not inflated (Fig 24–2). It would appear that expanding lung tissue normally provides an important constraint on the expansion of adjacent tissue. *Failure of adjacent tissue to expand effectively may increase the expansion due to an increase in AWP to a dangerous degree.* The larger change in local volume was associated with increased loss of radioactively labeled albumin into the alveolar space.[9] The clinical analogy might occur in patients in whom all bronchi but one are occluded while AWP is supplied that is normally well tolerated. The open lung region might have a similarly marked apparent increase in compliance and therefore in lung volume, with marked overdistention that can disrupt microvascular walls.

8. Any increase in oxygen consumption, which is likely to be 10%–50% in critically ill patients, will increase carbon dioxide production and minute ventilation requirement proportionately. Patients breathing spontaneously may experience a marked further increase in oxygen consumption and carbon dioxide production, and a need for increased minute ventilation as their compliance and Vd/Vt deteriorate.

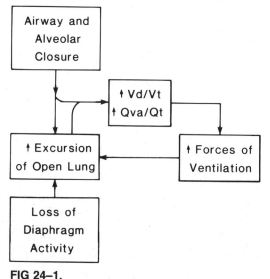

FIG 24–1.
Positive feedback of lung closure, overexpansion, and inefficient gas exchange.

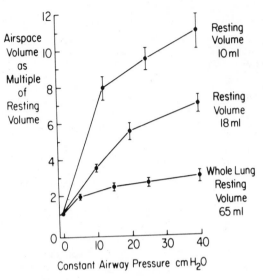

FIG 24–2.
In rabbits, transmission of increased AWP to a portion of lung can increase volume expansion by 300%–400% (to 12 times FRC) compared with when the entire lung expands, and the volume increases by a factor of only 2 or 3. The greater local expansion is an apparent change in local compliance, and is accompanied by increased microvascular permeability. (From Egan.[9] Reproduced by permission.)

The degree to which these factors together contribute to overexpansion during conventional ventilation in humans is unclear, but it would be significant even if it were only a fraction of that possible from the factors just discussed. Additional sequelae of local overexpansion are discussed in the following sections.

Lung Ventilation and Surfactant

Mechanical ventilation of the lungs with large volumes in several species in vivo and in vitro is accompanied by a loss of surfactant function and subsequently by greater surface tension, lower compliance, and pulmonary edema.[12, 16, 34, 63, 65, 68–70] Any increase in surface tension (attraction of surface molecules for each other) tends to collapse alveoli, decrease interstitial fluid pressure, and increase transudation (Fig 24–3).[36, 68] If the capacity for lymphatic drainage is overwhelmed, the resulting interstitial edema tends to cause alveolar and airway collapse; ventilatory effort must then be increased to maintain the same Vt; the Vt is then diverted to the lung still open, excursion increases, surfactant production increases to its

limit, and surfactant function is lost. This pathophysiologic cycle is diagramed in Figure 24–4.

The decrease in surfactant activity and therefore in compliance is related to pulmonary metabolic capacity: in rat lungs, recovery of normal compliance can occur quickly at 37° C but is impeded by hypothermia or cyanide,[12, 34] and the dysfunction is greater in cases of starvation.[62] Ventilation with Vt of 30% of maximal lung volume does not affect surfactant function at 37° C,[13] but significantly depresses surfactant function when surfactant production is slowed by hypothermia.[12]

The critical determinants of surfactant turnover and function appear to be the following: (1) Vt: the larger the Vt the more surfactant release is stimulated; (2) end-exhalation volume, or functional residual capacity (FRC): when the alveolus collapses or becomes very small with exhalation, either more surfactant is lost to the airway or more is disrupted during subsequent inspiratory expansions of the surface area; (3) the metabolic activity of type II cells; and (4) the rate and duration of mechanical ventilation. For compliance to deteriorate, the expiratory and inspiratory changes listed must recur with sufficient frequency and duration to deplete surfactant at a rate greater than it can be replaced. When surfactant production is normal, Vt must be about 60% of maximum lung volume to change surfactant function,[68] and a Vt of 15 ml/kg is only about 15% of maximum lung capacity. However, the capacity to produce surfactant may be impaired by many pulmonary insults, and local volume excursion may be grossly exaggerated above that calculated for the normal lung by the factors listed in the preceding section. Two other mechanisms of surfactant dysfunction should be mentioned. First, in clinical disease abnormal forms of surfactant may be produced.[25] Second, the material that gets into the alveolar space during a "capillary leak" may contain a protein that is a specific inhibitor of surfactant.[19]

Fariday and colleagues found that PEEP affects the increase in surface tension during mechanical ventilation of in vitro dog lungs over time: this increase was inversely related to end-expiratory pressure.[12] In this preparation the change in compliance was modified by 1 cm H_2O PEEP and completely prevented by 3 cm H_2O PEEP.[12] In another model, 10 cm H_2O PEEP protected in vivo rat lungs from loss of surfactant function.[65] This suggests that PEEP, in particular

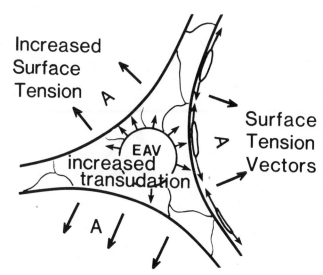

FIG 24–3.
Surface tension results from attraction of surface molecules. The net effect of increased surface tension is to collapse each alveolus, pulling the walls of the interstitial space away from each other and thus lowering interstitial fluid pressure. The result is increased transudation from the extra-alveolar vessel (EAV). *A*, alveolus. (From Snyder J.V., et al.: Mechanical ventilation: physiology and application. *Curr. Probl. Surg.*, vol. 21, 1984. © 1984, Year Book Medical Publishers, Inc., Chicago; reproduced by permission.)

circumstances, can help maintain the balance between increased surfactant production and increased surfactant loss during ventilation with large tidal volumes.[12, 65] Surfactant dysfunction has been suggested to have a role in ARDS.[17, 46] Recently the phospholipid pattern was noted to be normal in patients with mild to moderate ARF, but then deteriorate with decline in lung function in patients who died, compared with patients who were successfully weaned.[61] This deterioration may be related in part to the effect of ventilation pattern on surfactant activity.

Problems With Lung Closure

The consequences of overexpansion are closely related to the consequences of lung closure (Table 24–2). Cyclic opening of the alveoli causes surfactant dysfunction, the formation of hyaline membranes, and epithelial necrosis. Prolonged air space closure predisposes the lung to infection, partly because atelectasis impairs the antibacterial activity of the alveolar macrophages.[56] When some lung tissue fails to open, the lung that remains open is more readily overdistended. At the same time, the delivery of a fixed Vt

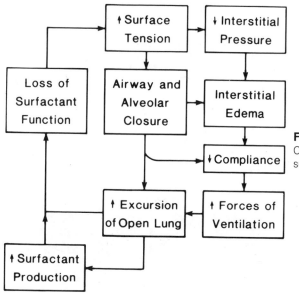

FIG 24–4.
Cyclic interaction between lung excursion, surfactant function, and pulmonary edema.

TABLE 24–2.

Consequences of Lung Closure*

Cyclic opening→early epithelial necrosis
Cyclic opening→surfactant depletion
Lung closure→ ↑ C_{local}, ↓ C_{lung}
↑ C_{lung}→ ↑ peak AWP, ↑ mean AWP
↑ Peak AWP + ↑ C_{local} → ↑ local expansion
  →capillary leak
  →compressed microvessels→blood flow diverted
    to closed lung→ ↑ Qva/Qt and ↑ Vd/Vt
  → ↑ surface tension, interstitial edema, lung
    closure

---

*C_{local} refers to the compliance of a small lung region; C_{lung} refers to total lung compliance.

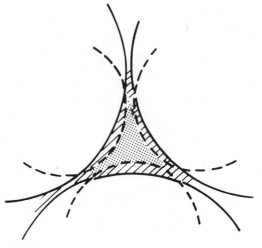

FIG 24–5.
Effect of lung inflation on interstitial fluid pressure (IFP) mechanisms. The space between spheres enlarges as the spheres enlarge. IFP decreases and transudation increases. This occurs whether lung inflation is spontaneous or mechanical, and occurs even in zone I (vascular pressure of 1 cm H_2O).[1] (From Snyder J.V., et al.: Mechanical ventilation: physiology and application. *Curr. Probl. Surg.* vol. 21, 1984. © 1984, Year Book Medical Publishers, Inc., Chicago; reproduced by permission.)

causes AWP to increase, so that overdistention of the now more compliant open lung is more likely. Thus it appears that with CMV, lung closure may be a primary cause of lung overexpansion, having multiple consequences.

Transudation

Interstitial fluid formation depends on the hydrostatic pressure gradient from the microvasculature (MVP) to the interstitial fluid (IFP), and on vessel permeability. The effects of lung expansion on interstitial fluid are likely mediated through direct and indirect influences on these factors, as summarized in Table 24–3.

Effects of Lung Expansion on Interstitial Fluid Pressure

If we think of the interstitial *space* as the area of immediate concern, any force that tends to separate the walls of the space will first cause vessels to fill, then decrease IFP and increase transudation; and any force that minimizes this distraction will minimize edema.[1, 20, 35, 44] IFP becomes less negative as interstitial fluid accumulates. These forces are diagramed in Figures 24–3, 24–5, and 24–6.

As the lung expands above normal FRC, some pulmonary vessels and surrounding interstitium are compressed by expanding alveoli (alveolar vessels). However, the same inspiration tends to expand extra-alveolar vessels, and to augment transudation by enlarging the extra-alveolar interstitial space and lowering IFP (see Fig 24–5). *Experimentally, increasing transpulmonary pressure from 0 to 30 cm H_2O decreases IFP by more than 30 cm H_2O.*[20] Edema formation is then significant even at a pulmonary microvascular pressure of only 10 cm H_2O. This occurs with positive pressure or spontaneous ventilation. The decrease in pleural pressure with spontaneous inspiration further decreases interstitial pressure, especially when airways are obstructed, elastic recoil is increased, or inspiratory effort is increased (see Fig 24–6).[20, 31, 35] Where the lung is locally collapsed, the decrease in IFP due to expansion of adjacent lung areas or to lower pleural pressure is apt to be even greater, owing to the forces of interdependence (see Fig 20–7 in chapter 20, "Pulmonary Physiology"). Low IFP during lung expansion appears to be the cause of pulmonary edema after reexpansion of atelectasis.[32, 40, 50, 57] More vigorous inspiratory efforts related to low compliance, inefficient gas exchange, J-receptor stimulation, and anxiety cause further decrease in interstitial pressure and increased transudation, establishing a cycle of deterioration. These cycles are diagramed in Figure 24–7. The negative IFP due to lung expansion and low pleural pressure may be sufficient to disrupt microvascular walls.

TABLE 24–3.

Mechanisms by Which Lung Inflation Influences Transudation*

IFP IS LOWERED BY:	MVP IS INCREASED BY:
↑ Lung volume (EAV)	↑ Microvascular compression, ↑ PVR (upstream bed)
↓ P_{pl} (with spontaneous inspiration)	↑ Systemic venous return (spontaneous ventilation)
↑ Elastic recoil (including surface tension)†	Iatrogenic fluid loading
↑ Airway obstruction†	Inhibition of left ventricular systole (spontaneous ventilation)
Local parenchymal collapse†	Hypoxic vasoconstriction (upstream bed)
PERMEABILITY IS INCREASED BY:	MVP IS DECREASED BY:
High transmural pressure gradients	↑ Microvascular compression (downstream bed)
AWP > 42 cm H_2O	↓ Systemic venous return (mechanical ventilation)

*From Snyder JV, et al: Mechanical ventilation: physiology and application. *Curr. Probl. Surg.* 1984, vol 21. Reproduced by permission of Year Book Medical Publishers, Inc., Chicago, copyright ©1984.
Abbreviations: EAV, extra-alveolar vessels; MVP, microvascular pressure; PVR, pulmonary vascular resistance; P_{pl}, pleural pressure.
†When factors that limit expansion exist, such as airway obstruction or increased surface tension, the drop in interstitial pressure can be greater.[31, 35] Interstitial pressure has a solid component and a fluid component. The latter is the important factor in determining fluid transudation.[20]

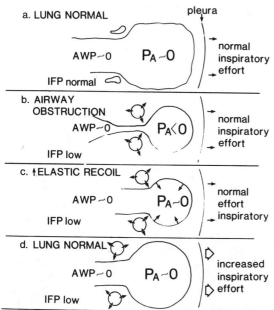

FIG 24–6.
With a normal inspiratory effort, rapid alveolar expansion prevents a significant decrease in pleural pressure or interstitial fluid pressure *(IFP)*. However, IFP is lower than normal *(a)* and transudation is facilitated *(arrows)* from microvasculature when alveolar filling is impaired by increased airway resistance *(b)* or by an increase in elastic recoil, such as that caused by higher alveolar surface tension *(c)*, and also when inspiratory effort is greater *(d)*. P_A, alveolar pressure. (From Snyder J.V., et al.: Mechanical ventilation: physiology and application. *Curr. Probl. Surg.* vol. 21. 1984. © 1984, Year Book Medical Publishers, Inc., Chicago; reproduced by permission.)

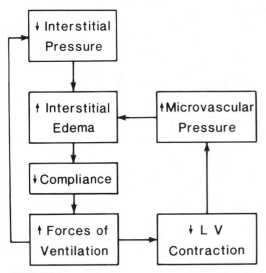

FIG 24–7.
Cyclic interaction between interstitial edema and mechanical ventilation *(clockwise)* and LV contraction; and the additional effect of spontaneous ventilation on LV contraction, and interstitial edema *(counterclockwise cycle).*

Effects of Lung Expansion on Microvasculature Pressure

1. At higher lung volumes, alveolar pressure directly compresses alveolar vessels, in which case upstream transmural vascular pressures (in the extra-alveolar arterial bed) may be increased and local downstream transmural pressures (in the extra-alveolar venous bed) may be decreased.[61]

2. When ventilation is spontaneous, lower pleural pressure elevates venous return, output from the right side of the heart, and pulmonary microvascular pressure.

3. At high lung volumes, pulmonary vascular compression can significantly compromise right ventricular function; left ventricular filling may then be impeded by a right-to-left septal shift (ventricular interdependence or left ventricular tamponade). The iatrogenic fluid loading needed to maintain cardiac output in this setting will raise microvascular pressure.

4. When positive airway pressure is used, transmural pulmonary capillary pressure may be decreased secondary to lower venous return; this decreased capillary pressure can be an important determinant of lung water.[53]

5. As noted in Figure 24–7 and in chapter 31, "Ventilatory Support of the Failing Circulation," the compromise of left ventricular systole by negative pleural pressure can be significant if the inspiratory effort is vigorous or if ventricular contractility is already impaired. Higher LV filling pressure (and therefore transmural microvascular pressure) may then be needed to maintain cardiac output.

6. Experimentally, hypoxic pulmonary vasoconstriction further increases transudation at a given blood flow.[38]

Thus, most of the effects of lung expansion on transmural microvascular pressure favor increased transudation. Combined with the increased venous return of spontaneous ventilation causing pulmonary vascular engorgement, these influences seem the likely mechanisms for pulmonary edema during attacks of asthma[43, 60] and in individuals with upper airway obstruction.[21, 37, 50, 64, 67] They also may be a basis for the pulmonary edema seen at high altitudes, especially in young and vigorous climbers.

The Effect of Lung Expansion on Microvascular Permeability

The decrease in interstitial pressure generated by lung expansion (see Fig 24–5) and low pleural pressure and exaggerated by interdependent forces (see Fig 20–7 in chapter 20, "Pulmonary Physiology") may be sufficient to disrupt the microvascular wall. Such disruption may have caused the leaking of albumin into the alveolar space that Egan saw when he experimentally produced regional lung overinflation by applying a pressure of 40 cm H_2O to a relatively small lung region.[9] The increased vascular permeability in lung reexpansion edema, seen experimentally[41] and in humans,[32, 51, 59] suggests the same mechanism. These forces may be disruptive when atelectatic lung is expanded by any means, but especially so when the relatively aggressive directed recruiting technique is used. It is important to note that microvascular damage related to lung expansion is not limited to expansion of collapsed lung. Parker and associates observed increased permeability every time normal dog lungs were ventilated with more than 42 cm H_2O at a respiration rate of 6/min for 20 min.[40]

"RESPIRATOR LUNG"

Most of the factors relating to increased transudation and edema discussed above occur in relatively normal lungs subjected to large volume changes, especially if exhalation is to a low volume. The effects may be exaggerated by high respiratory rates and by lung closure.

The tissue changes in ARDS are not homogeneous at first, and the severity of damage varies from one part of the lung to another.[8] In patients with nonhomogeneous acute pulmonary disease, maldistribution of ventilation is exaggerated and the lung remaining open undergoes a larger volume change per lung unit than would be predicted if Vt were calculated on a per-kilogram basis. The ill effects of excessive inflation on surface tension and the other determinants of transmural microvascular pressure described above are possible sequelae. When they are due to mechanical ventilation, the consequences of these multiple factors may properly be called a form of "respirator lung." *A ventilation pattern designed to avoid this problem would prevent any lung region from collapsing during exhalation, would avoid high transpulmonary inflation pressure, and would facilitate efficient gas exchange to minimize the required minute ventilation.* The pathophysiologic processes described may also occur when ventilation is spontaneous, as in IRDS.

Although it is tempting to attribute pulmonary parenchymal dysfunction in chronically ventilated ill patients to ventilator-derived processes such as excessive Vt, AWP, and hyperinflation, the situation is far from clear. Many patients requiring ventilator support for hypoxemic respiratory failure have on-going pathologic processes (such as sepsis, pneumonia, shock) that may produce pulmonary parenchymal damage independently of mechanical ventilation. That mechanical ventilation can produce lung injury in the appropriate settings as described in the previous section is clear. The problem lies at defining where, within the spectrum of disease processes, changes in ventilator management may primarily affect lung function. Since mechanical ventilation is often lifesaving and its withdrawal is occasion-

ally associated with cardiovascular collapse, very careful consideration of the interaction between the ventilator and lung function should occur prior to and while modifying effective artificial ventilation in an attempt to minimize "respirator lung."

IRDS Paradigm, and the Effect of CPAP

When we are seeking a relation between ventilation pattern and lung injury, the effect of CPAP on lung failure in IRDS is striking. The progression of lung dysfunction leading to hypoxic death is slowed, stopped, and reversed simply by an increase in expiratory (and inspiratory) AWP. It is possible that rapid respiratory efforts in early IRDS promote removal to the airways of more surfactant than can be replaced by premature type II cells. The resulting increase in surface tension causes airway and alveolar closure and, combined with increasing inspiratory efforts, causes sufficient decrease in IFP to promote fluid accumulation. The fluid accumulation in turn further decreases compliance and oxygenation, which stimulates stronger ventilatory efforts. The several cycles of deterioration that can result were described earlier and are illustrated in Figure 24–8.

Continuous positive airway pressure (CPAP) may interrupt this cyclic deterioration in several ways. CPAP can diminish the initial loss of surfactant function, as has been shown experimentally, perhaps by enlarging alveolar end-expiratory volume.[12, 65] IFP would increase and therefore transudation would decrease, by several mechanisms: the increase in alveolar pressure established by CPAP directly opposes the pressure reduction imposed on the interstitial space by alveolar surface tension, so IFP is higher. The effect of any given alveolar surface tension on IFP is attenuated by increasing alveolar size according to the Laplace relation. The surface tension itself decreases to the degree that CPAP prevents functional surfactant loss. As FRC is increased, pleural pressure (and therefore IFP) becomes less negative; and if regional compliance changes are such that overall lung compliance is improved, a less negative pleural pressure *change* (and less work) is needed to maintain the same ventilation. Oxygen consumption, carbon dioxide production, and the need for high minute ventilation decrease. If a more efficient distribution of ventilation (recruitment and ventilation of low $\dot{V}/\dot{Q}$ lung) is established, then a still lower minute vol-

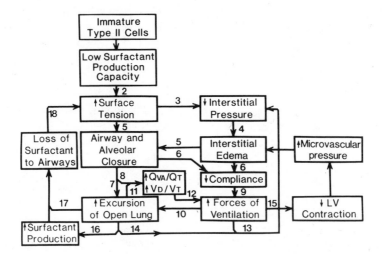

FIG 24–8.
Detrimental cycle in IRDS and the effect of CPAP. Immature alveolar cells have lower capacity to form surfactant *(1)*. Surface tension is higher when surfactant concentration is low *(2)*. High surface tension causes the alveoli to pull inward, creating a more negative pressure in the surrounding interstitium *(3)* (see Fig. 24–3). Greater transmural hydrostatic pressure promotes edema *(4)*. Interstitial edema and high surface tension promote air space closure *(5)*, and edema and air space closure both lower compliance *(6)*. Closure of airways requires greater excursion of lung remaining open *(7)*, both to maintain minute ventilation and because carbon dioxide elimination is less efficient (↑ Vd/Vt, *8)*. Lower compliance requires increased effort to maintain minute ventilation constant *(9)*. Greater respiration effort, such as due to J-receptor stimulation and hypoxia, also increases excursion of the lung remaining open *(10)*. If alveolar vessels are compressed, blood flow is diverted to closed lung, and both deadspace and venous admixture increase *(11)*. Inefficient carbon dioxide elimination requires higher minute ventilation *(12)*. Interstitial pressure is further decreased by more negative pleural pressure *(13)* and by enlargement of EAV interstitial space with lung distention *(14)*. More vigorous inspiratory effort impairs LV contraction *(15)*, which results in a need for higher microvascular pressure to sustain cardiac output. Lung distention stimulates surfactant production *(16)*, and exhalation to low volume enhances loss of surfactant *(17)*, resulting in higher surface tension *(18)*. Maintaining the lung open can counter these interactions, primarily at points 3, 5, and 6 in the cycle. Recruitment of closed airways counters forces *6, 7*, and *8*. Secondarily every other point in the cycle is interrupted except *1* and *2*. (From Snyder J.V., et al.: Mechanical ventilation: physiology and application. *Curr. Probl. Surg.,* 1984, vol 21. ©1984, Year Book Medical Publishers, Inc., Chicago; reproduced by permission.)

ume (and still less work) is required. The distal lung units are supported in exhalation until surfactant production is adequate. As that accumulates, high alveolar surface activity induces a further decrease in surface tension, which progressively increases IFP and opposes microvascular transudation. Several pathophysiologic cycles are broken, deterioration stops, accumulated edema dissipates, and the infant can be weaned from CPAP.

The ARDS Paradigm and the Effect of Keeping Lung Open

In ARF in adults, FRC might be decreased by an elevated diaphragm, pleural effusion, paralysis, straining, or other extrapulmonary factors, as well as by a decrease in pulmonary compliance. Ventilation is inefficient both when ventilated units are underperfused and when closed units are overperfused; surfactant is lost in excess of its production; inflation pressures are excessive and cause exaggerated volume changes in areas of the lung that remain open, with a resulting increase in transmicrovascular pressure, and edema is progressive. Thereby, interacting cycles comparable to those described in IRDS may be established (Fig 24–9); similarly, it may be possible to break those cycles by keeping the lung open.

The beneficial effects of a change in ventilatory support are less easily demonstrated in

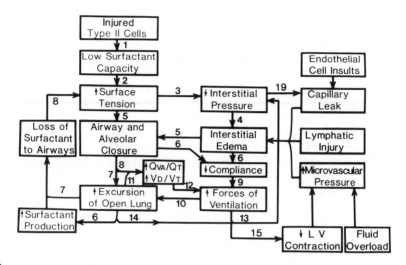

FIG 24–9.

Detrimental cycles in severe acute respiratory failure. Most of the influences diagramed are similar to those proposed for IRDS. In addition, use of mechanical ventilation with large Vt without first expanding closed lung may exaggerate expansion of open lung and divert more blood flow to closed lung, further increasing Qva/Qt and Vd/Vt, thus establishing a need for greater increase in minute ventilation; the cycle of forces *10*, *11*, and *12* is exaggerated. Overdistention of open lung may also exaggerate edema of EAV interstitial space *(13)*, thereby making parenchymal dysfunction more homogeneous. Capillary permea-bility also may be increased when hydrostatic forces are grossly exaggerated *(19)*.[9, 40] Recruitment of closed lung is effective at the same points as in Figure 24–8 (*3, 5, 6* and secondarily at almost every other interactive point). In addition, left ventricular *(LV)* contraction may be usefully augmented (reverse of *15*), and excessive venous return can be effectively retarded by an increase in pleural pressure due to both increased AWP and recruitment. (From Snyder J.V., et al.: Mechanical ventilation: physiology and application. *Curr. Probl. Surg.* vol 21. 1984. ©1984, Year Book Medical Publishers, Inc., Chicago; reproduced by permission.)

ARDS than in IRDS because of often subtle variations in chronic pulmonary conditions and because of the complex etiology and variable severity of the acute pulmonary insult in the adult. Subclinical cardiac dysfunction and associated surgical and medical diseases can complicate the analysis. A further distinction is that IRDS is self-limiting (if appropriate support is given), whereas ARDS is a label for many conditions of different etiology and mechanisms, only some of which are self-limiting. Therefore, even if some of the cycles described are broken, the outcome may not be different if the primary process continues. Another difference is the relative homogeneity of the pulmonary insult and of critical opening pressures in IRDS, compared with the disparate early lesions in ARDS. The multifocal nature of ARDS might justify directed recruiting efforts before the use of PEEP.

The Influence of PEEP in ARDS

The avoidance of excessive volume excursion, through the use of directed recruiting and PEEP, or the use of extra-corporeal CO_2 removal should interrupt the cycles that lead to respirator lung. The striking improvement in patients treated by Gattinoni and associates[15] with extracorporeal membrane support are compatible with the respirator lung concept. It is unlikely that the improvement they saw was due to exposure to the membrane lung, and alternative explanations, excepting severe bias in the data collection, are not apparent. There are several differences between that study and the multihospital extracorporeal membrane oxygenation project[71] that might explain the better response in Gattinoni's patients. In the latter study, mechanical ventilation was relinquished earlier, lung was more often splinted open, and bypass flow was limited to about one fourth of cardiac output. The "protection" provided by the support system was perhaps from mechanical ventilation and not from blood flow. However, we must recognize that while pulmonary dysfunction was comparably severe in the two studies, the findings of Gattinoni et al. were uncontrolled and have not been confirmed, so no final conclusion is yet justifiable. It is enticing to think that many of the ill effects of mechanical ventilation can be avoided by changing ventilation mode rather than by resorting to extracorporeal support. It may be possible that the pathophysiologic cycles can be avoided by establishing efficient patterns of ventilation in an open lung.

No mechanism has been described by which PEEP might have any direct influence on primary pathophysiologic processes. PEEP is a modification of only one part of the ventilation cycle, and therefore projection of the concepts presented here to the effects of PEEP on ARDS (without taking into account recruiting, peak AWP, Vd/Vt, and other important aspects of ventilatory support) must be limited. The application of relatively low levels of PEEP might result in an open lung when the pulmonary insult is uniform, or when PEEP is used prophylactically in patients at risk for ARDS. None of the available studies clearly supports or detracts from this concept. The paradigm presented in this chapter also makes one question whether the results of many clinical trials of early treatment[42, 54, 66] may have been inconclusive because the studies lacked an appropriate physiologic target. These questions need to be readdressed with more precisely targeted ventilatory protocols. Schmidt and colleagues[54] reported effective prophylaxis against ARDS, but the study has been criticized as lacking distinctive criteria,[41] and no physiologic criteria were used to determine the level of PEEP administered. Weigelt and co-workers[66] concluded that 45 patients at risk for ARDS who received PEEP early had a lower incidence of respiratory failure, lower pulmonary-related mortality, and lower overall mortality than did 34 patients randomly selected not to receive PEEP until it was required by hypoxemia. Pepe et al.,[42] in a well-defined and controlled study of 92 patients at risk for ARDS, found that the early application of 8 cm H_2O of PEEP had no effect on the incidence of ARDS or other associated complications and that the decrease in mortality that occurred was not significant. PEEP was adjusted by approximately the same criteria as Weigelt et al. used. The data of Pepe et al. suggest that using PEEP early shortens the duration of pulmonary dysfunction, but a more extensive study is needed to confirm this.

It would be preferable to adjust PEEP, and most therapy, according to physiologic criteria rather than to a rote prescription, and it is unclear how aspects of ventilation other than end-expiratory pressure were managed in this and other studies of PEEP. PEEP is more likely to be effective when it is used to keep open lungs that would otherwise close or collapse; but PEEP may have a less pronounced effect if excessive expansion of open lung is already being avoided, such as by lower frequency, lower Vt, adequate intravascular volume, and effective recruiting maneuvers and control of secretions. PEEP may have deleterious effects if closed lung regions are not opened as a result of its use, but blood flow is diverted from open to closed lung and increased ventilation is required because deadspace is increased.[3, 4] Pepe et al. provided a strong argument that application of PEEP per se was not a major deterrent to the ARDS in the patient group studied. This conclusion must be qualified, however, by recognition that no study to date has adequately controlled all of the factors currently thought to be mechanistically important in the development of respirator lung.

The pathophysiologic mechanisms discussed with respect to respirator lung would not be expected to exert any significant influence until pulmonary dysfunction (especially lung closure) is established. Early application of PEEP might reduce the incidence of lung closure, but until alveolar instability becomes established, so might other approaches to careful respiratory care, such as physical therapy, patient mobilization, or any increase in attention to respiratory activity. After ARDS has become established, the application of PEEP sufficient to open closed lung entails the risk of overexpanding open lung and causing barotrauma, and it may necessitate reduction of Vt and intravascular volume supplementation to avoid depression of venous return. Reports of the use of high levels of PEEP suggest that the outcome from ARDS can be improved with such treatment.[26, 27] It is noteworthy that low IMV rates are considered an important component of the approach in these reports, the goal being principally to reduce peak AWP. At the same time the benefits of lower volume excursion and more efficient distribution of ventilation to dependent low V/Q lung may be obtained. It is reasonable that the same effects could be obtained with lower levels of PEEP if directed recruiting efforts were successful in opening closed lung.

REFERENCES

1. Albert RK, Lakshiminarayan S, Kirk W, et al: Lung inflation can cause pulmonary edema in zone I of in situ dog lungs. *J Appl Physiol* 1980; 49:815.
2. Barber RE, Lee J, Hamilton WK: Oxygen toxicity in man: A prospective study in patients with irreversible brain damage. *N Engl J Med* 1970; 283:1478–84.
3. Bindslev L, Hedenstierna G, Santesson J, et al: Airway closure during anaesthesia, and its prevention by positive end expiratory pressure. *Acta Anaesthesiol Scand* 1980; 24:199–205.
4. Bindslev L, Hedenstierna G, Santesson J, et al: Ventilation-perfusion distribution during inhalation anaesthesia. *Acta Anaesthesiol Scand* 1981; 25:360.
5. Churg A, Golden J, Fligiel S, et al: Bronchopulmonary dysplasia in the adult. *Am Rev Respir Dis* 1983; 127:117–120.
6. Coalson JJ: Pathophysiological features of respiratory distress in the infant and adult, in Shoemaker WC (ed): *Critical Care: State of the Art.* Fullerton, Calif, Society for Critical Care Medicine, 1982, vol 13, pp 1–28.
7. Demling RH, Staub NC, Edmundo LH Jr: Effect of end-expiratory airway pressure on accumulation of extravascular lung water. *J Appl Physiol* 1975; 38:907.
8. Divertie MB: The adult respiratory distress syndrome. *Mayo Clin Proc* 1982; 57:371.
9. Egan EA: Lung inflation, lung solute permeability, and alveolar edema. *J Appl Physiol* 1982; 53:121.
10. Enhorning G, Robertson B: Lung expansion in the premature rabbit fetus after tracheal deposition of surfactant. *Pediatrics* 1972; 50:58–66.
11. Escobedo MB, Hillianr JL, Smith F, et al: A baboon model of bronchopulmonary dysplasia. *Exp Mol Pathol* 1982; 37:323–334.
12. Fariday EE, Perbutt S, Riley R: Effect of ventilation on surface forces in excised dogs' lungs. *J Appl Physiol* 1966; 21:1453.
13. Fariday EE: Effect of alterations in PO_2, PCO_2, pH, and blood flow on elastic behavior of dogs' lungs. *J Appl Physiol* 1969; 27:342.
14. Gallagher T, Civetti J: Normal pulmonary vascular resistance during acute respiratory insufficiency. *Crit Care Med* 1981; 9:647.
15. Gattinoni L, Pesenti A, Pellizola A, et al: Extracorporeal carbon dioxide removal in acute respiratory failure. *Ann Chir Gynaecol* 1982; 71(suppl 196):77.
16. Greenfield LJ, Ebert PA, Benson DW: Effect of positive pressure ventilation on surface tension properties of lung extracts. *Anesthesiology* 1964; 25:312.
17. Hallman M, Spragg R, Harrell JH, et al: Evidence of lung surfactant abnormality in respiratory failure. *J Clin Invest* 1982; 70:673.
18. Hamilton PP, Onayemi A, Smyth JA, et al: Comparison of conventional and high-frequency ventilation: Oxygenation and lung pathology. *J Appl Physiol* 1983; 55:131–138.
19. Ikegami M, Jacobs HC, Jobe AH: Inhibition of surfactant function in the respiratory distress syndrome (RDS) (abstract). *Pediatr Res* 1982; 16:292A.
20. Inoue H, Inque C, Hilderbrandt J: Vascular and airway pressures, and interstitial edema, affect peribronchial fluid pressure. *J Appl Physiol* 1980; 48:177.
21. Jenkins JG: Pulmonary edema following laryngospasm (letter). *Anesthesiology* 1984; 60:611.
22. Kao DK, Tierney DF: Air embolism with positive pressure ventilation of rats. *J Appl Physiol* 1977; 42:368.
23. Katz JA, Ozanne GM, Zinn SE, et al: Time course and mechanisms of lung volume increase with PEEP in acute pulmonary failure. *Anesthesiology* 1981; 54:9.
24. Katzenstein AA, Bloor CM, Leibow AA: Diffuse alveolar damage: The role of oxygen, shock, and related factors. *Am J Pathol* 1976; 85:210.
25. King RJ: Pulmonary surfactant. *J Appl Physiol* 1982; 53:1.
26. Kirby RR, Downs JB, Civetta JM, et al: High level positive end expiratory pressure (PEEP) in acute respiratory insufficiency. *Chest* 1975; 67:156.
27. Kirby R, Perry J, Calderwood H, et al: Cardiorespiratory effects of high positive end-expiratory pressures. *Anesthesiology* 1975; 43:533.
28. Kolton M, Cattran CB, Kent G, et al: Oxygenation during high-frequency ventilation compared with conventional mechanical ventilation in two models of lung injury. *Anesth Analg* 1982; 61:323–332.
29. Kuhn TS (ed): *The Structure of Scientific Revolutions.* Chicago, The University of Chicago Press, 1962, pp 10–12.

30. Lemaire F, Cerrina J, Lange F: PEEP-induced airspace overdistention complicating paraquat lung. *Chest* 1982; 81:654.

31. Macklem PT, Murphy B: The forces applied to the lung in health and disease. *Am J Med* 1974; 57:371.

32. Marland AM, Glauser FL: Hemodynamic and pulmonary edema protein measurements in a case of reexpansion pulmonary edema. *Chest* 1982; 81:250.

33. McAdams AJ, Coen R, Kleinman LI, et al: The experimental production of hyaline membranes in premature rhesus monkeys. *Am J Pathol* 1973; 70:277–284.

34. McClenahan JB, Urtnowski A: Effect of ventilation on surfactant and its turnover rate. *J Appl Physiol* 1967; 23:215.

35. Mead J, Takishima T, Leith D: Stress distribution in lungs: A model of pulmonary elasticity. *J Appl Physiol* 1970; 28:596.

36. Mellins RB, Levine OR, Skalak R, et al: Interstitial pressure of the lung. *Circ Res* 1969; 24:197.

37. Melnick BM: Postlaryngospasm pulmonary edema in adults (letter). *Anesthesiology* 1984; 70:516.

38. Mitzner W, Sylvester JT: Hypoxic vasoconstriction and fluid filtration in pig lungs. *J Appl Physiol* 1981; 51:1965.

39. Nilsson R, Grossman G, Robertson B: Lung surfactant and the pathogenesis of neonatal broncheolar lesion induced by artificial ventilation. *Pediatr Res* 1978; 12:249–255.

40. Parker JC, Townsley MI, Rippe B, et al: Increased microvascular permeability in dog lungs due to high peak airway pressures. *J Appl Physiol* 1984; 57:1809.

41. Pavlin DJ, Nessly ML, Cheney FW: Increased pulmonary vascular permeability as a cause of re-expansion edema in rabbits. *Am Rev Respir Dis* 1981; 124:442.

42. Pepe PE, Hudson LD, Carrico CJ: Early application of positive end-expiratory pressure in patients at risk for the adult respiratory-distress syndrome. *N Engl J Med* 1984; 311:281.

43. Permutt S: Relation between pulmonary arterial pressure and pleural pressure during the acute asthmatic attack. *Chest* 1973; 63:25S.

44. Permutt S: Mechanical influence on water accumulation in the lungs, in Fishman AP, Renkin EM (eds): *Pulmonary Edema*. Washington, DC, American Physiological Society, 1979, pp 175–193.

45. Pesenti A, Kolobow T, Buckhold DK, et al: Prevention of hyaline membrane disease in premature lambs by apneic oxygenation and extracorporeal carbon dioxide removal. *Intensive Care Med* 1982; 8:11–17.

46. Petty TL, Silvers GW, et al: Abnormalities in lung elastic properties and surfactant function in adult respiratory distress syndrome. *Chest* 1979; 75:571.

47. Pontoppidan H, Hedley-Whyte J, Bendixen HH: Ventilation and oxygen requirements during prolonged artificial ventilation in patients with respiratory failure. *N Engl J Med* 1965; 273:401.

48. Pontoppidan H, Geffin B, Lowenstein E (eds): *Acute Respiratory Failure in the Adult*. Boston, Little, Brown & Co, 1973, pp 52–53.

49. Pratt PC, Vollmer RT, Shelburne JD, et al: Pulmonary morphology in a multihospital collaborative extracorporeal membrane oxygenation project. *Am J Pathol* 1979; 95:191.

50. Price RD, Algren JT, Buchino JJ, et al: Pulmonary edema consequent to inspiratory obstruction in dogs (abstract). *Crit Care Med* 1984; 12:216.

51. Ray RJ, Alexander CM, Chen L, et al: Influence of the method of re-expansion of atelectatic lung upon the development of pulmonary edema in dogs. *Crit Care Med* 1984; 12:364.

52. Rennard SI, Bitterman PB, Crystal RG: Response of the lower respiratory tract to injury: Mechanisms of repair of the parenchymal cells of the alveolar wall. *Chest* 1983; 84:735.

53. Russell JA, Hoeffel J, Murray JF: Effect of different levels of positive end-expiratory pressure on lung water content. *J Appl Physiol* 1982; 53:9.

54. Schmidt G, O'Neill W, Kotb K, et al: Continuous positive airway pressure in the prophylaxis of the adult respiratory distress syndrome. *Surg Gynecol Obstet* 1976; 143:613.

55. Schoenberger CI, Rennard SI, Bitterman PB: Paraquat-induced pulmonary fibrosis: Role of the alveolitis in modulating the development of fibrosis. *Am Rev Respir Dis* 1984; 129:168.

56. Shennib H, Mulder DS, Chiu RC: The effects of pulmonary atelectasis and reexpansion on lung cellular immune defenses. *Arch Surg* 1984; 119:274.

57. Slavin G, Nunn JF, Crow J, et al: Bronchiolectasis: A complication of artificial ventilation. *Br Med J* 1982; 285:931.

58. Sprung CL, Loewenherz JW, Baier H, et al:

Evidence for increased permeability in reexpansion pulmonary edema. *Am J Med* 1981; 71:497.

59. Sprung CL, Elser B: Reexpansion pulmonary edema (letter). *Chest* 1983; 84:788.

60. Stalcup SA, Mellins RB: Mechanical forces producing pulmonary edema in acute asthma. *N Engl J Med* 1977; 297:592.

61. Tahvanainen J, Hallman M, Nikki P: The significance of surfactant deficiency in acute respiratory failure (abstract). *Crit Care Med* 1984; 12:330.

62. Taylor AE: Personal communication, 1982.

63. Thet LA, Alvarez H: Effect of hyperventilation and starvation on rat lung mechanics and surfactant. *Am Rev Respir Dis* 1982; 126:286.

64. Venus V, Takayoshi M, Capiozo JB, et al: Prophylactic intubation and continuous positive airway pressure in the management of inhalation therapy in burn victims. *Crit Care Med* 1981; 9:519.

65. Webb H, Tierney D: Experimental pulmonary edema due to intermittent positive pressure ventilation with high inflation pressures: Protection by positive end-expiratory pressure. *Am Rev Respir Dis* 1974; 110:556.

66. Weigelt JA, Mitchell RA, Snyder WH: Early positive end-expiratory pressure in the adult respiratory distress syndrome. *Arch Surg* 1979; 114:497.

67. Weissman C, Damask MC, Yang J: Noncardiogenic pulmonary edema following laryngeal obstruction. *Anesthesiology* 1984; 60(2):163.

68. Williams JV, Tierney DF, Parker HR: Surface forces in the lung, atelectasis, and transpulmonary pressure. *J Appl Physiol* 1966; 21:819.

69. Woo S.W., Berlin D, Buch U, et al: Altered perfusion, ventilation, anesthesia and lung-surface forces in dogs. *Anesthesiology* 1970; 33:411.

70. Wyszogrodski I, Kyei-aboagye K, Taeusch W, et al: Surfactant inactivation by hyperventilation: Conservation by end-expiratory pressure. *J Appl Physiol* 1975; 38:461.

71. Zapol WM, Snider MT, Hill JD: Extracorporeal membrane oxygenation in severe acute respiratory failure. *JAMA* 1979; 242:2193.

25   The Open Lung Approach: Concept and Application

James V. Snyder, M.D.

Alison Froese, M.D.

Recent discussions of optimal ventilatory support for the patient with acute hypoxemic respiratory failure have focused primarily on the level of airway pressure (AWP) remaining at the end of exhalation. It has been suggested that positive end-expiratory pressure (PEEP) has a beneficial effect on some aspects of pulmonary pathophysiology: colloquially, "PEEP heals." Our approach to ventilatory support emphasizes the importance of considering *all* aspects of the ventilation cycle along with ancillary support mechanisms such as recruitment of collapsed areas of the lung. In essence, our approach to ventilatory support can be summed up in the directive: maintain an open lung at minimal AWP. This approach has been derived significantly from the approaches of others* and is designed to incorporate all the major concepts presented in earlier chapters. Various changes in our perception of ventilator-patient interaction are emphasized. The "open lung" approach is loosely structured, emphasizing objectives rather than specific steps. We hypothesize that the "open lung" approach may minimize ventilator-induced pulmonary damage and decrease the time to recovery should such damage occur. The details of this approach will undoubtedly change over the next few years as concepts of ventilation and lung injury are refined and data from more controlled clinical trials accumulate.

INTRODUCTION

Patients often require mechanical ventilatory support (increased expiratory pressure and artificial ventilation) to maintain adequate oxygenation and

*References 5, 18, 28, 29, 32, 39, 45, 46, 58, 59, 60, 106, and 107.

carbon dioxide removal during the course of their disease. This requirement for artificial ventilation may be short term, as in the case of intraoperative and acute postoperative care or after drug overdosage. At the opposite extreme, patients can require ventilatory support for weeks, months, or even years because of a neuromuscular weakness, chronic obstructive lung disease, severe congenital abnormalities, or bronchopulmonary dysplasia. The indications for artificial ventilation of any kind are many and the pathophysiology of lung disease requiring mechanical support for the failing ventilatory system is diverse. A chapter attempting to define the specific ventilator settings for all patients would be doomed to fail. Artificial ventilation must be individualized. Accordingly, this chapter discusses certain basic concepts that are universal to all forms of lung disease and describes how to apply them in a rational fashion to treat appropriately patients who require ventilatory support. On the basis of the factors identified and discussed in the preceding chapters, in some cases we may suggest the optimal pattern of artificial ventilation for a given patient.

In general, artificial ventilators allow us to vary the tidal volume (Vt) delivered to the patient, the respiratory rate, the maximum AWP that can be achieved during inspiration, the fractional concentration of oxygen delivered (FI_{O_2}), the inspiratory flow rate, and the degree to which expiratory pressure exceeds atmospheric pressure (CPAP and PEEP). By manipulating these elements of ventilatory support, we attempt to maximize oxygen delivery to and carbon dioxide removal from the patient without causing hemodynamic compromise or pulmonary parenchymal damage, and, we hope, to aid in the repair processes necessary to wean the patient from mechanical ventilatory support.

It is useful to discuss oxygenation (which requires an open lung) separately from carbon dioxide elimination (which requires ventilation, optimally of an open lung) and from airway protection (which requires intact neuromuscular function or intubation). It is feasible and may be preferable to maintain the lung open without augmenting ventilation and without intubation (CPAP by mask). Thus, ventilatory support may consist of providing continuous positive pressure without intubation or mechanical ventilation. Clarification of related subjects is important: the work of breathing may be lower with CPAP than without; the mode of ventilatory support can significantly influence the efficiency of carbon dioxide elimination; and details of the ventilatory support circuit (demand valve threshold, expiratory and inspiratory limb resistance, reservoir bag compliance) can significantly alter the patient's tolerance of a given support system.

Certain concepts have emerged in our understanding of ventilatory support that should be summarized before we discuss the specific adjustments of the ventilator to the patient for a given condition. These concepts will be loosely grouped into three subsections: (1) the effect of Vt, AWP, and PEEP on shunt ($\dot{Q}s/\dot{Q}t$) and deadspace (Vd/Vt), (2) the relation between PEEP and cardiac output, and (3) the clearing of airway secretions. Subsequently we discuss the advantages and disadvantages of various modes of artificial ventilatory support, and conclude with a general discussion of the mechanisms necessary to optimize gas exchange during artificial ventilation and the weaning process.

THE EFFECT OF Vt, AWP, AND PEEP ON $\dot{Q}s/\dot{Q}t$ AND Vd/Vt

As a simplistic approach to artificial ventilation, one may attempt to match artificial positive pressure breathing patterns to those that occur with normal spontaneous ventilation. By this approach a normal Vt, respiration rate, inspiratory flow rate, and room air F_{IO_2} (0.21) without PEEP would be delivered to the patient. However, as described in Chapter 20, "The Development of Supported Ventilation: A Critical Summary," the constant delivery of a normal Vt (5–7 ml/kg) by mechanical ventilation results in progressive decreases in functional residual capacity (FRC), associated with collapsed airways and alveoli. High

Vt ventilation (10–15 ml/kg) will significantly impede this collapse when the lung is normal. When the stability of distal lung units (alveolus and alveolar duct) is impaired by disease (surfactant disruption or deficiency), collapse can occur immediately upon loss of inflation pressure even if a large Vt, or sigh, is used. This observation implies that when distal lung units are unstable, increased expiratory pressure (PEEP) is necessary to maintain the lung open. Progressive collapse of distal lung units is still related to the relation between FRC and critical closing volume, but the critical closing volume is much higher for the unstable lung units than for normal units. If high Vt opens previously closed lung units, then increasing end-expiratory transpulmonary pressure by increasing FRC may splint those alveoli open with a lower Vt. Subsequent recruiting maneuvers may open more alveoli, further increasing FRC without the need for additional PEEP.

Because critical opening pressure as well as regional lung compliance can vary widely in acute respiratory failure (ARF), sequential increases in PEEP may have several detrimental effects. PEEP may predominantly overdistend lung units that are already open without recruiting a significant proportion of closed lung units. As a result, peak AWP may increase more than expected for the amount of PEEP used. Also, because overdistention of the healthy lung will increase its selective pulmonary vascular resistance, blood flow will be diverted from open to still closed lung. Because blood flow to open lung is less, V/Q in open lung is higher, and carbon dioxide elimination is less efficient; because blood flow to closed lung is increased, $\dot{Q}s/\dot{Q}t$ is higher. The increase in Vd/Vt requires an increase in minute ventilation to maintain Pa_{CO_2} constant, further elevating mean AWP. In addition, peak AWP in excess of 40 cm H_2O can increase lung microvascular permeability, resulting in interstitial and alveolar edema, with impaired gas exchange, lower compliance, and higher AWP. When these are the consequences of increased PEEP, commonly considered therapeutic alternatives include (1) returning to the lower level of PEEP and accepting the consequences of leaving significant portions of the lung either closed or closing with each exhalation, and (2) continuing with sequential small increases in PEEP (2–3 cm H_2O), accepting some deterioration in gas exchange and some increase in AWP in hope of eventually reaching the critical opening pressure of the lung regions still closed, after which gas exchange will be improved again. To a certain extent, the increase in deadspace and shunt may be counteracted by intravascular volume infusion, which by increasing venous return will increase pulmonary arterial pressure and may maintain capillary perfusion in open lung. Also, the risk of barotrauma can be reduced by lowering the frequency and volume of mechanical Vt, and by incorporating a system by which capable patients can contribute spontaneous breaths. Dyspneic or weak patients or those in shock may be intolerant of these reductions in support. We prefer to avoid both these courses, and attempt instead to obtain the advantages of a sustained open lung while minimizing both PEEP and peak AWP by using directed recruiting techniques. That is, body position can be manipulated to optimize blood flow, ventilation, and distending pressure to improve gas exchange as well as facilitate postural drainage. Accordingly, closed lung may be opened and compliance increased, and $\dot{Q}s/\dot{Q}t$ and Vd/Vt may be decreased with minimal risk to open lung and little or no increase in PEEP. If sufficient lung alveoli are recruited, compliance may improve while peak AWP is decreased. If carbon dioxide elimination becomes more efficient as more low V/Q units are recruited, minute ventilation and peak and mean AWP can be reduced. Vd/Vt can be monitored efficiently using the P_{CO_2} of continuously mixed exhaled gas ($P\bar{e}_{CO_2}$) and values of Pa_{CO_2} (directly measured intermittently or estimated continuously by transcutaneous monitor methods), in the Enghoff-Bohr equation:

$$Vd/Vt = \frac{Pa_{CO_2} - P\bar{e}_{CO_2}}{Pa_{CO_2}} \quad \text{(Eq. 25–1)}$$

If alterations in ventilator settings significantly modify the efficiency of carbon dioxide elimination, then monitoring Vd/Vt might provide information important to the adjustment of ventilatory support.

Although oxygen in high concentrations is well known to be directly toxic to lung tissue, it also has undesirable effects at relatively low concentrations. However, the influence of these effects on morbidity and outcome is ill defined. The toxic effects of oxygen include impairment of ciliary function and macrophage function at F_{IO_2} of 0.4 and 0.6, reabsorption atelectasis, lung injury from oxygen free radical interactions, and possibly damage to surfactant. Accordingly, F_{IO_2}

should be kept as low as that necessary for adequate oxygen transport, and changes in ventilatory support pattern that enable lowering F_{IO_2} below 0.4, or even 0.3, may be justified.

Patients with air flow obstruction must be approached somewhat differently. Since ARF in this group of patients is often associated with hyperinflation because of the patient's inability to expire completely and resulting maldistribution of ventilation to perfusion (V/Q mismatch), both large Vt breaths and increased respiratory rates may be detrimental. Here, besides the appropriate pharmacologic therapy to reverse air flow obstruction (bronchodilators, antibiotics, pulmonary toilet, etc.), manipulation of the ventilator can minimize hyperinflation and decrease Vd/Vt.

PEEP is often considered contraindicated in patients with chronic air flow obstruction because the lung is already hyperinflated and FRC is greater than normal. However, if airways that close prematurely can be splinted open, areas that remain fully inflated during exhalation may then deflate more fully. They may also be perfused better at their lower volume. Because the inspiratory work of breathing is now recognized to contribute significantly to respiratory failure in acute and chronic air flow obstruction, the use of PEEP or CPAP to increase FRC may diminish the work of the inspiratory muscles and the risk of muscle exhaustion, as well as improve the distribution of V/Q. These physiologic effects are similar in many respects to those that occur when a patient with air flow obstruction sits up—and feels it is easier to breathe that way. Finding the balance of PEEP, Vt, and inspiratory flow rate that is appropriate to each patient with asthma or chronic air flow obstruction remains a problem of individual management, but our perception of the effects of those variables is clearly changing.

THE EFFECT OF MECHANICAL VENTILATION AND PEEP ON CARDIAC OUTPUT

All forms of positive pressure ventilation can decrease cardiac output by decreasing the pressure gradient for venous return. These points are discussed in detail in chapter 21, "Hemodynamic Effects of Artificial Ventilation." Increasing lung volume, by increasing pleural pressure, will passively increase central venous pressure (CVP), which acts as the downstream pressure to venous return. Any factor that increases pleural pressure will tend to decrease venous return. Such factors include an increased respiratory rate, which allows less time for passive exhalation; an increased Vt; a decreased expiratory time; and increased level of PEEP. In addition, increases in pulmonary vascular resistance as would occur with overdistention of the lung will increase CVP by impeding right ventricular ejection.

The potential for depression of venous return is of particular concern when oxygen transport is already compromised. However, the beneficial effects of mechanical ventilation on the distribution of oxygen supply, and on oxygen demand, must also be considered. Benefit may occur in the form of a reduction of the work of breathing with less competition by respiratory muscles for a limited oxygen supply. Similarly, in congestive heart failure states, cardiac output may be augmented rather than depressed. Compared to spontaneously breathing subjects, mechanical ventilatory support was associated with improved blood flow to liver, brain, and nonrespiratory muscle, and with lower levels of lactic acid, in a model of shock from cardiac tamponade.[9, 112] Cardiac output was equal with both forms of ventilation, but respiratory muscles received 21% of total blood flow during spontaneous breathing, compared to 3% when ventilation was controlled. Respiratory muscle failure and apnea were also characteristic in an endotoxin shock model.[52] A similar sequence of initial tachypnea, and then bradypnea due to inspiratory muscle fatigue, sometimes followed by apnea, has been described for patients with respiratory muscle fatigue.[7] This pattern and related observations are all compatible with muscle energy failure[93] and may be relieved by provision of ventilatory support if excessive reduction of venous return is avoided.

The decrease in cardiac output that is usually observed with increases in pleural pressure can be compensated for by intravenous fluid administration since the primary cause of the decrease in cardiac output is a decreased pressure gradient for venous return. Fluid loading in this fashion, however, results in an increase in mean capillary pressure in the peripheral vasculature and an increased tendency for peripheral edema. Thus, when fluid resuscitation is given to maintain cardiac output for a patient receiving PEEP, it may be necessary to give fluid continually to compensate for third space losses despite an initially good response to the fluid resuscitation. When ventricular function is severely compromised and

preload is adequate, increases in pleural pressure will not decrease cardiac output because in this condition (heart failure), ventricular function is relatively independent of preload. In heart failure states, the increase in pleural pressure, by decreasing the afterload for left ventricular ejection,[86] may augment cardiac output and thus improve oxygen delivery. On this basis it may be safer to increase PEEP to improve oxygenation, and maintain cardiac output by volume infusions if necessary—and to reduce Vt at the same time to lower peak AWP. If ventricular function is depressed and intravascular volume is adequate, increases in PEEP should improve oxygen delivery to the tissues by increasing both arterial P_{O_2} and cardiac output.

CLEARING SECRETIONS AND LUNG EXPANSION

It is fundamentally important to keep the lung open and clear of excess secretions. The combination of changing body position in bed and vigorous coughing is probably the most efficacious way to clear airway secretions in normal lungs.[27] Patients who cannot clear tracheal secretions when supine or sitting can often do so when turned semiprone. With the help of gravity to move mucus to the larynx, a minimal cough is then effective. Such patients are probably better served by being turned than by catheter insertion. In the patient who cannot or will not cough adequately, suctioning is useful to remove secretions and to stimulate coughing and subsequent inspiratory gasping, which expands the lungs. However, suctioning may cause hypoxia, mucosal damage, or decreased lung compliance if the secretions are not removed.[31] The nonintubated patient who is nasotracheally suctioned is also at risk for serious bleeding due to local trauma from the suction catheter. The suction catheter may also stimulate laryngospasm. In addition, nasotracheal suctioning causes transient bacteremia, which may put patients with heart valve lesions at risk for bacterial endocarditis.[62] Suctioning or forced exhalation may result in atelectasis[76] and should be followed by inspiratory sighing maneuvers. In the intubated patient the principal risk of suctioning is the suctioning-induced hypoxemia.[31] Use of a conventional[20] or jet ventilator[44] during suctioning or preoxygenation prior to suctioning may limit this problem.

Ultrasonic nebulization as it is routinely prescribed has not been shown to be efficacious in clearing secretions.[108] Since it can cause bronchospasm and overhydration, especially in young children, its use should be monitored to detect these complications. In some patients whose sputum production is minimal, prolonged (1 hour) continuous delivery of an ultrasonically generated aerosol can induce a considerable outpouring of secretions, including casts, and subsequent pulmonary clearing. Bronchodilator therapy should precede ultrasonic nebulization and the patient must be continuously observed for signs of deterioration related to increased volumes of retained secretions, pulmonary edema, or bronchoconstriction.

Since tracheal injection of small aliquots of saline may yield similar results without these complications, we favor the use of intermittent small-volume saline instillation directly into the endotracheal tube and brisk inspiratory support by "bagging" to aid in clearing secretions.

Narcotic agents used to minimize pain will depress such spontaneous airway clearing reflexes.[23] In patients who require analgesia, epidural anesthesia, intercostal block, and other regional anesthetic approaches can give pain relief without the respiratory depression of systemic narcotics.

Postural Drainage

Since the hydrostatic pressures in the pulmonary vessels are greater in the bases of the lung due to gravitational forces, greater transudation of fluid from the capillaries in dependent lung segments may also occur. Interstitial fluid accumulation, by causing distal lung units to collapse, may decrease compliance and compromise ventilation in dependent areas of the lung. Lung segments that are uppermost are more likely to be drained not only of secretions, but also of interstitial fluid. Drainage of the lung bases is better in the semiprone than in the lateral position. Patients who have pillows behind their backs to keep them in a lateral position usually have not been turned far enough. Mechanically rotating beds (Roto-Rest bed, Kinetic Concepts, Inc., San Antonio, Texas) are useful in many patients with pulmonary, brain, and spinal cord injuries. In patients with copious secretions, postural drainage used with coughing, sighing, and perhaps percussion and vibration is important. However, postural drainage and percussion may be associated with hypoxia, following as well as during treatment.

Lung Expansion and the Prevention of Atelectasis

Of the currently used techniques designed to prevent and treat atelectasis, none has been shown to be superior to the traditional "stir-up" regimen of frequent turning, coughing, and deep breathing.[74] Intermittent positive pressure breathing (IPPB) treatments do little to expand the lung,[1] deliver inhaled medication no more effectively than aerosol treatments,[54] and may have more side effects.[24] Since IPPB treatments have little indication and are expensive, it is appropriate that they are ordered much less often than in the past.[78] The exception may be the patient who cannot or will not take deep breaths with any other technique. For IPPB to be effective, machine Vt must be monitored so that the machine pressure can be set to deliver an adequate volume for the particular patient.[76]

Percussion, vibration, and postural drainage (chest physical therapy) may be useful in mobilizing secretions and thereby preventing atelectasis.[48] In patients with pneumonia, chest physical therapy has been documented not to lessen the severity of illness or to speed recovery,[42] in chronic obstructive pulmonary disease (COPD) patients it has little benefit,[91] and in patients with cystic fibrosis it may be no more effective than simple coughing.[27] Chest physical therapy can cause transient hypoxemia, so its risk/benefit ratio must be weighed in the individual patient.

A means of preventing airway closure that has become increasingly popular is incentive spirometry. Unlike "blow bottles," which provide expiratory resistance and only indirectly encourage the patient to inhale deeply, incentive spirometers function as a form of behavior modification by providing the patient with information about how deeply he or she has inhaled. Well-motivated and carefully instructed patients can use an incentive spirometer frequently on their own, freeing staff for other tasks. Incentive spirometry has been shown to be as effective as turning, coughing, and deep breathing regimens[13, 24] and has been associated with a shorter length of hospitalization after abdominal surgery.[24]

β agonists and theophylline enhance mucociliary function and ventilatory muscle function as well as providing bronchodilation, and are therefore very helpful in preventing and treating atelectasis in patients with asthma and COPD.

A new technique for the prevention and treatment of atelectasis is CPAP given by face mask. Experimentally, CPAP can be as effective as mechanical ventilation with PEEP in maintaining adequate oxygenation,[2] and clinical studies have shown it to be as effective as stir-up regimens and incentive spirometry; furthermore, many patients find it less painful than other modalities.[82, 103]

Treatment of Established Atelectasis

Neither an increase in venous admixture (intrapulmonary shunt) nor a decrease in pulmonary compliance is an adequate index of atelectasis.[15] Also, recall that atelectasis grossly apparent on direct examinaton of the lung, and presumably sufficient to cause dysfunction, may not be evident radiologically.[14] Therefore, an increase in venous admixture that is unexplained radiologically should be recognized as potentially due to atelectasis (or occlusion of airways), and appropriate therapeutic maneuvers should be undertaken. Once atelectasis has occurred, several forms of treatment are available. The conservative approach involves vigorous use of percussion, coughing, deep breathing, and incentive spirometry. While some advocate therapeutic bronchoscopy to selectively suction the affected area, Marini et al. have shown this to be no more effective than conservative treatment.[67] Their evidence shows that most atelectasis resolves quickly with either therapy, and that the small number of patients who will respond slowly to either mode can be predicted on the basis of air bronchograms on the chest radiograph. On the other hand, Lindholm and Grenvik described a series of 70 fiberoptic bronchoscopies in critically ill patients in whom routine respiratory therapy, including physiotherapy and tracheal suctioning, had failed to improve the pulmonary condition; radiographic densities were diminished in 67% of these.[64] Passage of the flexible bronchoscope into the endotracheal tube of a mechanically ventilated patient can markedly and abruptly alter tidal exchange and AWP.[64] We consider it mandatory that the bronchoscopist be aware of the potential pathophysiologic aspects of bronchoscopy in such patients, and we recommend that well-oriented assistants monitor chest excursion, vital signs, and patient response continually during the procedure. Specific catheter suctioning of the left lung without bronchoscopic direction is difficult, because even curved catheters tend to go down the right main stem.[33] Other techniques, such as balloon occlusion of the airway and reexpansion of the distal lung using the bronchoscope, have been described but not studied in a controlled fashion.[71]

In our opinion, when new lobar or segmental lung collapse is identified on the chest x-ray film, an effort should be made to reexpand the lung the same day. If conventional measures fail, then directed recruiting techniques may be useful. In an attempt to optimize reexpansion of collapsed lung units, we have incorporated many principles into a single technique called directed recruitment. This technique as it evolved at Presbyterian University Hospital has been detailed in an anecdotal report.[94] The physiologic principles are summarized below. There are several documented as well as theoretical risks to this approach, and no controlled data support its use. The technique is continually being improved as more clinical experience is gained.

Principles of Directed Recruitment

Directed recruitment attempts to combine the benefit of chest physiotherapy with a titrated application of manual mechanical expansion. Proper positioning of the patient protects some of the open lung areas from overdistention and maximizes the effect of a sustained high transpulmonary pressure on closed lung. Particular attention is paid to the effects of position, the manual application of transpulmonary (distending) pressure, preservation of venous return, and forceful exhalation.

Position.   Positioning affects regional transpulmonary pressure (TPP). Although alveolar pressure is equal in all regions of the lung at both end-exhalation and end-inspiration, pleural pressure is not. Since the pleural space must support the weight of the thoracic viscera, the pleural pressure will be greatest in the most dependent regions of the lung. Positioning the patient so that the lung segment to be recruited is uppermost and the more normal lung is dependent directs a maximum TPP across the closed lung and a minimum TPP across the open lung.[17] In this position gravity optimizes perfusion to the more functional dependent lung and also facilitates clearing of secretions from the uppermost lung. Thus, not only reexpansion of collapsed lung regions may occur, but better matching of ventilation to perfusion in the "good" dependent lung may improve gas exchange.

Transpulmonary Pressure and Time. Recruitment is maximal when TPP is greatest. After proper positioning, AWP is increased with the aim of reexpanding the collapsed lung. This might occur by three mechanisms: alveolar interdependence, collateral ventilation,[1] or ventilation of partially occluded bronchi. Alveolar interdependence refers to the increase in expansive force experienced by collapsed airways and lung parenchyma when adjacent open lung is further inflated. When airways remain closed, as by mucus, expansion may still occur via the pores of Cohn and channels of Lambert. The higher distending pressure may also combine with increased radial distending forces on collapsed and occluded airways to partially open them and inflate the distal lung directly. In a cooperative patient, it is often possible to combine patient inspiratory effort with an increased mean AWP to minimize the compromise of venous return while maximizing TPP. When the patient inspires, lung inflation is accompanied by a decrease in pleural pressure, and less of a simultaneous increase in AWP is needed for the same total lung expansion. Because AWP and pleural pressure are less elevated, venous return is less impaired. Even small increases in TPP, when sustained, can effectively expand collapsed lung by both airway and collateral ventilation.[1]

Preservation of Venous Return. Sustained high AWP may profoundly decrease arterial pressure by the elevation in right atrial pressure (RAP), decreasing the pressure gradient for venous return. This will depend to a large degree on both pulmonary compliance and the blood volume status of the patient. Transiently elevating AWP (for up to 3 seconds) by rapidly elevating RAP will often identify patients who cannot tolerate sustained elevation of AWP, as the transient elevations induce hypotension from decreased venous return during or immediately after the use of the recruiting maneuver. The pulse pressure is a more sensitive indicator of a reduction in stroke volume than is the mean arterial pressure (MAP) when AWP is elevated. This is because MAP may be factitiously maintained by a sustained increase in pleural pressure, as occurs during a Valsalva maneuver.[10] Compromise of cardiac output during the recruiting maneuver can be avoided or minimized by elevating the patient's legs and/or the foot of the bed with the patient still in the lateral position. Incorporating patient effort also preserves venous return, as described above.

Forceful Exhalation. Forceful exhalation may be required to expel occluding mucus into larger airways. This usually occurs spontaneously when the patient coughs. Less reactive individuals may need encouragement or suctioning to stimulate coughing. External chest compression helps to increase expiratory force in patients unable to cough. When distal lung units are unstable, as occurs with alveolar cell injury, it is preferable not to allow full exhalation at the end of the last sustained inflation of a series; instead, to prevent collapse of unstable lung units, the patient is returned to CPAP or ventilatory support with PEEP.

MECHANICAL VENTILATION: THE OPEN LUNG APPROACH

On the basis of the interactions summarized in the preceding text, we propose that supporting ventilation optimally with a minimum of complications requires the physician to balance the following *objectives:* (1) to maintain all lung units open with minimal peak AWP, avoiding barotrauma and increased right ventricular afterload; (2) to operate at the minimal possible increase in pleural pressure, avoiding decreased venous return; (3) to optimize patient work of breathing while avoiding exhaustion by the appropriate use of ventilatory modes; and (4) to minimize the use of tracheal intubation so as to avoid loss of FRC, laryngotracheal injury,[63, 65] and pulmonary infection. We call this method of mechanical support of respiration the "open lung approach." Some differences in this approach from conventional therapy are emphasized in Table 25–1. In the open lung approach, we pursue these objectives in the following way: *pulmonary secretions are cleared, closed lung areas are aggressively recruited, recruited lung is then splinted open, diaphragmatic activity is encouraged, and excessive inflation pressures are avoided.* We have found it useful to consider the goals of airway support, airway protection, and ventilatory assistance as three separate issues (Table 25–2).

Nonintubated Airway Support: CPAP by Mask

CPAP given by mask is appropriate to help the patient who is adequately ventilated but inadequately oxygenated and who is alert enough to protect his or her airway. The intermittent use of CPAP may be useful, especially following upper

TABLE 25–1.

Open Lung Approach Versus Conventional Approach

CONVENTIONAL APPROACH	OPEN LUNG APPROACH
1. Goal is adequate Pao_2 with nontoxic Fio_2	1. Goal is open lung with minimal AWP
2. Use assisted ventilation, Vt 10–15 ml/kg	2. Assist/IMV with PEEP, lower Vt
3. Increase PEEP to recruit closed lung	3. Directed recruiting to open lung, and PEEP to splint
4. Venous admixture is a total V/Q problem (i.e., FRC:CC)	4. Venous admixture is a regional V/Q problem
5. PEEP causes low cardiac output and barotrauma	5. Increased pleural pressure and peak AWP and intrathoracic hypovolemia, not PEEP per se, cause low cardiac output and barotrauma; increased pleural pressure can also augment cardiac output
6. CO_2 elimination is not a problem	6. CO_2 elimination may be a problem because increased Vd/Vt requires increased minute ventilation, necessitating increased AWP, which can lower cardiac output and cause barotrauma
7. Mechanical ventilation = security	7. Mechanical ventilation is inefficient and a cause of higher Vd/Vt and AWP, tracheal injury and increased incidence of nosocomial infection

abdominal surgery (as suggested in chapter 20, "Pulmonary Physiology"). Supporting data have been reported by Stocks et al.[104] If the closing and opening of distal airways is as destructive in adult humans as it is experimentally (see chapter 24, "Respirator Lung"),[45] then the splinting effect of CPAP in patients with alveolar instability is desirable independent of its effect on gas exchange. Since AWP is increased with CPAP, the work of breathing may also change. The work of breathing is not necessarily greater with CPAP, and it may be less, because of the mechanisms summarized in chapter 20, "Pulmonary Physiology." The potential risk associated with this technique is aerophagia. The resulting gastric distention increases the risk of emesis and stresses gastrointestinal suture lines. Because the risk of aspiration is greater, CPAP by mask is contrain-

TABLE 25–2.

Goals and Principal Techniques of Ventilatory Support*

AIRWAY PROTECTION	OXYGENATION	CO_2 ELIMINATION
1. Self-protection by alert patient	1. Remove secretions	1. Ventilate low V/Q (CO_2 rich) lung; recruit and splint (CPAP); use diaphragm
2. Self-protection by intact gag and cough reflexes	2. Increase $Fio_2 < .4$	
3. Body position (semiprone)	3. Open lung by recruiting and splinting (CPAP or PEEP)	2. Mechanical ventilation
4. Oral or nasopharyngeal airway	4. Further increase $Fio_2 > 0.4$	
5. Tracheal tube		

*From Snyder JV, et al.[101] Reproduced by permission. Goals and techniques are listed in approximate order of preference. Maintaining the lung open is an important aspect of efficiency in carbon dioxide elimination as well as in oxygenation.

dicated in unconscious and semicomatose patients. Prophylactic nasogastric suction may diminish this risk. The fit of the mask around the nasogastric tube can be improved with a commercially available adapter (Vital Signs, East Rutherford, New Jersey). We have applied 15 cm H_2O CPAP by mask without a gastric tube without complication. *Careful observation for gastric distention is advisable whether or not a gastric tube is in place. The first sign of a gas-filled stomach can be an unexpected eructation and emesis during a subsequent intubation attempt.* Light-weight equipment and a properly fitted mask are essential to the patient's acceptance.

> CASE 25–1.—A 37-year-old woman had a systolic arterial pressure of 80 torr after 6 hours of repeated syncope at home. An estimated 1,500 ml of blood was removed from the peritoneal cavity, and a cornual rupture from pregnancy was surgically repaired. Postoperatively the patient complained of shoulder pain with full inspiration, but her recovery seemed otherwise uncomplicated for 48 hours. She then noted the sudden onset (over 30 minutes) and rapid progression of respiratory distress. Pa_{O_2} was 40 torr on room air and increased only to 60 torr on FI_{O_2} of 1.0 with high flows of oxygen. A chest roentgenogram made within 1 hour of the onset of dyspnea showed bilateral diffuse infiltrates (Fig 25–1,A). Fluid overload was not thought to be present, and diuresis was not induced. The directed recruiting technique by mask was applied and Pa_{O_2} transiently increased to 200 torr with the same oxygen delivery. Pulmonary function continued to deteriorate and the lungs were more radiodense 12 hours later. Response to directed recruiting diminished until, 20 hours after the onset of respiratory distress, directed recruiting had no sustained effect. Respiratory rate was 40 to 60/min through most of this period. However, improvement in oxygenation and radiologic status could be maintained after recruitment if CPAP was applied by mask (Fig 25–1,B). Respirations remained about 20/min on CPAP. Pa_{O_2} then increased to 138 with FI_{O_2} of 0.5, and remained above 100 with FI_{O_2} of 0.3. Good pulmonary function continued to depend on maintenance of CPAP for the next 3 days, and deteriorated less with each trial removal of CPAP. When pulmonary function deteriorated it could always be restored to the previous level by CPAP and directed recruiting. The course of pulmonary function and response to recruiting and CPAP are summarized in Figure 25–2. The alterations in this patient's course are apparent in those data.

> *Comment.*—This patient developed a classic "shock lung" response, with pulmonary deterio-

ration becoming manifest 48 hours after the period of hypotension. Pulmonary function was severely compromised and less responsive to therapy until the lung was splinted open, after which gas exchange function improved and the deteriorating course was reversed.

INTUBATION CRITERIA AND PROBLEMS

The trachea may be intubated to protect the airway, to provide mechanical ventilation for carbon dioxide elimination, and for the application of positive pressure for oxygenation when positive pressure by mask is contraindicated and high FI_{O_2} is required.

The risks of intubation include hypoxia during the procedure; mucosal trauma; inhibition of mucociliary transport; colonization of tracheobronchial secretions and subsequent pulmonary infection; depression of the cough through discomfort, fear, or loss of laryngeal closure; increased resistance to air flow; a significant decrease in FRC;[3, 87] and the risk of pulmonary edema after intubation. The sudden onset of pulmonary edema is a challenging problem that seems related to loss of laryngeal approximation during exhalations (grunting), which may have been serving to splint the rather fragile pulmonary epithelium, or in some cases may have been augmenting ventricular systole by increasing pleural pressure (see chapter 21, "Hemodynamic Effects of Artificial Ventilation," and chapter 31, "Ventilatory Support of the Failing Circulation"). Several cases have been reasonably well documented.[55, 70, 111, 114] Technical problems following intubation may include right main-stem bronchus intubation if the tube is advanced too far and laryngeal damage.[65]

The physician must decide whether or not to intubate according to his or her understanding of the patient's probable clinical course. For example, patients with cardiogenic pulmonary edema or drug overdose may not need immediate intubation even when blood gas tensions are severely deranged if a rapid response to therapy seems likely, if adequate ventilation can be maintained by a bag-mask unit, and if the patient or personnel are able to protect against aspiration.

A commonly seen problem in the hour following intubation is *new hypotension*. The causes may include the vasodilating effect of sedatives,

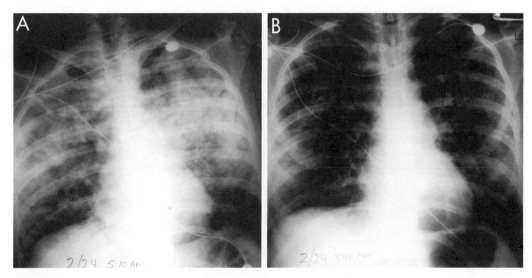

FIG 25–1.
Chest roentgenograms. **A,** diffuse infiltrates typical of ARDS. **B,** expanded lung shortly after directed re- cruiting and application of CPAP by mask. (From Scholten et al.[94] Reproduced by permission.)

which are often given at the time of intubation (morphine, diazepam), a decrease in plasma cate- cholamines as the work of breathing is dimin- ished and tissue oxygenation is improved, and an increase in pleural pressure impeding venous re- turn and thus reducing cardiac output.

APPLICATION OF PEEP

Most pulmonary insults, including intubation of the trachea,[25, 34, 87, 111] increase the tendency of otherwise healthy lungs to collapse, thereby in- creasing $\dot{Q}s/\dot{Q}t$. PEEP inhibits such changes. When PEEP is applied before lung collapse has occurred, it is appropriately called prophylactic. No study has documented that prophylactic PEEP affects outcome. Lungs that are unstable function better if splinted open. Although it is tempting to hypothesize that lung function might deteriorate less and heal more quickly when splinted open, this has not been proved. Accordingly, we prefer to base our therapy on more established princi- ples. Faced with choosing between treatment ap-

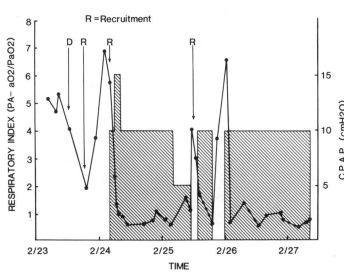

FIG 25–2.
Response of lung function to deep breaths and coughing *(D)*, recruiting *(R)*, and mask CPAP *(shaded areas)*. Respiratory index correlates roughly with severity of venous admixture; a value of 5 approximates a "shunt" of 25%. The initial good response to recruiting was not sustained unless CPAP was added.

proaches of apparently equal risk and gas exchange, we favor splinting the lung open. How does one accomplish this task? First, we categorize acute lung injury as homogeneous or nonhomogeneous disease. Homogeneous disease responds more predictably than nonhomogeneous disease to the application of PEEP. Unilateral lung disease is better treated with the good lung dependent. Since repeated lung collapse may be harmful, we are willing to use PEEP to splint regionally insulted lung in some cases with minimal gas exchange abnormalities as long as end-organ function (urine output, for example) remains adequate. However, there is no firm evidence to support using this aggressive approach. As in all clinical situations, many rational approaches may be attempted before the one best for a given patient is found.

Homogeneous Lung Disease

When no focal lesions are apparent radiologically, we often apply PEEP incrementally, without a recruiting maneuver. Thus, PEEP is routinely added in 3–5 cm H_2O increments, and organ perfusion, Pa_{O_2}, and $P\bar{v}_{O_2}$, when available, are evaluated between adjustments. When the insult appears homogeneous, PEEP is usually added until $\dot{Q}s/\dot{Q}t$ is less than 15%, or when systemic perfusion or organ function is compromised (indicated by reduced $P\bar{v}_{O_2}$ or decreased urine output, for example). At the same time we specifically attempt to keep peak AWP less than 40 cm H_2O by adjusting the gas flow and decreasing Vt when possible. Thus, in diffuse lung disease we use PEEP sufficient to keep the recruited lung open, though with concern regarding systemic perfusion and the level of peak pressure. Developments in the treatment of infant respiratory distress syndrome (IRDS) and in our technique of recruiting closed lung in adults have led us to modify our thinking somewhat. Therefore we diverge to summarize the IRDS experience.

On the basis of experiments by Kolton et al.[60] and Hamilton et al.,[46] it was suggested in 1982 that the new generation of high-frequency ventilators should be viewed as convenient tools with which to pursue an "open lung" approach.[36] High-frequency ventilators can sustain carbon dioxide elimination while applying much smaller pressure and volume swings to the lung

than a conventional ventilator (see chapter 23, "High-Frequency Ventilation"). Therefore, for any given mean AWP, the *minimum* AWP will be higher during high-frequency ventilation (HFV) than during conventional mechanical ventilation (CMV), and one has a better chance of keeping alveoli open once they are recruited. In a sense, HFV can be viewed as a way of giving PEEP with built-in carbon dioxide elimination.

However, with the small phasic pressure swings of HFV one loses the high peak pressures of CMV as well as the lower minimum pressures. Therefore, during HFV one must substitute some deliberate volume recruitment maneuver to open the atelectatic alveoli.[14, 19, 60] Once they are open, HFV at appropriate settings may hold them open for prolonged periods of time. Kolton et al. also demonstrated that the operating mean AWP must be selected carefully.[60] If the operating mean AWP was too low (presumably less than the closing pressure of many airways and alveoli) volume recruitment maneuvers became totally ineffectual. As discussed in chapter 23, "High-Frequency Ventilation," AWP within the trachea must be measured when HFV is used.

How should we assess whether or not we have reached our goal of the "open lung"? In diffuse lung disease the most logical end point appears to be calculated $\dot{Q}s/\dot{Q}t$, or venous admixture ($\dot{Q}va/\dot{Q}t$) if not at an Fi_{O_2} of 1.0. In the experience of Hamilton et al.,[45] successful volume recruitment was reflected immediately in oxygenation. In recent experience treating infants with IRDS using high-frequency oscillatory (HFO) ventilation, the clearest indication of the appropriateness of ventilator settings was a decrease in Fi_{O_2} requirement, followed, after a time, by increased aeration as assessed on chest x-ray film.

Using HFO Ventilation to Support Alveolar Patency

Recently, we have approached IRDS using HFO to pursue a structured protocol of early lung volume recruitment (in essence, an "open lung" approach) applied *as early as possible* in the course of ventilator treatment for the disease. Using a high-frequency oscillator (a form of HFV providing an active expiratory phase, called HFO-A), the operating frequency is fixed at 15 Hz and the stroke volume adjusted to achieve appropriate arterial P_{CO_2} levels.

The initial mean AWP is set a few cm H_2O higher than the value used on CMV prior to initiation of HFO-A. If oxygenation improves, $F_{I_{O_2}}$ is lowered appropriately. If there is only a modest improvement or no improvement in oxygenation, a sustained inflation (SI) is then applied by raising the mean AWP 5–10 cm higher than the operating mean AWP for 20 seconds, and then returning it to the previous level. On-line transcutaneous oxygen monitoring is used to assess the response to this volume recruitment maneuver. If the response is good but the improvement is not sustained [i.e., initial improvement is not sustained in transcutaneous oxygen (TC_{O_2})], then the mean AWP is raised stepwise in 2 cm H_2O increments. At each step, SI is applied again and the response assessed. The mean AWP is not considered to be appropriate until such time as the TC_{O_2} improvement gained by an SI (i.e., opening up new gas-exchanging units) is also *maintained* indefinitely (units are kept open). At this point, $F_{I_{O_2}}$ can be progressively reduced while the lung is held at an effective level of distending pressure. Volume recruitment maneuvers (SI) are repeated whenever there is reason to expect a drop in TC_{O_2} as the result of loss of operating lung volume (e.g., endotracheal tube disconnecting for any reason; suctioning; straining). Generally SI maneuvers are not required frequently unless the infant is being handled a lot. If SI is needed too frequently (every 5 or 10 minutes), we deduce that the operating mean AWP is inadequate and try a small increase in mean AWP instead.

It must be recognized that two goals are opposed in the open lung approach. On the one hand, we know that excessively high AWPs are dangerous, although we don't know precisely what level is too high. On the other hand, we cannot open up closed lung without using high AWPs. Our compromise is to expose the lung to the peak recruiting pressures as seldom as possible, but nonetheless to do so, but judiciously, and only if it proves effective. We view *some* exposure to pressure as a tolerable risk if it enables one to open up collapsed lung and achieve oxygenation at lower $F_{I_{O_2}}$ values.

Using this approach in a series of infants with IRDS we were able to reduce $F_{I_{O_2}}$ from a mean of 0.90 ± 0.14 to less than 0.40 in 18.9 ± 25 hours. In infants treated conventionally it took 64 ± 14 hours to lower the $F_{I_{O_2}}$ requirement from 0.66 ± 0.13 to less than 0.40. There was no evidence of an increase in incidence of either acute or chronic barotrauma despite the systematic use of volume recruitment maneuvers

in the HFO-A–treated infants, but the group was too small to yield conclusions about the incidence of long-term complications.[37]

Similar systematic approaches might also prove useful in acute diffuse lung injury in adults, utilizing CMV with low Vt (or perhaps HFV when appropriate guidelines for use are available), although these studies have not been performed. The critical level of PEEP at which most of the lung is splinted open without significant depression of cardiac output could be approximated by observing changes in arterial or transcutaneous P_{O_2}, and periodic $P\bar{v}_{O_2}$ (or continuous $S\bar{v}_{O_2}$) when adequacy of oxygen transport is in question. The efficacy of $S\bar{v}_{O_2}$ as a monitor of the effect of rapid PEEP titration on oxygen transport is shown in Figure 13–7 of chapter 13, "Assessment of Systemic Oxygen Transport." The need for recruiting maneuvers should be apparent from changes in arterial or skin P_{O_2} or oxygen saturation, and a need for frequent recruiting maneuvers may indicate the need for a change in level of PEEP. Changes in other factors may also be useful in diffuse lung disease. Suter showed that deadspace was lowest when oxygen transport was highest. Frequent or continuous monitoring of Vd/Vt or related indices can be performed easily and might be useful not only for estimating the "best PEEP" of Suter and associates, but also for evaluating the effect of all changes in ventilation pattern on the efficiency of ventilation. As a side benefit, we would be alerted more readily to spontaneous increases in Vd/Vt, as caused by progressive hypovolemia or pulmonary embolism. Continuous monitoring of Vd/Vt can be carried out simply by measuring P_{CO_2} in mixed exhaled gases and Pa_{CO_2} by intravascular or transcutaneous sensor, as described in chapter 22, "Technical and Semantic Aspects of Ventilator Support." The titration of PEEP according to observed changes in the arterial to end-tidal carbon dioxide gradient is based on similar logic and has been used experimentally in acute diffuse lung injury.[73] Because multiple factors in addition to the Vd/Vt alter the arterial to end-tidal carbon dioxide gradient or ratio in critically ill patients,[99] we would predict that monitoring Vd/Vt would prove of greater value.

Table 25–3 summarizes our current view of the relative indications for and contraindications to the use of PEEP. Some of these vary signifi-

TABLE 25–3.

Relative Indications for and Contraindications to Use of PEEP*

RELATIVE INDICATIONS	RELATIVE CONTRAINDICATIONS
Tracheal intubation	Right ventricular failure[†]
Paralysis or anesthesia	High peak airway pressure[†]
Local or diffuse loss of lung volume	Systemic hypoperfusion not due to myocardial failure
Settings in which ARDS is likely	Obstructive airways disease (if gas trapping decreases)[†]
Left ventricular failure	Increased intracranial pressure
	Intracardiac right-to-left shunt

*From Snyder JV, et al.[101] Reproduced by permission.
†Mechanical ventilation may be more strongly contraindicated than CPAP or PEEP.

cantly from the earlier opinions of Ashbaugh and Petty.[5]

Nonhomogeneous Acute Lung Injury

When the initial lung injury is disparate, as it is in most cases of adult respiratory distress syndrome (ARDS), increases in AWP may, by hyperexpanding the normal compliant lung, divert blood flow from open to still closed lung, increasing calculated $\dot{Q}va/\dot{Q}$. Although more lung tissue is open, gas exchange may deteriorate. This circumstance seems more likely to occur when PEEP is slowly increased sequentially, and less likely when closed areas are more aggressively recruited and then adequately splinted with PEEP. Even normal lungs inflate very unevenly from a completely collapsed state.[4] Therefore, when local collapse is known or suspected it is our practice to use directed recruiting efforts followed by only as much PEEP as is needed to keep the lung open, rather than using incremental increases in PEEP as the sole means of therapy.[58]

In nonhomogeneous lung disease we still beg the question, how much PEEP is enough? The therapeutic course is best selected by the characteristics of the individual case. For example, if an increase in PEEP resulted in unchanged or worse $\dot{Q}va/\dot{Q}t$ and the chest x-ray findings were compatible with bibasilar loss of volume (usually at least some atelectasis cannot be excluded), then recruiting maneuvers directed to both bases,

perhaps accompanied by an increase in PEEP, would be an appropriate trial. Obviously a decrease in $\dot{Q}va/\dot{Q}t$ would indicate that atelectasis within the diffuse opacity had been contributing to the dysfunction but could be reversed by a transient, directed increase in TPP, coupled with a minimal increase in PEEP. We perceive this approach as better than either leaving the lung closed or subjecting the lung already open to sustained higher increases in peak AWP and PEEP. On the other hand, what if our effort might have resulted in radiologic clearing with no change in $\dot{Q}va/\dot{Q}t$? According to the "respirator" lung hypothesis, in the preceding example we should still try to keep the newly reexpanded lung tissue splinted open with adequate PEEP, if no ill effect from the higher pressure is apparent, even though there is no improvement in $\dot{Q}va/\dot{Q}t$. We are more inclined to adopt this approach if peak AWP can be kept to less than 40 cm H_2O. We see then that, depending on acceptance of the unproved respirator lung concepts, the open lung approach can be extended to include the use of PEEP in some cases where other approaches would not. Finally, it is not uncommon to have to deal with a more subtle question. When we add PEEP, with or without prior recruiting, and do not see a change on chest x-ray film or in $\dot{Q}va/\dot{Q}t$, it is still possible that some additional lung units were opened. Should the increase in PEEP be maintained even without radiologic or blood gas evidence of improvement? In such cases we have no guidelines to offer.

LIMITATIONS OF THE OPEN LUNG APPROACH AS A TREATMENT FOR RESPIRATOR LUNG

There are several worrisome factors that might limit the value of an open lung strategy if the respirator lung concept is valid. Nonhomogeneity of the underlying disease process will work most directly to undermine the open lung approach, if it proves impossible to achieve single values for recruiting pressure and maintenance AWP that will succeed in keeping enough of the lung open to significantly ameliorate the pathophysiologic processes hypothesized.

Also, only a very short time (5 hours) may be needed for atelectasis to induce structural damage.[45] In Hamilton's study, late application (after >4 hours) of the open lung approach with HFO resulted in a much poorer response.[46] The increase in microvascular permeability from peak AWP of more than 40 cm H_2O observed by Parker and colleagues occurred within 20 minutes at rates of only 6/min.[81] We expect the emphasis on techniques to minimize peak AWP to preclude any increase in barotrauma from this approach. Only experience will prove whether systematic pursuit of an open lung rationale for ventilatory support can more successfully support gas exchange with less pulmonary damage in patients with respiratory failure.

INSPIRED OXYGEN CONCENTRATION

In the context of acute lung injury and repair and chronic ventilatory support we may need to reassess our target F_{IO_2}. In the 1970s the call went out to keep F_{IO_2} below 0.7 (or even below 0.5) to decrease the risk of oxygen toxicity. More recently some centers have advocated even lower F_{IO_2}.[89]

We prefer to decrease F_{IO_2} as rapidly as is tolerated, to 0.5–0.3 if possible, using recruiting maneuvers to open the lung and PEEP as needed to splint the lung open. Pa_{O_2} is usually kept at 60–100 torr. Although a Pa_{O_2} of 60–70 torr is adequate in most patients, allowing the F_{IO_2} to be kept lower by accepting that level, in patients who are likely to have tissue hypoxia we prefer to keep P_{O_2} close to 100 torr. This is both to increase oxygen content (by about 10%) and to provide a margin of safety, so that even if the venous admixture were to increase abruptly (from bronchial occlusion with mucus, for example) arterial oxygen saturation might still be adequate. A higher Pa_{O_2} is indicated when tissue hypoxia is due to severe anemia or abnormal hemoglobin (see chapter 1, "Oxygen Transport: The Model and Reality").

SPONTANEOUS VERSUS MECHANICAL VENTILATION

We prefer that the patient contribute to ventilation as much as is possible, because contraction of the diaphragm seems to minimize not only V/Q abnormalities, but the impedance of venous return and risk of barotrauma from high inflation pressures as well. Respiratory muscle power may also be better sustained. Our course is determined by balancing the factors discussed in the section on the spectrum of controlled to spontaneous ventilation in chapter 22, "Technical and Semantic Aspects of Ventilatory Support." Spontaneous ventilation, when allowed, is usually directed through a continuous flow intermittent mandatory ventilation (IMV) circuit. We provide enough mechanical breaths to prevent respiratory distress and maintain an arterial pH usually greater than 7.34. We increase mechanical support if oxygen transport is compromised and respiratory muscles might be "stealing" limited blood flow, or if fatigue is manifest in a respiratory rate over 30/min or there is palpable contraction of the scalene muscles on inspiration.[43, 50]

When controlled ventilation is indicated (by increased intracranial pressure or patient exhaustion, for example), the mechanical rate should be set high enough to satisfy the patient's respiratory drive. We recommend that the ventilator be left in the assist or the IMV mode so that the patient can increase minute ventilation should his or her requirements change. With the ventilator in the control mode, the patient has no access to gas for spontaneous breaths.

Muscle relaxants are rarely indicated. Paralysis decreases FRC[98] (which can be reversed with PEEP) and abates the selective ventilation of the dependent lung that occurs with diaphragmatic breathing.[35, 98] The paralyzed patient cannot cough, turn, or breathe deeply, so he or she is dependent on the ICU staff for pulmonary toilet. When the patient "fights the ventilator," we prefer to discover and alleviate the cause of discomfort. Sensitive manipulation of the ventilator can usually achieve comfortable support for the patient without risking death from inadvertent disconnection of a paralyzed patient from the ventilator. Patients who are given muscle relaxants should also be sedated.

WEANING

In general, patients are weaned from high $F_{I_{O_2}}$ first, from mechanical ventilation next, and from PEEP last. Recruiting maneuvers and PEEP can be used to maintain Pa_{O_2} while reducing $F_{I_{O_2}}$. As initially described by Kirby et al.,[58] patients are weaned from mechanical ventilation by decreasing IMV breaths as rapidly as the patient can tolerate. Alternatively, CPAP or T tube support with assisted ventilation can be used (see chapter 22, "Technical and Semantic Aspects of Ventilator Support").

When a high level of PEEP is necessary, it is important to recalculate $\dot{Q}va/\dot{Q}t$ (or simply to monitor paired arterial and venous blood gas tensions) as PEEP is withdrawn. A common error is to assume that a stable level of Pa_{O_2} after PEEP is reduced indicates that $\dot{Q}va/\dot{Q}t$ has not changed. The $\dot{Q}va/\dot{Q}t$ may have increased significantly but not be shown by the Pa_{O_2} level, because a higher cardiac output has increased $P\bar{v}_{O_2}$. A significant increase in venous admixture may warrant raising PEEP to its preweaning level even if the Pa_{O_2} has not changed. If restoration of PEEP does not reduce venous admixture to its preweaning level,[49, 66] recruiting maneuvers may recapture the lung expansion that has been lost by prematurely removing PEEP. Therefore, when the venous admixture increases on reduction of PEEP, a recruiting maneuver is often undertaken simultaneously when PEEP is restored. If the $\dot{Q}va/\dot{Q}t$ is satisfactorily reduced at the higher AWP, that pressure is maintained to allow time for further resolution of the underlying pathophysiology.

IMV Versus Assisted Ventilation/T Tube Program for Weaning

Once the patient's underlying disorder has improved, it is important to consider weaning the patient from ventilatory support. The more rap-idly support is withdrawn and the more unstable the patient's condition, the more closely the patient must be observed. Most patients can be weaned using either IMV or alternating assisted ventilation with periods of spontaneous breathing through a T tube or with CPAP. If IMV was used as the ventilatory mode from the time of intubation, which is more often the case when higher AWP is required, then IMV is used for weaning. When IMV is used to wean patients with minimal reserve, the work of breathing inherent in overcoming the resistance of the artificial ventilatory system is important. Because IMV allows weaning to be done in minute steps, less frequent observations may suffice for most of a prolonged weaning phase. Likewise, assisted ventilation permits less frequent observation than does low IMV ventilation. *Occasionally, weaning (either IMV or T tube) proceeds more slowly than necessary when it is done according to formula or habit rather than according to the patient's capacity and needs.* The patient should usually be allowed to resume spontaneous ventilation as soon as he or she can, without delay of extubation. The values identified by Pardee and associates to indicate continued need for mechanical ventilation are helpful in the weaning process.[80] These are: "pulse over 120 or under 70 beats per minute, respiratory rate of over 30, palpable scalene muscle recruitment in inspiration, palpable abdominal tensing in expiration, presence of irregular irregularity of respiratory rhythm with apneic pauses of varying duration, and coma or any condition preventing a patient from responding appropriately to commands aimed at producing ventilatory movements like those needed for vital capacity testing."[80]

Patients may be taken abruptly from assisted ventilation to a T tube, but they must be closely observed during the transition, especially if PEEP is removed simultaneously. Maintenance of CPAP diminishes the threat of lung closure and excessive increase in venous return. Patients are routinely extubated from 5 cm H_2O CPAP.[3, 34, 87, 113]

Newly extubated patients are at risk of aspiration for hours or days because of persistent laryngeal anesthesia and motor dysfunction.[21]

SPECIAL CASES

Fulminant Pulmonary Edema

Fulminant pulmonary edema is diagnosed when light yellow to quite red foam pours from the endotracheal tube. Foam may be so profuse that tracheal suctioning is of little value. Hypoxic arrest may be imminent. Foaming can almost invariably be controlled within a few breaths by manual ventilation with low Vt and PEEP, but up to 60 cm H_2O PEEP may be needed. Usually, sustained high AWP rapidly improves arterial oxygenation. Low Vt minimizes peak pressure and the risk of barotrauma.

As the lung opens and compliance is improved, AWP is increasingly transmitted to the pleural space, impeding venous return.[22] If the patient is hypovolemic, hypotension may occur at AWPs that were well tolerated by the patient only minutes before. Reduction of PEEP at that time may restore arterial pressure while maintaining oxygenation.

In some patients, no level of PEEP can be found at which both venous return is adequate and venous admixture is kept low, without intravenous volume loading being undertaken. In our experience, rapid administration of 200–800 ml of crystalloid solution, in all but one case, has permitted administration of high PEEP and low Vt without serious hypotension. The exception was a patient with a pulmonary interstitial hemorrhage.

We continually reassess the patient and change the ventilatory and intravenous support as needed to optimize oxygenation and cardiac output. This titration is based primarily on assessment of foam in the airway, arterial pressure waveform, and frequent arterial and mixed venous blood gas analyses. Measuring of cardiac output and $\dot{Q}va/\dot{Q}t$ is time-consuming and impractical during such rapid physiologic changes. Continuous recording of mixed venous oxygen saturation (Oximetrix, Mountainview, Calif.) can be exceptionally helpful in such rapidly changing cases.

Obstructive Pulmonary Disease

In obstructive lung disease, intubation by removing the glottic closure mechanism can increase compression of the airways on exhalation, resulting in gas trapping. Mechanical ventilation can then result in both an increase in intrathoracic expiratory pressure ("occult PEEP")[83] and a decrease in ventricular filling pressure. In this setting, bullous lung can progressively overdistend and eventually rupture. Cardiac output and arterial pressure may be low due to less venous return and compression of the heart by the inflated lung. Because of this, sufficient expiratory time is an important concern in mechanical ventilation of such patients. When gas trapping is suspected as a cause of hypotension the ventilator should be disconnected. A fall in wedge pressure accompanied by a rising arterial pressure confirms the diagnosis.

Traditional teaching of mechanical ventilation in patients with obstructive pulmonary disease includes the caveat that PEEP is contraindicated in patients with emphysema or asthma. The argument has been that such patients already have increased FRC, have little to gain from increasing it further with PEEP, and are at increased risk of barotrauma from overdistention.[5, 18] However, the addition of PEEP to ventilatory support can have more subtle effects than simply increasing FRC, and it is becoming apparent that PEEP and CPAP may be useful in managing the care of these patients, both when the acute disease process impairs oxygenation and when chronically unstable airways need support. It has been observed that PEEP can move the critical closing point proximally in the airway toward the trachea, relieving gas trapping and allowing FRC to decrease, minimizing the probability of barotrauma. Indeed, a case can be made for using PEEP to open small airways, to improve the distribution of ventilation, and to decrease pulmonary edema, as suggested by Barach et al. in 1938.[11] FRC might even become lower on PEEP in this special case. As with an expiratory retard, the increased AWP may compensate for the changes in tissue elastic recoil that allow airways to collapse in emphysematous or bronchospastic lungs, such that a larger FRC is required to increase the forces of interdependence[69] and keep airways open. Although lung regions with previously open airways will be larger at end-exhalation when PEEP is added, regions with PEEP-splinted airways may actually reach a lower FRC. These regions are likely to be lower in the lung, and contain a higher Pco_2. Splinting them open may therefore decrease Vd/Vt. Several observations support this approach. Pursed-lip breathing seems helpful to emphysematous patients. Motoyama et al. have shown reducton in the trapped gas volume in patients with cystic fibrosis given 2.5 cm H_2O PEEP.[72] Similarly, Barach et al. found that chronic OPD patients obtained relief from exertional dyspnea and improved efficiency of ventilation with CPAP.[12] Our study of PEEP in a single patient with large bullae, using nonradioactive xenon-enhanced CT scanning, showed no change in size or ventilation of bullae.[100] The effect of CPAP to improve efficiency of ventilation and lower the pressure-time product of inspiratory muscles in asthma (see below) may also occur in COPD.

Indirectly, PEEP may contribute to barotrauma if the bursting strength of the weakest part of the lung is not exceeded by the peak pressure before the use of PEEP but is exceeded by the higher peak after PEEP is added. The same is true of lung necrotic from ischemia or infection. Therefore, it might be desirable to reduce Vt in order to keep the peak pressure constant when PEEP is added.

Air trapping may increase in some patients with obstructive pulmonary disease when PEEP is added or expiratory time is decreased, resulting in increased pleural pressure, decreased cardiac output, and risk of barotrauma. *Manifestations of air trapping during mechanical ventilation include a progressive increase in peak AWP, CVP, and wedge pressure and a decrease in arterial pressure.*[83] Nevertheless, as reviewed here, positive pressure during exhalation can distinctly improve exhalation when gas trapping occurs.

The cardiovascular benefits of mechanical ventilation in chronic respiratory insufficiency have been well reviewed;[92] some of these apply to PEEP.

Additional considerations in the management of the patient with COPD have recently been presented by Hudson.[50] Among these, inhaled atropine (.02 mg/kg) has been rediscovered as an effective bronchodilator with tolerable side effects in patients unresponsive to conventional therapy,[50] and glycopyrrolate (1.3 mg) was shown to have a comparable effect on airway conductance, with fewer side effects.[56] Aminophylline improves the contractility of the diaphragm in patients with COPD as well as in normal individuals, and the effect is long-lasting.[8] Discussions of the work of breathing and exercise of respiratory muscles in chapter 20, "Pulmonary Physiology," and chapter 22, "Technical and Semantic Aspects of Ventilatory Support," also relate to the patient with obstructive pulmonary disease.

In the treatment of asthma, the primary goal is relieving bronchospasm. Yet it now seems clear that the work of breathing in asthma is largely inspiratory work,[105] and that ventilation is inefficient because of impaired perfusion of overdistended alveoli.[38] Therefore we should consider how CPAP might influence the distribution of ventilation and the work of inspiration. Airways that intermittently close with ventilation do not reopen until a certain lung volume and TPP (critical opening pressure) are reached.[84] Maintaining FRC closer to the lung volume at which dependent airways open may thus decrease the work of breathing in several ways: (1) by decreasing the inspiratory volume required to open closed airways; (2) by changing the distribution of the inspired volume to more efficient (dependent) lung areas, thereby decreasing required minute ventilation; (3) by relieving wasteful persistence of inspiratory tone throughout exhalation; and (4) by inducing decreased airway resistance,[68] perhaps by means of bronchodilation from prostaglandin release.[16] If inspiratory muscle tone is relieved and pleural pressure increases, CPAP should also increase interstitial pressure, and fluid transudation (edema) might diminish.[53, 105] These potential benefits of CPAP in asthma would have to overcome several mechanical disadvantages of higher FRC, as Roussos and Macklem have recently elaborated;[93] several observations suggest that the net effect of CPAP in asthma can indeed be beneficial.

High levels of PEEP have been reported to reverse the course of two patients moribund with severe asthma.[88] An average CPAP of 12 cm H_2O in eight patients with induced asthma raised FRC by only 0.27 L while improving the efficiency of ventilation and lowering the pressure-time product of the inspiratory muscles.[68] In another preliminary report of 20 asthmatics, CPAP was associated with reduced inspiratory work of breathing and increased expiratory flow at low lung volumes.[96] Two patients with severe asthma who were hypercarbic and could not be weaned from mechanical ventilation were able to lower their own $Paco_2$ by 12 torr to 44 and 46 torr after 20 minutes on CPAP; hypercarbia recurred when mechanical ventilation was restored.[109] There appear to be a sufficient rationale and experimental support for the cautious application of PEEP or CPAP in patients with chronic or acute obstructive pulmonary disease when due attention is paid to reduction of peak AWP and to the resultant effects on work of breathing and efficiency of carbon dioxide elimination.

Flail Chest

The major components of flail chest injury are mechanical instability, parenchymal injury, excessive respiratory drive, and pain.[90, 95, 110] Stabilization of the chest wall is not necessary in most cases. Flailing results not only from multiple fractures, but also from increased inspiratory effort and lower lung compliance. Thus the condition of a patient breathing quietly with minimal flail may deteriorate to gross and painful flailing as pulmonary congestion develops or secretions accumulate. The increase in flailing represents greater than normal change in pleural pressure, owing not only to decreased static pulmonary compliance, but also to increased respiratory drive from any cause. Thus, keeping the airways open and lungs expanded and free of secretions is important. Also, ventilatory support systems that allow unrestricted spontaneous ventilation will require less effort by the patient and cause less flailing. Active contributions from the patient (coughing and changing posture, for example) are facilitated when the patient has minimal pain. This can be achieved with firm supportive coaching and the use of epidural and intercostal analgesia. Intubation and mechanical ventilation are indicated by the same criteria as in other pulmonary insults.

REFERENCES

1. Ali J, Serrette C, Wood LDH, et al: Effect of postoperative intermittent positive pressure breathing on lung function. *Chest* 1984; 85:192.
2. Anderson JB, Zvist J, Kann T: Recruiting collapsed lung through collateral channels with positive end-expiratory pressure. *Scand J Respir Dis* 1979; 60:260.
3. Annest SJ, Gottlieb M, Paloski WH, et al: Detrimental effects of removing end-expiratory pressure prior to endotracheal extubation. *Ann Surg* 1980; 191:539.
4. Anthonisen NR: Effect of volume and volume history of the lungs on pulmonary shunt flow. *Am J Physiol* 1964; 207:235.
5. Ashbaugh DG, Petty TL: Positive end-expiratory pressure: Physiology, indications, and contraindications. *J Thorac Cardiovasc Surg* 1973; 65:165.
6. Askanazi J, Weissman C, Rosenbaum SH, et al: Nutrition and the respiratory system. *Crit Care Med* 1982; 10:163.
7. Aubier M, Trippenbach T, Roussos C: Respiratory muscle fatigue during cardiogenic shock. *J Appl Physiol* 1981; 51:499.
8. Aubier M, Murciano D, Lecocguic Y, et al: Effects of aminophylline on diaphragmatic strength and fatigue in patients with chronic obstructive pulmonary disease. *Chest* 1984; 85:59S.
9. Aubier M, Vires N, Syllie G, et al: Respiratory muscle contribution to lactic acidosis in low cardiac output. *Am Rev Respir Dis* 1982; 126:648.
10. Baehrendtz S, Santesson J, Bindslev L, et al: Differential ventilation in acute bilateral lung disease: Influence on gas exchange and central hemodynamics. *Acta Anaesthesiol Scand* 1983; 27:270.
11. Barach AL, Martin J, Eckman M: Positive pressure respiration and its application of the treatment of acute pulmonary edema. *Ann Intern Med* 1938; 12:754.
12. Barach AL, Bickerman HA, Rodgers J: Continuous positive pressure breathing in chronic obstructive lung disease: Effect on minute ventilation and blood gases. *Ann Allergy* 1973; 31:72.
13. Bartolome R, Rodriquez K, Snider G: A controlled trial of IPPB, incentive spirometry, and deep breathing exercises in preventing pulmonary complications after abdominal surgery. *Am Rev Respir Dis* 1984; 130:12–15.
14. Bell RE, Kuehl TJ, Coalson JJ, et al: High-frequency ventilation compared to conventional positive pressure ventilation in the treatment of hyaline membrane disease in primates. *Crit Care Med* 1984; 12:764–768.
15. Bendixen HH, Hedley-Whyte J, Chir B, et al: Impaired oxygenation in surgical patients during general anesthesia with controlled ventilation. *N Engl J Med* 1963; 269:991.
16. Berend N, Christopher KL, Voekel NF: The effect of PEEP on functional residual capacity of prostaglandin production. *Am Rev Respir Dis* 1982; 126:646.
17. Bindslev L, Hedenstierna G, Santesson J, et al: Airway closure during anaesthesia, and its prevention by positive and expiratory pressure. *Acta Anaesthesiol Scand* 1980; 24:199.
18. Bone RC: Treatment of severe hypoxemia due to the adult respiratory distress syndrome. *Arch Intern Med* 1980; 140:85.

19. Boynton BR, Mannino F, Davis RF, et al: Combined high-frequency oscillatory ventilation and intermittent mandatory ventilation in critically ill neonates. *J Pediatr* 1984; 105:297–302.

20. Brown SE, Stansburg DW, Merrill E, et al: Prevention of suctioning-related arterial oxygen desaturation. *Chest* 1983; 83:621–627.

21. Burgess GE, Cooper JR, Marino RJ: Laryngeal competence after tracheal extubation. *Anesthesiology* 1979; 51:73.

22. Chapin JC, Downs JB, Douglas ME, et al: Lung expansion, airway pressure transmission, and positive end-expiratory pressure. *Arch Surg* 1979; 114:1193.

23. Catley DM, Thornton C, Jordan C, et al: Pronounced, episodic oxygen desaturation in the postoperative period: Its association with ventilatory pattern and analgesic regimen. *Anesthesiology* 1985; 63:20.

24. Celli BR, Rodriquez KS, Snider GL: A controlled trial of intermittent positive pressure breathing, incentive spirometry, and deep breathing exercises in preventing pulmonary complications after abdominal surgery. *Am Rev Respir Dis* 1984; 130:12–15.

25. Dammann JF, McAslan TC: PEEP: Its use in patients with apparently normal lungs. *Crit Care Med* 1979; 7:14.

26. Dantzker DR, Brook CJ, Dehart P, et al: Ventilation-perfusion distributions in the adult respiratory distress syndrome. *Am Rev Respir Dis* 1979; 120:1039.

27. Deboeck C: Cough versus chest physiotherapy. *Am Rev Respir Dis* 1984; 129:182.

28. Downs JB, Klein EF, Desautels D, et al: Intermittent mandatory ventilation: A new approach to weaning patients from mechanical ventilators. *Chest* 1973; 64:331.

29. Downs JB, Klein EF, Modell JH: The effect of incremental PEEP on Pao_2 in patients with respiratory failure. *Anesth Analg* 1973; 52:210.

30. Driver AG, McAlevy MT, Smith JL: Nutritional assessment of patients with chronic obstructive pulmonary disease and acute respiratory failure. *Chest* 1982; 5:569.

31. Egbert LD, Laver MB, Benedixen HH: Intermittent deep breaths and compliance during anesthesia in man. *Anesthesiology* 1963; 24:57.

32. Enhorning G, Robertson B: Lung expansion in the premature rabbit fetus after tracheal

33. Freedman AP, Goodman L: Suctioning the left bronchial tree in the intubated adult. *Crit Care Med* 1982; 10:43–45.

34. Feeley TW, Klick JM, Saumarez R, et al: Positive end-expiratory pressure in weaning patients from controlled ventilation: A prospective randomised trial. *Lancet* 1975; 2:725.

35. Froese AB, Bryan AC: Effects of anesthesia and paralysis on diaphragmatic mechanics in man. *Anesthesiology* 1974; 41:243.

36. Froese AB: High frequency ventilation: An update, in *33rd Annual Refresher Course Lectures*. Las Vegas, CA, American Society of Anesthesiologists, Inc, 1982, vol 216, p 1.

37. Froese AB: Unpublished data.

38. Freyschuss U, Hedlin G, Hedenstierna G: Ventilation-perfusion relationships during exercise-induced asthma in children. *Am Rev Respir Dis* 1984; 130:888.

39. Gallagher TJ, Civetta JM: Goal-directed therapy of acute respiratory failure. *Anesth Analg* 1980; 59:831–834.

40. Gallagher T, Civetti J: Normal pulmonary vascular resistance during acute respiratory insufficiency. *Crit Care Med* 1981; 9:647.

41. Grace MP, Greenbaum DM: Cardiac performance in response to PEEP in patients with cardiac dysfunction. *Crit Care Med* 1982; 10:358.

42. Graham WGB, Bradley DA: Efficacy of chest physiotherapy and intermittent positive pressure breathing in the resolution of pneumonia. *N Engl J Med* 1978; 299:624–627.

43. Grassino A, Bellemare F, Laporta D: Diaphragm fatigue and the strategy of breathing in COPD. *Chest* 1984; 85(6):51S.

44. Guntapalli K, Sladen A, Klain M: High frequency jet ventilation and tracheobronchial suctioning. *Crit Care Med* 1984; 12:791.

45. Hamilton PP, Onayemi A, Smyth JA, et al: Comparison of conventional and high-frequency ventilation: Oxygenation and lung pathology. *J Appl Physiol* 1983; 55:131–138.

46. Hamilton PP: Unpublished data.

47. Hedley-Whyte J, Burgess GE, Feeley TW, et al (eds): *Applied Physiology of Respiratory Care*, ed 1. Boston, Little, Brown & Co, 1976.

48. Holody B, Goldberg HS: The effect of mechanical vibration physiotherapy on arterial

oxygenation in acutely ill patients with atelectasis or pneumonia. *Am Rev Respir Dis* 1981; 124:372–375.

49. Hudson LD: Ventilatory management of patients with adult respiratory distress syndrome. *Semin Respir Med* 1981; 2:128.

50. Hudson LD: Management of COPD: State of the art. *Chest* 1984; 85:76S.

51. Hunker FD, Bruton CW, Hunker EM, et al: Metabolic and nutritional evaluation of patients supported with mechanical ventilation. *Crit Care Med* 1980; 8:628.

52. Hussain SNA, Simkus G, Roussos C: Respiratory muscle fatigue: A course of ventilatory failure in septic shock. *J Appl Physiol* 1985; 58:2033.

53. Inoue H, Inque C, Hilderbrandt J: Vascular and airway pressures, and interstitial edema, affect peribronchial fluid pressure. *J Appl Physiol* 1980; 48:177.

54. IPPB Trial Group: Intermittent positive pressure breathing therapy of chronic obstructive pulmonary disease. *Ann Intern Med* 1983; 99:612.

55. Jenkins JG: Pulmonary edema following laryngospasm (letter). *Anesthesiology* 1984; 60:611.

56. Johnson BE, Suratt PM, Gal TJ, et al: Effect of inhaled glycopyrrolate and atropine in asthma precipitated by exercise and cold air inhalation. *Chest* 1984; 85:325.

57. Katz JA, Ozanne GM, Zinn SE, et al: Time course and mechanisms of lung volume increase with PEEP in acute pulmonary failure. *Anesthesiology* 1981; 54:9.

58. Kirby RR, Downs JB, Civetta JM, et al: High level positive end expiratory pressure (PEEP) in acute respiratory insufficiency. *Chest* 1975; 67:156.

59. Kolton M, Perry J, Calderwood H, et al: Cardiorespiratory effects of high positive end-expiratory pressures. *Anesthesiology* 1975; 43:533.

60. Kolton M, Cattran CB, Kent G, et al: Oxygenation during high-frequency ventilation compared with conventional mechanical ventilation in two models of lung injury. *Anesth Analg* 1982; 61:323–332.

61. Larca L, Greenbaum DM: Effectiveness of intensive nutritional regimes in patients who fail to wean from mechanical ventilation. *Crit Care Med* 1982; 10:297.

62. Lefrock JC, Klainer AS, Wuy W, et al:

Transient bacteremia associated with nasotracheal suctioning. *JAMA* 1976; 236:1610–1611.

63. Lindholm CE, Grenvik A: Tracheal tube and cuff problems. *Int Anesthesiol Clin* 1982; 20:3.

64. Lindholm CE, Ollman B, Snyder JV, et al: Cardiorespiratory effects of flexible fiberoptic bronchoscopy in critically ill patients. *Chest* 1978; 74:362.

65. Lindholm CE, Grenvik A: Intubation and tracheostomy, in Sprung C, Grenvik A (eds): *Invasive Procedures in Critical Care*. New York, Churchill Livingstone (in press).

66. Luterman A, Horovitz JH, Carrico CJ, et al: Withdrawal from positive end-expiratory pressure. *Surgery* 1978; 83:328.

67. Marini JJ, Pierson DJ, Hudson LD: Acute lobar atelectasis: A prospective comparison of fiberoptic bronchoscopy and respiratory therapy. *Am Rev Respir Dis* 1979; 119:971.

68. Martin JG, Shore S, Engel LA: Effect of continuous positive airway pressure on respiratory mechanics and pattern of breathing in induced asthma. *Am Rev Respir Dis* 1982; 126:812.

69. Mead J, Takishima T, Leith D: Stress distribution in lungs: A model of pulmonary elasticity. *J Appl Physiol* 1970; 28:596.

70. Melnick BM: Postlaryngospasm pulmonary edema in adults (letter). *Anesthesiology* 1984; 60:516.

71. Millen JE, Vandree J, Glauser FL: Fiberoptic bronchoscopic balloon occlusion and reexpansion of refractory unilateral atelectasis. *Crit Care Med* 1978; 6:50–55.

72. Motoyama EK, Hen J, Tamas L, et al: Spirometry with positive airway pressure: A simple method to evaluate obstructive lung disease in children. *Am Rev Respir Dis* 1982; 126:766.

73. Murray IP, Modell JH, Gallagher TJ, et al: Titration of PEEP by the arterial minus end-tidal carbon dioxide gradient. *Chest* 1984; 85(1):101.

74. National Heart, Lung, and Blood Institute: Conference on the scientific basis of in-hospital respiratory therapy. *Am Rev Respir Dis* 1980; 122:1–161.

75. Nunn JF, Coleman AJ, Sachithanadan T, et al: Hypoxaemia and atelectasis produced by forced expiration. *Br J Anaesth* 1965; 37:3.

76. O'Donohue WJ: Maximum volume IPPB for

the management of pulmonary atelectasis. *Chest* 1979; 76:683–687.

77. O'Donohue WJ: Position and positive end-expiratory pressure in lobar atelectasis (letter). *Chest* 1979; 75:764.

78. O'Donohue WJ Jr: National survey of the usage of lung expansion modalities for the prevention and treatment of postoperative atelectasis following abdominal thoracic surgery. *Chest* 1985; 87:76–80.

79. Pace NL, East TD, Westenskow DR, et al: Differential lung ventilation after unilateral hydrochloric acid aspiration in the dog. *Crit Care Med* 1983; 11:17.

80. Pardee NE, Winterbauer RH, Allen JD: Bedside evaluation of respiratory distress. *Chest* 1984; 85:203.

81. Parker JC, Townsley MI, Rippe B, et al: Increased microvascular permeability in dog lungs due to high peak airway pressures. *J Appl Physiol* 1984; 57:1809.

82. Paul WL, Downs JB: Postoperative atelectasis. *Arch Surg* 1981; 116:861–863.

83. Pepe PE, Marini JJ: Occult positive end-expiratory pressure in mechanically ventilated patients with airflow obstruction. *Am Rev Respir Dis* 1982; 126:166.

84. Permutt S: Relation between pulmonary arterial pressure and pleural pressure during the acute asthmatic attack. *Chest* 1973; 63:25S.

85. Petty TL (ed): *Intensive and Rehabilitative Respiratory Care,* ed 3. Philadelphia, Lea & Febiger, 1982.

86. Pinsky MR, Summer WR: Cardiac augmentation by phasic high intrathoracic support (PHIPS) in man. *Chest* 1985; 84:370–375.

87. Quan SF, Faltrick RT, Schlobohm RDM: Extubation from ambient or expiratory positive airway pressure in adults. *Anesthesiology* 1981; 55:53.

88. Qvist J, Andersen JB, Pemberton M, et al: High level PEEP in severe asthma (letter). *N Engl J Med* 1982; 307:1347.

89. Register SD, Downs JB: Is 50% oxygen harmful? (abstract). *Crit Care Med* 1984; 12:327.

90. Richardson JD, Adams L, Flint LM: Selective management of flail chest and pulmonary contusion. *Ann Surg* 1982; 196:481.

91. Rivington-Law BA, Epstein SW, Thompson GL, et al: Effect of chest wall vibrations on pulmonary function in chronic bronchitis. *Chest* 1984; 85:378–381.

92. Robotham J: Cardiovascular disturbances in chronic respiratory insufficiency. *Am J Cardiol* 1981; 47:941.

93. Roussos C, Macklem PT: The respiratory muscles. *N Engl J Med* 1982; 307:786.

94. Scholten DJ, Novak R, Snyder JV: Directed manual recruitment of collapsed lung in intubated and nonintubated patients. *Am Surg* 1985; 51:330.

95. Shackford S, Virgilio R, Peters R: Selective use of ventilator therapy in flail chest injury. *J Thorac Cardiovasc Surg* 1981; 81:194.

96. Shivaram U, Donath J, Khan F, et al: Continuous positive airway pressure (CPAP) in the treatment of acute bronchial asthma: Clinical study of 20 patients (abstract). *Am Rev Respir Dis* 1984; 129:A41.

97. Sladen A, Arnett CW: The ambulatory bird ventilator. *Anesthesiology* 1970; 33:666.

98. Schmid E, Rehder K: General anesthesia and the chest wall. *Anesthesiology* 1981; 55:668.

99. Snyder JV: Capnography, in Spence AA (ed): *Respiratory Monitoring in Intensive Care.* New York, Churchill Livingstone, 1982, pp 100–121.

100. Snyder JV, Pennock B, Herbert D, et al: Local lung ventilation in critically ill patients using non radioactive xenon-enhanced transmission computed tomography. *Crit Care Med* 1983; 12:46–51.

101. Snyder JV, Carroll GC, Schuster DP. et al: *Mechanical Ventilation: Physiology and Application. Curr Probl Surg,* vol 21, 1984.

102. Snyder JV, Powner DJ, Grenvik A: Neurologic intensive care, in Cottrell JE, Turndorf H (eds): *Anesthesia and Neurosurgery,* ed 3. St Louis, CV Mosby Co (in press).

103. Stocks MC, Downs JB, Cooper RB, et al: Comparison of continuous positive airway pressure, incentive spirometry, and conservative therapy of cardiac operations. *Crit Care Med* 1984; 12:969–971.

104. Stocks MC, Downs JB, Gauer PK, et al: Prevention of postoperative pulmonary complications with CPAP, incentive spirometry, and conservative therapy. *Chest* 1985; 87:151.

105. Stalcup SA, Mellins RB: Mechanical forces producing pulmonary edema in acute asthma. *N Engl J Med* 1977; 297:592.

106. Suter PM, Fairley HB, Isenberg MD: Optimum end-expiratory airway pressure in patients with acute pulmonary failure. *N Engl J Med* 1975; 292:284.

107. Suter PM, Fairley HB, Isenberg MD: Effect of tidal volume and positive end-expiratory pressure on compliance during mechanical ventilation. *Chest* 1978; 73:158.

108. Swift DL: Aerosols and humidity therapy: Generation and respiratory deposition of therapeutic aerosols. *Am Rev Respir Dis* 1980; 122(5):71.

109. Tenaillon A, Salmona J-P, Burdin M: Continuous positive airway pressure in asthma (letter). *Am Rev Respir Dis* 1983; 127:658.

110. Trinkle J, Richardson D, Franz J, et al: Management of flail chest without mechanical ventilation. *Ann Thorac Surg* 1975; 19:355.

111. Venus V, Takayoshi M, Copiozo JB, et al: Prophylactic intubation and continuous positive airway pressure in the management of inhalation therapy in burn victims. *Crit Care Med* 1981; 9:519.

112. Viires N, Sillye G, Aubier M, et al: Regional blood flow distribution in dog during induced hypotension and low cardiac output. *J Clin Invest* 1983; 72:935.

113. Visick WD, Fairley HB, Hickey RF: The effects of tidal volume and end-expiratory pressure on pulmonary gas exchange during anesthesia. *Anesthesiology* 1973; 39:285.

114. Weissman C, Askanazi J, Rosenbaum S, et al: Amino acids and respiration. *Ann Intern Med* 1983; 98:41.

26 Cellular Mechanisms in Adult Respiratory Distress Syndrome

Jean E. Rinaldo, M.D.

Acute respiratory failure (ARF) characterized by noncardiogenic pulmonary edema frequently complicates critical illness in medical and surgical intensive care units (ICUs). Regardless of the underlying illness that predisposes to the development of this complication, ARF is usually a major contributor to derangement in oxygen delivery. This chapter reviews the current understanding of the basic pathophysiologic concepts thought to underlie adult respiratory distress syndrome (ARDS), a generic term used to describe ARF characterized by noncardiogenic pulmonary edema.

DEFINITION AND CLINICAL PREDISPOSITIONS

In 1967 Ashbaugh and associates described a syndrome of sudden respiratory distress in 12 adult patients without known underlying lung disease.[2] They termed the disorder "the adult respiratory distress syndrome" and defined it as the concurrence of dyspnea, severe hypoxemia refractory to a high inspired oxygen concentration, reduced respiratory system compliance, and diffuse alveolar infiltrates that resemble pulmonary edema, without clinical evidence of congestive heart failure. Although described quite recently, the syndrome has since been found to be both common and lethal, affecting an estimated 150,000 persons per year in the United States. Initially, the mortality was said to be 90%, but it appeared to decrease to about 50% if positive end-expiratory pressure (PEEP) was used. Since that time, despite technological innovations in intensive care, the mortality from "well-established ARDS" has remained approximately the same, according to recent clinical series.[19, 41] However,

it should be noted that "well-established ARDS" is defined by rigorous criteria in most of the published reports; these include low compliance, profound and protracted hypoxemia despite therapy, and pulmonary capillary wedge pressure (WP) that is documented to be normal by measurement with a pulmonary arterial (PA) catheter. These criteria may distinguish a small and perhaps shrinking subset of patients with intractable ARDS, the tip of the iceberg. As supportive care for patients with milder or earlier ARDS has improved, it is possible that the published series of well-established (i.e., advanced) ARDS cases have diverged from the common experience of more typical cases, which resolve before meeting the criteria for "well-established ARDS." If this has occurred, the finding that outcome in well-established ARDS has not changed may be misleading and overly pessimistic.

A large number of clinical predispositions to ARDS have been described. The most common are septicemia, primary bacterial or nonbacterial pneumonias, aspiration of gastric contents, direct chest trauma, prolonged or profound shock, fat embolism, massive blood transfusion, cardiopulmonary bypass, oxygen toxicity, acute hemorrhagic pancreatitis, toxemia of pregnancy, and amniotic fluid embolus. Recent careful epidemiologic studies suggest that the incidence of ARDS differs greatly among these predisposed groups.[19, 41] The highest incidence appears to occur in patients with the so-called sepsis syndrome, described as a combination of leukocytosis or leukopenia, a known source of infection, fever or hypothermia, and hypotension, whether or not blood cultures are positive for a bacterial pathogen. More than one third of such patients develop ARDS. The second most common predisposition appears to be aspiration of gastric contents, which has an incidence rate of approximately 30%. The risk of developing ARDS increases dramatically if more than one predisposing feature is present. The low incidence rates for ARDS in many of the predisposed groups suggest that the combination of factors that results in pathophysiologic events causing well-established ARDS occurs infrequently in patients predisposed by a single risk. The high incidence rates in patients with several predisposing conditions suggest that some of the pathophysiologic events causing ARDS may be facilitated in the lung that has already been mildly injured.

The management of ARDS in respiratory ICUs is discussed in other chapters. In recent years, new information pertinent to the basic mechanisms that cause lung injury in ARDS[9, 47, 57] has supplanted the previous exclusive emphasis on empirical life support technology. This chapter summarizes several new concepts that have emerged from this basic research.

CONCEPTS OF PATHOPHYSIOLOGY OF ARDS

Pulmonary Edema in ARDS

When ARDS was described in 1967, the attention of both physiologists and clinical investigators was directed toward the genesis and treatment of lung edema. This was a natural focus because of the prominence of the roentgenologic infiltrates and the other clinical similarities to pulmonary edema caused by heart failure.

Several varieties of experimentally induced acute lung injury resembling ARDS were developed using the singularly important animal model developed by Staub.[56] In this model, the caudal mediastinal lymph duct of a sheep was cannulated, making it possible to collect lymph from the lung. From the assumption that no lymph from other viscera was present in the "lung lymph," it followed that in the steady state the composition of the "lung lymph" would be identical to the composition of the net flux of water, electrolytes, and proteins traversing the pulmonary endothelium. Therefore, alterations in the amount of lung lymph and in the concentration and molecular radii of the constituent proteins were assumed to reflect either changes in the hydrostatic and oncotic driving pressures for filtration or changes in the membrane permeability coefficients. These permeability coefficients describe the sizes of the theoretical "pores" in the capillary walls of the lung. In several landmark papers, intravenous infusions of bacteria, endotoxin, histamine, fibrin degradation products, and microemboli were given.[6-8, 20, 37] These produced evidence of altered lung microvascular permeability and in several models also produced pulmonary edema and hypoxemia. Thus these animal models were taken to be analogous to ARDS in humans.

It has been difficult to demonstrate conclusively in clinical studies that lung microvascular permeability is altered in ARDS in humans, although the assumption seems to follow logically from the radiologic appearance of lung edema despite low microvascular hydrostatic pressures documented by the use of flow-directed PA catheters. Several techniques have been developed to study microvascular permeability in humans with ARDS. Elevated edema fluid to serum protein ratios were described in patients with ARDS: a ratio of less than 0.3 was said to reflect heart failure, and a ratio of more than 0.7 was said to reflect ARDS. However, there are difficulties with this measurement. Extreme values may be useful, but the ratio was sometimes as high as 0.8 in heart failure and as low as 0.5 in ARDS. Most measurements fell into an intermediate, nondiagnostic range.[55] Furthermore, measurements based on the protein content in aspirated edema fluid did not clearly distinguish altered capillary permeability from exudation of protein in proximal airways due to tracheobronchial inflammation. More recently, Brigham et al.[10] described the use of a multiple radiolabeled indicator dilution technique in humans that provided more evidence of altered lung microvascular permeability in patients with severe ARDS. In patients with milder forms of the disease, however, altered microvascular permeability could not be demonstrated using this technique.

Despite the difficulties in making conclusive measurements of driving pressures and permeability coefficients in the lung in patients, the assumption that ARDS is associated with altered lung microvascular permeability at the alveolar level was widely accepted. The concept resulted initially in therapeutic approaches to ARDS that were based almost entirely on manipulation of hydrostatic and oncotic driving forces for filtration, using the Starling equation as the basis for therapy. Coincident with the growth of a body of experimental data that described ARDS as a derangement of the permeability coefficients in the Starling equation, technological advances facilitated the application of this concept at the bedside. The rapid and widespread acceptance of the use of flow-directed PA catheters permitted the measurement of pulmonary capillary WP routinely in the ICU. This allowed clinicians to distinguish more clearly between "permeability edema" and "hydrostatic edema" in patients with suspected ARDS, by measuring pulmonary WP.[59] (The assumption that WP is equivalent to capillary pressure is not entirely accurate, as is discussed in chapter 15, "Technical Problems in Data Acquisition"). The use of PA catheters also permitted rapid and reliable determination of mixed venous oxygen content and of cardiac output by thermodilution. These additional data made possible rapid and complex calculations of derived physiologic indices such as systemic and pulmonary vascular resistance, intrapulmonary shunt fraction, oxygen consumption and delivery, and others that could be monitored as therapy was titrated. Also, the measurement of serum colloid osmotic pressure in clinical laboratories became possible, allowing measurements of another allegedly important component of the Starling equation, intravascular oncotic pressure, which could also be "titrated" by the therapeutic administration of albumin and diuretics.

Unfortunately, recent clinical studies[19, 41] document the apparent failure of a therapeutic approach to ARDS that is based on manipulation of Starling forces to significantly influence survival. In retrospect we can see that such failure was inevitable, because the conceptual description of ARDS as a simple capillary leak syndrome of noncardiogenic pulmonary edema was greatly simplified. Although lung water is clearly elevated, the derangement of oxygenation in patients with ARDS is poorly correlated with the quantity of edema fluid that is present.[10] Lung water is not the central pathophysiologic factor causing respiratory failure in patients with ARDS. Rather, a series of complex sequential morphological and physiologic abnormalities occur after acute lung injury. The result is a severe dysfunction in pulmonary gas exchange and mechanics that arises from a complex series of structural and physiologic mechanisms in addition to alveolar flooding. These mechanisms are not likely to be influenced by hydrostatic or oncotic forces.

Morphological Derangements of the Lung in ARDS

Between 1974 and 1977, the National Heart, Lung, and Blood Institute (NHLBI) undertook a multicenter prospective collaborative study of extracorporeal membrane oxygenation (ECMO) in patients with ARDS.[40] This study had profound effects on the understanding and subsequent investigation of ARDS, and the "ECMO study" remains an important historic landmark. It was the first large multicenter clinical series in which epidemiologic, histologic, and physiologic data about a large group of ARDS patients were collected. It prompted a major shift in investigative attention because the study demonstrated that severe derangements in the architecture of the lung developed rapidly in ARDS.[43] Although lung edema, which had been emphasized exclusively by most investigators until that time, was shown to be present initially, it was apparent that with adequate ventilatory support this early phase evolved to secondary and tertiary phases in which virtually all structural elements and cell types within the lung were affected. The attenuated alveolar type I cells, which line alveoli and provide a thin surface for gas exchange, were lost and replaced within 72 hours by cuboidal and rapidly proliferating alveolar type II cells. These cells may ultimately differentiate to become type I cells and may ultimately restore the attenuated epithelial surface, but during the proliferative phase the structural impairment of the lung impedes gas exchange. Simultaneously, the interstitium is rapidly infiltrated with mesenchymal cells and inflammatory cells.[3, 31, 34] Pulmonary fibrosis follows, alveoli and alveolar ducts are obliterated, and the interstitium is replaced with sheets of collagen. In addition, the pulmonary vasculature is profoundly altered. The capillary bed is obliterated, which diminishes the surface available for gas exchange and contributes to pulmonary hypertension and right ventricular failure. The NHLBI ECMO study and subsequent studies also demonstrated that superinfection with bacterial and fungal pathogens occurs frequently in ARDS. The alveolar infiltrates that occur in ARDS due to edema, cell proliferation, and fibrosis are difficult to distinguish from superimposed pneumonia using clinical criteria such as fever and leukocytosis.[1, 4]

Another late but important finding of the

NHLBI ECMO study was the apparent reversal of severe lung fibrosis in ARDS patients who survived. It had been thought previously that lung fibrosis was irreversible. Follow-up evaluation of pulmonary function studies in survivors of ARDS demonstrated definitively that in the majority of cases, even severe lung fibrosis resolved almost totally after many months.[16, 33, 50]

The current methods of cardiopulmonary support do not appear to prevent the relentless progression of alveolar and interstitial injury in ARDS. Although refinements in modes of mechanical ventilatory support may diminish the progression of ARDS in some cases, it now seems likely that drug therapy aimed at the cellular mechanisms causing lung injury and the fibrotic response to injury will be necessary to improve the outcome of ARDS in many others. Therefore, there has been a growing interest in the cellular pathophysiology of lung injury and repair.

The Role of Polymorphonuclear Leukocytes in Lung Injury in ARDS

Considerable experimental evidence has accumulated to implicate polymorphonuclear leukocytes as inducing the initial pulmonary capillary injury that leads to increased permeability edema in ARDS and also as potentially mediating the subsequent interstitial fibrosis.

Insight into the possible role of neutrophil-mediated endothelial injury in ARDS arose from the observation that sudden transient neutropenia occurred in patients undergoing cellophane membrane hemodialysis.[30] In later studies, it became apparent that the neutrophils "disappeared" transiently from the circulation because they aggregated in visceral vascular beds, especially in the lung.[13, 14, 29] Infusion of activators of complement and of complement fragments reproduced the neutropenia. The peptide fragment C5A was found to be the probable mediator. It was then recognized that many clinical predispositions to ARDS, including endotoxemia, trauma, and pancreatitis, involve the action of the intravascular complement cascade. Using the "lung-lymph" preparation in sheep, Craddock and associates infused complement-activated plasma and showed increased lung microvascular permeability similar to what is seen in ARDS; leukocytes were found aggregated in the lung.[13] From these and other observations the hypothesis was advanced that ARDS is caused by complement activation, which causes leukocyte aggregation in the lung. The activated neutrophils were thought to injure pulmonary endothelial cells by generating toxic oxygen radicals, releasing neutral proteases from lysosomes, and releasing other mediators such as prostaglandins and leukotrienes. In support of this concept, it was shown that in several animal models of ARDS, neutropenia produced by administering antineoplastic chemotherapeutic agents prevented or diminished the severity of "ARDS" in animal models caused by endotoxemia, microemboli, oxygen toxicity, or other insults to the lung.[18, 26, 53]

Despite convincing animal studies, evidence supporting the role of leukocytes in humans with ARDS is inconclusive. Hammerschmidt et al.[22] reported that complement activation was a sensitive and specific predictor of ARDS. However, others have been unable to confirm this observation.[62] Zimmerman et al.[64] found increased activation of the circulating neutrophils in patients with ARDS. Thommasen et al.[58] found a predictive relation between an acute fall in circulating neutrophils and the onset of ARDS in septic patients, and Harris et al.[23] found an inverse correlation between circulating neutrophils and both microvascular permeability and the alveolar-arterial oxygen tension difference in patients with ARDS. Recently, several groups have reported increased numbers of neutrophils and their proteolytic enzymes in the bronchoalveolar lavage (BAL) fluid from patients with ARDS.[11, 35, 36]

Several objections to these clinical studies can be raised. Both the reported abnormalities in the state of activation of the circulating neutrophils and such abnormalities as their decreased number may well be markers of more severe predispositions to ARDS, such as overwhelming sepsis, rather than of sequestration of the neutrophils in the lung, as has been inferred. Neutrophils and neutrophil-associated enzymes reported in the BAL fluid of ARDS patients could have resulted at least in part from superimposed pneumonia.[1, 4] At present, although there is substantial circumstantial evidence linking leukocytes to lung injury in ARDS, no causal relationship has been proved.

Coagulation Abnormalities and Fibronectin in ARDS

There is evidence that ARDS, intravascular coagulation, and activation of circulating platelets are related, but the exact nature of their pathophysiologic interaction is unclear. Pulmonary thrombi can frequently be visualized angiographically in the vasculature of patients with ARDS.[21] Platelet and fibrin thrombi are found in the lungs of these patients, and frank disseminated intravascular coagulation occurs in 23% of patients.[5] Thrombocytopenia complicates ARDS in 50% of cases.[52] Even if disseminated intravascular coagulation cannot be diagnosed by the usual chemical criteria, purpura fulminans may occur and progress to frank peripheral gangrene.[46] Platelet kinetic studies have been performed in these patients and suggest that there is a reduced platelet life span with deposition of platelets in the lungs, in the liver, and in the spleen.[52]

A recent emphasis on the possible role of fibronectin deficiency in ARDS is partly related to the role of intravascular coagulation.[28] There appears to be reticuloendothelial system suppression in most patients with ARDS, due to decreased levels of fibronectin, the cold-insoluble plasma opsonin. The reticuloendothelial system and plasma opsonin (fibronectin) play a major role in the clearance of fibrin aggregates, fibrin degradation products, aggregated or injured platelets, leukocytes, erythrocytes, and other particulate debris from the circulation. Thus these particulate products may circulate for prolonged periods in ARDS patients, which amplifies their injurious effects on the pulmonary microvasculature. However, a pathogenetic role for fibronectin deficiency in ARDS remains unproved in clinical studies.[38]

Role of Products of Arachidonic Acid in the Pathogenesis of ARDS

Production of both prostaglandins and leukotrienes accompanies infusion of endotoxin in sheep, an alleged animal model of ARDS.[54] Inhibition of cyclo-oxygenase using indomethacin, meclofenamate, ibuprofen, or other cyclo-oxygenase inhibitors of prostaglandin function diminishes several manifestations of pulmonary dysfunction that occur in that model, including pulmonary hypertension, hypoxemia, and bronchoconstriction. Thus it has been proposed that cyclo-oxygenase inhibitors may be of clinical value in ARDS. At this time there are no clinical data to support the value of cyclo-oxygenase inhibitors in ARDS patients. Furthermore, aspirin, a cyclo-oxygenase inhibitor, has been shown to

impair bactericidal responses in pneumococcal pneumonia,[17] and ibuprofen, another cyclo-oxygenase inhibitor, was shown to enhance endotoxin-induced alveolar inflammation when given in low doses.[49] Thus, cyclo-oxygenase inhibitors may have risks as well as benefits in ARDS. This emphasizes the need for carefully controlled prospective clinical trials if such agents are to be used.

Bronchoalveolar Inflammation: Links to Fibrosis in ARDS

Severe lung fibrosis may be a sequela of ARDS. Prevention of this complication may be essential to improving survival. To elucidate the pathogenesis of lung fibrosis in ARDS, recent clinical investigations have attempted to employ segmental BAL using fiberoptic bronchoscopy, a technique that has been used extensively to study the more chronic forms of lung fibrosis, such as idiopathic pulmonary fibrosis (IPF) and sarcoidosis. BAL permits recovery from the diseased lung of inflammatory cells, which can be enumerated and further studied in tissue culture. In both chronic lung fibrosis and ARDS, BAL fluid is frequently neutrophil rich. There is evidence to suggest that these neutrophils contribute to lung fibrosis. It should be noted parenthetically that IPF and ARDS are similar in several respects. Both initially show morphological evidence of acute alveolar injury that is characterized by interstitial inflammation, hemorrhage, and edema. Both are followed by a hypercellular proliferative phase, which is followed, in turn, by the loss of alveolar units due to the appearance of obliterative fibrosis. This occurs within 2–3 weeks in patients with ARDS but takes months or years to develop fully in patients with IPF. BAL fluid in ARDS is characterized by neutrophil-rich inflammatory cell populations, which appear to release leukocyte elastase and to inactivate α_1-antitypsin.[11, 35, 36] However, despite the recent proliferation of BAL studies in ARDS, no evidence is available confirming that clear-cut pathophysiologic mechanisms link bronchoalveolar neutrophilic inflammation with the pathogenesis of fibrosis in patients with ARDS. Studies are in progress to determine whether alveolar macrophages from the lungs of ARDS patients secrete factors that stimulate the growth of lung fibroblasts, as in silicosis and IPF, but to date these studies are inconclusive.

Oxygen Toxicity

There is evidence that oxygen toxicity superimposed on acute lung inflammation may accelerate lung fibrosis during ventilatory support for ARDS.

Oxygen in high concentrations is toxic to the lungs of all species. Shortly after ARDS was clinically described, and before there was widespread acceptance of the early aggressive use of PEEP, overt iatrogenic oxygen toxicity may have occurred often in the respiratory ICUs. Older series suggest that the use of inspired oxygen concentrations of 70% or more was common, and ventilation with 100% oxygen for many hours was not infrequent.[39] Currently there is much greater awareness of the problem of oxygen toxicity, and physicians can usually avoid prolonged use of frankly cytotoxic oxygen concentrations (greater than 70%) while treating ARDS by using PEEP.

It should not be concluded that oxygen toxicity is no longer a significant clinical problem. Recent clinical and experimental observations suggest that lower concentrations of oxygen than were previously found to be toxic to the normal lung may in fact cause damage and enhance fibrosis in the injured lung. In reviewing morphological findings in the NHLBI ECMO study, Pratt et al. found that the intensity of lung fibrosis significantly correlated with the duration of respiratory support received by the patients rather than with the duration or severity of their underlying disease.[43] Furthermore, Pratt et al. asserted that the histologic pattern of concentric fibrosis of alveolar ducts observed in the NHLBI ECMO study was pathognomonic for oxygen toxicity. In a recent confirmatory study, Collins et al. found that the number of days that a patient breathed an inspired oxygen concentration greater than 0.4 was the strongest predictive factor associated with the quantity of collagen measured in the lungs of ARDS patients who died.[12] Recent studies in animal models strongly support the conclusion that breathing 40%–60% oxygen for less than 72 hours promotes lung fibrosis in previously injured lungs, although it causes no apparent injury to normal lungs.[24, 25, 45] Also, Rinaldo et al. showed that previous oxygen toxicity that is so mild as to be inapparent histologically accelerates and intensifies the acute pulmonary neutrophilic inflammatory response to endotoxin in rats.[48]

Because of the subtlety of these interactions among oxygen toxicity, inflammation, and fibrosis of the lungs of patients with ARDS, it is impossible to define what concentration of oxygen, if any, is completely safe for critically ill patients. Therefore, meticulous efforts must be made to minimize the exposure to oxygen. A therapeutic goal of arterial PO_2 of 60–70 torr usually ensures adequate hemoglobin saturation. Scrupulous attention should be directed to the inspired oxygen concentrations in use, and they should be minimized to the lowest levels that achieve that goal.

Effect of PEEP on Pathogenesis of ARDS

PEEP improves arterial oxygenation by opening closed lung units that are characteristic of ARDS. Other chapters have addressed in detail the rationale for the clinical use of PEEP and the methods of its application. Because of its unquestioned benefit as a life support technique that permits the minimization of inspired oxygen concentrations, it has been tempting to assert that PEEP directly prevents or reduces lung injury in ARDS. Several groups have advocated the use of PEEP as a prophylactic measure based on the notion that early PEEP might prevent ARDS[51, 60, 61] by "aborting or reversing the primary pathophysiologic processes producing acute respiratory failure."[32] However, an excellently designed recent prospective controlled clinical trial appeared to definitively refute this concept.[42] The early emphasis on edema in ARDS and the clinical efficacy of PEEP also prompted the misconception that PEEP decreases lung edema by hydrostatic mechanisms. However, observations using several techniques have shown that PEEP does not decrease the amount of edema fluid in the lung.[15, 27, 44] The sole proved value of PEEP, in subjects who are not hypervolemic, is to permit the minimization of inspired oxygen concentrations and diminish the many deleterious cytotoxic effects of high inspired oxygen concentrations. Viewed in this way, PEEP clearly does decrease lung injury and promote healing. The possibility that other aspects of ventilatory support might influence lung injury is discussed in chapter 24, "Respirator Lung," and chapter 25, "The Open Lung Approach: Concept and Application."

IMPLICATIONS FOR THERAPY

On the basis of the pathophysiologic concepts outlined here, several novel forms of therapy for ARDS have been proposed or tried anecdotally. These include (1) corticosteroids to inactivate leukocytes; (2) cryoprecipitate (fibronectin) to promote opsonization of circulating particulates; (3) antioxidants to minimize both oxygen toxicity and superoxide-mediated cellular injury caused by leukocytes; (4) analogues of collagen precursors to prevent fibrosis; and (5) cyclo-oxygenase inhibitors to restore the ventilation/perfusion balance in injured areas of the lung. Although excellent rationales can be constructed and case reports, animal studies, or in vitro evidence marshalled in each case, no prospective controlled clinical trial has proved that any of these agents improves survival in ARDS. Such controlled studies of clinical outcome are excruciatingly difficult to perform but are essential to demonstrate that the benefits exceed the risks of these agents in critically ill patients.

At this time it must be concluded that the only proved therapy for ARDS is supportive. Important elements of support aimed at cellular mechanisms of lung injury include nutritional support, adequate attention to systemic oxygen delivery to maintain the functional integrity of other organs, scrupulous avoidance of oxygen toxicity, and the detection and treatment of new infections that might perpetuate ARDS. These measures are critically important to minimize ongoing lung injury and to promote healing of the previously injured lung.

REFERENCES

1. Andrews CP, Coalson JJ, Smith JD, et al: Diagnosis of nosocomial bacterial pneumonia in acute, diffuse lung injury. *Chest* 1980; 80:254–257.
2. Ashbaugh DG, Bigelow DB, Petty TL, et al: Acute respiratory distress in adults. *Lancet* 1967; 2:319–323.
3. Bachofen M, Weibel ER: Alterations of the gas exchange apparatus in adult respiratory insufficiency associated with septicemia. *Am Rev Respir Dis* 1977; 116:589–615.
4. Bell RC, Coalson J, Smith JD, et al: Multiple organ system failure and infection in adult respiratory distress syndrome. *Ann Intern Med* 1983; 99:293.
5. Bone RC, Francis PB, Pierce AK: Intravascular coagulation associated with the adult respiratory distress syndrome. *Am J Med* 1976; 61:585–589.
6. Brigham KL, Woolverton WC, Blake LH, et al: Increased sheep lung vascular permeability caused by pseudomonas bacteremia. *J Clin Invest* 1974; 54:792–804.
7. Brigham KL, Owen PJ: Increased sheep lung vascular permeability caused by histamine. *Circ Res* 1975; 37:647–657.
8. Brigham KL, Bowers RE, Haynes J: Increased sheep lung vascular permeability caused by *Escherichia coli* endotoxin. *Circ Res* 1979; 45:292–297.
9. Brigham KL: Mechanisms of lung injury. *Clin Chest Med* 1982; 3:9–24.
10. Brigham KL, Kariman K, Harris TR, et al: Correlation of oxygenation with vascular permeability surface area but not with lung water in humans with acute respiratory failure and pulmonary edema. *J Clin Invest* 1983; 72:339–349.
11. Cochrane CG, Spragg R, Revak SD: Pathogenesis of the adult respiratory distress syndrome. *J Clin Invest* 1983; 71:754–761.
12. Collins JF, Smith JD, Coalson JJ, et al: Variability of lung collagen amounts after prolonged support of acute respiratory failure. *Chest* 1984; 85:641–646.
13. Craddock PR, Fehr J, Dalmasso AP, et al: Hemodialysis leukopenia: Pulmonary vascular leukostasis resulting from complement activation by dialyzer cellophane membrane. *J Clin Invest* 1977; 59:879–888.
14. Craddock PR, Hammerschmidt DE, White JG, et al: Complement (C5a)-induced granulocyte aggregation in vitro: A possible mechanism of complement-mediated leukostasis and leukopenia. *J Clin Invest* 1977; 60:260–264.
15. Demling RH, Staub NC, Edmunds LH Jr: Effect of end-expiratory airway pressure on accumulation of extravascular lung water. *J Appl Physiol* 1975; 38:907–912.
16. Elliott CG, Morris AH, Cengiz M: Pulmonary function and exercise gas exchange in survivors of adult respiratory distress syndrome. *Am Rev Respir Dis* 1981; 123:492–455.
17. Esposito AL: Aspirin impairs antibacterial mechanisms in experimental pneumococcal pneumonia. *Am Rev Respir Dis* 1984; 130:857–862.
18. Flick MR, Perel G, Staub NC: Leukocytes are

required for increased lung microvascular permeability after microemboli in sheep. *Circ Res* 1981; 48:344–351.

19. Fowler AA, Hamman RF, Good JT, et al: Adult respiratory distress syndrome: Risk with common predispositions. *Ann Intern Med* 1983; 98:593–597.

20. Gerdin B, Saldeen T: Effect of fibrin degradation products on microvascular permeability. *Thromb Res* 1978; 13:995–1006.

21. Greene R, Zapol W, Snider M, et al: Early bedside detection of pulmonary vascular occlusion during acute respiratory failure. *Am Rev Respir Dis* 1981; 124:593–601.

22. Hammerschmidt DE, Weaver LJ, Hudson LD, et al: Association of complement activation and elevated plasma-C5a with adult respiratory distress syndrome: Pathophysiological relevance and possible prognostic value. *Lancet* 1980; 1:947–949.

23. Harris TR, Bernard GR, Brigham KL: Lung vascular permeability correlates with alveolar-arterial oxygen difference and inverse of neutrophil count in adult respiratory distress patients (abstract). *Am Rev Respir Dis* 1984; 129:102.

24. Hascheck WM, Witschi H: Pulmonary fibrosis: A possible mechanism. *Toxicol Appl Pharmacol* 1979; 51:475–487.

25. Haschek WM, Reiser KM, Klein-Szanto AJP, et al: Potentiation of butylated hydroxytoluene-induced acute lung damage by oxygen: Cell kinetics and collagen metabolism. *Am Rev Respir Dis* 1983; 127:28–34

26. Heflin AC Jr, Brigham KL: Prevention by granulocyte depletion of increased vascular permeability of sheep lung following endotoxemia. *J Clin Invest* 1981; 68:1253–1260.

27. Hopewell PC: Failure of positive end-expiratory pressure to decrease lung water content in alloxan-induced pulmonary edema. *Am Rev Respir Dis* 1979; 120:813–819.

28. Hyers TM: Pathogenesis of adult respiratory distress syndrome: Current concepts. *Semin Respir Med* 1981; 2:104–108.

29. Jacob HS, Craddock PR, Hammerschmidt DE, et al: Complement-induced granulocyte aggregation: An unsuspected mechanism of disease. *N Engl J Med* 1980; 302:789–794.

30. Kaplow LS, Goffinet JA: Profound neutropenia during the early phase of hemodialysis. *JAMA* 1968; 203:1135–1137.

31. Katzenstein A-LA, Bloor CM, Leibow AA: Diffuse alveolar damage: The role of oxygen, shock, and related factors. *Am J Pathol* 1976; 85:210–228.

32. Kirby RR, Downs JB, Civetta JM, et al: High level positive end-expiratory pressure (PEEP) in acute respiratory insufficiency. *Chest* 1975; 67:156–163.

33. Lakshminarayan S, Stanford RE, Petty TL: Prognosis after recovery from adult respiratory distress syndrome. *Am Rev Respir Dis* 1976; 113:7–16.

34. Lamy M, Fallat RJ, Koeniger E, et al: Pathologic features and mechanisms of hypoxemia in adult respiratory distress syndrome. *Am Rev Respir Dis* 1976; 114:267–284.

35. Lee CT, Fein AM, Lippman M, et al: Elastolytic activity in pulmonary lavage fluid from patients with adult respiratory distress syndrome. *N Engl J Med* 1981; 304:192–196.

36. McGuire WW, Spragg RG, Cohen AB, et al: Studies on the pathogenesis of the adult respiratory distress syndrome. *J Clin Invest* 1982; 69:543–553.

37. Malik AB, van der Zee H: Mechanism of pulmonary edema induced by microembolization in dogs. *Circ Res* 1978; 42:72–79.

38. Maunder RJ, Harlan JM, Pepe PE, et al: Measurement of plasma fibronectin in patients who develop the adult respiratory distress syndrome. *J Lab Clin Med* 1984; 104(4):583–590.

39. Nash G, Pontoppidan H: Pulmonary lesions associated with oxygen therapy and artificial ventilation. *N Engl J Med* 1967; 276:368–374.

40. National Heart Lung and Blood Institute, Division of Lung Diseases: *Extracorporeal Support for Respiratory Insufficiency.* Bethesda, Md, National Institutes of Health, 1979; pp 243–245.

41. Pepe PE, Potkin RT, Reus DH, et al: Clinical predictors of the adult respiratory distress syndrome. *Am J Surg* 1982; 144:124–130.

42. Pepe PE, Hudson LD, Carrico CJ: Early application of positive end-expiratory pressure in patients at risk for the adult respiratory-distress syndrome. *N Engl J Med* 1984; 311:281–286.

43. Pratt PC, Vollmer RT, Shelburne JD, et al: Pulmonary morphology in a multihospital collaborative extracorporeal membrane oxygenation project: 1. Light microscopy. *Am J Pathol* 1979; 95:191–214.

44. Prewitt RM, McCarthy J, Wood LDH: Treatment of acute low pressure pulmonary edema in dogs: Relative effects of hydrostatic and on-

cotic pressure, nitroprusside, and positive end-expiratory pressure. *J Clin Invest* 1981; 67:409–418.

45. Rinaldo JE, Goldstein RH, Snider GL: Modification of oxygen toxicity after lung injury by bleomycin in hamsters. *Am Rev Respir Dis* 1982; 126:1030–1033.

46. Rinaldo JE, Perez H: Ischemic necrosis of both lower extremities as a result of the microembolism syndrome complicating the adult respiratory distress syndrome caused by Escherichia coli pneumonia and septicemia. *Am Rev Respir Dis* 1982; 126:932–936.

47. Rinaldo JE, Rogers RM: Medical Progress. Adult respiratory-distress syndrome: Changing concepts of lung injury and repair. *N Engl J Med* 1982; 306:900–909.

48. Rinaldo JE, Dauber JH, Christman J, et al: Neutrophil alveolitis following endotoxemia: Enhancement by previous exposure to hyperoxia. *Am Rev Respir Dis* 1984; 130:1065–1071.

49. Rinaldo JE, Dauber JH: Effect of methylprednisolone and of ibuprofen, a non-steroidal anti-inflammatory agent, on bronchoalveolar inflammation following endotoxemia. *Circ Shock* 1985; 16:195–203.

50. Rotman HH, Lavelle TF Jr, Dimcheff DG, et al: Long-term physiologic consequences of the adult respiratory distress syndrome. *Chest* 1977; 72:190–192.

51. Schmidt GB, O'Neill WW, Kotb K, et al: Continuous positive airway pressure in the prophylaxis of the adult respiratory distress syndrome. *Surg Gynecol Obstet* 1976; 143:613–618.

52. Schneider RC, Zapol WM, Carvalho AC: Platelet consumption and sequestration in severe acute respiratory failure. *Am Rev Respir Dis* 1980; 122:445–451.

53. Shasby DM, Fox RB, Harada RN, et al: Reduction of the edema of acute hyperoxic lung injury by granulocyte depletion. *J Appl Physiol* 1982; 52:1237–1244.

54. Snapper JR, Hutchison AA, Ogletree ML, et al: Effects of cyclooxygenase inhibitors on the alterations in lung mechanics caused by endotoxemia in the unanesthetized sheep. *J Clin Invest* 1983; 72:63–76.

55. Sprung CL, Rackow EC, Fein IA, et al: The spectrum of pulmonary edema: Differentiation of cardiogenic, intermediate, and noncardiogenic forms of pulmonary edema. *Am Rev Respir Dis* 1981; 124:718–722.

56. Staub NC: Steady state pulmonary transvascular water filtration in unanesthetized sheep. *Circ Res* 1971; 28(suppl 1):I135–I139.

57. Tate RM, Repine JE: Neutrophils and the adult respiratory distress syndrome. *Am Rev Respir Dis* 1983; 128:552–559.

58. Thommasen HV, Russell JA, Boyko WJ, et al: Transient leucopenia associated with adult respiratory distress syndrome. *Lancet* 1984; 1:809–812.

59. Unger KM, Shibel EM, Moser KM: Detection of left ventricular failure in patients with adult respiratory distress syndrome. *Chest* 1975; 67:8–13.

60. Valdes ME, Powers SR Jr, Shah DM, et al: Continuous positive airway pressure in prophylaxis in adult respiratory distress syndrome in trauma patients. *Surg Forum* 1978; 29:187–198.

61. Weigelt JA, Mitchell RA, Snyder WH III: Early positive end-expiratory pressure in the adult respiratory distress syndrome. *Arch Surg* 1979; 114:497–501.

62. Weinberg PF, Matthay MA, Webster RO, et al: Biologically active products of complement and acute lung injury in patients with the sepsis syndrome. *Am Rev Respir Dis* 1984; 130:791–796.

63. Witschi HR, Hascheck WM, Klein-Szanto AJP, et al: Potentiation of diffuse lung damage by oxygen: Determining variables. *Am Rev Respir Dis* 1981; 123:98–103.

64. Zimmerman GA, Renzetti AD, Hill HR: Functional and metabolic activity of granulocytes from patients with adult respiratory distress syndrome: Evidence for activated neutrophils in the pulmonary circulation. *Am Rev Respir Dis* 1983; 127:290–300.

PART 6 —————— Circulatory Support

27 _____ Principles of Circulatory Support and the Treatment of Hemorrhagic Shock

Andrew Peitzman, M.D.

Shock is a clinical syndrome resulting from tissue dysfunction secondary to inadequate perfusion. Although histotoxic factors may play a role, the final common denominator in all forms of shock is low blood flow to vital organs associated with certain pathophysiologic mechanisms of negative feedback. In the clinical setting we are often confronted with a patient in shock, the origin of which is not initially apparent. Since shock may progress rapidly to cardiovascular collapse, it is often treated empirically while the specific cause is sought. Since shock is caused by dysfunction of the normal cardiovascular homeostatic mechanisms, it is important to understand these processes before addressing shock management. The reader is referred to chapters 3 through 6 and 8 for a discussion of the determinants of cardiovascular regulation. The components of this system fall into two categories: factors related primarily to cardiac pump function, vasomotor tone, and circulating blood volume; and microcirculatory factors such as viscosity and cellular aggregation. Derangement of any one or a combination of these factors may result in the clinical syndrome of shock. The major etiologic categories of shock are cardiogenic, septic, neurogenic, obstructive, and hypovolemic.[9, 95] These differ in their pathophysiology and various aspects of their treatment; each will be reviewed briefly, with the goal of defining common principles of resuscitation.

THE ETIOLOGY OF SHOCK

Hypovolemic shock is shock caused by inadequate intravascular volume. Therapy for this form of shock should not focus on restoring blood pressure alone but rather on increasing both blood pressure and flow.[89] In practice this can usually be accomplished by intravascular volume replacement. It is clear that vasoconstrictor therapy alone in hypovolemic shock can actually worsen the low flow state.

Cardiogenic shock is failure of the heart as a pump and may be due to many factors, including acute myocardial infarction and arrhythmias. Since by the Starling mechanism preload is a primary determinant of cardiac output, the adequacy of preload is fundamental in the treatment of all forms of shock, including cardiogenic shock. Specific drug therapy will be discussed in chapter 29, ''Pharmacologic Treatment of Cardiogenic Shock.'' It is clear that pharmacologic treatments work optimally in patients with adequate blood volume.

Neurogenic shock can be due to vasovagal responses, spinal cord trauma, or spinal anesthesia and is characterized by an overall loss of sympathetic tone. The clinical picture of neurogenic shock includes hypotension, a slow heart rate, and warm, dry skin. There is a decrease in cardiac output due to a decrease in arterial and venous tone. The primary circulatory problem in neurogenic shock is a previously normal blood volume inadequately filling an acutely dilated vascular bed. Therapy consists of avoiding orthostasis, administering intravenous volume infusion, and the selective use of vasopressors to increase vasomotor tone.

Septic shock is an infection-induced loss of the ability of the vasculature to regulate flow according to metabolic needs. In addition, reserve blood volume may fail to drain from vascular capacitance beds such as the gut; and often vascular membrane permeability increases, causing profound loss of intravascular volume. Mortality for septic shock is high, and its prevention by prompt treatment of local infections before the onset of clinical septic shock should be a primary goal. When shock occurs, therapy optimally consists first of adequate volume resuscitation, antibiotic administration, and drainage of any abscess. Volume resuscitation and drug therapy may induce transient recovery but usually do not change the outcome unless the septic nidus is eliminated.

Obstructive shock is due to vascular mechanical blockage, such as that caused by pericardial tamponade, tension pneumothorax, or massive pulmonary embolization. Obstructive shock is treated by removing the obstruction. However, volume administration is still the initial therapy. In cardiac tamponade, increasing preload will increase cardiac output and "buy time" before definitive therapy can be established. Similarly, increasing blood volume may be important to maintain left ventricular (LV) filling in the setting of massive pulmonary embolism. Early use of vasoconstricting agents in patients with pulmonary embolism and systemic hypotension may also be important in this condition to sustain right ventricular perfusion pressure since right ventricular systolic pressure is greatly increased.

Hypovolemic shock is the form of shock most commonly encountered clinically and the most studied experimentally.[9, 82] When it is profound enough and lasts long enough, it results in generalized tissue dysfunction.[18, 28, 42, 68, 70, 83] Many of the microvascular changes and serologic cascades associated with this deterioration are also seen in other forms of shock. Therefore, the physiology and treatment of hypovolemic shock will be summarized to illustrate the major principles in the management of shock. Features related to other etiologic forms of shock will be mentioned where relevant.

NORMAL RESPONSE
TO HYPOVOLEMIA

The circulatory system has a complex homeostatic mechanism to control blood flow to various tissues. These interrelated controls include (1) autonomic control of cardiac contractility and peripheral vascular tone; (2) hormonal, adrenergic, and nonadrenergic response to stress and volume depletion supplementing this autonomic control;

and (3) local organ-specific mechanisms that fine-tune regulation of local blood flow. The loss of blood is the primary disturbance in hemorrhagic shock, and low cardiac output and hypotension are the consequences. Since arterial blood pressure is a function of these homeostatic mechanisms, the posthemorrhagic arterial pressure depends on their effectiveness. This varies from individual to individual and from species to species, and also depends on the individual's nutritional status and hydration before the hemorrhagic insult.[41]

Neural Regulation

Two characteristics of the autonomic nervous system's regulation of the circulation are important to this discussion.[12, 13, 23, 41] First, sympathetically mediated vasoconstrictor responses occur almost immediately after hypovolemia or pain. Second, the autonomic nervous system provides a pathway by which blood flow in large components of the circulatory system can be simultaneously affected in a coordinated effort to maintain adequate blood flow to vital organs. The mechanisms involved in these responses are discussed in more detail in chapter 6, "Neurohumoral Regulation of Cardiovascular Function."

The sensor for this control system resides primarily in the baroreceptors located in the carotid sinus and aortic arch. They respond rapidly to changes in blood pressure induced by alterations in blood flow, by adjusting sympathetic tone to maintain blood pressure within an acceptable range. Changes in blood pressure change afferent impulses from arterial baroreceptors, which are integrated primarily in the medulla. In hypotension, the baroreceptors decrease their rate of firing. This withdraws the inhibition on the vasoconstriction center of the medulla, increasing sympathetic discharge, and also inhibits the vagal center, reducing parasympathetic tone. Hypoperfusion of the brain induces additional and more potent activation of the vasomotor center of the medulla, further increasing sympathetic output. This "last ditch effort," as Guyton refers to it,[41] becomes active when arterial pressure falls to 50 torr and is maximal when arterial pressure is less than 15 torr.

This sympathetic response to acute hypovolemia has three major cardiovascular effects: (1) arterioles constrict in most areas, thus increasing total peripheral resistance; (2) capacitance veins increase their drainage, augmenting venous return; and (3) cardiac performance (both rate and inotropy) increases. The arterial vasoconstriction is not homogeneous throughout the systemic circulation, and thus causes a marked redistribution of blood flow.[5, 11, 13, 35, 48] Sympathetic stimulation causes constriction of cardiac and cerebral vessels,[11] but metabolic vasoregulation in these organs prevents excessive local vasoconstriction. On the other hand, blood flow to nonvital tissues decreases significantly. Renal blood flow may be reduced to as little as 5%–10% of normal, and flow to the splanchnic circulation, skin, and resting skeletal muscle may decrease greatly.[11, 41]

Approximately two thirds of the circulating blood volume is within the venous circulation.[41] The venous system is thus the capacitance side of the circulation. Emptying of these capacitance vessels preserves cardiac filling pressures by returning more blood to the heart as circulating blood volume falls. The constrictor responses in early hypovolemic shock are mediated by norepinephrine and epinephrine, released into the circulation from the adrenal medulla as well as through direct effects of local sympathetic activity on the vascular walls. This sympathetic discharge also has potent inotropic effects.[11–13, 23, 41]

Hormonal Influences

Hypovolemia also initiates complex endocrine responses. Plasma levels of adrenocorticotropin (ACTH), growth hormone, glucagon, and cortisol increase.[36, 41, 75] The renin-angiotensin-aldosterone axis is stimulated by hypovolemia via hypoperfusion of the juxtaglomerular apparatus. Hypovolemia is also a potent stimulus for the release of antidiuretic hormone (ADH).[36] ADH acts on the distal tubule to increase resorption of water. ADH also causes splanchnic vasoconstriction. Growth hormone opposes the effects of insulin by promoting gluconeogenesis and lipolysis.[20] Glucagon promotes gluconeogenesis, glycogenolysis, and lipolysis. In addition, glucagon has a direct inotropic cardiovascular effect.[34, 56] Gluconeogenesis, glycogenolysis, and inhibition of insulin release by epinephrine and norepinephrine result in hyperglycemia. There may also be a tissue resistance to insulin.[19] Catecholamines, glucagon, growth hormone, and insulin resistance combine to increase blood sugar and osmolality, which tends to shift fluid from the cells and interstitium to the vascular bed.[24, 41, 72] The sympathetic cardiovascular mechanisms operative in hypovolemic shock are facilitated by ADH, glucagon, and angiotensin. Hormonal effects also limit further loss of fluids or salt via the kidneys. These hormonal responses serve to maximize cardiovascular function, conserve salt and water, and provide nutrients and oxygen to the heart and brain.[36]

Microcirculatory Changes

An equally important mechanism in the maintenance of central blood volume is autoregulation of local blood flow. Autoregulation is regulation of microvascular tone by local tissue mediators in response to pressure change or tissue metabolic needs.[11, 13, 35] These microcirculatory changes are a major component of the homeostatic response to hemorrhagic shock. When microcirculatory autoregulation fails, shock becomes irreversible.[11, 13, 35]

Blood flow through the capillaries is normally intermittent rather than continuous. This is due to the intermittent contraction of the metarterioles and precapillary sphincters (vasomotion). The tone of these sphincters is inversely proportional to the oxygen concentration in the tissue.[11, 27, 35]

In hemorrhagic shock, the sympathetic response causes vasoconstriction of the 90- to 150-μ arterioles. There is also early dilation of the 20- to 50-μ arterioles. The constriction of the larger arterioles and dilation of the smaller arterioles lowers hydrostatic pressure within the capillary. This causes a flux of fluid from the extracellular space into the capillary. This is probably the prime mechanism of the capillary refilling and hemodilution that is observed 3–4 hours after hemorrhage. Hyperglycemia increases the osmotic gradient, promoting the influx of fluid from the interstitium into the capillary by altering Starling forces.[24, 41, 72] The net result of these mechanisms is partial restoration of vascular volume by relative depletion of interstitial volume.

These compensatory mechanisms—neural, hormonal, and autoregulatory—allow a patient to sustain substantial blood loss (approximately 15%) and recover without treatment. In this compensated stage of hypovolemia, tissue perfusion may be lower than normal, and anaerobic metabolism may be apparent as lactic acidosis, but the microcirculation is not blocked irreversibly and is not so deficient that progressive tissue dysfunction occurs. Any dysfunction that does occur can be reversed by intravascular volume replacement. If volume loss continues a vicious cycle may result: further depression in cardiac output causes further tissue and microcirculatory changes, which feed back negatively on the heart, causing further cardiac decompensation. This transition from simple hypovolemia to reversible dysfunction (progressive shock) to irreversible shock is often subtle and ill-defined. Therefore, fluid resuscitation should be given promptly and aggressively to most patients that present in shock.

PROGRESSIVE SHOCK

Wiggers first suggested that myocardial failure is a major component of progressive hemorrhagic shock.[97] Several studies support the concept that progressive cardiac deterioration occurs in hemorrhagic shock.[3, 6, 58, 63, 85] As venous return diminishes, cardiac output falls.[41, 46] Archie and Mertz demonstrated that in spite of responses that tend to protect coronary blood flow, there is a decline in myocardial blood flow in progressive hemorrhagic shock.[6] This may be compounded by decreased myocardial oxygen diffusion. The net result is subendocardial ischemia during shock. MacDonald et al. reported depressed LV function in irreversible shock, which they thought was due to decreased cardiac contractility.[58] Recently, Alyono et al. found that LV contractility was limited only in late (preterminal) shock.[3] The authors concluded that the apparently depressed LV function seen in prolonged shock was due to decreased LV diastolic compliance, not to impaired contractility.[3] Thus, myocardial dysfunction may be a late component of progressive hemorrhagic shock. Myocardial dysfunction may be due to sympathetic exhaustion, or to myocardial depressant factor released from ischemic tissue. However, Downing states that "there is no evidence in this system for the appearance of a depressant substance from the splanchnic bed that reduces the performance of hearts with adequate coronary flow."[33]

Fluid Shifts and Cellular Changes

As mentioned earlier, a decrease in capillary perfusion pressure promotes resorption of interstitial fluid into the capillary lumen, decreasing extracellular fluid (ECF) volume.[64, 80, 81, 82] Early laboratory studies by Shires et al. demonstrated that this ECF volume deficit persisted only when shed blood or shed blood plus additional plasma was used in volume resuscitation of these animals. In addition, returning the shed blood alone resulted in 80% mortality at 24 hours, and returning shed blood plus plasma caused 70% mortality at 24 hours.[80–82] Infusing shed blood plus lactated Ringer's solution returned the measured ECF volume to near control levels and decreased mortality to 30% at 24 hours.

The reduction in ECF volume associated with prolonged hemorrhagic shock was greater than could be accounted for by simply the vascular refilling from the interstitial space.[64, 80] This led investigators to propose that cellular dysfunction occurs in prolonged shock and that interstitial fluid uptake by the cells results in cellular edema.[4, 28, 81] Studies of cell membrane integrity and transport across the cell membrane have since elucidated cell membrane dysfunction in hemorrhagic shock.[28, 29, 49, 70, 81]

In hemorrhagic shock, skeletal muscle potential difference (PD) decreases.[18, 68, 81] This reduction in PD is proportional to the degree and the duration of the shock state. Intracellular sodium, chloride, and water levels increase in prolonged shock, associated with membrane depolarization. Consistent with these findings, there is a marked decrease in extracellular water volume in hemorrhagic shock. Skeletal muscle cells (50% of body mass) may be the principal site of cellular fluid and electrolyte sequestration after severe hemorrhagic shock.[81, 82]

These findings are further corroborated by the electron microscopic observations of Holden et al.[47] In this study, ultrastructural changes in the skeletal muscle of animals subjected to hemorrhagic shock demonstrated intracellular edema with spreading of myofibrils and distortion of the mitochondria. Since mitochondria are the primary source of adenosine triphosphate (ATP) production, their impairment results in profound loss of cellular function. Lysosomal disruption also occurs in shock states, with resultant release of lysosomal enzymes and intracellular autodigestion.[37, 47] After volume resuscitation in baboons (with shed blood and lactated Ringer's solution), not only was hypotension reversed and muscle PD returned to baseline, but abnormal electrolyte and water shifts were also corrected.[82] These data suggest that a defect in Na-K active transport occurs in hemorrhagic shock. Because Na-K active transport depends on ATP, intracellular energy depletion has been suggested as a cause of the persistent cellular dysfunction.[21, 22, 52] However, recent studies have shown that membrane dysfunction can occur despite normal ATP stores in both muscle and red blood cells (RBCs) and that lower ATP in cells is not the initial cause of membrane instability.[49, 67–69, 77] Widespread membrane dysfunction occurs in progressive shock. It causes fluid shifts and tissue dysfunction. However, the mechanism responsible for this dysfunction remains unclear. The only treatment that has been documented to consistently reverse these changes is adequate volume, including crystalloid, resuscitation.[81, 82] Rapid assessment and volume resuscitation are mandatory to abort the microcirculatory damage that results in irreversible shock.

IRREVERSIBLE SHOCK

If the shock state is profound enough and lasts long enough, what was previously adequate resuscitation therapy may fail to reverse the process. This condition is referred to as irreversible shock. The clinical distinction between progressive and irreversible shock is difficult to make, except retrospectively. The irreversible stage of hemorrhagic shock can be created in a dog model by the spontaneous uptake of a set volume (30%–50%) of previously shed blood after an interval of shock.[41, 97] Despite the return of all shed blood and further fluid resuscitation, survival usually is not possible after this "uptake stage."[97] The mechanisms responsible for the irreversibility of the process are unclear. However, increased capillary permeability, with leakage of fluid from the vascular tree, is probably only a late event and not a cause of irreversible shock.

Even brief experimental hemorrhage may be followed by nearly complete cessation of blood flow in skeletal muscle for 5–20 minutes.[5] The primary site of this constriction is in the larger arterioles. When shed blood was restored after only 5 minutes of hypoperfusion, 50% of the capillaries still remained closed.[5] Thus maldistribution of flow occurs in the muscle bed during the resuscitation phase, which may contribute to the progression of the shock state. Sludging of RBCs, WBCs, or platelets and increasing microvascular viscosity also play major roles in the progression of hemorrhagic shock. Flow may stop in some microvessels and continue in adjacent bypass capillaries. The normal "winking" on and off of capillary flow may be converted to halted flow in some vessels and persistent flow (due to mediators from hypoxia) in neighboring

vessels.[5, 11, 27, 48] Thus, measured overall resistance to tissue flow may not change even when local tissue perfusion is severely decreased. This problem complicates any analysis of pressure and flow data during shock.

The uptake of blood that marks the onset of irreversibility occurs at a constant arterial pressure, and therefore indicates loss of vasomotor tone. Several studies have suggested that loss of vasomotor tone is due either to local mediator release or to vasomotor paralysis.[10, 11, 13, 35] Flint et al.[35] found that in irreversible shock arteriolar dilation occurred despite continued hypovolemia and high circulatory levels of norepinephrine. The 90- to 150-μ arterioles showed a persistent constriction response and a lower sensitivity to norepinephrine. Smaller arterioles and all venules dilated in irreversible shock. Local tissue acidosis further compounds these mechanisms.[10, 27] Bond et al. have also confirmed that vasomotor failure may be an important component of hemorrhagic shock.[11, 13] Thus, vasomotor failure (loss of autoregulation), possibly due to resistance to catecholamines, may be a major determinant in irreversible shock.

The physician faced with a patient in shock is often unsure of the etiology, the mechanisms, and the reversibility of the process in his patient. The multiple microvascular and cellular processes on which outcome will depend are poorly understood in principle and often resistant to analysis in the individual patient. Thus a certain degree of empirical therapy is warranted in the management of shock.

TREATMENT OF HEMORRHAGIC SHOCK

Resuscitation consists of simultaneous evaluation and treatment. Because pathophysiologic cascades become more established with time, resulting in further cardiovascular dysfunction, resuscitation measures should be instituted quickly. Rapid restoration of adequate blood flow may avoid the microcirculatory cascade that results in myocardial, cerebral, splanchnic, or renal insult. Delay in aggressive volume resuscitation may result in irreversible organ injury. Resuscitation that is initiated prior to diagnosis must be directed toward those elements common to most forms of shock. During initial therapy the patient is evaluated primarily for signs of adequate tissue perfusion, which is most easily done today by assessing organ system function.

First a patent airway and adequate breathing are assured, then therapy is directed at rapid restoration of central and then adequate total blood volume. The primary treatment for hemorrhagic shock is control of the hemorrhage and replacement of the blood.

In the treatment of hypotension, the lower extremities are often elevated and the patient is placed in the Trendelenburg position to increase central blood volume and arterial pressure. However, the Trendelenburg position was found to have no consistent effect on venous return or systemic vascular resistance in a recent study of normotensive and hypotensive patients.[87] In addition, cerebral perfusion and pulmonary function may be compromised in patients in the Trendelenburg position.

The military antishock trousers (MAST) are widely used in the emergency field treatment of hemorrhagic shock. The MAST suit consists of a pair of trousers with three inflatable bladders. The abdominal portion and each leg may be controlled individually. Until recently, it was thought that MAST use caused an autotransfusion of blood from the periphery to the central circulation by squeezing blood out of the capacitance vessels in the legs and abdomen. However, recent data demonstrate that only a minimal autotransfusion, to 4 ml/kg, occurs with inflation of the MAST suit.[8, 15, 50, 54, 66] The primary mechanism for the maintenance of central blood pressure with the use of the MAST suit is by decreasing the size of the perfused vascular bed and by increasing total peripheral resistance. Other beneficial effects of the MAST suit in trauma patients are hemostasis in vessels under the garment and stabilization of fractures. MAST treatment may also have utility in the early resuscitation of patients with septic shock, neurogenic shock, and hypotension secondary to vasodilators. Contraindications to use of the MAST suit include pulmonary edema, pregnancy, and tension pneumothorax. Proper application and removal of the garment are critical.[50]

If the volume lost includes RBCs, they may be replaced with packed RBCs or whole blood. With prolonged blood bank storage, RBCs lose their ability to transport oxygen.[25] This is thought to be due to progressive depletion of intracellular 2,3-diphosphoglyceric acid (DPG) and ATP. These effects may be clinically significant in

blood preserved with acid-citrate-dextrose for 3 weeks and after a slightly longer time in blood preserved with citrate-phosphate-dextrose. The low ATP levels increase RBC fragility and decrease their deformability. The low 2,3-DPG levels increase RBC affinity for oxygen, decreasing oxygen release in the capillary. After transfusion, RBC 2,3-DPG levels return to normal in 6–24 hours.

How much blood and crystalloid solution are necessary for adequate volume replacement? Restoring normal tissue perfusion, rather than simply maintaining an adequate blood pressure, should be emphasized. Because the body's homeostatic mechanisms keep systemic arterial pressure constant over a wide range of flow, a patient may not become hypotensive in the supine position until approximately 25%–30% of the blood volume has been lost. Thus, if one used only blood pressure as an index of volume resuscitation, inadequate amounts of volume would be given. More appropriate clinical indicators of adequate fluid resuscitation include a good urine output (0.5–1.0 ml/kg/hr), normal heart rate, brisk capillary refill, and normal sensorium, in addition to restoration of blood pressure. Normal organ system function is a more reliable sign of adequate resuscitation than are normal hemodynamic indices alone.

Central (cardiac) filling pressures are often used as end points in volume resuscitation. Several recent studies have indicated that central filling pressures, specifically central venous pressure (CVP) and the pulmonary artery occlusion pressure (wedge pressure, WP) may not reliably predict preload in critically ill patients. Furthermore, a study by McNamara et al. found that direct measurements of left atrial pressure (LAP) may not even reliably indicate optimal fluid resuscitation in hemorrhagic shock. When sufficient volume was given to baboons in hemorrhagic shock to return LAP to baseline, large volumes of crystalloid solution were required and resulted in equally large urinary output.[14, 16, 17, 53, 78, 79] Furthermore, fluid resuscitation to either a normal blood pressure or normal LAP did not restore blood volume to normal 18 hours after shock.[62] Thus, the vasoconstrictive and inotropic reflex mechanisms that protect the organism during shock are still in effect 18 hours after "adequate" resuscitation. Since LAP may not be a reliable index of adequate resuscitation in shock, it is not surprising that WP is also a poor predictor of intravascular volume status in critically ill patients. Because hemodynamic monitoring is unreliable in the management of patients in shock, monitoring some metabolic functional index might be beneficial. Oxygen consumption,[85] tissue pH,[10, 51, 55] transmembrane potential difference,[81] or transcutaneous oxygen content are such variables that are being investigated. Currently, adequate urine output, clear sensorium, adequate capillary filling, and normal heart rate remain our most reliable indices.

The hematocrit does not indicate the volume status of the patient. It is merely an indication of the balance between RBCs and nonsanguinous fluid in the vascular space. Enough RBC mass must be present to optimize oxygen delivery. However, if the hematocrit is too high ($> 45\%$) with a resultant increase in viscosity, resistance to flow increases. A hematocrit lower than 30% decreases oxygen delivery substantially and increases patient mortality. Thus, the optimal hematocrit is probably between 30% and 45%.[30] Optimal hematocrit was discussed in further detail in chapter 1, "Oxygen Transport: The Model and Reality."

Dilutional thrombocytopenia is commonly seen after massive blood replacement and is roughly proportional to the volume of RBCs infused.[60] In the actively bleeding patient, a platelet count of more than 50,000–100,000/mm^3 is needed to control bleeding. A count of 20,000/mm^3 is usually sufficient once bleeding has been controlled. Thus platelet transfusion may be required in the hemorrhagic patient if massive quantities of blood products are given. Levels of factors V and VIII correlate poorly with the volume of blood transfused.[26, 60] Thus, unless coagulation times are prolonged, transfusion of fresh frozen plasma is not indicated. Coagulation times should be checked after approximately every ten units of RBCs infused. Besides dilutional thrombocytopenia, the complications of massive blood replacement include altered oxygen transport (low 2,3-DPG and ATP levels), hypothermia, hyperkalemia, citrate intoxication, transfusion incompatibility, and acidosis.[25, 26, 60, 61, 74, 90]

Studies have shown that infusion of asanguinous fluid, in addition to RBCs, is necessary for maximal survival after hemorrhagic shock. The basic choice of nonsanguinous fluid is between a crystalloid solution and a colloid solution—a choice that has generated considerable comment.

The premise for giving albumin-containing solutions is based on the Starling equation and presumes that with the increase in plasma colloid osmotic pressure (PCOP) caused by albumin infusion, fluid will be drawn from the interstitium, particularly within the lung. This should make resuscitation more effective with fewer pulmonary complications.[38, 40, 86, 96] Two assumptions are implicit here: first, that the alveolar capillary membrane is impermeable to albumin, and second, that there is no mechanism for rapid removal of albumin from the lung interstitium. However, the albumin content in the lung interstitium may be 70% of that in plasma.[44, 93] Thus, changes in PCOP cause little change in the osmotic gradient between the lung interstitium and the capillary. Also, under normal conditions the pulmonary lymphatics efficiently clear albumin and fluid from the lung interstitium.[41, 44, 93] Interstitial fluid formation must increase about tenfold before this lymphatic system is overwhelmed and pulmonary edema results.[32, 44] Animal studies have shown that the hypoproteinemia that occurs with crystalloid volume resuscitation is usually compensated for by a transient increase in lung lymph flow and decrease in the protein content of the pulmonary interstitium that return to baseline within 4 hours of volume resuscitation.[32, 44] Furthermore, reducing the PCOP to 25% of normal will not result in pulmonary edema if normal filling pressures are maintained.[98] Hypoproteinemia alone does not lead to pulmonary edema.[32, 44, 93] Although it is likely that low PCOP may contribute to an increase in lung water when hydrostatic pressure is high, the use of colloid (beyond that given with RBCs) for acute volume replacement or resuscitation has never been shown in a controlled study to be beneficial, and the 20-fold increase in cost of colloid solutions argues against their routine use.[57, 65] Independent of the type of fluid administered, if the infusion is rapid enough, the LV will dilate and filling pressure will transiently increase.[71] In the setting of increased capillary permeability, this may lead to the development of pulmonary edema.[71] This will be true even when the total volume administered is not excessive. Thus, although the volume and rate of fluid administration must be sufficient to restore circulation, an excess of either may be detrimental.

Clinical studies in trauma patients or patients undergoing aortic reconstructive surgery indicate that successful volume resuscitation can be achieved with crystalloid or colloid solution in addition to packed RBCs.[84, 88, 94] Pulmonary function tests in trauma patients studied for 5 days after injury were identical for crystalloid- and colloid-treated groups.[65] In patients undergoing aortic surgery, either blood plus lactated Ringer's solution or blood plus colloid restored cardiac indices.[84, 94] Intrapulmonary shunt fraction, compliance, need for ventilatory support, and extravascular lung water (EVLW) measurements were similar for the two groups. These and other studies found no correlation between the PCOP-WP gradient and EVLW, shunt fraction, or any other pulmonary index.[84, 93, 94] Elevated filling pressure dictated the development of pulmonary dysfunction. Thus, in hemorrhagic shock, successful resuscitation may be achieved with RBCs plus salt solution or RBCs plus colloid solution.

ADJUVANT STUDIES

The key to successful resuscitation in hemorrhagic shock is early and adequate volume repletion. This may avoid progressive organ dysfunction and microcirculatory changes that lead to irreversible injury. Adjuvant treatments have been reported for hemorrhagic shock. However, these agents should not be given in lieu of appropriate volume resuscitation. Many experimental studies in particular have used adjuvant treatments of hemorrhagic shock in animals without first adequately restoring volume. The clinical significance of such studies is difficult to interpret.

Several studies have advocated the administration of steroids in the treatment of hemorrhagic shock.[1, 59, 73, 92] The ability of steroids to stabilize lysosomal membranes and their positive effects on cardiac output may be beneficial. However, the evidence for the efficacy of steroids in the treatment of hemorrhagic shock is inconclusive at best.

Cellular energy depletion has been proposed as a component of cellular failure in prolonged hemorrhagic shock. Several studies have reported beneficial effects from the administration of ATP–magnesium chloride (ATP-MgCl$_2$) in hemorrhagic shock.[22, 52] However, amelioration of cell membrane dysfunction in hemorrhagic shock was not found in animals given ATP-MgCl$_2$.[69, 77] Furthermore, ATP was found to rapidly degrade in whole blood.[69, 77] Thus, its suggested benefit

in preservation of cell function by increasing energy substrates available to the cells has not been supported.

Endorphins are released from the CNS during hemorrhagic shock. They may have an important role in the pathophysiology of hemorrhagic shock. Elevated levels of endorphins have been found in various shock states.[39, 43, 76] Improved survival has been reported following the administration of naloxone, a β-endorphin inhibitor. A study by Albert et al.[2] found that maintenance of cellular function and hemodynamics were improved when naloxone was given to rats in hemorrhagic shock. The beneficial cellular effect seemed to be independent of naloxone's beneficial effect on the circulation. Furthermore, Gurll et al.[39] have demonstrated that naloxone has a dose-dependent effect in the treatment of hemorrhagic shock.

Prostaglandins play a role in the pathophysiology of hemorrhagic shock.[45, 59] Some of their interactions have been discussed in detail in chapter 9, "Role of Prostacyclin, Thromboxane A$_2$, and Leukotrienes in Cardiovascular Function and Disease." Elevated thromboxane A$_2$ (TXA$_2$) levels have been reported in various shock states.[45] The actions of TXA$_2$ include vasoconstriction, breakdown of lysosomes, and platelet aggregation. A study by Hock and Lefer[45] demonstrated that administration of a thromboxane synthetase inhibitor in hemorrhagic shock depressed levels of TXA$_2$, maintained mean arterial pressure, and prolonged survival time in rats.

All these agents (naloxone, steroids, prostaglandin inhibitors) are still experimental and at best only adjuvant measures in the treatment of hemorrhagic shock. Models used to assess their benefit should include volume resuscitation if they are to have clinical relevance. The primary basis of successful treatment in hypovolemic shock is aggressive and appropriate volume replacement. There is no substitute for it. The end points of resuscitation are improved organ and tissue function, not simply restoration of blood pressure or central filling pressure.

REFERENCES

1. Abel FL: Effects of glucocorticoids on ventricular performances and capillary permeability during hemorrhagic shock. *Circ Shock* 1977; 4:345.
2. Albert SA, Shires GT III, Illner H, et al: Effects of naloxone in hemorrhagic shock. *Surg Gynecol Obstet* 1982; 155:326.

3. Alyono E, Ring WS, Chao RYN, et al: Characteristics of ventricular function in severe hemorrhagic shock. *Surgery* 1983; 94:250.

4. Amundson B, Haljamae H: Skeletal muscle metabolites as possible indicators of imminent death in acute hemorrhage. *Eur Surg Res* 1976; 8:311.

5. Amundson B, Jennische E, Haljamae H: Correlative analysis of microcirculatory and cellular metabolic events in skeletal muscle during hemorrhagic shock. *Acta Physiol Scand* 1980; 108:147.

6. Archie JP, Mertz WR: Myocardial oxygen delivery after experimental hemorrhagic shock. *Ann Surg* 1978; 187:205.

7. Bellamy RF, Pederson DC, DeGuzman LR: Organ blood flow and the cause of death following massive hemorrhage. *Circ Shock* 1984; 14:113.

8. Bivins H, Knopp R, Tiernan C, et al: Blood volume displacement with inflation of anti-shock trousers. *Ann Emerg Med* 1982; 11:409.

9. Blalock A: *Principles of Surgical Care, Shock and Other Problems*. St Louis, CV Mosby Co, 1940.

10. Bond RF, Manning ES, Peissner LC: Skeletal muscle pH, O_2, CO_2, and electrolyte balance during hemorrhagic shock. *Circ Shock* 1977; 4:115.

11. Bond RF, Green HD: Peripheral circulation, in Altura BM, Lefer AM, Schumer W (eds): *Handbook of Shock and Trauma*. Vol 1: *Basic Science*. New York, Raven Press, 1983, pp 29–49.

12. Bond RF, Johnson G III: Cardiovascular adrenoreceptor function during compensatory and decompensatory hemorrhagic shock. *Circ Shock* 1984; 12:9.

13. Bond RF, Johnson G III: Vascular adrenergic interactions during hemorrhagic shock. *Fed Proc* 1985; 44:281.

14. Brisman R, Parks LC, Benson DW: Pitfalls in the clinical use of central venous pressure. *Arch Surg* 1967; 95:902.

15. Burchard KW, Zippe C, Gann DS: Trendelenburg versus PASG application in hemorrhagic hypoperfusion, in *Program of the American Association for the Surgery of Trauma*, 1984, p 46.

16. Calvin JE, Driedger AA, Sibbald WJ: The hemodynamic effect of rapid fluid infusion in critically ill patients. *Surgery* 1981; 90:61.

17. Calvin JE, Driedger AA, Sibbald WJ, et al: Does the pulmonary capillary wedge pressure predict left ventricular preload in critically ill patients? *Crit Care Med* 1981; 9:437.

18. Campion DS, Lynch LJ, Rector FC Jr, et al: Effect of hemorrhagic shock on transmembrane potential. *Surgery* 1969; 66:1051.

19. Carey LC, Lowery BD, Cloutier CT: Blood sugar and insulin response in humans in shock. *Ann Surg* 1970; 172:342.

20. Cerchio GM, Moss GS, Popovich PA, et al: Serum insulin and growth hormone response to hemorrhagic shock. *Endocrinology* 1971; 88:138.

21. Chaudry EH, Sayeed MM, Bane AE: Alterations in adenosine nucleotides in hemorrhagic shock. *Surg Forum* 1972; 23:1.

22. Chaudry IH, Sayeed MM, Baue AE: Depletion and restoration of tissue ATP in hemorrhagic shock. *Arch Surg* 1974; 108:208.

23. Chien S: Role of the sympathetic nervous system in hemorrhage. *Physiol Rev* 1967; 47:214.

24. Civetta JM: A new look at the Starling equation. *Crit Care Med* 1979; 7:84.

25. Collins JA: Problems associated with the massive transfusion of stored blood. *Surgery* 1974; 75:274.

26. Counts RB, Haisch C, Simon TL, et al: Hemostasis in massively transfused trauma patients. *Ann Surg* 1979; 190:91.

27. Cryer HM, Kaebnick H, Harris PD, et al: Effects of tissue acidosis on skeletal muscle microcirculatory responses to hemorrhagic shock in unanesthetized rats, in *Program of the Association for Academic Surgery*, 1984, p 43.

28. Cunningham JN Jr, Shires GT, Wagner Y: Cellular transport defects in hemorrhagic shock. *Surgery* 1971; 70:215.

29. Cunningham JN Jr, Shires GT, Wagner Y: Changes in intracellular sodium and potassium content of red blood cells in trauma and shock. *Am J Surg* 1971; 122:650.

30. Czer LSC, Shoemaker WC: Optional hematocrit value in critically ill postoperative patients. *Surg Gynecol Obstet* 1978; 147:363.

31. Davis JM, Stevens JM, Peitzman AB, et al: Neutrophil migratory activity in severe hemorrhagic shock. *Circ Shock* 1983; 10:199.

32. Demling RH: Correlation of changes in body weight and pulmonary vascular pressures with lung water accumulation during fluid overload. *Crit Care Med* 1979; 7:153.

33. Downing SW: The heart in shock, in Altura BM, Lefer AM, Schumer W (eds): *Handbook of Shock and Trauma*. New York, Raven Press, 1983, vol 1, pp 1–18.

34. Drucker MR, Pindyck F, Brown RS, et al: The interaction of glucagon and glucose on cardiorespiratory variables in the critically ill patient. *Surgery* 1974; 75:487.

35. Flint LM, Cryer HM, Simpson CJ, et al: Microcirculatory norepinephrine constriction response in hemorrhagic shock. *Surgery* 1984; 96:240.

36. Gann DS: Endocrine and metabolic responses to injury, in Schwartz SI (ed): *Principles of Surgery*. New York, McGraw-Hill Book Co, 1984, pp 1–44.

37. George BC, Ryan NT, Ullrick WC, et al: Persisting structural abnormalities in liver, kidney, and muscle tissues following hemorrhagic shock. *Arch Surg* 1978; 113:289.

38. Granger DN, Gabel JC, Drake RE, et al: Physiologic basis for the clinical use of albumin solutions. *Surg Gynecol Obstet* 1978; 146:97.

39. Gurll NJ, Vargish T, Reynolds DG, et al: Opiate receptors and endorphins in the pathophysiology of hemorrhagic shock. *Surgery* 1981; 89:364.

40. Guyton AC, Lindsey AW: Effect of elevated left atrial pressure and decreased plasma protein concentration on the development of pulmonary edema. *Circ Res* 1959; 7:649.

41. Guyton AC: *Textbook of Medical Physiology*. Philadelphia, WB Saunders Co, 1981.

42. Haljamae H: "Hidden" cellular electrolyte responses to hemorrhagic shock and their significance. *Rev Surg* 1970; 27:315.

43. Handal KA, Schauben JL, Salamone FR: Naloxone. *Ann Emerg Med* 1983; 12:438.

44. Harms BA, Kramer GC, Bodai BI, et al: Effect of hypoproteinemia on pulmonary and soft tissue edema formation. *Crit Care Med* 1981; 9:503.

45. Hock CE, Lefer AM: Beneficial effect of a thromboxane synthetase inhibitor in traumatic shock. *Circ Shock* 1984; 14:159.

46. Holcroft JW: Impairment of venous return in hemorrhagic shock. *Surg Clin North Am* 1982; 62:17.

47. Holden WD, DePalma RG, Drucker WR, et al: Ultrastructural changes in hemorrhagic shock: Electron microscopic study of liver, kidney, and striated muscle cells in rats. *Ann Surg* 1965; 162:517.

48. Hutchins PM, Goldstone J, Wells R: Effects of hemorrhagic shock on the microvasculature of skeletal muscle. *Microvasc Res* 1973; 5:131.

49. Illner HP, Cunningham JN Jr, Shires GT: Red blood cell sodium content and permeability changes in hemorrhagic shock. *Am J Surg* 1982; 143:349.

50. Kaback KR, Sanders AB, Meislin HW: MAST suit update. *JAMA* 1984; 252:2598.

51. Kost GJ: Surface pH of the medial gastrocnemius and soleus muscles during hemorrhagic shock and ischemia. *Surgery* 1984; 95:183.

52. Kraven TB, Rush BF Jr, Ghosh A, et al: Improved survival and metabolic changes in rat shock model produced by ATP-MgCl$_2$. *Curr Surg* 1979; 36:435.

53. Ledgerwood AM, Lucas CE: Postresuscitation hypertension: Etiology, morbidity and treatment. *Arch Surg* 1974; 108:531.

54. Lee H, Blank W, Massion W, et al: Venous return in hemorrhagic shock after application of military antishock trousers. *Am J Emerg Med* 1983; 1:7.

55. Lemiux MD, Smith RN, Couch NP, et al: Surface pH and redox potential of skeletal muscle in graded hemorrhage. *Surgery* 1969; 65:457.

56. Lindberg B, Haljamae H, Jonsson O, et al: Effect of glucagon and blood transfusion on liver metabolism in hemorrhagic shock. *Ann Surg* 1978; 187:103.

57. Lowe RJ, Moss GS, Jilek J, et al: Crystalloid vs colloid in the etiology of pulmonary failure after trauma: A randomized trial in man. *Surgery* 1977; 81:676.

58. MacDonald JAE, Milligan GF, Mellon A, et al: Ventricular function in experimental hemorrhagic shock. *Surg Gynecol Obstet* 1975; 140:572.

59. Machiedo GW, Rush BF Jr: Comparison of corticosteroids and prostaglandins in treatment of hemorrhagic shock. *Ann Surg* 1979; 190:735.

60. Maier RV: The consequences of massive blood transfusion. *Surg Rounds* 1984; 7:57.

61. McClellan B, Reid R, Lane P: Massive blood transfusion causing hypomagnesemia. *Crit Care Med* 1984; 12:146.

62. McNamara JJ, Suehiro GT, Suehiro A, et al: Resuscitation from hemorrhagic shock. *J Trauma* 1983; 23:552.

63. Merin G, Eimerl D, Raz S, et al: Preservation of myocardial contractility in hemorrhagic shock with methylprednisolone. *Ann Thorac Surg* 1978; 25:536.

64. Middleton ES, Mathews R, Shires GT: Radio-

sulphate as a measure of the extracellular fluid in acute hemorrhagic shock. *Ann Surg* 1969; 170:174.

65. Moss GS, Lowe RJ, Jilek J, et al: Colloid or crystalloid in the resuscitation of hemorrhagic shock: A controlled clinical study. *Surgery* 1981; 89:434.

66. Niemann J, Stapczynski S, Rosborough J, et al: Hemodynamic effects on pneumatic external counterpressure in canine hemorrhagic shock. *Ann Emerg Med* 1983; 12:661.

67. Pass LJ, Schloerb PR, Chow FT, et al: Liver adenosine triphosphate (ATP) in hypoxia and hemorrhagic shock. *J Trauma* 1982; 22:730.

68. Peitzman AB, Corbett WA, Illner H, et al: Correlation of transmembrane potential with high energy phosphate levels in hemorrhagic shock in primates. *Surg Forum* 1980; 31:5.

69. Peitzman AB, Shires GT III, Illner H, et al: Effect of intravenous ATP-MgCl₂ on cellular function in liver and muscle in hemorrhagic shock. *Curr Surg* 1981; 38:300.

70. Peitzman AB, Corbett WA, Shires GT III, et al: Cellular function in liver and muscle during hemorrhagic shock in primates. *Surg Gynecol Obstet* 1985; 161:419.

71. Peters RM, Hogan JS: Mechanism of death in massive fluid infusion. *J Trauma* 1980; 20:452.

72. Peters RM, Hargens AR: Protein vs. electrolytes and all of the Starling forces. *Arch Surg* 1981; 116:1293.

73. Pinilla J, Wright CJ: Steroids and severe hemorrhagic shock. *Surgery* 1977; 82:489.

74. Robinson NB, Heimback DM: Ventilation and perfusion alterations following homologous blood transfusion. *Surgery* 1982; 92:183.

75. Russel RCG, Pardy BJ, Carruthers ME, et al: Plasma glucagon levels in haemorrhagic shock. *Br J Surg* 1977; 64:285.

76. Salerno TA, Milne B, Jhamandas KH: Hemodynamic effects of naloxone in hemorrhagic shock in pigs. *Surg Gynecol Obstet* 1981; 152:773.

77. Schloeb PR, Sieracki L, Botwin AJ, et al: Intravenous adenosine triphosphate (ATP) in hemorrhagic shock in rats. *Am J Physiol* 1981; 240:R52.

78. Sheldon CA, Balik E, Dhanalal D, et al: Peripheral postcapillary venous pressure: A new hemodynamic monitoring parameter. *Surgery* 1982; 92:663.

79. Sheldon CA, Cerra FB, Bohnhoff N, et al: Pe-

ripheral postcapillary venous pressure: A new, more sensitive monitor of effective blood volume during hemorrhagic shock. *Surgery* 1983; 94:379.

80. Shires T, Coln D, Carrico J, et al: Fluid therapy in hemorrhagic shock. *Arch Surg* 1964; 88:688.

81. Shires GT, Cunningham JN, Baker CRF, et al: Alterations in cellular membrane function during hemorrhagic shock in primates. *Ann Surg* 1972; 176:288.

82. Shires GT, Carrico CJ, Canizaro PC: *Shock*. Philadelphia, WB Saunders Co, 1973.

83. Shires GT III, Peitzman AB, Illner H, et al: Change in red blood cell transmembrane potential in hemorrhagic shock. *Surg Forum* 1981; 32:5.

84. Shires GT III, Peitzman AB, Albert SA, et al: Response of extravascular lung water to intraoperative fluids. *Ann Surg* 1983; 197:515.

85. Shoemaker WC, Lim L, Boyd DR, et al: Sequential hemodynamic events after trauma to the unanesthetized patient. *Surg Gynecol Obstet* 1971; 132:651.

86. Shoemaker WC, Hauser CJ: Critique of crystalloid versus colloid therapy in shock and shock lung. *Crit Care Med* 1979; 7:117.

87. Sibbald WJ, Patterson N, Holliday R, et al: The Trendelenburg position: Hemodynamic effects in hypotensive and normotensive patients. *Crit Care Med* 1979; 7:218.

88. Skillman JJ, Restall DS, Salzman EW: Randomized trial of albumin vs electrolyte solutions during abdominal aortic operations. *Surgery* 1975; 78:291.

89. Snyder JV, Carroll GC: Tissue oxygenation: A physiologic approach to a clinical problem. *Curr Probl Surg* 1982, vol 19.

90. Sohmer P, Dawson B: Transfusion therapy in trauma: A review of the principles and techniques used in the MIEMS program. *Ann Surg* 1979; 45:109.

91. Sweadner KJ, Goldin SM: Active transport of sodium and potassium ions. *N Engl J Med* 1980; 302:777.

92. Trachte GJ, Lefer AM: Preservation of cellular integrity as a protective mechanism of dexamethasone in hemorrhagic shock. *Arch Int Pharmacodyn* 1978; 232:309.

93. Tranbaugh RF, Lewis FR: Mechanisms and etiologic factors of pulmonary edema. *Surg Gynecol Obstet* 1984; 158:193.

94. Virgilio RW, Rice CL, Smith DE, et al: Crys-

talloid vs. colloid resuscitation: Is one better? *Surgery* 1979; 85:129.

95. Weil MH: Current understanding of the mechanisms and treatment of circulatory shock caused by bacterial infections. *Ann Clin Res* 1977; 9:181.

96. Weil MH, Henning RJ, Puri VK: Colloid oncotic pressure: Clinical significance. *Crit Care Med* 1979; 7:113.

97. Wiggers CJ: The present status of the shock problem. *Physiol Rev* 1942; 22:74.

98. Zarins CK, Rice CL, Peters PM, et al: Lymph and pulmonary response to isobaric reduction in plasma oncotic pressure in baboons. *Circ Res* 1978; 43:925.

28

Pathophysiology and Treatment of Septic Shock

Andrew Peitzman, M.D.

Michael R. Pinsky, M.D.

James V. Snyder, M.D.

Fulminant sepsis is a major cause of mortality in intensive care unit (ICU) patients.[3, 49, 58, 85, 92, 94, 135, 145] Its clinical expression is that of septic shock. Septic shock is usually due to gram-negative or gram-positive bacteria, but it may be caused by fungi, viruses, parasites, or rickettsia.[3, 135, 148] Many patients are presumed to have sepsis on clinical grounds when no organisms can be cultured from the bloodstream.[74, 85, 140] Over the past few years, presumably owing to the widespread use of antibiotics and the increased incidence of immunocompromised patients, the proportion of patients with septic shock due to gram-negative organisms has increased.[3, 145] Despite major advances in physiologic monitoring and antibiotic chemotherapy, the mortality from septic shock remains 50%–70%.[3, 49, 85, 92, 135, 145, 148] Patients who ultimately succumb to sepsis rarely do so during the clinical episode of hypotension. Most die later after recurrent bouts of sepsis have progressed to the syndrome of multiple system organ failure.[12, 41, 49, 94, 128] Accordingly, sepsis is the most frequent cause of adult respiratory distress syndrome (ARDS).[46, 71, 145]

Septic shock presents in many forms. Commonly a patient in septic shock may be seen initially with hypotension, high cardiac output, warm skin, altered mental status, and respiratory alkalosis. This hyperdynamic condition is the classic presentation of sepsis. However, many septic patients have low cardiac output and signs of vasoconstriction (hypodynamic sepsis) indistinguishable from hypovolemic shock. It appears that these two presentations represent a continuum of disease, with the modifying variables being intravascular volume status and peripheral vasomotor tone, since the hypodynamic state is commonly seen when intravascular volume is inadequate[24] and also late in the course when therapy has failed and peripheral vascular tone is lost.[72] We will review the various experimental models used in the study of septic shock and their relevance, and then discuss current therapeutic options.

EXPERIMENTAL MODELS

Experimental animal models of sepsis have helped our understanding of the mechanisms involved in septic shock in humans, but direct extrapolation to human sepsis is difficult. The primary difficulties involved in interpreting results from animal models are species differences in response to sepsis, the unclear role of endotoxin in the development of septic shock,[62, 118, 127, 149] and the lack of appropriate volume resuscitation in models assessing treatments.

Species differences in the response to endotoxic shock are important in understanding the results from different animal models. Infusion of endotoxin in dogs causes splanchnic pooling of blood from hepatic venous constriction and a prompt reduction in cardiac output[17, 82, 135] that does not occur in other species.[17, 62, 82] Endotoxemia in humans may produce (1) no reaction, (2) an increase in cardiac output and vasodilation, or (3) vasoconstriction with fever.[135]

Although septic shock may present as a hyperdynamic, hypotensive circulatory derangement (hyperdynamic sepsis), most animal models of sepsis induced by intravenous (IV) infusion of live gram-negative bacteria generally result in hypodynamic sepsis. Previous studies have demonstrated that both the total dose of bacteria and the rate of infusion affect the cardiovascular response in these animal models.* A rapid injection of a large bolus of live bacteria usually results in the rapid development of cardiovascular collapse and death. However, infusion of up to 400 times this lethal dose (LD_{100} dose) of *E. coli* into monkeys pretreated with large volume expansion only reduced cardiac output from high to near-normal levels.[24] If intravascular volume is adequate, slower infusions of bacteria can result in a hemodynamic state similar to human hyperdynamic sepsis.[24, 50, 67, 83, 118, 123]

Gahhos et al. proposed that a nidus of infection was the key to developing hyperdynamic sepsis.[50] Presumably such a nidus would cause intermittent episodes of moderate bacteremia with which the patient's immune system could initially cope. Later, with repeated episodes of bacteremia, exhaustion of the immune defense mechanisms would result in tissue dysfunction, including cardiac depression, leading to a hypodynamic state. Studies in experimental models more closely mimicking human experience have been reported.[16, 149, 151] Numerous models of intraperitoneal sepsis have been studied. Intraperitoneal instillation of either feces[83, 144] or cultured organisms[44, 84] often results in minimal systemic response. Ligation of the biliary tract can result in hyperdynamic sepsis.[33, 113] Cecal ligation and perforation cause a predictable septic hemodynamic response that has been extensively studied.[7, 26, 51, 149] However, many of these studies have not adequately controlled for changes in intravascular volume or vascular capacitance, and the similarity of sepsis so induced to clinical sepsis remains unclear. Unlike hemorrhagic shock, septic shock is not a static event with a known start and progression. Thus, despite similar methods, studies often do not generate the same degree of shock. To date, no one model of septic shock stands out for its ability to duplicate human sepsis.

FACTORS PREDISPOSING TO SEPSIS

Many factors predispose to the development of septic shock. The extremes of age, the use of broad-spectrum antibiotics, better early care of

---

*References 4, 15, 24, 65, 67, 116–118, and 133.

multiple trauma patients, and wider use of immunosuppression all increase the incidence of sepsis.[3, 4, 27, 35, 66, 78, 126, 145]

The immune system is central in the prevention and reversal of sepsis. The components of the immune system include circulatory cellular and humoral factors, such as white blood cells, complement, and immunoglobins, as well as fixed tissue factors, such as local monocytes and macrophages and the reticuloendothelium system (RES). Drug-induced suppression of the immune system increases the likelihood of sepsis.[4, 91, 126] Patients receiving chemotherapy, patients with acquired immunodeficiency syndrome (AIDS), and transplantation patients receiving immunosuppression therapy are at increased risk of developing sepsis.[66, 91, 108, 126, 148] Not only are these patients more susceptible to infection, but diagnosis and successful treatment are much more difficult in the immunosuppressed patient population.

Reticuloendothelial System

Decreased effectiveness of the immune system is a common condition in patients predisposed to sepsis.[4, 27, 66, 78, 91, 98, 99, 126, 142] The RES is a major arm of the immune system. The RES functions to clear the blood of bacteria, platelet aggregates, and other particulate matter. This function is impaired after trauma, burns, and sepsis.[35, 84, 91, 98, 128, 129, 131, 132] Septic animals and patients with impaired RES function are more likely to die.[84, 91, 98, 102, 128, 129, 131, 132]

The RES can be overwhelmed in previously healthy patients by physiologic stress. For example, RES function is depressed after trauma, burns, and fluorocarbon or lipid infusion. In patients with liver disease, uremia, diabetes mellitus, old age, starvation, or malignancies RES function is also impaired.[3, 4, 9, 27, 102, 103, 145, 148] The spleen functions as a reticuloendothelial filter, clearing bacteria and debris from the circulation.[40] Previous splenectomy predisposes to overwhelming septicemia.[40] If RES function is impaired, there is decreased clearance of bacterial and antigenic material, and the ability of the host to neutralize toxins from the bloodstream is decreased. Normal homeostasis is impaired and there is increased release of lysosomal enzymes with resulting cellular destruction, and abnormal vascular tone and vasomotion.[4, 6] Besides being a prognosticator of the patient's response to sepsis, RES function can be used as a diagnostic index of sepsis.[129] Once RES integrity is lost, all tissues can be exposed to the toxic effects of the circulatory products of sepsis.[41, 49, 71, 74, 85, 94, 128] Thus, RES exhaustion may be pivotal in the development of overwhelming sepsis and multiple organ failure, including ARDS.

Normal RES function requires sufficient levels of circulating fibronectin. Fibronectin is an opsonin that binds to circulating particles, facilitating their uptake and removal by the RES. Saba and co-authors have found fibronectin deficiency in burn and trauma patients to be important in their predisposition to sepsis.[84, 128, 129, 131, 132] Adequate RES function has been proposed as a critical determinant of host survival in sepsis.[84, 128, 129, 131, 132] The difference between lethal and sublethal injections of live organisms in experimental animal models may depend on the degree to which the RES can clear these organisms. In support of this hypothesis, Coalson et al.[30] have demonstrated that after sublethal and lethal sepsis in primates induced by live *E. coli* infusion, the Kupffer (RE) cells contain massive amounts of bacteria. Since bacterial phagocytosis by Kupffer cells is limited, massive or persistent bacteremia may exhaust the RES. Thus, RES exhaustion may precede fulminant sepsis. A similar mechanism may be responsible for the development of multiple system organ failure or ARDS during sepsis. According to this hypothesis, as the RES is overwhelmed in fulminant sepsis, fewer bacteria, byproducts of infection and cellular debris may be cleared from the bloodstream. These products will progressively lodge in the capillary beds of the lungs, kidneys, and other organs. Local inflammation and toxin tissue damage may result, leading to the capillary leak syndrome of ARDS or to the generalized anasarca of sepsis, depending on which vascular beds are primarily affected.

Underlying Diseases

Certain systemic diseases may predispose to the development of infection by their associated impairment of the immune system.[3, 4, 135, 145] Patients with diabetes mellitus demonstrate abnormal neutrophil chemotaxis and impaired lymphocyte function.[4, 145] Their microvascular disease may impede the response of components of the immune system. Patients with malignancies have a depressed immune responsiveness greater than can be ascribed to their chemotherapeutic agents. Uremia also predisposes to infection.[4] Cirrhosis is a poor prognostic factor if associated with infection.[9, 104, 145] Patients with

multiple trauma or burns are more likely to develop infection.[84, 91, 98, 128, 129, 131, 132] Abnormal neutrophil chemotaxis has been reported in these patients, and depressed lymphocyte responsiveness may have a role in this patient population as well.[35, 78]

Other important immune system deficiency conditions include those associated with depressed neutrophil chemotaxis and blocking agents. For example, burn patients have elevated levels of suppressor lymphocytes with a reversed helper-to-suppressor ratio. On the basis of this observation, delayed hypersensitivity skin testing, as a marker of T lymphocyte function, was initially thought to be predictive of both sepsis and outcome in at-risk patients. Meakins et al.[27, 98] stated that anergy, or failure of delayed hypersensitivity reaction, was a marker for host resistance in surgical patients. Brown et al.[18] found a higher mortality in anergic surgical patients than in those with normal response. Unfortunately, the anergy usually followed, rather than preceded, the onset of major complications. Subsequent studies have suggested that responsiveness to skin antigens after injury is not useful in a quantitative or predictive sense,[4, 18, 78] However, recent data suggest that lymphocyte responsiveness may be used for serial monitoring of critically ill patients.[78]

Nutritional Factors

Nutritional factors may be important in the development of sepsis, primarily by the way in which they affect the immune system. Several investigators have found an association between malnutrition and anergy.[27, 145] Neutrophil chemotaxis may be abnormal in malnourished patients.[4, 145] Zinc deficiency and vitamin C deficiency suppress wound healing.[4, 145] Abnormal immune function occurs with deficiencies of phosphate, copper, iron, zinc, vitamin A, vitamin B_{12}, or pyridoxine.[4, 145] Although the precise role of nutritional repletion remains unclear, it now seems appropriate to attempt adequate nutritional support in all septic patients to minimize the role of malnutrition in the progression of sepsis.

PATHOPHYSIOLOGY OF SEPTIC SHOCK

The initiating mechanism of hemorrhagic shock is decreased blood volume resulting in depressed cardiac output and decreased organ perfusion.

Loss of vasoregulation is a late phenomenon related to prolonged inadequate tissue perfusion. In contrast, loss of autoregulation and tissue dysfunction occur early in septic shock and persist despite normal or supranormal cardiac output. Proposed mechanisms for the observed impairment of vasoregulation include histotoxicity, arteriovenous shunting, and vasoderegulation (see chapter 5, "Patterns of Hemodynamic Response"). Histotoxicity implies that, unlike the hypovolemic shock state, septic shock represents a primary cellular disease in which subsequent circulatory dysfunction occurs. Alternatively, the high cardiac output and organ dysfunction could be due to dysfunction of vasoregulatory mechanisms, such that the blood flow is not directed primarily to the metabolically active tissues.*

There is evidence for histotoxicity in the progression of septic shock.† Infusion of live *E. coli* in baboons results in a decline in skeletal muscle transmembrane potential difference (PD) prior to a significant fall in blood pressure.[112] Hepatocellular PD also declines, and abnormalities in liver function occur with normal or increased hepatic blood flow in early sepsis.[97, 99, 106, 112] The red blood cell (RBC) membrane, which is not dependent on a microcirculation for its energy requirements, also shows increased permeability early in *E. coli* sepsis.[136] These studies suggest that widespread cell dysfunction occurs prior to hypotension in septic shock and support the concept that histotoxicity may be a primary factor initiating organ dysfunction in sepsis despite a relatively high cardiac output. On the other hand, the infusion of large numbers of bacteria (up to 400 times the LD_{100}) into subhuman primates does not cause depression of oxygen consumption when cardiac output is kept above normal.[24] Therefore, sepsis can cause histotoxicity in the form of cell membrane changes and liver dysfunction, and it is possible that such changes can progress to the point of disturbing oxygen metabolism, but there is no evidence that oxygen consumption is depressed early in sepsis other than by disturbance of circulation.

The pathophysiology of the progression from hyperdynamic sepsis to hypodynamic sepsis remains unresolved. Several factors probably play a role in this transition, including relative hypovolemia, right ventricular dysfunction secondary to a transient increase in pulmonary vascular resistance, impaired left ventricular (LV) function, and resistance of the cardiovascular system to catecholamines.[22, 53, 81, 88, 116] The heart will eventually fail in all progressive forms of shock. In primate models of lethal bacterial sepsis, ventricular function is significantly depressed within 3–6 hours.[60]

A humoral myocardial depressant factor has been proposed as responsible for the fall in cardiac output seen in late sepsis.[22, 37, 53, 56, 87, 93, 96] Although these studies could not be duplicated in another laboratory,[59, 64] such a cardiodepressant factor has recently been isolated from septic humans.[109]

Resistance of the microcirculation to catecholamines has also been demonstrated.[8, 119] Such decreases in mean arterial pressure may decrease coronary blood flow as well.

Recent studies have indicated that circulatory disturbances such as arteriovenous shunting are not the cause of the small arteriovenous oxygen difference.[5, 16, 24, 45, 151] Using radiolabeled microspheres in a monkey model of live *E. coli* sepsis, Carroll and Snyder[24] demonstrated that there was no increase in systemic anatomical shunting when cardiac output was elevated. Wright et al.[151] found no abnormal arteriovenous shunting of blood in the skeletal muscle in a canine cecal ligation model, and found a strong correlation between the increase in cardiac output and muscle capillary blood flow.[151] Similarly, Archie[5] found that anatomical arteriovenous shunting was not the cause of the elevated cardiac output and decreased arteriovenous oxygen difference seen in sepsis. In a study of human sepsis,[45] [133]Xe was used to measure muscle capillary blood flow in high output sepsis.[45] Capillary blood flow increased in direct proportion to cardiac output. Thus, the dysfunction of shock appears to be due either to hypoperfusion of some capillary beds, with the high output state maintained by excessive perfusion of open capillaries, or to a generalized inability of the periphery to metabolize oxygen.

Furthermore, Carroll and Snyder found that except for an occasional transient change at the start of bacterial infusion, a hyperdynamic septic state could be achieved only with volume loading. Also, when a hyperdynamic state was induced by volume administration before infusion of bacteria, the introduction of bacteria always

---

*References 4–6, 16, 24, 45, 72, and 124.
†References 22, 26, 37, 52, 53, 56, 73, 87, 93, and 112.

depressed cardiac output. Therefore, the elevated cardiac output in their monkey model was not due to sepsis per se, but primarily reflected adequate intravascular volume in a stressed but vasodilated animal. Thal et al. also found that volume status was critical in septic shock.[147] They demonstrated that septic dogs quickly decompensated when minimal blood loss was superimposed on their sepsis. Thus, adequate venous return supported by volume loading seems mandatory in the development of hyperdynamic sepsis.

It appears that a primary circulatory derangement of sepsis is the loss of vasoregulation. As a result, areas of hyperperfusion and hypoperfusion may exist simultaneously and even in adjacent microvascular beds. Because severe dysfunction has not been shown to occur when perfusion is normal, the establishment of microvascular hypoperfusion seems a fundamental component of septic shock. Whether the patient survives or proceeds through organ dysfunction to death may depend on the persistence and extension of microcirculatory failure due to vasoderegulation, local toxic factors, enhanced coagulation, cell toxicity, and inadequate resuscitation. The reversal of this microcirculatory process may be critical in the management of sepsis.

ORGAN FAILURE IN SEPSIS

Presumably because of aggressive acute resuscitation, patients rarely die during the acute hypotensive episode of sepsis. Most patients who die do so subsequently of multiple system organ failure. Late mortality from septic shock is related to the number of organ systems involved (Table 28–1). The systems commonly involved are the lung, liver, kidney, gut, coagulation, and heart. Sepsis is the most frequent cause of both multiple organ system failure and ARDS.[12, 41, 49, 71, 94, 128, 145]

TABLE 28–1.

Mortality Associated With Organ System Failure*

NUMBER OF FAILED ORGAN SYSTEMS	% MORTALITY
1	30
2	60
3	85
4	100

*Data from Fry et al.[49]

TREATMENT

Operative Intervention

To date, the most effective way to reduce mortality from sepsis is to adequately treat the infection prior to the onset of septic shock. The mortality from septic shock remains more than 50%. For infections amenable to surgical drainage mortality is 50%, whereas only 23% of patients with infections not amenable to surgical drainage can be expected to survive.[92] In part this discrepancy represents different patient populations. Once shock occurs, if surgical drainage of the infectious source is possible, it becomes a critical component of therapy.

In the surgical ICU setting, the abdomen is the usual source of occult infection in a septic patient. Early reexploration should be undertaken in septic postoperative patients, sometimes without definitive localization of a source. These patients may have "soft" signs of sepsis without obvious localization: prolonged ileus, guaiac-positive nasogastric drainage, subtle CNS changes, or glucose intolerance.[58, 74, 85, 140] Computed tomography may be useful in localizing an intraabdominal abscess. Gallium scanning and sonography have been found to be less reliable in this application.[58, 140] In addition, multiple organism bacteremia, the development of ARDS, or multiple system organ failure in the ICU patient should alert the physician to the possibility of an intraabdominal source of infection.[74]

Fluid Resuscitation

During an episode of septic shock, volume resuscitation should be given to restore adequate blood flow as manifested by restoration of normal sensorium, blood pressure, heart rate, and urine output. However, urinary output is not as useful a monitor of fluid therapy as it is during treatment of hemorrhagic shock, because renal tubular injury related to sepsis can impair concentrating function and increase urine volume despite decreases in blood flow.[36, 123, 150] The pulmonary artery occlusion pressure (wedge pressure, WP) is often monitored to assess the adequacy of intravascular volume and cardiac function in critically ill patients. In septic patients, however, the WP is a poor predictor of LV preload.[1, 19, 20, 77, 86, 107, 110] This may be because of changes in LV diastolic compliance or an altered relation between WP and left atrial pressure in septic patients.[141]

Krausz et al.[81] evaluated the relation between central venous pressure (CVP) and WP during volume loading in patients who were septic but still had adequate urine output. When the initial CVP was higher than the WP, volume infusion increased blood pressure and cardiac output without significantly changing CVP, WP, or heart rate. When the initial WP was higher than the CVP, infusion of smaller volumes of fluid increased signs of fluid overload without elevating blood pressure or cardiac output. They suggest that when WP is less than CVP, fluid resuscitation should improve left heart filling, and, to the extent that decreased LV preload was responsible for the shock state, cardiovascular status should improve.

In another study of volume resuscitation in 28 critically ill patients, Calvin et al.[16] found that 20 patients responded to fluid infusion with an increase in stroke volume. This was secondary to an increase in LV end-diastolic volume in 11 and to an increase in LV ejection fraction in nine.[16] Stroke volume did not increase in eight patients. The response of a given patient to fluid challenge was not predictable before treatment. Thus, initial assessment of WP as an isolated value may not accurately predict the response to volume infusion. Different hemodynamic responses to volume infusion from similar WP could reflect differences in LV diastolic compliance, or contractility. Similarly, during sepsis the discrepancy between WP and LAP may increase.[123] Right ventricular function also may be important in the response to volume infusion, since sepsis often increases pulmonary vascular resistance and acute cor pulmonale may result.

Whether the patient presents in high or low output sepsis, immediate volume resuscitation is central to the management of these patients. Consideration of fluid overload should rarely take precedence over volume resuscitation.

Siegel, Shoemaker, and others have proposed that oxygen consumption ($\dot{V}O_2$) may be the critical end point in the volume resuscitation of critically ill patients.[65, 119, 120] A low $\dot{V}O_2$ is a poor prognostic sign, but is usually preceded by hemodynamic deterioration. However, increases in $\dot{V}O_2$ may be reliable indicators of appropriate resuscitative therapy in septic shock. Unfortunately, the measurement of a supranormal $\dot{V}O_2$ at a single point in time during sepsis does not correlate with survival.[1, 72]

Drug Therapy

Vasoactive and Inotropic Drugs

Volume expansion alone will improve the hemodynamic status of most septic patients. Addition of an inotropic agent may enhance hemodynamic performance at a lower WP.[29] Both dopamine and dobutamine have been shown to be effective in supporting the circulation in septic shock.[36, 75, 150] Dopamine may have a beneficial effect on renal function in septic patients, in addition to its systemic hemodynamic changes.[150] It is tempting to administer vasoactive drugs to septic patients, especially when they are hypotensive. Administration of vasoconstricting agents to enhance perfusion of the brain and heart may be necessary in acute hypotensive crises, but it compromises overall systemic perfusion.

Certain assumptions are implicit in the use of vasoactive agents in the treatment of septic shock. Giving vasoconstrictors to improve the distribution of systemic perfusion implies that the drugs will selectively affect the overperfused vessels and not those supplying ischemic tissue. Similarly, vasodilating agents are assumed to work selectively on hypoperfused vessels. Progress in our understanding of local differences in vascular receptors and drug response (see chapter 9, "Role of Prostacyclin, Thromboxane A_2, and Leukotrienes in Cardiovascular Function and Disease," and chapter 30, "Pharmacologic Manipulation of Regional Blood Flow") suggests that therapeutic control of this sort might be achievable in the future. However, there are currently no data to direct such specific vasoactive drug therapy. Table 28–2 lists guidelines for dilution and dosage of common vasoactive drugs. At the bedside, evaluation of the immediate (within minutes) response of oxygen consumption and oxygen transport to any vasoactive drug regimen may be useful in assessing the response of a patient to a specific agent (see chapter 5, "Patterns of Hemodynamic Response"). Increases in $\dot{V}O_2$ after a change in vasoactive drug therapy may be due to improved perfusion of ischemic tissue. The increase in $\dot{V}O_2$ also may be due to increased work and oxygen consumption by the heart, or may represent increased systemic oxygen consumption due to metabolic arousal, as from increased stress. Thus the isolated measurement of $\dot{V}O_2$ in the management of the septic patient is of limited value in assessing the adequacy of therapy.

TABLE 28–2.

Guidelines for Administration of Vasoactive Drugs*

DRUG	RECOMMENDED ROUTE OF ADMINISTRATION	DOSAGE RANGE	STANDARD SOLUTION	FLUID RESTRICTION SOLUTION
Sympathetic Amines				
Norepinephrine (Levophed)	Central line	2–16 μg/min	4 mg (1 ampule) in 500 ml D5W or D5NS (not NS); 8 μg/ml	8 mg in 500 ml D5W; 16 μg/ml
Epinephrine (various)	Central line	0.005–0.02 μg/kg/min for β effect, > 0.02 μg/kg/min for mixed α and β effect	1 mg (1 ml 1:1,000 solution) in 250 ml D5W; 4 μg/ml	
Dopamine† (various)	Central line	0.5–3 μg/kg/min for dilation of renal and mesenteric arteries; 5–12 μg/kg/min for increased cardiac contractility; > 20 μg/kg/min for potent vasoconstriction	200 mg (1 ampule) in 250 ml D5W; 800 μg/ml	400 mg in 250 ml D5W; 1,600 μg/ml
Isoproterenol (Isuprel)	Central line	0.5–8 μg/min	2 mg (2 ampules) in 500 ml D5W; 4 μg/ml	4 mg in 500 ml D5W; 8 μg/ml
Dobutamine (Dobutrex)	Central line	2.5–20 μg/kg/min	250 mg (1 ampule) in 250 ml D5W; 1,000 μg/ml	500 mg in 250 ml D5W; 2,000 μg/ml
Systemic Vasodilator				
Sodium nitroprusside‡ (Nipride)	Peripheral line	0.25–8 μg/kg/min	50 mg (1 vial) in 250 ml D5W *only*; 200 μg/ml	50 mg in 100 ml D5W; 500 μg/ml

*Modified from Pinsky,[115] by permission; original data by Marilyn Hravnak, R.N., Nursing Inservice Department, Presbyterian-University Hospital, University of Pittsburgh. D5W, 5% dextrose in water; NS, normal saline solution.
†Dopamine and dobutamine are compatible.
‡Must be protected from light. Effective for 4 hr from time of reconstitution.

Antibiotics

Since bacteremia often occurs in sepsis, and since organism-specific antibiotic therapy is associated with the least mortality in such patients, blood should be drawn for culture (even as IV access is obtained) in the septic patient. Urine and sputum likewise should be obtained for culture. The patient should be carefully examined for localizing signs of infection. Wounds should be examined and cultured. Changing an intravascular catheter over a wire to culture the tip is undesirable but is a practical recognition of limited vascular access, and the predicted resulting increase in infection ratio has not been shown.[13, 100] Changing central venous catheters over a guide wire was reported to reduce catheter-related sepsis from 11% to zero.[13] Cerebrospinal fluid may need to be examined for cells and bacteria if altered mental status or neurologic signs accom-

pany the septic state. Aggressive therapy requires that antibiotics be given before bacterial culture and sensitivity reports are available. Such antibiotic therapy should not be "blind" but rather should be based on the probable source of sepsis.[31, 103] Altemeier et al. have shown that mortality doubles when inappropriate antibiotics are used in septic patients.[3] The selection and dosage of antibiotics are emphasized in current practice, but drug timing and distribution may still be suboptimal.

Adjuvant Therapy in Sepsis

That minimal improvement in mortality results from any treatment regimen is testimony to our still inadequate understanding of the processes that lead to death from sepsis. Fluids, antibiotics, and elimination of any nidus of infection are not enough to ensure a favorable outcome. New and potentially effective experimental therapies are currently being studied. However, we do not yet recommend any for clinical practice.

Steroids. The use of steroids in sepsis was first supported by Schumer's clinical study in 1976.[130] He showed that improved survival was associated with the early use of steroids in septic shock. However, steroids have also been reported to be of no benefit, and they may actually increase mortality.[7, 30, 42] Lucas and Ledgerwood[90] showed in a clinical study of steroids in septic shock that steroids produced a transient cardiovascular benefit. However, intrapulmonary shunt fraction and $Pa_{O_2}/F_{I_{O_2}}$ ratio deteriorated in the steroid-treated group. These differences resolved when the steroids were discontinued. There was no difference in survival between the steroid- and non-steroid-treated groups.

Sprung et al. showed that bolus administration of methylprednisolone (30 mg/kg) or dexamethasone (6 mg/kg) was more likely to cause reversal of shock than placebo, especially when given within 4 hours from the onset of shock.[143] The drug was repeated only once, 4 hours later, if shock persisted. The differences in reversal of shock did not persist past 48 hours, and overall mortality was not different between the two groups. This study was interpreted in different ways in the literature.[34, 76] It may be that the timing of specific therapies and their rate of infusion affect survival in septic shock. Hinshaw refers to observed important therapeutic benefits achieved

with large doses of corticosteroids combined with antibiotics when primates are previously given massive infusions of *E. coli* (LD_{100}). Hinshaw and colleagues have used a 2-hour infusion of *E. coli* to establish a model of hyperdynamic septic shock in both dogs and baboons. Their data are of considerable interest because their models include volume loading in addition to adjuvant therapy, and because they focus on outcome rather than course. By trials of various antibiotics and steroid schedules, they have increased long-term survival in the baboon model to 100% (Table 28–3).[70]

In a similar model, when the administration of methylprednisolone was switched from bolus to continuous infusion, survival increased from 57% to 100%.[11] Hinshaw and associates have observed an interesting difference in central venous versus peripheral venous concentration of antibiotics in surviving versus nonsurviving dogs and baboons. Central venous antibiotic levels are much higher than peripheral venous antibiotic levels in nonsurviving animals, whereas central antibiotic concentrations are much lower in surviving animals.[69] Hinshaw et al. have also observed lower blood levels of gentamicin when higher doses of steroids were given earlier,[63] and less nephrotoxicity from gentamicin when it was given concomitantly with corticosteroids.[63, 70] Thus, the continuous infusion of corticosteroids may be important to their effect, and their useful effects may have more to do with distribution of systemic blood flow and uptake of antibiotic than previously considered.[2] Because steroids might

TABLE 28–3.

Experimental Septic Shock: Treatment With Steroid Plus Antibiotic*

STUDY GROUP	SHOCK MODEL†	TREATMENT (INFUSION; STEROID DOSE)‡	TIME MPSS BEGUN (HR)	% SURVIVAL (> 7 DAYS)
Hinshaw et al.	Dog: LD_{100} *E. coli* (1-hr infusion)	MPSS (60 mg/kg) + GS	0.25	100
		GS alone		20
		MPSS alone		0
Hinshaw et al.	Baboon: LD_{100} *E. coli* (2-hr infusion)	MPSS (75 mg/kg) + GS	0.5	100
		GS alone		0
Hinshaw et al.	Baboon: LD_{100} *E. coli* (2-hr infusion)	MPSS (75 mg/kg) + GS	2.0	85
Hinshaw et al.	Baboon: LD_{100} *E. coli* (2-hr infusion)	MPSS (75 mg/kg) + GS	4.0	65
Beller et al.	Dog: LD_{100} *E. coli* (1-hr infusion)	MPSS (60 mg/kg) + GS	0.25	100
		MPSS (60 mg/kg) + NS		83

*From Hinshaw.[70] Reproduced by permission.
†LD_{100} *E. coli* = 2.6 ± 0.7 × 10^{10} organisms. Crystalloid, 6–7 ml/kg/hr.
‡MPSS, methylprednisolone sodium succinate; GS, gentamicin sulfate; NS, netilmicin sulfate.

impair the response to sepsis, a similar model has been used to test the effect of high-dose corticosteroids on the immune response to bacteremia. The immune response was normal or increased when corticosteroids were given for 2 days prior to a bacterial infusion, but impaired when the corticosteroid infusion prior to bacterial injection was increased to 8 days.[70] These observations from Hinshaw and associates have strengthened the support for high-dose steroids in sepsis. Many of the therapeutic principles suggested by these findings were incorporated into a controlled clinical trial now underway in ten VA hospitals (VA Cooperative Study No. 209, Evaluation of Corticosteroids in Severe Sepsis).

The Eicosanoids. Blockade of prostaglandin synthesis by indomethacin or ibuprofen has been recommended in the treatment of septic shock. As discussed in chapter 9, "Role of Prostacyclin, Thromboxane A$_2$, and Leukotrienes in Cardiovascular Function and Disease," changes in prostanoid levels do occur in clinical and experimental septic shock. Preliminary data indicate that blockade of prostaglandin synthesis (indomethacin, ibuprofen) may be beneficial in the treatment of septic shock,[23, 32, 44, 48] although clinically relevant outcome studies and controlled studies in humans have not been published. Nonsteroidal acute inflammatory drugs may increase susceptibility to bacterial infection. Such increased susceptibility has been demonstrated experimentally.[43]

Naloxone. Septic shock has been associated with β-endorphin release.[121] β-Endorphins depress cardiovascular function and reduce the sympathetic response to pain, similarly to morphine. Treatment with the opiate antagonist naloxone has been reported to improve cardiovascular function in clinical and canine sepsis.[54, 114, 119–122, 125] In a canine model of endotoxemia, naloxone increased survival time.[119] Treatment with naloxone in a live *E. coli* infusion canine model demonstrated attenuation of the hypotension and acidosis without changing cardiac output or total peripheral resistance.[120] Naloxone has also been reported to diminish myocardial depression in sepsis.[120] Interestingly, Hinshaw et al. found that naloxone increased survival in dogs given live *E. coli* and gentamicin, but not in baboons treated similarly.[68] Thus, differences in responses among species and experimental models

limit the significance of these studies on the efficacy of naloxone in treatment of septic shock. Clinical studies have produced conflicting results.[54, 114, 125] Further studies are necessary before the role of β-endorphins in sepsis can be clearly described.

Fibronectin. Depression of RES function by fibronectin deficiency occurs during sepsis, and treatment with fibronectin infusion not only reverses the fibronectin and opsonic deficiency in trauma patients,[128, 129, 131] but also improves pulmonary and metabolic function.[84, 128, 129] However, excessive fibronectin therapy impairs RES function, and appropriate titration of therapy remains unclear.

In summary, sepsis remains a major cause of morbidity and mortality in the critically ill patient. Septic shock is seen more frequently today owing to the extensive use of immunosuppressive agents and advanced life-support systems. Although major advances have been made with antibiotic therapy, mortality from sepsis remains high. Adequate removal of the focus of infection is central to the treatment of septicemia. The ideal therapy is to treat the infection before septic shock develops. We are slowly beginning to understand more about the pathophysiology of septic shock. On the basis of this understanding, volume replacement has become central to resuscitation. The WP and CVP values must be carefully interpreted. Similarly, the effects of adjuvant treatments should be judged in clinically relevant models and should be associated with improvement in survival before they are incorporated into routine clinical practice. At present, there are no proved adjuvant therapies for septic shock beyond the administration of fluids and antibiotics.

REFERENCES

1. Abraham E, Bland RD, Cobo JC, et al: Sequential cardiorespiratory patterns associated with outcome in septic shock. *Chest* 1984; 85:75.
2. Alexander JW: Emerging concepts in control of surgical infections. *Surgery* 1974; 75:934–946.
3. Altemeier WA, Todd JC, Inge WW: Gram-negative septicemia: A growing threat. *Ann Surg* 1967; 166:530.
4. Altura BM: Endothelium, reticuloendothelial cells, and microvascular integrity: Roles in

host defense, in Altura BM, Lefer AM, Schumer W (eds): *Handbook of Shock and Trauma.* Vol 1: *Basic Science.* New York, Raven Press, 1983, pp 51–95.

5. Archie JP Jr: Anatomic arterial-venous shunting in endotoxic and septic shock in dogs. *Ann Surg* 1977; 186:171.

6. Baker CH: Effects of endotoxin on microvascular flow velocity and indicator dispersion. *Circ Shock* 1980; 7:387.

7. Baker CC, Chaudry IH, Gaines HO, et al: Evaluation of factors affecting mortality rate after sepsis in a murine cecal ligation and puncture model. *Surgery* 1983; 94:331.

8. Baker CH, Wilmoth FR: Microvascular responses to *E. coli* endotoxin with altered adrenergic activity. *Circ Shock* 1984; 12:165.

9. Banks JG, Foulis AK, Ledingham I McA, et al: Liver function in septic shock. *J Clin Pathol* 1982; 35:1249.

10. Bell H, Thal A: The peculiar hemodynamics of septic shock. *Postgrad Med* 1970; 48:106.

11. Beller BK, Archer LT, Passey RB, et al: Effectiveness of modified steroid-antibiotic therapies for lethal sepsis in the dog. *Arch Surg* 1983; 118:1293.

12. Borzotta AP, Polk HC Jr: Multiple system organ failure. *Surg Clin North Am* 1983; 63:315.

13. Bozzetti F, Terno G, Bonfanti G, et al: Prevention and treatment of central venous catheter sepsis by exchange via a guidewire. *Ann Surg* 1983; 198:48.

14. Brigham KL, Bowers RE, Haynes J: Increased sheep lung vascular permeability caused by *Escherichia coli* endotoxin. *Circ Res* 1979; 45:292.

15. Brigham KL, Woolverton WC, Blake LH, et al: Increased sheep lung vascular permeability caused by *Pseudomonas* bacteremia. *J Clin Invest* 1974; 54:792.

16. Broadie TA, Homer L, Herman CM: Effect of endotoxin on oxygen consumption by a flow-controlled canine hind-limb preparation. *Surgery* 1980; 88:566.

17. Brobmann GF, Ulano HB, Hinshaw LB, et al: Mesenteric vascular responses to endotoxin in the monkey and dog. *Am J Physiol* 1970; 219:1464.

18. Brown R, Bancewicz J, Hamid J, et al: Delayed hypersensitivity skin testing does not influence the management of surgical patients. *Ann Surg* 1982; 196:672.

19. Calvin JE, Driedger AA, Sibbald WJ: The hemodynamic effect of rapid fluid infusion in critically ill patients. *Surgery* 1981; 90:61.

20. Calvin JE, Driedger AA, Sibbald WJ, et al: Does the pulmonary capillary wedge pressure predict left ventricular preload in critically ill patients? *Crit Care Med* 1981; 9:437.

21. Cameron DE, Chaudry IH, Schleck S, et al: Hepatocellular dysfunction in early sepsis despite increased hepatic blood flow. *Adv Shock Res* 1981; 6:65.

22. Carli A, Auclair MC, Bleichner G, et al: Inhibited response to isoproterenol and altered action potential of beating rat heart cells by human serum in septic shock. *Circ Shock* 1978; 5:85.

23. Carmona RH, Tsao TC, Trunkey DD: The role of prostacyclin and thromboxane in sepsis and septic shock. *Arch Surg* 1984; 119:189.

24. Carroll GC, Snyder JV: Hyperdynamic severe intravascular sepsis depends on fluid administration in cynomolgus monkey. *Am J Physiol* 1982; 243:R313.

25. Chaudry IH, Schleck S, Clemens MG, et al: Altered hepatocellular active transport: An early change in peritonitis. *Arch Surg* 1982; 117:151.

26. Chaudry IH, Wichterman KA, Baue AE: Effect of sepsis on tissue adenine nucleotide levels. *Surgery* 1979; 85:205.

27. Christou NV, Meakins JL: Neutrophil function in anergic surgical patients: Neutrophil adherence and chemotaxis. *Ann Surg* 1979; 190:557.

28. Clowes GHA, O'Donnell TF, Ryan NT, et al: Energy metabolism in sepsis: Treatment based on different patterns in shock and high output stage. *Ann Surg* 1974; 179:684.

29. Coalson JJ, Greenfield LJ, Hinshaw LB: Effects of digoxin on myocardial ultrastructure in endotoxin shock. *Surg Gynecol Obstet* 1972; 135:908–912.

30. Coalson JJ, Benjamin BA, Archer LT, et al: A pathologic study of *Escherichia coli* shock in the baboon and the response to adrenocorticosteroid treatment. *Surg Gynecol Obstet* 1978; 147:726.

31. Conte JE, Barriere SL: Empiric antibiotic therapy pending results of appropriate cultures, in Conte JE, Barriere SL (eds): *Manual of Antibiotics and Infectious Diseases.* Philadelphia, Lea & Febiger, 1984, pp 92–105.

32. Cook JA, Wise WC, Butler RR, et al: The potential role of thromboxane and prostacyclin in endotoxic and septic shock. *Am J Emerg Med* 1983; 2:28.

33. Corbett WA, Peitzman AB, Shires GT: Production of a canine model of chronic sepsis by biliary tract ligation: Parallel with a patient problem. *Eur Surg Res* 1981; 13:88.

34. Corticosteroids for septic shock (letters). *N Engl J Med* 1985; 312:509–512.

35. Davis JM, Stevens JM, Peitzman AB, et al: Neutrophil migratory activity in severe hemorrhagic shock. *Circ Shock* 1983; 10:199–204.

36. DeLaCal MA, Miravalles E, Pascual T, et al: Dose-related hemodynamic and renal effects of dopamine in septic shock. *Crit Care Med* 1984; 12:22.

37. Demeules JE: A physiologic explanation for cardiac deterioration in septic shock. *J Surg Res* 1984; 36:553.

38. Demling RH, Proctor R, Grossman J, et al: Lung injury and lung lysosomal enzyme release during endotoxemia. *J Surg Res* 1981; 30:135.

39. Demling RH, Wong C, Wenger H: Effect of endotoxin on the integrity of the peripheral (soft tissue) microcirculation. *Circ Shock* 1984; 12:191.

40. Dickerman JD: Bacterial infection and the asplenic host: A review. *J Trauma* 1976; 16:662.

41. Eiseman B, Beart R, Norton L: Multiple organ failure. *Surg Gynecol Obstet* 1977; 144:323.

42. Elinger JH, Seyde WC, Longnecker DE: Methylprednisolone plus ibuprofen increases mortality in septic rats. *Circ Shock* 1984; 14:203.

43. Esposito AL: Aspirin impairs anti-bacterial mechanisms in experimental pneumonia. *Am Rev Respir Dis* 1984; 130:857.

44. Fink MP, MacVittie TJ, Casey LC: Inhibition of prostaglandin synthesis restores normal hemodynamics in canine hyperdynamic sepsis. *Ann Surg* 1984; 200:619.

45. Finley RJ, Duff JH, Holliday RL, et al: Capillary muscle blood flow in human sepsis. *Surgery* 1975; 78:87.

46. Finley RJ, Holliday RL, Lefcoe M, et al: Pulmonary edema in patients with sepsis. *Surg Gynecol Obstet* 1975; 140:851.

47. Fischer P, Millen JE, Glauser FL: Endotoxin-induced increased alveolar capillary membrane permeability. *Circ Shock* 1977; 4:387.

48. Flynn JT: Endotoxic shock in the rabbit: The effects of prostaglandin and arachidonic acid administration. *J Pharmacol Exp Ther* 1978; 206:555.

49. Fry DE, Perlstein L, Fulton RL, et al: Multiple system organ failure. *Arch Surg* 1980; 115:136.

50. Gahhos FN, Chiu RCJ, Bethune D, et al: Hemodynamic responses to sepsis: Hypodynamic versus hyperdynamic states. *J Surg Res* 1981; 31:475.

51. Garrison RN, Ratcliffe DJ, Fry DE: Hepatocellular function and nutrient blood flow in experimental peritonitis. *Surgery* 1982; 92:713.

52. Gibson WH, Cook JJ, Gatipon G, et al: Effect of endotoxin shock on skeletal muscle membrane potential. *Surgery* 1977; 81:571.

53. Goldfarb RD: Characteristics of shock-induced circulating cardiodepressant substances: A brief review. *Circ Shock* 1979; 1:23.

54. Groeger JS, Carlon GC, Howland WS: Naloxone in septic shock. *Crit Care Med* 1983; 11:650.

55. Guillem JG, Clemens MG, Chaudry IH, et al: Hepatic gluconeogenic capability in sepsis is depressed before changes in oxidative capability. *J Trauma* 1982; 22:723.

56. Haglund E, Myrvold H, Lundgren O: Cardiac and pulmonary function in regional intestinal shock. *Arch Surg* 1978; 113:963.

57. Hastings PR, Skillman JJ, et al: Antacid titration in the prevention of acute gastrointestinal bleeding. *N Engl J Med* 1978; 298:1041.

58. Hinsdale JG, Jaffe BM: Re-operation for intra-abdominal sepsis: Indications and results in a modern critical care setting. *Ann Surg* 1984; 199:31.

59. Hinshaw LB, Archer LT, Block MR, et al: Myocardial function in shock. *Am J Physiol* 1974; 226:357.

60. Hinshaw LB, Archer LT, Spitzer JJ, et al: Effects of coronary hypotension and endotoxin on myocardial performance. *Am J Physiol* 1974; 227:1051.

61. Hinshaw LB: Concise review: The role of glucose in endotoxin shock. *Circ Shock* 1976; 3:1.

62. Hinshaw LB, Benjamin B, Holmes DD, et al: Responses of the baboon to live *Escherichia*

coli organisms and endotoxin. *Surg Gynecol Obstet* 1977; 145:1.

63. Hinshaw LB, Beller-Todd BK, Archer LT: Current management of the septic shock patient: Experimental basis for treatment. *Circ Shock* 1982; 9:543–553.

64. Hinshaw LB: Myocardial function in endotoxin shock. *Circ Shock* 1979; 1:43.

65. Hinshaw LB, Beller BK, Archer LT, et al: Recovery from lethal *Escherichia coli* shock in dogs. *Surg Gynecol Obstet* 1979; 149:545.

66. Hinshaw LB, Archer LT, Beller-Todd BK: Hematologic disturbances during sepsis: Platelets and leukocytes. *Adv Shock Res* 1982; 7:1.

67. Hinshaw LB, Brackett DJ, Archer LT, et al: Detection of the "hyperdynamic state" of sepsis in the baboon during lethal *E. coli* infusion. *J Trauma* 1983; 23:361.

68. Hinshaw LB, Beller BK, Chang ACK, et al: Evaluation of naloxone for therapy of *Escherichia coli* shock: Species differences. *Arch Surg* 1984; 119:1410.

69. Hinshaw LB: Unpublished data.

70. Hinshaw LB: Corticosteroids in shock. *Semin Respir Med* 1985; 7:24.

71. Horovitz JH, Carrico CJ, Shires GT: Pulmonary response to major injury. *Arch Surg* 1974; 108:349.

72. Houtchens BA, Westershaw DR: Oxygen consumption in septic shock: Collective review. *Circ Shock* 1984; 13:361.

73. Illner H, Shires GT: Membrane defect and energy status of rabbit skeletal muscle cells in sepsis and septic shock. *Arch Surg* 1981; 116:1302.

74. Ing AFM, McLean APH, Meakins JL: Multiple organism bacteremia in the surgical intensive care unit: A sign of intraperitoneal sepsis. *Surgery* 1981; 90:779.

75. Jardin F, Gurdjian F, Desfonds P, et al: Effect of dopamine on intrapulmonary shunt fraction and oxygen transport in severe sepsis with circulatory and respiratory failure. *Crit Care Med* 1979; 7:273.

76. Kass EH: High dose corticosteroids for septic shock. *N Engl J Med* 1984; 311:1178.

77. Kaufman BS, Rackow EC, Falk JL: The relationship between oxygen delivery and consumption during fluid resuscitation of hypovolemic and septic shock. *Chest* 1984; 85:336.

78. Keane RM, Birmingham W, Shatney CM, et al: Prediction of sepsis in the multitraumatic patient by assays of lymphocyte responsiveness. *Surg Gynecol Obstet* 1983; 156:163.

79. Kohler JP, Rice CL, Moseley P, et al: Sepsis reduces the threshold hydrostatic pressure necessary for pulmonary edema in baboons. *J Surg Res* 1981; 30:129.

80. Kass EH: High dose corticosteroids for septic shock. *N Engl J Med* 1984; 311:1178.

81. Krausz MM, Perel A, Eimerl D, et al: Cardiopulmonary effects of volume loading in patients in septic shock. *Ann Surg* 1977; 185:429.

82. Kuida H, Gilbert RP, Hinshaw LB, et al: Species differences in effect of gram-negative endotoxin on circulation. *Am J Physiol* 1961; 200:1197.

83. Lang CH, Bagby GJ, Bornside GH, et al: Sustained hypermetabolic sepsis in rats: Characterization of the model. *J Surg Res* 1983; 35:201.

84. Lanser ME, Saba TM: Opsonic fibronectin deficiency and sepsis. Cause or effect? *Ann Surg* 1982; 195:340.

85. Ledingham I McA, McArdle CS: Prospective study of the treatment of septic shock. *Lancet* 1978; 1:1194.

86. Lefcoe MS, Sibbald WJ, Holliday RL: Wedged balloon catheter angiography in the critical care unit. *Crit Care Med* 1979; 7:449.

87. Lefer AM: Mechanisms of cardiodepression in endotoxin shock. *Circ Shock* 1979; 1:1.

88. Levison MA, Tsao TC, Trunkey DD: Altered potassium flux and myocardial dysfunction during sepsis. *J Surg Res* 1984; 37:295.

89. Lucas CE, Suzawa C, Friend W, et al: Therapeutic implications of disturbed gastric physiology in patients with stress ulcerations. *Am J Surg* 1972; 123:25.

90. Lucas CE, Ledgerwood AM: Cardiopulmonary response to massive doses of steroids in patients with septic shock. *Arch Surg* 1984; 119:537.

91. MacLean LD, Meakins JL, Jaguchi K, et al: Host resistance in sepsis and trauma. *Ann Surg* 1975; 182:207.

92. MacLean LD, Mulligan WG, McLean APH, et al: Patterns of septic shock in man: A detailed study of 56 patients. *Ann Surg* 1967; 166:543.

93. Maksad AK, Cha CJ, Stuart RC, et al: Myo-

cardial depression in septic shock: Physiologic and metabolic effects of a plasma factor on an isolated heart. *Circ Shock* 1979; 1:35.

94. Manship L, McMillin RD, Brown JJ: The influence of sepsis and multisystem and organ failure on mortality in the surgical intensive care unit. *Ann Surg* 1984; 50:94–101.

95. McAlhany JC Jr, Czaja AJ, Pruitt BA Jr: Antacid control of complications from acute gastroduodenal disease after burns. *J Trauma* 1976; 16:645.

96. McConn R, Greineder JK, Wasserman F, et al: Is there a humoral factor that depresses ventricular function in sepsis? *Circ Shock* 1979; 1:9.

97. McDougal WS, Heimburger S, Wilmore DW, et al: The effect of exogenous substrate on hepatic metabolism and membrane transport during endotoxemia. *Surgery* 1978; 84:55.

98. Meakins JL, Pietsch JB, Bubeniko O, et al: Delayed hypersensitivity: Indicator of acquired failure of host defenses in sepsis and trauma. *Ann Surg* 1977; 186:241.

99. Nakatani T, Tanaka J, Sato T, et al: The pathophysiology of septic shock: Studies of reticuloendothelial system function and liver high-energy metabolism in rats following sublethal and lethal *Escherichia coli* injection. *Adv Shock Res* 1982; 7:147.

100. Newsome HH, Armstrong CW, Mayhall GC, et al: Mechanical complications from insertion of subclavian venous feeding catheters: Comparison of de novo percutaneous venipuncture or change of catheter over guidewire. *J Parenter Enter Nutr* 1984; 8:560–562.

101. Nicholas GG, Mela LM: Protection against the effects of endotoxemia by glucocorticoids. *J Surg Res* 1975; 19:321.

102. Niehaus GD, Schumacker PR, Saba TM: Reticuloendothelial clearance of blood-borne particulates: Relevance to experimental lung microembolization and vascular injury. *Ann Surg* 1980; 191:479.

103. Norrby SR, Geddes AM: Management of septicaemia. *Scand J Infect Dis* 1982; 31(suppl):112–117.

104. Norton L, Moore G, Eueman B: Liver failure in the postoperative patient: The role of sepsis and immunologic deficiency. *Surgery* 1975; 78:6.

105. Nylander WA Jr, Hammon JW, Roselli RJ, et al: Comparison of the effects of saline and homologous plasma infusion on lung fluid balance during endotoxemia in the unanesthetized sheep. *Surgery* 1981; 90:221.

106. Nxumalo JL, Teranaka M, Schenk WG Jr: Hepatic blood flow measurement: III. Total hepatic blood flow measured by ICG clearance and electromagnetic flowmeters in a canine septic shock model. *Ann Surg* 1978; 187:299.

107. O'Quin R, Marini JJ: Pulmonary artery occlusion pressure: Clinical physiology, measurement, and interpretation. *Am Rev Respir Dis* 1983; 128:319.

108. Pape JW, Liautaud B, Thomas F, et al: Characteristics of the acquired immunodeficiency syndrome (AIDS) in Haiti. *N Engl J Med* 1983; 309:945.

109. Parrillo JE, Burch C, Roach P, et al: Septic shock patients with a reduced left ventricular ejection fraction have a circulating factor that depresses in vitro myocardial cell performance. *Crit Care Med* 1985; 13:340.

110. Parker MM, Shelhamer JH, Bacharach SL: Profound but reversible myocardial depression in patients with septic shock. *Ann Intern Med* 1984; 100:483.

111. Peitzman AB, Shires GT III, Corbett WA, et al: Measurement of lung water in inhalation injury. *Surgery* 1981; 90:305.

112. Peitzman AB, Shires GT III, Illner H, et al: Cellular function in liver and muscle with intravenous *E. coli* sepsis in primates. *Surg Gynecol Obstet* (in press).

113. Perbellini A, Shatney CH, MacCarter DJ, et al: A new model for the study of septic shock. *Surg Gynecol Obstet* 1978; 147:68.

114. Peters WP, Friedman PA, et al: Pressor effect of naloxone in septic shock. *Lancet* 1981; 1:529.

115. Pinsky MR: Cause-specific management of shock. *Postgrad Med* 1983; 73:127.

116. Postel J, Schloerb PR: Cardiac depression in bacteremia. *Ann Surg* 1977; 186:74.

117. Postell J, Schloerb PR: Metabolic effects of experimental bacteremia. *Ann Surg* 1977; 185:475.

118. Postel J, Schloerb PR, Furtado D: Pathophysiologic alterations during bacterial infusions for the study of bacteremic shock. *Surg Gynecol Obstet* 1975; 141:683.

119. Raymond RM, Harkema JM, Stoffs WV, et al: Effects of naloxone therapy on hemodynamics and metabolism following a superlethal dosage of *Escherichia coli* endotoxin in dog. *Surg Gynecol Obstet* 1981; 152:159.

120. Rees M, Bowen JC: Hemodynamic response to naloxone during live *Escherichia coli* sepsis in splenectomized dogs. *Ann Surg* 1984; 200:614.

121. Rees M, Bowen JC, Payne JG, et al: Plasma β-endorphin immunoreactivity in dogs during anesthesia, surgery, *Escherichia coli* sepsis and naloxone therapy. *Surgery* 1983; 93:386.

122. Rees M, Payne JG, Bowen JC: Naloxone reverses tissue effects of live *Escherichia coli* sepsis. *Surgery* 1982; 91:81.

123. Richmond JM, Walker JF, Avila A, et al: Renal and cardiovascular response to nonhypotensive sepsis in a large animal model with peritonitis. *Surgery* 1985; 97:205.

124. Robin ED: Of men and mitochondria: Coping with hypoxic dysoxia. *Am Rev Respir Dis* 1980; 122:517.

125. Rock P, Silverman H, Plump D, et al: Efficacy and safety of naloxone in septic shock. *Crit Care Med* 1985; 13:28.

126. Rosenberg JC, Kaplan MP, Lysz K: Mechanisms of steroid suppression of immune function: Effect of methylprednisolone and lymphocyte activation and proliferation. *Surgery* 1980; 88:193.

127. Rutherford RB, Balis JV, Trow RS, et al: Comparison of hemodynamic and regional blood flow changes at equivalent stages of endotoxin and hemorrhagic shock. *J Trauma* 1976; 16:886.

128. Saba TM: Reversing multiple organ failure. *J Trauma* 1979; 19:883.

129. Saba TM, Blumenstock FA, Shah DM, et al: Reversal of fibronectin and opsonic deficiency in patients: A controlled study. *Ann Surg* 1984; 199:87.

130. Schumer W: Steroids in the treatment of clinical septic shock. *Ann Surg* 1976; 184:333.

131. Scovill WA, Saba TM, Blumenstock FA, et al: Opsonic α2 surface binding glycoprotein therapy during sepsis. *Ann Surg* 1978; 188:521.

132. Scovill WA, Saba TM, Kaplan JE, et al: Deficits in reticuloendothelial humoral control mechanisms in patients after trauma. *J Trauma* 1976; 16:898.

133. Shaw JHF, Wolfe RR: A conscious septic dog model with hemodynamic and metabolic responses similar to responses of humans. *Surgery* 1984; 95:553.

134. Schennib H, Chiu RCJ, Mulder DS, et al: Pulmonary bacterial clearance and alveolar macrophage function in septic shock lung. *Am Rev Respir Dis* 1984; 130:444.

135. Shires GT, Canizaro PC, Carrico JC: Shock, in Schwartz SI (ed): *Principles of Surgery*. New York, McGraw-Hill Book Co, 1984, pp 115–164.

136. Shires GT III, Peitzman AB, Illner H, et al: Changes in red blood cell transmembrane potential, electrolytes, and energy content in septic shock. *J Trauma* 1983; 23:769.

137. Shoemaker WC, Hauser CJ: Critique of crystalloid versus colloid therapy in shock and shock lung. *Crit Care Med* 1979; 7:117.

138. Siegel JH, Giovanni I, Coleman B: Ventilation: Perfusion maldistribution secondary to the hyperdynamic cardiovascular state as the major cause of increased pulmonary shunting in human sepsis. *J Trauma* 1979; 19:432.

139. Simonian SJ, Curtis LE: Treatment of hemorrhagic gastritis by antacids. *Ann Surg* 1976; 184:429.

140. Sinanan M, Maier RV, Carrico CJ: Laparotomy for intra-abdominal sepsis in patients in an intensive care unit. *Arch Surg* 1984; 119:652.

141. Snyder JV: Cardiac function in septic shock (letter). *Ann Intern Med* 1984; 101:879.

142. Solomkin JS, Jenkins MK, Nelson RD, et al: Neutrophil dysfunction in sepsis: II. Evidence for the role of complement activation products in cellular deactivation. *Surgery* 1981; 90:319.

143. Sprung CL, Caralis PV, Marcial EH, et al: The effects of high-dose corticosteroids in patients with septic shock. *N Engl J Med* 1984; 311:1137.

144. Sugerman HJ, Austin G, Newsome HH, et al: Hemodynamics, oxygen consumption and serum catecholamine changes in progressive, lethal peritonitis in the dog. *Surg Gynecol Obstet* 1982; 154:8.

145. Sugerman HJ, Peyton JWR, Greenfield LJ: Gram-negative sepsis. *Curr Probl Surg* 1981, vol 18.

146. Teule GJJ, Lingen AV, Voght MAAJ, et al: Role of peripheral pooling in porcine *Escherichia coli* sepsis. *Circ Shock* 1984; 12:1145.

147. Thal AP, Robinson RG, Nagamine T, et al:

The critical relationship of intravascular blood volume and vascular capacitance in sepsis. *Surg Gynecol Obstet* 1976; 143:17.

148. Weil MH: Current understanding of the mechanisms and treatment of circulatory shock caused by bacterial infections. *Ann Clin Res* 1977; 9:181.

149. Wichterman KA, Bane AE, Chaudry IH: Sepsis and septic shock: A review of laboratory models and a proposal. *J Surg Res* 1980; 29:189.

150. Wilson RF, Sibbald WJ, Jaanimagi JL: Hemodynamic effects of dopamine in critically ill septic patients. *J Surg Res* 1976; 20:163.

151. Wright CJ, Duff JH, McLean APH, et al: Regional capillary blood flow and oxygen uptake in severe sepsis. *Surg Gynecol Obstet* 1971; 132:637.

29

Pharmacologic Treatment of Cardiogenic Shock

Barry F. Uretsky, M.D.

Christine E. Lawless, M.D.

Cardiogenic shock may be considered any condition in which the cardiac pump cannot support the body's needs, that is, provide adequate nutritive tissue flow. By this definition, shock secondary to acute myocardial infarction represents the acute paradigm of this problem. In its pathophysiology, prognosis, and to a certain extent therapy, it may be contrasted to cardiogenic shock secondary to chronic myocardial dysfunction. Both types of cardiogenic shock are the subject of this chapter.

The exact definition of cardiogenic shock differs in various studies. The Myocardial Infarction Research Unit (MIRU) study group has defined cardiogenic shock secondary to myocardial infarction as follows:[31] (1) systolic blood pressure less than 90 torr, or 30 torr less than baseline in a hypertensive patient; (2) cold, clammy, cyanotic skin; (3) urine flow less than 20 ml/hour; and (4) alteration of mental state. The criteria for cardiogenic shock are less well defined in the setting of chronic heart failure. Frequently the patient with chronic heart failure will have a systolic blood pressure less than 90 torr when still compensated. Decompensation or incipient shock in chronic heart failure becomes apparent when azotemia and oliguria develop, often with some alteration in mental state. This situation frequently occurs insidiously, obscuring the moment when chronic compensation deteriorates to incipient shock.

CARDIOGENIC SHOCK SECONDARY TO MYOCARDIAL INFARCTION

Mortality from cardiogenic shock secondary to acute myocardial infarction is extremely high,

ranging from 80% to 100% in various studies.[85, 93] Pharmacologic interventions have improved hemodynamics, but mortality has not clearly been affected. The marginal salvage from pharmacologic therapy in acute cardiogenic shock has led various investigators to recommend certain drugs or drug combinations on the basis of hemodynamic changes, improvement in regional blood flow, favorable changes in myocardial oxygen supply/demand ratio, or improvement in clinical or laboratory findings of shock. Such a multiplicity of drug regimens attests to the relative inefficacy of any of them. The intra-aortic balloon pump (IABP)[31, 35, 73, 102] and the left ventricular (LV) assist and other devices[76, 78] may be able to stabilize the patient with shock (see chapter 31, "Mechanical Circulatory Assistance"). It is unlikely that such devices will greatly improve overall survival by themselves, although individual patients may benefit.[73] In contrast is our experience at the University of Pittsburgh (1981–1984) with patients in cardiogenic shock secondary to acute myocardial infarction on pharmacologic and/or IABP therapy, who subsequently underwent cardiac transplantation. Of five such patients, all have lived longer than 6 months.

Pathophysiology of Cardiogenic Shock Secondary to Acute Myocardial Infarction

Cardiogenic shock secondary to acute myocardial infarction is a result of the loss of a critical mass (approximately 35%–40%) of LV myocardium.[74] In the setting of decreased pump function, cardiac compensatory mechanisms to maintain nutritive organ flow include increased heart rate, sympathetic stimulation, increased preload, cardiac dilation, LV hypertrophy, and increased LV compliance. The latter three mechanisms require time to develop. Thus, in cardiogenic shock secondary to acute myocardial infarction, these mechanisms have not been fully developed, whereas in the chronic state they have (Fig 29–1). The absence of dilation in heart failure and shock secondary to acute myocardial infarction may be illustrated by the difference in ejection fraction (EF) between a group of patients with cardiogenic shock secondary to myocardial infarction and a cohort with chronic severe heart failure who subsequently died of terminal myocardial dysfunction. In the former group, EF was 27% ± 11%,[88] whereas in the chronic heart failure group at a time of cardiac compensation, EF was lower, 16% ± 8%. We attribute the ability of the patient to survive at a lower EF in the chronic state in part to adequate cardiac dilation and increase in LV compliance, mechanisms that cannot fully develop acutely after myocardial infarction.

The pathophysiology of cardiogenic shock has been likened to a "vicious cycle."[82] Because of impaired pump function and the subsequent drop in cardiac output, several mechanisms to increase peripheral vasoconstriction come into play to maintain systemic blood pressure. Stimulation of the sympathetic nervous system causes norepinephrine release, thus provoking arteriolar vasoconstriction, increased heart rate, increased venous tone, and increased myocardial contractility. Increased renal sympathetic activity and decreased renal perfusion pressure stimulate renin release and angiotensin II production. The latter agent is an important peripheral vasoconstrictor. It is clear, also, that hypotension will provoke release of arginine vasopressin, a potent vasoconstrictor, which may play a role in maintaining blood pressure during cardiogenic shock.

During the attempt to maintain blood pressure, these mechanisms increase afterload and may further impede the ejection of blood.[67] Increased impedance will further depress cardiac performance, which will further stimulate these vasoconstrictor mechanisms. Thus, the vicious cycle continues until death ensues. Coupled to this increased afterload are tachycardia, increased contractility, and an increase in ventricular volume, all of which increase myocardial oxygen utilization. Thus, little by little, in the peri-infarction zone, where oxygen supply cannot keep up with myocardial oxygen demand, cell necrosis ensues, enlarging the infarct and weakening the pump further. If this schema is correct, it is not surprising that mortality in this setting approximates 100%.

Diagnostic Considerations in Cardiogenic Shock Secondary to Acute Myocardial Infarction

The pharmacologic therapy discussed refers specifically to shock due to a decreased effective muscle mass from a single large infarct or cumulative multiple infarcts. Several diagnostic possibilities should be entertained before one concludes that shock is secondary to infarction alone. These include (1) acute mitral regurgitation secondary to papillary muscle dysfunction or rupture,[26] (2) ventricular septal rupture,[26] (3) right ventricular (RV) infarction,[25] (4) LV aneurysm,[26] (5) free wall ventricular rupture,[20, 26, 72] (6) active ischemia superimposed on acute myocardial infarction, and (7) hypovolemia.

Acute mitral regurgitation should be considered when a new apical murmur develops in the setting of pulmonary edema and shock. Occasionally, the degree of mitral regurgitation is so severe that equilibration of left atrial (LA) and LV pressure occurs early in systole and the mur-

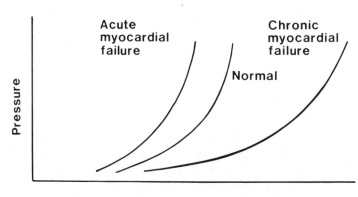

FIG 29–1.
The left ventricular diastolic pressure-volume relationship is shown in normal subjects, in patients with acute heart failure secondary to myocardial infarction, and in patients with chronic heart failure. In chronic heart failure ventricular compliance may increase, whereas the opposite occurs during acute myocardial infarction.

mur is inconsequential. Figure 29–2 shows LA and LV tracings in a patient in whom sudden severe hypotension and shock developed 10 days after an uncomplicated myocardial infarction and 1 hour after a routine predischarge submaximal stress test. The patient had a trivial murmur because of near equilibration of LA and LV pressures during early systole. The patient was stabilized on dobutamine and nitroprusside and underwent uncomplicated mitral valve replacement. In general, however, prognosis must remain guarded in this disorder, which has a reported mortality, with or without surgery, of more than 50%.[26]

Acute ventricular septal rupture also has a high mortality with or without surgical intervention.[26, 63] It may be diagnosed by sudden decompensation associated with a new murmur and oxygen saturation step-up at the RV level. There are few convincing cases reporting surgery to be lifesaving once cardiogenic shock has developed. In our experience, early surgery has a mortality approaching 100%. On the other hand, candidates thought to be in extremis treated medically have fared at least as poorly as those treated operatively. It appears that patients able to survive several weeks after rupture are self-selected and represent a better group for operative repair. It should be added, however, that at least two operative series have reported higher survival in patients not in shock operated on within 2 weeks of rupture than in those operated on at a later time.[63, 69]

RV infarction often accompanies inferior wall LV myocardial infarction.[25] Hypotension in this setting appears to be secondary to RV dysfunction and relatively inadequate filling pressure of the less compliant, damaged RV. LV compliance may be lowered by septal shift, and LV end-diastolic volume (LVEDV) may be lower than suggested by the wedge pressure (WP). It is important to recognize this entity, because its treatment and prognosis are different from those of cardiogenic shock secondary solely to LV infarction. Pulmonary capillary WP may be relatively low in this setting and volume loading may produce dramatic improvement in the clinical state. It is interesting to note in this regard that in patients surviving this problem who do not develop LV failure, there have not been any reports of chronic RV failure on the basis of a previous RV infarction.

The definition of ventricular aneurysm remains problematic.[99] Rarely can one demonstrate a true aneurysmal bulge during acute myocardial infarction severe enough to be designated the etiology of shock. Although it has been demonstrated that aneurysmectomy in the immediate postinfarction period (8 weeks) may be performed without prohibitive mortality,[101] there are few convincing cases in which removal of an aneurysm has improved the patient's shock state. The difficulty of assessing operative intervention is illustrated by the following case.

Case 29–1.—A previously healthy 67-year-old woman was given 1.5 million units of streptokinase intravenously (IV) and underwent successful emer-

FIG 29–2.
Left atrial *(LA, lower trace)* and left ventricular *(LV, upper trace)* pressure recordings for a patient with papillary muscle rupture after myocardial infarction. The systolic murmur in this patient was unimpressive, probably relating to near equilibration of LA and LV pressures during systole.

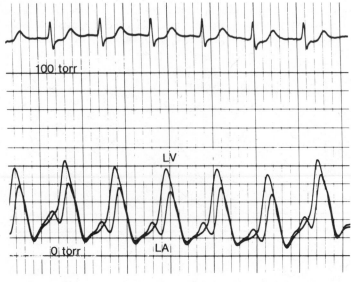

gency coronary angioplasty of the proximal left anterior descending coronary artery within 3 hours of the development of chest pain and precordial ST elevation. Nevertheless, enzymatic and electrocardiographic (ECG) evidence of an acute myocardial infarction developed. Echocardiography revealed hypokinesis of the anteroseptal, anterior, and anterolateral walls with hyperkinesis of the remainder of the ventricle. The patient was in pulmonary edema over the first 3 days despite diuretics and low-dose dobutamine (5 μg/kg/min). On the third postinfarction day, oliguria and hypotension (as low as 60 torr systolic) developed. High doses of dobutamine (20 μg/kg/min) and dopamine (15 mg/kg/min) and IABP were required to stabilize the systolic blood pressure in the 80–90 torr range. After 12 hours on this regimen, urine output, blood pressure, and pulmonary congestion improved. Consideration was given to aneurysmectomy at this point. Contrast angiography revealed akinesis, as previously noted, with vigorous contraction of the other segments. EF on pressors and IABP therapy was 41%. Two surgical teams were consulted, and both thought continued observation without surgery to be the most prudent course. Over a period of 10 days, the patient was weaned from drug and IABP therapy and was discharged 6 weeks after the myocardial infarction, in stable condition.

Comment.—Although we have reserved the term "aneurysm" for an obvious ballooning of the LV myocardium, many observers would have classified this case an aneurysm. If the patient had survived an aneurysmectomy, success might have been attributed to surgery. This case demonstrates that with good residual LV function, survival may be possible without surgery in this setting.

Free wall rupture is usually a sudden, fatal catastrophe. Occasionally several minutes may elapse between sudden decompensation and death. Signs of decompensation are those related to cardiac tamponade. Consideration of the diagnosis and rapid diagnostic measures (right heart catheterization, pericardiocentesis) may reveal the source of the decompensation and temporarily stabilize the patient. A few successful heroic surgical corrective procedures have been reported.[20, 72]

In occasional cases reversible ischemia of viable muscle appears to contribute to the patient's myocardial dysfunction and shock. This possibility should be considered if chest pain and ischemic ECG changes are components of the shock state. Under such circumstances, urgent coronary arteriography must be considered, although diagnostic choices will remain difficult and uncertain,

as will the value of techniques to augment coronary flow (diastolic balloon augmentation) or to relieve obstruction (streptokinase, angioplasty, coronary artery bypass surgery).

Volume losses from profuse diaphoresis, vomiting, diuretics, or lack of intake may occur in the setting of acute myocardial infarction. Volume losses may produce hypotension and signs of shock. This problem is important to recognize as it is the most treatable of the conditions noted. Intravenous administration of normal saline solution, usually with pressure monitoring, is often adequate to resolve this problem.

Pharmacologic Therapy for Cardiogenic Shock Secondary to Acute Myocardial Infarction

General Principles

Once the diagnosis of cardiogenic shock is firmly established, the chance of the patient's dying, no matter what the therapy is, approximates 80%–100%. Stated another way, the salvage from therapy must be relatively small. Therapy should thus utilize a central Hippocratic principle: "Primum non nocere." In this setting, this would include not performing sins of commission, such as overmedicating with vasodilators or sedatives and thus worsening hypotension, or sins of omission, such as withholding therapy while trying to insert monitoring devices (pulmonary artery catheter, intra-arterial line). In this setting, the physician should gather all the diagnostic material and proceed in the usual manner, that is, create a priority list and execute procedures in order of importance. On the other hand, clinical estimates of hemodynamic parameters in this setting are usually incorrect and invasive monitoring is frequently indicated (see chapter 14, "Invasive Hemodynamic Assessment Compared With Clinical Evaluation"). The approaches available to the physician should be aimed at maintaining organ perfusion and maintaining cardiac viability by providing a favorable myocardial oxygen supply/demand ratio. An ideal agent would combine a decrease in cardiac work with an increase in cardiac output and coronary perfusion and no change in blood pressure. A potentially salvageable area of myocardium is the so-called peri-infarction zone. This area appears to be highly vulnerable, and thus an area that should be considered in deciding on therapy. A major determinant of myocardial oxygen consumption is myocardial wall tension. An equation may be written as follows: wall tension = Pr/2h, where P denotes pressure at any time during the cardiac cycle, r is the LV radius, and h denotes LV wall thickness. Thus, a potential method of decreasing wall tension would be to decrease the LV radius. If this is to be accomplished with diuretics, such volume depletion must occur only to a level that will drop LVEDP to less symptomatic levels without dropping cardiac output and blood pressure. Data reported by several investigators[29, 94] suggest that optimal filling pressures in this setting range from 15 to 20 torr. Therapies to decrease outflow impedance (vasodilators), improve contractility (positive inotropic therapy), and improve blood pressure by peripheral vasoconstriction (vasoconstrictors) will be discussed separately.

Finally, it is worth noting that in this relatively bleak setting, medical personnel can play an important role in providing comfort and support to both the family and the patient.

Inotropic Therapy in Cardiogenic Shock Secondary to Myocardial Infarction

Although these agents may improve hemodynamic parameters, convincing evidence of improved survival has not been forthcoming. Inotropic stimulation alone will increase oxygen consumption and may jeopardize ischemic tissue. Furthermore, tachycardia is an undesirable side effect with most of these agents. Tachycardia increases oxygen consumption and in so doing, jeopardizes myocardial tissue viability. The general rule therefore is to use as little of any agent as possible to provide hemodynamic stability.

Isoproterenol. Isoproterenol, a pure β-adrenergic agonist, was once widely used in the treatment of cardiogenic shock.[47, 54, 70] Today, with superior sympathomimetic agents available, this agent is generally not recommended. It increases both heart rate and myocardial contractility, as well as causing peripheral vasodilation. It is not useful in cardiogenic shock with hypotension because the fall in systemic vascular resistance exceeds the increase in cardiac output, resulting in a further drop in mean arterial pressure (MAP).[54] In experimental models, isoproterenol has been shown to increase the area of ischemia and infarction.[66] In patients, myocardial lactate production may increase, signifying worsening myocardial ischemia despite increases in cardiac performance and coronary blood flow.[70] Other adverse effects include development of ventricular arrhythmias.

Epinephrine. Epinephrine is an endogenous catecholamine that directly stimulates α- and β-adrenoreceptors. Typically, in both animal and human studies, epinephrine produces increases in heart rate and contractility.[7, 28, 41, 43] The peripheral action of the drug varies and depends on the type of receptor present in a specific vascular bed and the dosage of the drug used. At low doses (< 0.1 μg/kg/min) the β vasodilatory effect predominates.[21] At higher doses the α constrictor effect predominates.[21] In animal and human studies, it appears that β-adrenoreceptor stimulation results in vasodilation and consequent increases in skeletal muscle and hepatosplanchnic blood flow,[2, 6, 8, 15, 21] while α-adrenoreceptor stimulation results in vasoconstriction of the renal and cutaneous vascular beds.[2, 45, 91] It has been concluded that epinephrine-induced increases in myocardial contractility result in increased coronary blood flow from autoregulation rather than a direct effect on the coronary vasculature.[30, 46] It has been suggested that in man, pressor doses of epinephrine cause increases in cerebral blood flow, an effect related to systemic blood pressure.[52] In addition to the systemic arterial effects, epinephrine also causes constriction of the systemic veins. There is experimental evidence that such constriction may shift appreciable quantities of blood centrally.[34] Because of these vascular effects and the tendency to produce tachycardia, other catecholamines such as norepinephrine, dopamine, and dobutamine have been more frequently employed in cardiogenic shock. On the other hand, epinephrine has improved cardiac performance in some of our post-cardiopulmonary bypass patients when other drugs have failed.

Epinephrine can be infused at rates as low as 0.05 μg/kg/min and titrated to as high as 3 μg/kg/min until the desired effect is attained or untoward side effects occur. These include reduced urine output, tachycardia, ventricular arrhythmias, and excessive vasoconstriction.

Norepinephrine. Norepinephrine, a naturally occurring catecholamine, increases myocardial contractility by stimulating β_1-receptors and causes arteriolar constriction by stimulating α-receptors. Since norepinephrine stimulates both central and peripheral α- and β-receptors, its hemodynamic effects are variable and depend on the dosage given in the clinical setting. In one animal study, increases in heart rate, stroke volume, cardiac output, and blood pressure occurred at low doses (0.5–1.0 μg/min).[55] In a human study, at higher doses, a marked increase in systemic vascular resistance and an eventual fall in cardiac output resulted.[14, 90] It is possible that this adverse hemodynamic effect can occur when norepinephrine is given in lower doses to patients with initially high systemic vascular resistance. Because the vasoconstrictive effects of norepinephrine are most pronounced in the cutaneous, skeletal muscle, and splanchnic beds, blood flow may be redistributed to the heart and brain.[33] The vasoconstrictor effects generally result in reduced renal perfusion and a subsequent decrease in urine flow.

Early hemodynamic studies by Binder[14] and Shubin and Weil[89, 90] in patients with shock following acute myocardial infarction showed a 40% mean increase in arterial pressure and a 32% increase in cardiac output with norepinephrine infusion. Gunnar and Loeb demonstrated that when MAP was less than 50 torr, norepinephrine increased cardiac output by 34%.[47] However, when initial MAP was 70 torr, cardiac output increased by only 16%. Raising MAP above 80 torr does not appear to be indicated, since this may result in excessive cardiac work without further improvement in cardiac output.[90]

The increases in inotropy and afterload that occur with norepinephrine may result in worsening of myocardial oxygen balance. On the other hand, one would anticipate that the rise in coronary perfusion pressure due to the rise in MAP to 50–80 torr would improve coronary blood flow, favorably affecting myocardial oxygen balance. This effect was apparent in an animal study that showed reduction of infarct size in response to pharmacologic support of arterial pressure.[66] In addition, in patients with shock due to acute myocardial infarction, norepinephrine has been shown to increase coronary blood flow and myocardial lactate extraction,[70] thereby favorably altering myocardial metabolism.

Dosage of norepinephrine should begin at 0.025–0.1 μg/kg/min. In one clinical study, dosages of 12–40 μg/min were used to achieve the desired clinical effect.[70] Adverse effects include tachycardia, ventricular arrhythmias, renal vasoconstriction and oliguria, and reduced cardiac output at high doses. The drug must be administered through a large vein, preferably a central vein, since extravasation can result in tissue necrosis.

Because of the undesirable vasoconstrictive properties and because norepinephrine does not appear to regularly improve survival, it has been suggested that its use be restricted to patients who are profoundly hypotensive.

Dopamine.   Dopamine is a naturally occurring precursor of norepinephrine. Dopamine not only is a β₁-adrenoreceptor agonist, but it also acts indirectly by entering the sympathetic nerve terminal and releasing endogenous stores of norepinephrine into the synapse.[10, 42] The released norepinephrine will cause α- and β₁-adrenoreceptor activation. β₁ stimulation causes a positive inotropic effect, with a resulting increase in stroke volume and cardiac output. As a consequence of α₁-adrenoreceptor stimulation, vasoconstriction occurs in nonvital vascular beds, that is, skeletal muscle and skin. This potentially allows for diversion of blood to more vital organs. Postsynaptic dopaminergic receptors have been demonstrated in the renal, mesenteric, cerebral, and coronary vasculature.[40, 68] When stimulated, they produce vasodilation, thus improving vital organ perfusion pressure, renal blood flow, and urinary output. In an early clinical paper, four of six patients with cardiogenic shock who were oliguric during treatment with epinephrine and metaraminol showed improved urine flows during dopamine infusion.[64]

The precise cardiovascular effects of dopamine are dose dependent. At low doses (1–4 μg/kg/min) the dopaminergic effects predominate, causing renal vasodilation and increased renal blood flow. At moderate doses (5–10 μg/kg/min), the predominant hemodynamic effects include an augmentation in cardiac output, accompanied by a moderate decrease in systemic vascular resistance and little to no change in LV filling pressure.[13, 62, 71] At higher doses α-adrenoreceptor activity predominates, resulting in generalized vasoconstriction. This effect may counteract the beneficial effects of dopaminergic stimulation seen at lower doses. Adverse effects of dopamine include ventricular arrhythmias, gastrointestinal upset, tachycardia, and angina.

Dopamine has been used extensively in cardiogenic shock. In 13 patients with shock after acute myocardial infarction, dopamine caused a 10% increase in heart rate, a 40% increase in cardiac output, a 30% increase in stroke volume, and a 20% fall in systemic vascular resistance.[62] MAP rose slightly. However, these patients were not severely hypotensive (mean predrug systemic pressure, 75 ± 5 torr), and the same effects may not be seen with more profound shock. In the same study, dopamine was compared with iso-proterenol and norepinephrine, and its hemody-namic effects appeared superior in that cardiac output rose more with dopamine than with nor-epinephrine and the heart rate increased less than with isoproterenol. Thus, in patients who are not profoundly hypotensive, dopamine may be a pre-ferred sympathomimetic drug. One should con-sider a drug's effect on myocardial oxygen sup-ply/demand as well as its systemic hemodynamic effect. In a clinical study, dopamine in doses of 8–26 µg/kg/min improved systemic hemody-namics but increased myocardial oxygen con-sumption and lactate production.[71] It was con-cluded in that study that dopamine in the doses required to increase MAP exerts effects that are detrimental to the ischemic myocardium and should therefore be used with caution in patients in shock after acute myocardial infarction. For these reasons, dopamine should be infused at the lowest dose possible to achieve a clinical re-sponse.

Dobutamine. Dobutamine, a synthetic catecholamine, is most often referred to as a se-lective β_1-adrenergic agonist.[92] In actuality, its mechanism of action may be much more complex in man. Direct stimulation of cardiac β_1-adreno-receptors results in an increase in cardiac output through increased inotropy and augmentation of stroke volume. A decrease in total peripheral vas-cular resistance probably results from a reflex withdrawal of sympathetic tone and possibly a di-rect effect.[84] None of dobutamine's effects ap-pear to be mediated through release of endoge-nous norepinephrine, and it has not been shown to stimulate renal dopaminergic receptors.[81]

Recent studies have identified cardiac α_1-adrenoreceptors that cause a positive inotropic re-sponse with little to no chronotropic response.[87] Dobutamine has been shown to activate these re-ceptors. Two stereoisomers of dobutamine have been identified. α_1-Agonist activity resides in the (−) isomer, while β_1-agonist activity resides in the (+) and (−) isomer. The commercially available preparation of dobutamine is a racemic mixture of the two isomers. Thus, it has been postulated that the inotropic activity is the result of both α_1- and β_1-adrenoceptor stimulation, whereas the chronotropic effect results only from β_1-adrenoceptor stimulation.[84] That result could explain the apparent inotropic versus chrono-tropic selectivity of the drug.[51] In the peripheral

vasculature, the β_2-adrenoceptor-mediated vaso-dilation is balanced by α-adrenoceptor-mediated constriction. Thus, there is little or no effect of dobutamine on systemic blood pressure, although individual patients may show a hypertensive or hypotensive response.[59, 98]

Francis and colleagues[39] have tried dobuta-mine in the setting of cardiogenic shock. Al-though none of their patients was profoundly hy-potensive, dobutamine (10 µg/kg/min) raised the heart rate by 18%, the MAP by 15%, and the cardiac index by 53%. In this study LV filling pressures did not increase with dobutamine but did with dopamine. In an attempt to retain the advantages of each agent, yet avoid the deleteri-ous effects, Richard et al. infused both drugs at doses of 7.5 µg/kg/min each. With this combi-nation, MAP increased and LV filling pressure was unchanged.[80] These authors found that hy-poxemia increased with dopamine alone, which they attributed to increases in LV filling pressure; this deleterious effect was not observed with the combination.

Thus, it appears that dobutamine or a com-bination of dobutamine and dopamine may be used in the mildly hypotensive patient with shock secondary to acute myocardial infarction. Coro-nary flow increases in proportion to the increased oxygen demand, related to increased inotropy.[61] After coronary occlusion in dogs, dobutamine in-creased myocardial blood flow to both ischemic and nonischemic regions of the heart and reduced infarct size.[61] However, reduction of blood flow may occur if dobutamine is used in doses high enough to cause tachycardia.[83] In the few avail-able human studies, dobutamine has occasionally caused myocardial lactate production and angina pectoris in patients with coronary artery dis-ease.[27, 79] These effects have been thought to be related more to the chronotropic than to the ino-tropic effects of the drug.[83] In patients without coronary disease, the drug appears to have a fa-vorable effect on myocardial oxygen balance.[65]

Dobutamine is administered IV starting at 2–5 µg/kg/min, with the dosage increased incre-mentally by 2–5 µg/kg/min until the desired clin-ical or hemodynamic effect is achieved or untow-ard effects occur. The optimal maintenance dosage is usually 7.5–15 µg/kg/min, although dosages as high as 40 µg/kg/min have been used.[92] The onset of action is rapid (2 minutes), and the peak effect occurs by 10 minutes. The short half-life of the drug (2.5 minutes) allows rapid elimination in the event that side effects occur. These include sinus tachycardia, supraventricular and ventricular tachyarrhythmias, tremors, anxiety, nausea, headaches, and anginal pain. Hemodynamic effects are reduced by about 35% at 72 hours after the start of infusion and about 50% at 96 hours.[96] This attenuation is thought to be due to "downregulation" of myocardial β_1-receptors.[56, 96] Upward dose titration may, at least temporarily, restore drug efficacy.

Amrinone. Amrinone is a bipyridine derivative with both inotropic and vasodilator properties.[3, 4] The agent is one of a class of phosphodiesterase inhibitors, all of which produce elevated levels of intracellular cAMP. The increased level of cAMP is the putative mechanism through which increased inotropy eventuates,[36, 49] although some studies have cast doubt on this mechanism as the cause of improved contractile state.[48, 95] Amrinone may also increase contractility by increasing membrane calcium conductance.[1] It does not affect sodium-potassium ATPase, its action is not blocked by propranolol or reserpine, and its effect does not depend on release of myocardial catecholamines or stimulation of β-adrenoceptors. In patients with severe heart failure, it produces dose-related increases in cardiac output and decreases in filling pressures.[11] Decreases in systemic blood pressure and increases in heart rate are usually small (approximately 10%). Its effect in cardiogenic shock is unknown. In the compensated patient with severe heart failure the improvement seen with this drug is comparable to that seen with dobutamine.[53] In one study the beneficial effects of dobutamine were attenuated after 8 hours, whereas improvement with amrinone in the same group of patients was sustained.[53] In addition, IV amrinone does not increase myocardial oxygen consumption, an effect that is probably related to reduction of wall tension that more than offsets the effect of enhanced contractility to increase oxygen consumption.[12, 50] Side effects of amrinone include arrhythmias, thrombocytopenia, hypotension, gastrointestinal upset, and liver enzyme elevations.

Therapy is initiated with a 0.75 mg/kg IV bolus given over 2–3 minutes. This is followed by a maintenance infusion of 5–10 μg/kg/min. Based on the clinical response, an additional 0.75 mg/kg bolus may be repeated 30 minutes after initiation of therapy.

Digitalis. Although digitalis is frequently given, its efficacy in acute myocardial infarction with heart failure and/or shock remains controversial.[16] This controversy probably relates to digitalis being a weak inotropic agent and to its having a low therapeutic:toxic ratio. Although stroke work has been shown to improve with this agent in patients with acute myocardial infarction and heart failure, neither cardiac output, stroke volume, nor pulmonary capillary WP consistently improves.[44] In one study, digoxin showed minimal improvement in cardiac output when compared with dobutamine. The latter decreased both preload and afterload in this setting, whereas digoxin did not.[44] These data suggest that digitalis has a limited role in cardiac power failure.

Experimental Inotropic Agents

Several experimental inotropic phosphodiesterase inhibitors have hemodynamic effects similar to amrinone and may be available in the future. These drugs include milrinone,[5] MDL 17,043,[100] and MDL 19,205.[77]

Vasodilator Therapy

Although vasoconstrictive mechanisms are compensatory for maintaining systemic pressure in shock, excessive vasoconstriction can result in decreased tissue perfusion. The rationale for using vasodilator therapy in patients in shock is to break the progressive cycle of vasoconstriction and decreased cardiac output due to increased afterload. However, the major problem with this form of therapy is that it can further reduce arterial pressure, thereby potentially decreasing systemic and coronary tissue perfusion.

Vasodilators cannot be recommended routinely for cardiogenic shock. They may be of use, however, in the patient with excessive vasoconstriction and poor tissue perfusion with marginal (90–100 torr systolic) blood pressure. When initial preload is high, a reduction in wall tension may improve ventricular function and stroke volume sufficiently to compensate for the lower vascular resistance, so that arterial pressure does not drop (see Fig 29–1 and Fig 15–17 in chapter 15, "Technical Problems in Data Acquisition"). Vasodilators may also be useful in combination with an inotropic agent, such as dopamine or dobutamine.

Nitroprusside. The agent most commonly used has been sodium nitroprusside, which acts directly on vascular smooth muscle to cause arteriolar and venous dilation.[23, 75] Clinical studies with nitroprusside in cardiogenic shock and heart failure following myocardial infarction have demonstrated hemodynamic improvement in selected patients.[17] However, as with inotropic therapy, there has been no clear beneficial effect on mortality.[24, 32] The effect of nitroprusside on myocardial oxygen balance in metabolism is controversial. In some clinical studies, sodium nitroprusside has improved myocardial metabolism,[17] whereas in others, ECG changes have suggested worsening of myocardial oxygen balance.[18] In some experimental studies, nitroprusside has actually increased infarct size by redistributing flow away from the ischemic region.[9] These effects may override the reduction in oxygen consumption that is afforded by the reduction in afterload. It must be mentioned that vasodilators, in particular nitroprusside, have been extremely useful in shock due to mitral regurgitation or ventricular septal defect. In these situations, a decrease in peripheral vascular resistance reduces the amount of regurgitation or left-to-right shunting, thereby enhancing forward cardiac output. Nitroprusside is administered IV, beginning at 0.5 μg/kg/min, and titrating upward to achieve the desired hemodynamic and clinical response.

Nitroprusside decomposes to cyanide in the blood. Cyanide is converted to thiocyanate, which is excreted by the kidney. Cyanide interrupts aerobic metabolism and increases lactate production. Thus, one indicator of cyanide toxicity is metabolic acidosis. Neurologic signs (e.g., confusion, seizures, hyperreflexia) are indicative of thiocyanate toxicity. Toxicity generally occurs during high (> 3 μg/kg/min) or prolonged (> 72 hours) nitroprusside infusions.

Thiocyanate levels can be monitored. A level of 10 mg/dl should not be exceeded. Mild toxicity may be treated by stopping the infusion. Severe toxicity should be treated with more aggressive therapy. This includes hemodialysis and agents such as hydroxycobalamine and sodium nitrite, which convert cyanide to a nontoxic substance.

Nitroglycerin. Although in low doses nitroglycerin is predominantly a venodilator, in high doses it has significant arteriolar vasodilating capacity.[37] In fact, its hemodynamic profile in high doses in patients with heart failure is similar to that of nitroprusside.

In the past, sublingual nitroglycerin was not recommended for use in patients with acute myocardial infarction because of the risk of hypotension or reflex tachycardia. However, stable IV preparations are now available and infusion rates can be titrated to the desired hemodynamic parameter. Thus, nitroglycerin may be used cautiously in a patient with cardiogenic shock who is not profoundly hypotensive. It has a theoretical[37] and perhaps real advantage over nitroprusside as an unloading agent in this situation. In experimental animal studies, nitroprusside has been demonstrated to shunt blood away from ischemic areas ("coronary steal"), whereas nitroglycerin has not.[18] Thus, nitroprusside may actually have a detrimental effect in this setting. Also, if active ischemia of viable myocardium is suspected of contributing to myocardial failure, nitroglycerin may reverse this ischemia. IV nitroglycerin is usually begun at 10 μg/min (0.15 μg/kg/min) and titrated upward in 10-μg increments every 5–10 minutes, according to both hemodynamic and clinical responses. A vasodilator effect is usually obtained with 50–100 μg/min, but up to 400 μg/min can be given if clinically indicated.[75a]

Limitation of Myocardial Infarct Size

Multiple interventions have been studied experimentally and clinically in an attempt to limit infarct size and in so doing decrease the possibility of cardiogenic shock. They include modalities that decrease myocardial oxygen consumption, increase myocardial oxygen supply, and decrease inflammation.[104] Difficulties in evaluating any modality clinically include the inability to accurately size an infarct by existing diagnostic methods, as well as difficulty in acquiring an adequate sample size to determine whether the incidence of shock after intervention is decreased, relative to a control group. It is fair to conclude that at present, no form of therapy has been shown to decrease the incidence of cardiogenic shock after myocardial infarction.

Combined Use of Drug Therapy and Intra-aortic Balloon Pumping

Frequently pharmacotherapy and IABP are used together. IABP provides afterload reduction during systole and augmentation of coronary blood flow during diastole. The combined use may afford further improvement in clinical and hemodynamic status than either modality alone until operative intervention is possible or resolution occurs.

CARDIOGENIC SHOCK SECONDARY TO CHRONIC MYOCARDIAL DYSFUNCTION

Clinical Picture

Typically, the patient with chronic heart failure of any cause (ischemic, end-stage valvular or hypertensive, alcohol, or other toxic, or idiopathic) and acute decompensation presents with symptoms of "low cardiac output," that is, the patient is fatigued at rest, lethargic, and hypotensive. There is usually evidence of right-sided failure (elevated neck veins and peripheral edema) as well as left-sided failure. Dyspnea is usually present, but often not as prominent as in acute pulmonary edema. Urine output is scanty, with a low urine sodium concentration, hyponatremia, and elevations in the blood urea nitrogen and creatinine levels. Chest roentgenogram shows cardiomegaly, but pulmonary edema may not be present.

Whereas the situation is usually dominated by lethargy and low output, occasionally a patient may present in more unusual ways. We recently saw a chronic heart failure patient who decompensated with hypotension and acute pulmonary edema that was unresponsive to diuretics and vasodilators but improved during an 8-hour dobutamine infusion. We have also seen two patients who presented with hepatic encephalopathy and severe right heart failure who responded to lactulose and dobutamine infusions. The point at which low output, chronic compensated heart failure decompensates to the point of inadequate nutritive blood flow is often obscure. It is clear, however, that such a sequence of events occurs frequently in chronic heart failure. Death from terminal myocardial dysfunction has occurred within 1 year in approximately 50% of patients we have studied. The figure is representative of other series as well.[38, 103] It has not yet been established how frequently any particular therapeutic agent can temporarily reverse the spiral of dysfunction that leads to death. Most observers believe, however, that at least in some cases such a temporary improvement is possible. The final section will discuss specific therapies in this setting.

Pathophysiology of Cardiogenic Shock Secondary to Chronic Heart Failure

As opposed to shock secondary to acute myocardial infarction, compensatory mechanisms in this setting are relatively fully developed in the individual patient. LV dilation, hypertrophy, and increased compliance have developed, in addition to tachycardia, an increase in preload, and increased sympathetic drive, which are also seen after acute myocardial infarction and shock. Limitation in coronary blood flow does not appear to be a problem, except possibly in an occasional case of ischemic cardiomyopathy. Rather, intrinsic myocardial failure progresses to a critical drop in contractile power.

Therapy

General Principles

Unlike post-myocardial infarction shock, in which invasive monitoring is the rule, invasive monitoring in the chronic setting is less necessary if the diagnosis is secure. Often the hemodynamics of the patient with chronic heart failure during a period of stability are known. Typically, filling (right atrial, pulmonary artery wedge) pressures are high, cardiac output is low, systemic arteriovenous oxygen extraction is widened, and arterial blood pressure is low with a narrow pulse pressure. Such patients may slip insidiously into a low output state inadequate to meet the body's needs ("shock"). Usually the cause of the worsening of heart failure is unclear, but the progressive nature of the myocardial dysfunction is obvious. Under these circumstances, prompt therapy is of prime importance. Valuable treatment time may be lost to the insertion of hemodynamic monitoring catheters, which in this setting provide little diagnostic or management help. If a therapeutic agent does not rapidly ameliorate signs of shock or if management or diagnostic considerations arise, then invasive monitoring is more important.

The primary defect in chronic heart failure is poor myocardial function. Secondarily, increases in systemic vascular resistance and fluid retention develop. When the pump cannot provide adequate flow to vital organs, decompensation occurs. In the chronic setting, decompensation probably relates to relatively minor perturbations in the system. This fact may be used to advantage in treatment. If small changes have disrupted this tenuous equilibrium, then relatively limited therapeutic interventions such as short-term IV positive inotropic or vasodilator therapy may restore the system to an acceptable balance. This is one reason why we recommend prompt institution of therapy without elaborate invasive studies before a more profound state of myocardial dysfunction develops.

Pharmacologic Therapy for Cardiogenic Shock Secondary to Chronic Heart Failure

Vasodilators

Although many vasodilators have been demonstrated to produce dramatic acute hemodynamic effects, their use in the setting of severe decompensated heart failure appears to be limited by low blood pressure. An increase in cardiac output may compensate for a decrease in peripheral resistance, thus maintaining systemic blood pressure. However, this phenomenon does not always occur. Systolic blood pressure is frequently in the range of 70–90 torr. Even a small dose of IV vasodilator may produce decreases in blood pressure that may further compromise tissue perfusion and glomerular filtration and negate the beneficial effects of an increase in cardiac output. Thus, if an IV vasodilator is used, it should be given with extreme care, and usually with invasive monitoring. Similar precautions should be taken with the transcutaneous route of administration.

Nitroprusside.   This agent is both an arteriolar and venous dilator. The duration of action is brief (1–3 minutes). Limitation in dosing is related to the fall in systemic blood pressure or reaching a therapeutic end point. In patients with LV dysfunction and elevated filling pressures, this agent will predictably increase cardiac output and lower cardiac filling pressures. Because patients with chronic decompensated heart failure usually have relatively low blood pressure, these agents are difficult to titrate and frequently require invasive monitoring for safety purposes. Nitroprusside is usually begun at 0.5 μg/kg/min and titrated upward according to both hemodynamic and clinical responses.

Positive Inotropic Therapy

This modality is the most direct since it attacks the underlying defect. It has the advantage of not producing hypotension, as may occur with vasodilators. On the other hand, the increased inotropy will directly increase myocardial oxygen consumption, in some cases to the detriment of the patient.

Dobutamine.   Dobutamine has been widely used for treatment of chronic heart failure. It will predictably improve cardiac output and produce small decreases in cardiac filling pressures. Mean systemic arterial pressure is unchanged, or slightly decreased as a result of little to no increase in systolic arterial pressure and slight decreases in arterial diastolic pressure. Infusion of dobutamine will produce increases in urine flow and excretion of urine sodium, a decrease in blood urea nitrogen and creatinine levels, and an increase in serum sodium.[57] Unverferth et al. have demonstrated an increase in the ATP/creatine ratio in myocardial biopsy specimens after a 3-day infusion of dobutamine, suggesting an improvement in cell viability.[97] This group[58] and others[60] have also shown that repeated short infusions of dobutamine produce an improvement in exercise tolerance.

We have used dobutamine extensively at the University of Pittsburgh, both as a "holding action" prior to cardiac transplantation and as definitive therapy for patients with chronic heart failure who have decompensated.

A problem with dobutamine is drug tolerance or attenuation, as described in the section on cardiogenic shock secondary to acute myocardial infarction.

Dopamine.   Dopamine in low doses has the theoretical advantage of activating dopaminergic receptors in the kidney to increase urine flow and sodium excretion. In low doses it may dilate arterial beds of the mesentery and kidneys. However, in higher doses, vasoconstriction from α-receptor stimulation occurs (see previous section on dopamine). Tolerance to dopamine probably occurs, which may be related to its effect on the β-receptor.[57] Dopamine in the setting of chronic heart failure has a theoretical disadvantage of working in part through the release of myocardial stores of norepinephrine. In advanced heart failure, these stores may be depleted,[19] thereby limiting the usefulness of this agent. Additionally, the vasoconstriction seen with higher doses of dopamine would appear detrimental in a setting of already elevated peripheral vascular resistance.

Amrinone. Amrinone may prove to be a useful agent in the short-term treatment of cardiac decompensation in chronic heart failure because of its favorable effect on myocardial oxygen consumption, because the drug effect is not attenuated over prolonged infusion periods, and because tachycardia usually does not develop. However, studies have not been performed in this group of patients, and thus conclusions regarding the usefulness of amrinone in the reversal of decompensated chronic heart failure should be reserved until these studies have been performed.

Acknowledgment

We thank Mrs. Elsie F. Eberman for secretarial assistance in the preparation of this work.

REFERENCES

1. Adams HR, Rhody J, Sutko JL: Amrinone activates K^+-depolarized atrial and ventricular myocardium of guinea pigs. *Circ Res* 1982; 51:662.

2. Ahlquist RP: A study of the adrenotropic receptors. *Am J Physiol* 1948; 153:586.

3. Alousi AA, Farah AE, Lesher GY, et al: Cardiotonic activity of amrinone (WIN 40680):5-amino-3,4'-bipyridin-6(1H)-one (abstract). *Fed Proc* 1978; 37:914.

4. Alousi AA, Helstrosky A: Amrinone: A positive inotropic agent with a direct vasodilatory activity in the canine isolated perfused hind limb preparation (abstract). *Fed Proc* 1980; 39(3 part 2):855.

5. Baim DS, McDowell AV, Cherniles J, et al: Evaluation of a new bipyridine inotropic agent—milrinone—in patients with severe congestive heart failure. *N Engl J Med* 1983; 309:748.

6. Barcroft H, Konzett H: On the actions of noradrenaline, adrenaline, and isopropylnoradrenaline on the arterial blood pressure, heart rate, and muscle blood flow in man. *J Physiol* 1949; 110:194.

7. Barcroft H, Starr I: Comparison on the actions of adrenaline and noradrenaline on the cardiac output in man. *Clin Sci* 1951; 10:295.

8. Bearn AG, Billing B, Sherlock S: Effect of adrenaline and noradrenaline on hepatic blood flow and splanchnic carbohydrate metabolism in man. *J Physiol (London)* 1951; 115:430.

9. Becker LC: Conditions for vasodilatory-induced coronary steal in experimental myocardial ischemia. *Circulation* 1978; 57:1103.

10. Bejrablaya D, Burn JH, Walker JM: The action of sympathomimetic amines on heart rate in relation to the effect of reserpine. *Br J Pharmacol* 1958; 13:461.

11. Benotti JR, Grossman W, Braunwald E, et al: Hemodynamic assessment of amrinone: A new inotropic agent. *N Engl J Med* 1978; 299:1373.

12. Benotti JR, Grossman W, Braunwald E, et al: Effects of amrinone on myocardial energy metabolism and hemodynamics in patients with severe congestive heart failure due to coronary artery disease. *Circulation* 1980; 62:28.

13. Beregovich J, Bianchi C, Rubler S, et al: Dose-related hemodynamic and renal effects of dopamine in congestive heart failure. *Am Heart J* 1974; 87:550.

14. Binder MJ: Effect of vasopressor drugs on circulatory dynamics in shock following myocardial infarction. *Am J Cardiol* 1965; 16:834.

15. Bowman WC, Nott MW: Actions of sympathomimetic amines and their antagonists on skeletal muscle. *Pharmacol Rev* 1969; 21:27.

16. Chatterjee K, Parmley WW: Acute chronic heart failure: Use of digitalis. *Primary Cardiol* 1983; 2:139.

17. Chatterjee K, Parmley WW, Ganz W, et al: Hemodynamic and metabolic responses to vasodilator therapy in acute myocardial infarction. *Circulation* 1973; 48:1183.

18. Chiarello M, Gold HK, Leinbach RC, et al: Comparison between the effects of nitroprusside and nitroglycerin on ischemic injury during acute myocardial infarction. *Circulation* 1976; 54:766.

19. Chidsey CA, Braunwald E, Morrow AG, et al: Myocardial norepinephrine concentration in man: Effects of reserpine and of congestive heart failure. *N Engl J Med* 1963; 269:653.

20. Cobbs BW Jr, Hatcher CR, Robinson PH: Cardiac rupture. *JAMA* 1973; 112:532.

21. Coffin LH, Ankeney JL, Beheler EM: Experimental study and clinical use of epinephrine for the treatment of low cardiac output syndrome. *Circulation* 1966; 33(suppl I):79.

22. Cohn JN: Comparative cardiovascular effects of tyramine, ephedrine and norepinephrine in man. *Circ Res* 1965; 16:174.

23. Cohn JN, Burke LP: Nitroprusside. *Ann Intern Med* 1979; 91:752.

24. Cohn JN, Franciosa JA, Francis GS, et al:

Effect of short term infusion of sodium nitroprusside on mortality rate in acute myocardial
infarction complicated by left ventricular failure. *N Engl J Med* 1982; 306:1129.

25. Cohn JN, Guiha NH, Broder MJ, et al: Right
ventricular infarction: Clinical and hemodynamic features. *Am J Cardiol* 1974; 33:209.

26. Cohn LH: Surgical management of acute and
chronic cardiac mechanical complications due
to myocardial infarction. *Am Heart J* 1981;
102:1049.

27. Coté P, Bourassa MG, Tubau JF, et al: Effects of dobutamine on left ventricular performance and myocardial metabolic demands in
patients with ischemic heart disease. *Clin
Cardiol* 1984; 7:14.

28. Cotten MdeV, Pincus S: Comparative effects
of a wide range of doses of *l*-epinephrine and
of *l*-norepinephrine on the contractile force of
the heart in situ. *J Pharmacol Exp Ther*
1955; 114:110.

29. Crexells C, Chatterjee K, Forrester JS, et al:
Optimal level of filling pressure in the left
side of the heart in acute myocardial infarction. *N Engl J Med* 1973; 289:1263.

30. Dempsey PJ, Cooper T: Pharmacology of the
coronary circulation. *Annu Rev Pharmacol*
1972; 12:99.

31. Dunkman WB, Leinbach RC, Buckley MJ, et
al: Clinical and hemodynamic results of intra-
aortic balloon pumping and surgery for cardiogenic shock. *Circulation* 1972; 46:465.

32. Durrer JD, Lie KI, Van Capell FJL, et al:
Effect of sodium nitroprusside on mortality in
acute myocardial infarction. *N Engl J Med*
1982; 306:1121.

33. Eckstein JW, Abboud FM: Circulatory effects
of sympathomimetic amines. *Am Heart J*
1962; 63:119.

34. Eckstein JW, Hamilton WK: The pressure-
volume responses of human forearm veins
during epinephrine and norepinephrine infusions. *J Clin Invest* 1957; 36:1663.

35. Ehrich DA, Biddle TA, Kronenberg MW, et
al: The hemodynamic response to intra-aortic
balloon counterpulsation in patients with cardiogenic shock complicating acute myocardial
infarction. *Am Heart J* 1977; 93:274.

36. Endoh M, Shuji Y, Nario T: Positive inotropic effect of amrinone in relation to cyclic
nucleotide metabolism in the canine ventricular muscle. *J Pharmacol Exp Ther* 1982;
221:775.

37. Flaherty J: Comparison of intravenous nitroglycerin and sodium nitroprusside in acute
myocardial infarction. *Am J Med* 1983;
53:60.

38. Franciosa JA, Wilson J, Ziesche S, et al:
Survival in man with severe chronic left ventricular failure due to either coronary heart
failure or idiopathic detected cardiomyopathy.
Am J Cardiol 1983; 51:831.

39. Francis GS, Sharma B, Hodges M: Comparative hemodynamic effects of dopamine and
dobutamine in patients with acute cardiogenic
circulatory collapse. *Am Heart J* 1982;
103:995.

40. Goldberg LI: Cardiovascular and renal actions
of dopamine: Potential clinical applications.
Pharmacol Rev 1972; 24:1.

41. Goldberg LI, Bloodwell RD, Braunwald E, et
al: The direct effects of norepinephrine, epinephrine, and methoxamine on myocardial
contractile force in man. *Circulation* 1960;
11:1125.

42. Goldberg LI, Talley RC, McNay JL: The potential role of dopamine in the treatment of
shock. *Prog Cardiovasc Dis* 1969; 12:40.

43. Goldenberg M, Pines KL, Baldwin E, et al:
The hemodynamic response of man to norepinephrine and epinephrine and its relation to
the problem of hypertension. *Am J Med*
1948; 5:792.

44. Goldstein RA, Passamani ER, Roberts R: A
comparison of digoxin and dobutamine in patients with acute infarction and cardiac failure. *N Engl J Med* 1980; 303:846.

45. Gombos EA, Hulet WH, Bopp P, et al:
Reactivity of renal and systemic circulations
to vasoconstrictor agents in normotensive and
hypertensive subjects. *J Clin Invest* 1962;
41:203.

46. Gregg DE, Fisher LC: Blood supply to the
heart, in Hamilton WF (ed): *Handbook of
Physiology*. Washington, DC, American
Physiological Society, 1963, vol 2, pp 1517–
1584.

47. Gunnar RM, Loeb HS: Use of drugs in cardiogenic shock due to acute myocardial infarction. *Circulation* 1972; 45:1111.

48. Henry PD, Dobson JG Jr, Sobel BE: Dissociation between changes in myocardial cyclic
adenosine monophosphate and contractility.
Circ Res 1975; 36:392.

49. Honejager P, Schafer-Kort MY, Reiter M:
Involvement of cyclic AMP in the direct ino-

tropic action of amrinone. *Naunyn Schmiedebergs Arch Pharmacol* 1981; 318:112.

50. Jentzer JH, LeJemtel TH, Sonnenblick EH, et al: Beneficial effect of amrinone on myocardial oxygen consumption during acute left ventricular failure in dogs. *Am J Cardiol* 1981; 48:75.

51. Kenakin TP: An in-vitro quantitative analysis of the alpha-adrenoreceptor partial agonist activity of dobutamine and its relevance to inotropic selectivity. *J Pharmacol Exp Ther* 1981; 216:210.

52. King BD, Sokoloff L, Wechsler RL: The effects of *l*-epinephrine and *l*-norepinephrine upon cerebral circulation and metabolism in man. *J Clin Invest* 1952; 31:273.

53. Klein NA, Siskind SJ, Frishman WH, et al: Hemodynamic comparison of intravenous amrinone and dobutamine in patients with chronic congestive heart failure. *Am J Cardiol* 1981; 48:170.

54. Kuhn LA, Kline HJ, Goodman P, et al: Effects of isoproterenol on hemodynamic alterations, myocardial metabolism and coronary flow in acute myocardial infarction with shock. *Am Heart J* 1969; 77:772.

55. Laks M, Callis G, Swan HJC: Hemodynamic effects of low doses of norepinephrine in the conscious dog. *Am J Physiol* 1971; 220:171.

56. Lefkowitz RJ, Caron MD, Stiles GL: Mechanisms of membrane-receptor regulation. *N Engl J Med* 1984; 310:1570.

57. Leier CV, Heban PT, Huss P, et al: Comparative systemic and regional hemodynamic effects of dopamine and dobutamine in patients with cardiomyopathic heart failure. *Circulation* 1978; 58:466.

58. Leier CV, Huss P, Lewis RP, et al: Drug-induced conditioning in congestive heart failure. *Circulation* 1982; 65:1382.

59. Leier CV, Webel J, Bush CA: The cardiovascular effects of the continuous infusion of dobutamine in patients with severe heart failure. *Circulation* 1977; 56:468.

60. Liang C-S, Sherman LG, Doherty JV, et al: Sustained improvement of cardiac function in patients with congestive heart failure after short-term infusion of dobutamine. *Circulation* 1984; 69:113.

61. Liang C-S, Yi JM, Sherman LG, et al: Dobutamine infusion in conscious dogs with and without acute myocardial infarction: Effects on systemic hemodynamics, myocardial blood flow and infarct size. *Circ Res* 1981; 49:170.

62. Loeb HS, Winslow EBJ, Rahimtoola SH, et al: Acute hemodynamic effects of dopamine in patients with shock. *Circulation* 1971; 44:163.

63. Loisance DY, Cochera JP, Poulain H, et al: Ventricular septal defect after acute myocardial infarction: Early repair. *J Thorac Cardiovasc Surg* 1980; 80:61.

64. MacCannell KL, McNay JL, Meyer MB, et al: Dopamine in the treatment of hypotension and shock. *N Engl J Med* 1966; 275:1389.

65. Magorien RD, Unverferth DV, Brown GP, et al: Dobutamine and hydralazine: Comparative influences of positive inotropy and vasodilation on coronary blood flow and myocardial energetics in nonischemic congestive heart failure. *J Am Coll Cardiol* 1983; 1:499.

66. Maroko PR, Kjekshus JK, Sobel BE, et al: Factors influencing infarct size following experimental coronary artery occlusions. *Circulation* 1971; 43:67.

67. Mason DT: Afterload reduction and cardiac performance. *Am J Med* 1978; 65:1006.

68. McGiff JC, Burns CR: Separation of dopamine natriuresis from vasodilatation: Evidence for dopamine receptors. *J Lab Clin Med* 1967; 70:892.

69. Montoya A, McKeever L, Scanlon P, et al: Early repair of ventricular septal rupture after infarction. *Am J Cardiol* 1980; 45:345.

70. Mueller H, Ayres SM, Gregory JJ, et al: Hemodynamics, coronary blood flow, and myocardial metabolism in coronary shock: Response to *l*-norepinephrine and isoproterenol. *J Clin Invest* 1970; 49:1885.

71. Mueller HS, Evans R, Ayres SM: Effect of dopamine on hemodynamics and myocardial metabolism in shock following acute myocardial infarction in man. *Circulation* 1978; 57:361.

72. O'Rourke MF: Subacute heart rupture following myocardial infarction. *Lancet* 1973; 2:124.

73. O'Rourke MF, Sammel N, Chang VP: Arterial counterpulsation in severe refractory heart failure complication in acute myocardial infarction. *Br Heart J* 1979; 41:308.

74. Page DL, Caulfield JB, Kastor JA, et al: Myocardial changes associated with cardiogenic shock. *N Engl J Med* 1971; 285:133.

75. Palmer RF, Lasseter KC: Drug Therapy: so-

dium nitroprusside. *N Engl J Med* 1975; 292:294.

75a. Parrillo JE: Vasodilator therapy in, Chernow B (ed): *The Pharmacologic Approach to the Critically Ill Patient.* Baltimore, Williams & Wilkins Co, 1983, pp 283–302.

76. Pennington DG, Codd JE, Merjavy JP, et al: The expanded use of ventricular bypass systems for severe cardiac failure and as a bridge to cardiac transplantation. *Heart Transplant* 1983; 3:38.

77. Petein M, Levine B, Cohn J: Hemodynamic effects of a new inotropic agent, piroximone (MDL 19,205), in patients with chronic heart failure. *J Am Coll Cardiol* 1984; 4:364.

78. Pierce WS, Parr GVS, Myers JL, et al: Ventricular-assist pumping in patients with cardiogenic shock after cardiac operation. *N Engl J Med* 1981; 305:1606.

79. Pozen RG, DiBianco R, Katz RJ, et al: Myocardial metabolic and hemodynamic effects of dobutamine in heart failure complicating coronary artery disease. *Circulation* 1981; 63:1279.

80. Richard C, Ricome JL, Rinailho A, et al: Combined hemodynamic effects of dopamine and dobutamine in cardiogenic shock. *Circulation* 1983; 67:620.

81. Robie NW, Nutter DO, Moody C, et al: In vivo analysis of adrenergic receptor activity of dobutamine. *Circ Res* 1974; 34:663.

82. Ross RS, Lesch M, Braunwald E: Acute myocardial infarction, in Thorn CW, Adams RO, Braunwald E, et al (eds): *Principles of Internal Medicine,* ed 8. New York, McGraw-Hill Book Co, 1977, p 1278.

83. Rude RE, Bush LR, Izquierdo C, et al: Effects of inotropic and chronotropic stimuli on acute myocardial ischemic injury. III. Influence of basal heart rate. *Am J Cardiol* 1984; 53:1688.

84. Ruffolo RR Jr, Spradlin TA, Pollock D, et al: Alpha and beta adrenergic effects of the stereoisomers of dobutamine. *J Pharmacol Exp Ther* 1981; 219:447.

85. Scheidt S, Ascheim R, Killip T: Shock after myocardial infarction: A clinical and hemodynamic profile. *Am J Cardiol* 1970; 26:556.

86. Schuelke DM, Mark AL, Schmid PG, et al: Coronary vasodilatation produced by dopamine after alpha adrenergic blockade. *J Pharmacol Exp Ther* 1971; 176:320.

87. Schumann HJ, Wagner J, Knorr A, et al:

Demonstration in human atrial preparations of alpha-adrenoreceptors mediating positive inotropic effects. *Naunyn Schmiedebergs Arch Pharmacol* 1978; 302:333.

88. Shah PK, Pichler M, Berman DS, et al: Left ventricular ejection fraction determined by radionuclide ventriculography in early stages of first transmural myocardial infarction. *Am J Cardiol* 1980; 45:542.

89. Shubin H, Weil MH: Hemodynamic alterations in patients after acute myocardial infarction, in Mills LC, Moyer JH (eds): *Shock and Hypotension.* New York, Grune & Stratton, 1965, p 499.

90. Shubin H, Weil MH: The hemodynamic effects of vasopressor agents in shock due to myocardial infarction (abstract). *Am J Cardiol* 1965; 15:147.

91. Smythe C McC, Nickel JF, Bradley SE: The effect of norepinephrine (USP), epinephrine, and *l*-norepinephrine on glomerular filtration rate, renal plasma flow, and the urinary excretion of sodium, potassium, and water in normal man. *J Clin Invest* 1952; 31:499.

92. Sonnenblick EH, Frishman WH, LeJemtel TH: Dobutamine: A new synthetic cardioactive sympathetic amine. *N Engl J Med* 1979; 300:17.

93. Swan HJC, Forrester JS, Danzig R, et al: Power failure in acute myocardial infarction. *Prog Cardiovasc Dis* 1970; 12:568.

94. Swan HJC, Ganz W, Forrester JS, et al: Catheterization of the heart in man with the use of a flow directed balloon-tipped catheter. *N Engl J Med* 1970; 283:447.

95. Tsien RW: Cyclic AMP and contractile activity in heart. *Adv Cyclic Nucleotide Res* 1977; 8:363.

96. Unverferth DV, Blanford M, Kates RE, et al: Tolerance to dobutamine after a 72 hour continuous infusion. *Am J Med* 1980; 69:262.

97. Unverferth DV, Magorien RD, Altschuld R, et al: The hemodynamic and metabolic advantages gained by a three-day infusion of dobutamine in patients with congestive cardiomyopathy. *Am Heart J* 1983; 106:29.

98. Uretsky BF: Is inotropic therapy appropriate for patients with chronic congestive heart failure? *Postgrad Med* (in press).

99. Uretsky BF: Left ventricular aneurysm by angiogram: A problem of definition. *Am J Cardiol* 1983; 51:918.

100. Uretsky BF, Generalovich T, Reddy PS, et

al: The acute hemodynamic effects of a new agent MDL 17,043, in the treatment of congestive heart failure. *Circulation* 1983; 67:823.

101. Walker WE, Stoney WS, Alford WC Jr, et al: Results of surgical management of acute left ventricular aneurysms. *Circulation* 1980; 62(suppl I):75.

102. Weintraub RM, Thurer RL: The intra-aortic balloon pump: A ten-year experience. *Heart Transplant* 1983; 3:8.

103. Wilson JR, Schwartz JS, Sutton MStJ, et al: Prognosis in severe heart failure: Relation to hemodynamic measurements and ventricular ectopic activity. *J Am Coll Cardiol* 1980; 2:403.

104. Willerson JT, Buja LM: Cause and course of acute myocardial infarction. *Am J Med* 1980; 69:903.

30

Robert R. Ruffolo, Jr., Ph.D.

Joseph D. Fondacaro, Ph.D.

Blanche Levitt, Ph.D.

Richard M. Edwards, Ph.D.

Lewis B. Kinter, Ph.D.

Pharmacologic Manipulation of Regional Blood Flow

In critical vascular beds, local blood flow is changed by a complex interplay between local autoregulatory factors and neurogenically induced adjustments in vascular tone, both of which may be affected by global hemodynamic alterations such as changes in cardiac output. In addition, many drugs have the capacity to elicit changes in regional blood flow by stimulating or antagonizing specific drug, neurotransmitter, and hormone receptors, which may be differentially distributed in these critical vascular beds. In order to understand and predict regional blood flow changes likely to result from drug administration or likely to induce specific pharmacologic manipulation in local blood flow, it is important to understand the function of receptors present in the key vascular beds, and the responses (vasodilatory or vasoconstrictor) they mediate. In the present chapter, the important drug, neurotransmitter, and hormone receptors in crucial vascular beds are discussed. Since a detailed presentation of all vascular beds is not within the scope of this review, the most important are discussed: coronary, pulmonary, cerebral, renal, and splanchnic circulatory beds. The receptors present in these beds and responses of the vascular beds to certain drugs commonly used in the care of the critically ill are discussed.

CORONARY CIRCULATION

Blood flow through the coronary circulation is heavily influenced by autoregulatory factors that generally predominate over neural influences. The major innervation to the coronary circulation is provided by the sympathetic nervous system which, in contrast to most other vascular beds, mediates vasodilation via stimulation of β_1-adrenoceptors under normal conditions. However, in the presence of a limiting stenosis, sympathetic nerve stimulation can be shown to mediate a vasoconstrictor response, similar to that observed in other vascular beds. Furthermore, many drugs and circulating hormones have the capacity to alter coronary blood flow by direct stimulation of specific receptors on coronary blood vessels.

Receptors in the Coronary Circulation

α-Adrenoceptors

Stimulation of α-adrenoceptors in large epicardial vessels and small resistance coronary arteries leads to vasoconstriction.[193] α-Adrenoceptor-mediated coronary artery vasoconstriction can functionally antagonize metabolic coronary artery vasodilation[128] as well as β-adrenoceptor-mediated vasodilation, such that coronary artery resistance is determined by the net balance between these opposing actions. If a limiting stenosis is present in the coronary circulation, distal coronary arteries dilate to compensate for the stenosis. Under these conditions of maximal coronary artery vasodilation, α-adrenoceptor-mediated coronary artery vasoconstriction is increased[82] and may contribute to the genesis of coronary arterial vasospasm[85] and myocardial ischemia.[131]

Recent studies have demonstrated that α_1-

and α_2-adrenoceptors coexist postsynaptically in the coronary circulation and that both α-adrenoceptor subtypes mediate coronary artery vasoconstriction.[83] It has been proposed that the larger epicardial coronary arteries possess predominantly α_1-adrenoceptors, whereas the smaller subendocardial resistance vessels contain predominantly α_2-adrenoceptors.[83] This is consistent with the observation that a greater increase in coronary vascular resistance is mediated by α_2-adrenoceptors than by α_1-adrenoceptors.[82] In contrast to most peripheral arterial beds, in which postsynaptic vascular α_1-adrenoceptors are innervated by sympathetic neurons and postsynaptic vascular α_2-adrenoceptors are extrajunctional and noninnervated[157] (see also chapter 6, "Neurohumoral Regulation of Cardiovascular Function"), evidence suggests that in the resistance coronary arteries postsynaptic vascular α_2-adrenoceptors reside junctionally and may be innervated to a greater extent than the α_1-adrenoceptors.[82, 163] Because of the differential distribution of α_1- and α_2-adrenoceptors in the coronary circulation, it has been suggested that α_1-adrenoceptor-mediated vasoconstriction of large epicardial coronary arteries may be a cause of coronary artery vasospasm, which is consistent with the observation that in patients with Prinzmetal's variant angina, the frequency and severity of anginal attacks are often reduced by treatment with the selective α_1-adrenoceptor antagonist, prazosin. In contrast, postsynaptic vascular α_2-adrenoceptors on smaller distal resistance coronary arteries have been implicated as a possible cause of myocardial ischemia when there is a proximal coronary stenosis; this is a situation in which cardiac sympathetic nerve stimulation can induce poststenotic vasoconstriction.[82]

β-Adrenoceptors

If coronary vascular resistance is elevated, stimulation of sympathetic nerves produces coronary artery vasodilation, and this effect is mediated by β-adrenoceptors in coronary resistance vessels.[30] Although most vascular β-adrenoceptors in the peripheral circulation are of the β_2 subtype (see chapter 6, "Neurohumoral Regulation of Cardiovascular Function"), those present in the resistance vessels of the coronary circulation appear to be predominantly of the β_1 subtype. This accounts for the fact that exogenously or neuronally released norepinephrine, which is markedly selective for β_1-adrenoceptors, elicits a vasodilator response in the coronary circulation.[30]

There is also evidence, obtained from in vitro studies of large epicardial coronary arteries, for the existence of β_2-adrenoceptors, which, like the β_1-adrenoceptors in the resistance coronary vessels, mediate vasodilation.[74] These β_2-adrenoceptors are likely extrajunctional in distribution and may respond to circulating epinephrine acting as a blood-borne hormone, thereby augmenting coronary blood flow.

Muscarinic Cholinergic Receptors

Effects mediated by muscarinic cholinergic receptors in the coronary circulation are complex. When there are no metabolic effects, administering acetylcholine or stimulating parasympathetic nerves to the coronary circulation produces a net vasodilatory response.[52] Cholinergically mediated coronary artery vasodilation is believed to result primarily from an endothelium-derived relaxant factor, the release of which is activated by muscarinic cholinergic receptors on the endothelial surface.[192] The endothelium-derived relaxant factor subsequently interacts with vascular smooth muscle in the coronary circulation to decrease coronary vascular resistance and increase coronary blood flow. In addition, there are muscarinic cholinergic receptors on the smooth muscle of the coronary vasculature, and when activated these receptors mediate vasoconstriction. Thus, muscarinic cholinergic receptors in the coronary circulation produce a mixed response: indirect coronary artery vasodilation involving the endothelium and direct coronary artery vasoconstriction. The net effect reflects the balance of these two opposing responses, and in general the endothelium-mediated coronary vasodilator response predominates.[192]

Prostaglandin Receptors

A variety of prostaglandin receptors exist in the coronary circulation. Some of these receptors mediate coronary artery vasodilation and others mediate coronary artery vasoconstriction. Both prostaglandin E_1 (PGE$_1$) and prostacyclin (PGI$_2$) are potent coronary artery vasodilators,[172] and both agents have been used to treat unstable angina with some success. Prostacyclin has also been shown to limit infarct size in animals and humans (see chapter 9, "Role of Prostacyclin, Thromboxane A_2, and Leukotrienes in Cardiovascular Function and Disease"). PGE$_1$ and prostacyclin both inhibit platelet aggregation, which may play a role in their antianginal effects[129] and in their improving the balance between myocardial oxygen supply and demand.

In contrast, $PGF_{2\alpha}$ and thromboxane A_2 (TXA_2) interact with specific receptors in the coronary circulation to produce coronary artery vasoconstriction.[20, 30] TXA_2 in particular has been implicated as a causative factor in a number of pathologic states involving the coronary circulation, such as myocardial ischemia, variant angina, myocardial infarction, and sudden death syndrome.[87, 112]

Leukotriene Receptors

Leukotrienes C_4, D_4, and E_4 are potent mediators of coronary artery vasoconstriction. It has been proposed that the coronary vasoconstrictor effect of the leukotrienes contributes indirectly to the negative inotropic effects of these compounds. (For a more detailed discussion of the effects mediated by leukotrienes in the coronary circulation, refer to chapter 9, "Role of Prostacyclin, Thromboxane A_2, and Leukotrienes in Cardiovascular Function and Disease.")

Serotonin (5-HT) Receptors

Serotonin receptors, like muscarinic cholinergic receptors, mediate a complex response in the coronary circulation: one response may involve the coronary endothelium. Furthermore, 5-HT_1 and 5-HT_2 receptors coexist in coronary arteries, and it appears that these serotonin receptor subtypes mediate opposing responses.

Serotonin has been shown in vitro to dilate coronary arteries when vascular tone is elevated.[27] This dilation is seen only in vessels with intact endothelium and is not sensitive to 5-HT_2 receptor antagonists, which suggests that endothelial 5-HT_1 receptors mediate coronary artery vasodilation. Endogenous serotonin can also interact with endothelial 5-HT_1 receptors, since the vasoconstrictor response of coronary arteries induced by aggregating platelets (which release serotonin) is significantly potentiated by removal of vascular endothelium.[29]

In a perfused coronary artery preparation with intact endothelium, serotonin can have opposite effects when administered extraluminally (adventitial side) or intraluminally (intimal surface).[29] Extraluminal administration of serotonin, which selectively exposes 5-HT_2 receptors located on coronary artery smooth muscle to serotonin, produces a contractile response, whereas intraluminal administration of serotonin, in which endothelial 5-HT_1 receptors are preferentially exposed, commonly produces relaxation. In fact, intraluminal administration of serotonin can relax contractions induced by extraluminally applied serotonin. Relaxation can also be produced in this preparation by endogenous serotonin released from aggregating platelets intraluminally.[29]

Dopamine Receptors

Dopamine receptors have recently been identified in the coronary circulation, where they mediate a vasodilatory response. These receptors, which are of the DA_1 subtype, are associated with the smooth muscle layer of coronary arteries, where they produce direct vascular smooth muscle relaxation,[17] decreasing coronary vascular resistance.

Vasopressin Receptors

Vasopressin is a potent direct coronary artery vasoconstrictor that acts on V_1 (vascular) vasopressin receptors. It has been demonstrated in the coronary circulation that exogenously administered vasopressin decreases coronary blood flow by increasing coronary vascular resistance.[84] Additionally, endogenous release of vasopressin has been shown to promote an increase in coronary vascular resistance.[164] Vasopressin-induced increases in coronary vascular resistance and the resulting reductions in coronary blood flow in humans have been implicated as causative factors in specific pathologic states, such as myocardial ischemic injury, myocardial infarction,[127] anginal pain,[175] ventricular arrhythmias, and sudden death.[127]

Purinergic Receptors

The coronary circulation contains purinergic receptors that mediate coronary artery vasodilation in response to purine nucleotides. Vasodilation produced by adenosine triphosphate (ATP) and adenosine in the coronary circulation has been studied extensively, largely because of the possible implications for coronary occlusion and the potential relevance to the treatment of angina.[11, 21] Smaller coronary vessels are more sensitive to adenosine than are larger vessels.[165]

ATP and adenosine diphosphate (ADP) are the most potent of the adenyl compounds that relax coronary vessels; adenosine monophosphate (AMP) and adenosine are from one fourth to one third as potent as ATP. Adenine, hypoxanthine, guanine, cytosine, and uracil are either inactive or of low potency. Uridine nucleotides may dilate (UTP, UDP) or constrict (UMP) coronary resistance vessels.[21]

Stimulation of adenosine receptors may result in the influx of Ca^{++},[81] possibly via elevation of intracellular cAMP after stimulation of adenylate cyclase.[81, 110] As in cardiac muscle, the vasodilatory action of adenosine on coronary arteries is blocked by theophylline, aminophylline, and caffeine,[81] which is consistent with activation of the P_1 subtype of purinergic receptors.[81]

Effects of Various Drugs on the Coronary Circulation

Dobutamine

In animal studies, dobutamine increases blood flow to all regions of the myocardium, with a disproportionately greater increase to the subendocardium than is observed with isoproterenol.[187] The increase in coronary blood flow elicited by dobutamine may be secondary to the increase in myocardial work (i.e., contractility and heart rate) produced by the drug, since doses of dobutamine below those required to improve left ventricular (LV) function do not significantly increase regional myocardial blood flow.[204]

Dopamine

The doses of dopamine required to augment LV performance increase coronary blood flow.[102] The effects of dopamine on coronary blood flow reflect a complex interplay between direct and systemic hemodynamic responses and autoregulatory factors at the level of the myocardium. Dopamine may produce direct coronary arterial vasodilation by stimulating β_1-adrenoceptors and dopamine DA_1 receptors in the coronary circulation. Furthermore, the increase in LV minute work and stroke work produced by dopamine[159] will elicit an indirect vasodilatory response as the coronary circulation responds to an increase in myocardial oxygen demand by dilating resistance vessels (metabolic vasodilation). Finally, since the α-adrenoceptor-mediated vasoconstrictor properties of dopamine elevate blood pressure,[160] myocardial perfusion pressure (i.e., diastolic blood pressure) increases, further augmenting coronary blood flow.

Isoproterenol

Isoproterenol produces a complex response in the coronary circulation. At low doses, it increases coronary blood flow. Both subepicardial and subendocardial blood flows are increased, but the increase in the ratio of subendocardial to subepicardial blood flow is less for isoproterenol than for dobutamine.[187] At higher doses of isoproterenol, myocardial blood flow may decrease, owing to the significant decreases in diastolic perfusion pressure that result from hypotension and the decrease in diastolic perfusion time from tachycardia.

Norepinephrine and Epinephrine

In doses that augment LV function, both norepinephrine and epinephrine increase coronary blood flow. The effects of these catecholamines on coronary blood flow are complex and, like those of dopamine, result from a number of different mechanisms. Because they stimulate β_1-adrenoceptors in the coronary circulation, norepinephrine and epinephrine produce direct coronary artery vasodilation. Furthermore, because norepinephrine and epinephrine both augment LV function, coronary blood flow is indirectly increased by autoregulatory factors to supply sufficient oxygen to support the elevated myocardial oxygen demand. Finally, an increase in diastolic blood pressure produced by norepinephrine and epinephrine serves to increase coronary perfusion pressure, which further augments myocardial blood flow.

Nitroglycerin/Nitroprusside

When injected directly into the coronary circulation, nitroglycerin is a potent coronary artery vasodilator. The increase in coronary blood flow produced by nitroglycerin is secondary to a reduction in coronary vascular resistance.[150] In animals, nitroglycerin increases blood flow to the ischemic myocardium, induces a favorable redistribution of blood flow toward the ischemic endocardium, and does not decrease blood perfusion to the nonischemic myocardium.[37] Although with intracoronary administration nitroglycerin is a potent coronary arterial vasodilator, with systemic (sublingual or intravenous) administration, the antianginal effect appears to be secondary to the systemic hemodynamic effects of the compound. Thus, nitroglycerin decreases myocardial oxygen demand by reducing preload, afterload, and thereby myocardial wall tension.

Like nitroglycerin, nitroprusside can dilate the coronary arterial circulation. It appears that coronary arteries located more proximally dilate less with nitroprusside than do the more distal segments.

Calcium Channel Antagonists

The calcium channel antagonists increase coronary artery blood flow even when coronary perfusion pressure is reduced by a decrease in systemic arterial blood pressure.[156] These results indicate that calcium channel antagonists produce coronary artery vasodilation and decrease coronary vascular resistance to an extent great enough to offset reduced perfusion pressure. In patients with congestive heart failure, nifedipine has been demonstrated to reduce coronary vascular resistance and to increase coronary blood flow at rest in the absence of a change in myocardial oxygen consumption.[119] When there is a limiting stenosis, coronary vasoconstriction distal to the stenosis induced by cardiac sympathetic nerve stimulation, which is mediated by postsynaptic vascular α_2-adrenoceptors,[82] is effectively inhibited by calcium channel antagonists.[82] The resulting decrease in regional myocardial contraction and the increase in net lactate production are inhibited as well.

Propranolol

Although β-adrenoceptor antagonists reduce myocardial oxygen consumption and reduce the symptoms of myocardial ischemia in patients with angina, β-blockers have on occasion been observed to exacerbate coronary artery spasm in patients with variant angina. Propranolol augments the increase in coronary vascular resistance observed during the cold pressor test.[100] It has been proposed that by blocking coronary β-adrenoceptors, which mediate vasodilation, the unopposed α-adrenoceptor-mediated coronary artery vasoconstriction will predominate and lead to the observed increase in coronary artery resistance.

PULMONARY CIRCULATION

All of the cardiac output is received by the pulmonary circulation. As such, changes in pulmonary vascular resistance can have profound consequences, with significant increases resulting in pulmonary edema. Elevated pulmonary pressures can markedly affect the transport of oxygen across the pulmonary epithelium, and thereby the delivery of oxygen to systemic organs. The predominant innervation to the pulmonary circulation is sympathetic, in which both α-adrenoceptor-

mediated increases and β-adrenoceptor-mediated decreases in pulmonary vascular resistance may be observed. The response obtained depends largely on resting vascular tone in the pulmonary circulation. As expected, many drugs and circulating hormones have the capacity to alter pulmonary hemodynamics, and often the response observed is dependent on the degree of spontaneous vascular tone in this bed.

Receptors in the Pulmonary Circulation

α-Adrenoceptors

Stimulation of α-adrenoceptors in the pulmonary vascular bed produces a vasoconstrictor response, increasing pulmonary vascular resistance and pulmonary artery pressure. As in the peripheral arterial circulation, α_1- and α_2-adrenoceptors coexist in the pulmonary circulation, and both α-adrenoceptor subtypes mediate vasoconstriction.[89] However, large pulmonary arteries studied in vitro demonstrate only α_1-adrenoceptor-mediated responses,[16] suggesting that postsynaptic vascular α_2-adrenoceptors may be localized on the smaller pulmonary resistance vessels.[89]

β-Adrenoceptors

β-Adrenoceptors are present in the pulmonary circulation and mediate a vasodilator response, decreasing pulmonary vascular resistance and pulmonary artery pressure. The β-adrenoceptor-mediated pulmonary vasodilator response is especially marked when pulmonary vascular resistance is high. Pharmacologic studies indicate that the β-adrenoceptor present in the pulmonary circulation is of the β_2 subtype.[90] There is evidence to suggest that the β_2-adrenoceptors mediating vasodilation in the pulmonary circulation may be innervated by the sympathetic nervous system,[90] in contrast to other systemic vascular beds, in which β_2-adrenoceptors are noninnervated and located extrajunctionally (see chapter 6, "Neurohumoral Regulation of Cardiovascular Function").

Muscarinic Cholinergic Receptors

The responses mediated by muscarinic cholinergic receptors in the pulmonary circulation are complex. Acetylcholine actively constricts lobar small veins but not large veins, and possibly produces vasoconstriction of lobar arteries.[88] These responses to acetylcholine cause both pulmonary arterial and venous pressor responses secondary to increases in pulmonary arterial and venous resistance. However, in the presence of high pulmonary vascular resistance, stimulation of muscarinic cholinergic receptors may mediate a vasodilator response, possibly secondary to the release of an endothelium-derived relaxant factor.[88]

Prostaglandin Receptors

A variety of prostaglandins produce vascular responses in the pulmonary circulation. Prostaglandins E_2, $F_{2\alpha}$, and D_2, TXA_2, and the endoperoxide analogue, PGH_2, increase lobar arterial pressure by increasing pulmonary arterial resistance. Likewise, these prostaglandins produce vasoconstrictor responses in pulmonary vein in vitro.[96] In contrast, prostacyclin produces vasodilation and decreases pulmonary vascular resistance, and this response is particularly marked when pulmonary vascular resistance is elevated.

Leukotriene Receptors

Injection of LTC_4 into the right atrium in monkeys acutely raises pulmonary artery pressure by increasing pulmonary vascular resistance. Following the acute pulmonary pressor response is a decrease in pulmonary artery pressure that is likely due to a reduction in venous return and subsequently low output from the right ventricle.[176] It has been proposed that the LTC_4-induced increase in pulmonary artery resistance may limit LV filling and thereby also contribute to the observed reduction in output from the LV.

Serotonin (5-HT) Receptors

Serotonin produces a vasoconstrictor response in isolated intrapulmonary arteries and veins.[76] It has been suggested that the pulmonary pressor response to thromboembolism results, at least in part, from serotonin released by aggregating platelets. The pulmonary pressor response to serotonin results directly from an increase in pulmonary vascular resistance.

Histamine Receptors

Histamine receptors mediate an increase in lobar arterial pressure secondary to an increase in pulmonary vascular resistance.[98] Histamine receptors also mediate an increase in pressures of small intrapulmonary veins.[98] The pulmonary pressor response mediated by histamine receptors is due exclusively to the histamine H_1 receptor subtype.

Effects of Various Drugs on the Pulmonary Circulation

Dobutamine

Infusion of dobutamine generally decreases central venous pressure, right and left atrial pressures, pulmonary arterial pressure and resistance, and pulmonary capillary wedge pressure.[114, 178] As a direct consequence, LV filling pressure (i.e., LV end-diastolic pressure) and LV end-diastolic volume are reduced, allowing the hypertrophied myocardium characteristic of congestive heart failure to decrease to a size more suitable for efficient LV function.[158]

Dopamine

When dopamine and dobutamine are infused in doses that produce equivalent increases in cardiac output, dopamine is associated with significantly smaller reductions in LV filling pressure and pulmonary capillary wedge pressure.[117] In fact, dopamine commonly does not change or may even increase pulmonary arterial pressure, pulmonary capillary wedge pressure, and LV end-diastolic pressure. Increases in pulmonary arterial pressure observed with dopamine have been attributed to the greater net α-adrenoceptor-mediated vasoconstrictor activity of dopamine relative to dobutamine and to the relative lack of agonist activity of dopamine at β_2-adrenoceptors[160] that mediate vasodilation in the pulmonary circulation.[90]

Isoproterenol

Isoproterenol reduces pulmonary vascular resistance, thereby reducing pulmonary arterial pressure, pulmonary capillary wedge pressure, and LV end-diastolic pressure. The mechanism responsible for the reduction in pulmonary vascular resistance is stimulation of β_2-adrenoceptors in the pulmonary vasculature.

Norepinephrine

Norepinephrine causes vasoconstriction in the pulmonary circulation. The increase in pulmonary vascular resistance produced by norepinephrine elevates pulmonary arterial pressure, which may result in pulmonary edema.[9] The norepinephrine-induced pulmonary edema is caused by both elevated pulmonary vascular resistance and increased venous return, the latter being a direct consequence of α-adrenoceptor-mediated vasoconstriction of venous capacitance vessels.

Pressure in intrapulmonary small arteries and veins is increased by norepinephrine.[96]

Epinephrine

The effects of epinephrine on pulmonary hemodynamics are variable: both increases and decreases in pulmonary blood flow are observed in patients.[171] The variability observed with epinephrine in relation to the response of norepinephrine is likely because epinephrine can activate α-adrenoceptors to cause vasoconstriction in the pulmonary circulation and β_2-adrenoceptors to produce vasodilation, whereas norepinephrine can stimulate only α-adrenoceptors. Studies in animals have shown that in the presence of α-adrenoceptor blockade, epinephrine produces no effect during normoxia, but produces significant vasodilation in the pulmonary circulation during hypoxia.[116] Also, during hypoxia, β-adrenoceptor blockade converts the vasodilatory response of epinephrine in the pulmonary circulation to vasoconstriction, which indicates that under resting conditions, α-adrenoceptor-mediated vasoconstriction is counterbalanced by β_2-adrenoceptor-mediated vasodilation in the pulmonary circulation. It also appears that the response to epinephrine in the pulmonary circulation depends on resting vascular tone. Thus, at low pulmonary arterial pressures, epinephrine primarily increases pressure in the pulmonary circulation, presumably by an α-adrenoceptor-mediated vasoconstriction, whereas when pulmonary vascular pressures are elevated, epinephrine reduces pressure by producing β_2-adrenoceptor-mediated vasodilation.[90]

Nitrates

Nitroglycerin and nitroprusside reduce pulmonary arterial pressure by decreasing pulmonary vascular resistance. The effects of the nitrates on pulmonary vascular resistance are small under normal conditions but become marked when pulmonary vascular resistance is elevated. Both nitroglycerin and nitroprusside reduce lobar arterial and small-vein pressures.[96] The effect of the nitrates on the pulmonary circulation may be predominantly to dilate intrapulmonary veins and upstream segments.[96]

Hydralazine

Hydralazine is a direct arterial vasodilator that reduces pulmonary arterial pressure and pulmonary vascular resistance in animals. In the clinical setting, the effects of hydralazine on pulmonary arterial pressure are more variable and depend on the initial levels of pulmonary vascular resistance and the degree to which these vessels can dilate.[97] When pulmonary arterial pressures are elevated, as in congestive heart failure, hydralazine commonly decreases pulmonary vascular resistance and pulmonary arterial pressure.

Captopril

Angiotensin converting enzyme inhibitors, such as captopril, have pronounced effects on pulmonary hemodynamics. In patients with congestive heart failure, captopril reduces pulmonary arterial pressure and pulmonary capillary wedge pressure at doses that increase cardiac index. The effect of captopril on pulmonary hemodynamics appears to result not from reductions in pulmonary vascular resistance, but rather from a reduction in LV afterload in patients with high renin activity.

Calcium Channel Antagonists

Blockade of calcium channels in the pulmonary circulation is the logical treatment of pulmonary hypertension since these agents, such as verapamil, diltiazem, and nifedipine, exert direct vasodilator effects in the highly constricted pulmonary circulation.[141] Verapamil has been shown to decrease mean pulmonary arterial pressure without changing systemic vascular resistance in patients with pulmonary hypertension.[141] However, verapamil can have direct depressant effects on right ventricular function, as evidenced by reductions in right ventricular stroke work index and an increase in right ventricular filling pressure. This myocardial depressant effect is less likely with nifedipine. The ability of calcium channel antagonists to produce pulmonary arterial vasodilation is more pronounced when pulmonary vascular resistance is high.[95]

CEREBRAL CIRCULATION

The regulation of cerebral blood flow is controlled by many diverse substances including neurotransmitters, circulating hormones, autocoids, and metabolic factors that act on specific receptors located on cerebrovascular smooth muscle cells. Furthermore, several of these substances can have opposing effects on blood flow, depending on the initial degree of vascular tone and/or the presence of an intact vascular endothelium. Although many factors can affect cerebral blood flow, the prime determinant of cerebral blood flow is metabolic autoregulation.

Receptors in the Cerebral Circulation

α-Adrenoceptors

Cerebral blood vessels have a dense sympathetic innervation[46] which, when stimulated, causes vasoconstriction of large pial arteries via the interaction of norepinephrine with α-adrenoceptors. However, because of compensatory autoregulatory mechanisms, cerebral blood flow does not fall.[23] Isolated cerebral arteries respond poorly to either electrical stimulation or to norepinephrine, which suggests that the density and/or sensitivity of α-adrenoceptors is lower in cerebral arteries than in peripheral arteries.[126, 185] Although interspecies differences have been reported in the subtypes of α-adrenoceptors that mediate contraction in cerebral vessels, it is evident that α_1-adrenoceptors predominate in human cerebral arteries.[185]

Despite the observation that stimulation of α-adrenoceptors has minimal effect on cerebrovascular tone under normal conditions, it is thought that the sympathetic vasoconstrictor response may be important in preventing disruption of the blood-brain barrier during severe arterial hypertension.[107] In fact, several investigators have shown that sympathetic nerves protect against stroke and seizures in stroke-prone spontaneously hypertensive rats.[132, 162]

β-Adrenoceptors

When vascular tone is high, stimulating β-adrenoceptors by isoproterenol or norepinephrine dilates cerebral arteries in vitro. This vasodilation is mediated by β_1-adrenoceptors.[207] In vivo studies on the effects of β-adrenoceptor stimulation on pial arterial resistance have produced conflicting results;[169, 196] hence, the role of the β-adrenoceptor in regulating cerebral blood flow in the intact animal has not been firmly established.

In addition to β_1-adrenoceptors, β_2-adrenoceptors have been identified in rat cerebral microvessels.[103] This may have some physiologic relevance to the human cerebral circulation, particularly since this receptor subtype may be involved with oxygen consumption and cerebral glucose uptake.[118] It may also be important in the pathology of malignant hypertension, since it has

been shown that the density of β_2-adrenoceptors is decreased in rats with hypertension.[118]

Muscarinic Cholinergic Receptors

Histochemical and biochemical studies indicate that cholinergic nerves are present in the cerebral blood vessels of many species.[35] However, cholinergic nerve stimulation in vivo has no effect on cerebral blood flow.[22] Acetylcholine has been shown to have either vasoconstrictor or vasodilatory effects on isolated cerebral vessels. In the presence of active tone, acetylcholine induces relaxation, which depends on an intact endothelium.[41, 111] This is consistent with the observation that acetylcholine stimulates the release of an endogenous relaxing substance from endothelial cells in many vascular beds.[63] When vascular tone is low in cerebral blood vessels, or if the endothelium is damaged, acetylcholine will produce a dose-dependent vasoconstrictor response. High doses of acetylcholine will also contract cerebral blood vessels with an intact endothelium.[41, 111] Both the vasoconstricting and vasodilating actions of acetylcholine are blocked by atropine, indicating that these effects are mediated by muscarinic cholinergic receptors.

Although acetylcholine can relax cerebral blood vessels in vitro, there is considerable evidence to suggest that this neurotransmitter is not the mediator of neurogenic cerebral vasodilation in vivo.[35] In addition, cholinergic nerves do not appear to play a role in the autoregulation of cerebral blood flow.[22] Thus, the role of cholinergic nerves in the cerebral circulation is not established.

Dopamine Receptors

Stimulation of dopamine receptors by dopamine or selective dopamine receptor agonists mediates relaxation of cerebral blood vessels.[17] Results from pharmacologic studies on isolated human cerebral blood vessels suggest that these dopamine receptors are of the dopamine DA_1 subtype,[43, 61] similar to the receptors that are linked to adenylate cyclase and are located post-synaptically in selected peripheral vascular beds.[17] The existence of DA_1 receptors in the cerebral vasculature is supported by recent studies that have shown that dopamine selectively increases cAMP levels in pial arteries.[3]

Serotonin Receptors

Serotonin (5-HT) produces an intense vasoconstriction of cerebral blood vessels via activation of serotonergic receptors on vascular smooth muscle cells.[39] This vasoconstriction appears to be mediated by the 5-HT$_2$ receptor subtype,[73] which is the same receptor subtype that mediates vasoconstriction in the peripheral circulation.[29] As in peripheral tissues, activation of 5-HT$_2$ receptors may amplify the cerebral vasoconstrictor responses to a variety of other endogenous compounds, including norepinephrine and angiotensin II. In isolated cerebral arteries with induced vascular tone, serotonin also produces relaxation via inhibitory serotonergic receptors.[62, 191] Serotonin-induced vasodilation has been shown to be endothelial dependent and to be mediated by 5-HT$_1$ receptors in other vascular beds; however, this has not yet been addressed in studies of cerebral blood vessels.

Serotonin may have both a hormonal and a neurotransmitter role in the cerebral circulation, since evidence for a serotonergic innervation to the cerebrovascular bed has been reported, and serotonin can also be released into the circulation from platelets on aggregation.[39] Serotonin may be important in the etiology of migraine and cerebral vasospasm following subarachnoid hemorrhage. This is supported by studies that have shown that serotonin antagonists may provide effective prophylactic therapy in some forms of migraine.[149]

Histamine Receptors

Histamine can affect cerebrovascular resistance when released from a variety of sources, including perivascular mast cells, histaminergic nerves, blood basophils, and a non-mast cell store within cerebrovascular smooth muscle.[42] Histamine dilates pial vessels in situ and relaxes precontracted vessels in vitro by stimulating histamine H$_2$ receptors, which are located in the outer layers of the vascular smooth muscle. In addition, intra-arterial infusion of histamine increases cerebral blood flow[42, 75] and increases the permeability of the blood-brain barrier by stimulating the histamine H$_2$ receptor subtype. In contrast, pial veins do not respond to histamine, which suggests that receptors for histamine are sparsely populated or absent in cerebral venous smooth muscle.[75] In addition to the vasodilatory effects of histamine, several investigators have observed a histamine H$_1$ receptor–mediated vasoconstriction of pial vessels in vitro.[42, 120] However, it appears that vasodilation is the predominant response to histamine in the cerebral circulation in vivo. This may suggest that histamine H$_2$ receptors dominate over histamine H$_1$ receptors in this vascular bed.

Since blood levels of histamine can increase in some pathologic conditions, this amine may be an etiologic factor in several cerebrovascular disorders. Histamine has been implicated as a cause of cluster headache, in which large extracranial vessels are dilated during a headache attack. Extracranial vessels of patients with cluster headache are more sensitive to histamine-induced vasodilation than are extracranial vessels of controls.

Prostaglandin Receptors

Prostaglandins are synthesized in cerebrovascular smooth muscle[121] and may participate in the normal regulation of cerebral blood flow, as well as in cerebral vasospasm and migraine.[203] Various prostanoids produce either a contractile or a relaxant response in cerebrovascular smooth muscle. Prostaglandin-induced contractions in human pial arteries appear to be mediated via a TXA$_2$-sensitive receptor, whereas relaxant effects seem to be mediated by a receptor sensitive to prostacyclin.[190] TXA$_2$ is one of the most potent cerebral arterial vasoconstrictors known and has been considered to be one of the endogenous substances responsible for coronary and cerebral arterial vasospasm.[189, 195] PGF$_{2\alpha}$ and PGE$_2$ have weaker contractile effects on pial arteries than does TXA$_2$.[190] In contrast, prostacyclin is a potent vasodilator in the cerebral circulation. Prostacyclin has been shown to antagonize contractions induced by a variety of spasmogenic agents, which suggests that this prostanoid, or analogues of it, is a potential treatment of cerebral vasospasm.[143]

Purinergic Receptors

Adenosine may be an important metabolic factor in the autoregulation of cerebral blood flow, since increased cerebral adenosine levels are found during conditions such as ischemia, hypotension, and hypoxia.[12] Adenosine dilates cerebral arteries both in vitro and in situ, with smaller pial vessels being more reactive than larger vessels. Furthermore, in vivo studies have demonstrated that adenosine can also increase cerebral blood flow.[206] The vasodilatory effects of adenosine and related nucleotides are mediated via P_1 purinergic receptors. In addition to its relaxant effects on precontracted vessels, ATP has been shown to constrict some cerebral vessels; this effect is mediated via P_2 purinergic receptors.[133]

Opiate Receptors

Recent evidence demonstrates that opiates can affect cerebrovascular resistance by acting directly on vascular smooth muscle. Phencyclidine and its analogues can produce spasm of cerebral arterioles, arteries, and venules by interacting with specific σ opiate receptors.[2] In contrast, there are specific benzomorphan κ opiate receptors that mediate relaxation of precontracted cerebral blood vessels.[1]

Vasopressin Receptors

Recent studies have demonstrated that vasopressin exerts a powerful vasoconstrictor action on isolated human cerebral arteries by directly stimulating specific receptor sites for this neuropeptide.[115] In certain pathologic conditions in which vasopressin is released in large amounts, such as subarachnoid hemorrhage and hypertension, it is conceivable that vasopressin concentrations may occur sufficient to compromise cerebral blood flow.

Angiotensin Receptors

Both angiotensin I and II have been shown to produce concentration-related contraction of isolated cerebral arteries by stimulating angiotensin II receptors. Angiotensin I is converted to angiotensin II via the angiotensin converting enzyme, which is localized on the luminal surface of vascular endothelial cells.[202] Results from recent studies with captopril suggest that angiotensin II has a physiologic role in the autoregulation of cerebral blood flow. Chronic treatment with this angiotensin converting enzyme inhibitor produces cerebral vasodilation and a subsequent increase in cerebral blood flow in rats. In addition, IV infusion of captopril can decrease the pressure range over which cerebral blood flow can be autoregulated.[5, 104]

Bradykinin Receptors

Bradykinin is the most powerful cerebral vasodilator known. It is more potent and produces greater maximal cerebral vasodilation than either adenosine or histamine. Bradykinin relaxes human cerebral vessels in vitro by stimulating bradykinin B_2 receptors. In contrast, bradykinin has been shown to constrict cerebral arteries of other species via activation of bradykinin B_1 receptors.[189, 202]

Other Peptidergic Receptors

There are a number of recently discovered neuropeptides that are located within nerve terminals associated with cerebral blood vessels. Vasoactive intestinal polypeptide (VIP) has been shown to relax preconstricted cerebral vessels in vitro and to increase regional cerebral blood flow in vivo.[35, 205] These findings have led several investigators to propose that VIP is the transmitter responsible for the neurogenic vasodilator response in cerebral arteries.[36]

Substance P is a putative neurotransmitter of sensory pathways involved in pain perception.[19] This peptide has been shown to produce concentration-dependent relaxation of cerebral arteries and arterioles in vitro and in situ, and these effects are mediated via specific substance P receptors.[45] Due to its sensory role and vasodilatory effects, substance P may contribute to the genesis of headache pain.

Neuropeptide Y, a newly discovered peptide associated with adrenergic nerve terminals, is a potent vasoconstrictor of isolated cerebral arteries and has been shown to enhance the contractile response of the cerebral vasculature to other vasoactive substances.[40] These effects of neuropeptide Y on cerebrovascular tone appear to be species-specific and have not yet been examined in human cerebral arteries.

Effects of Various Drugs on the Cerebral Circulation

Dobutamine

Although both vasoconstrictor and vasodilator effects of dobutamine have been reported in the peripheral vasculature,[161] results from studies on isolated canine cerebral arteries demonstrate that cerebral vessels do not respond to dobutamine.[140] Therefore, direct effects of dobutamine on cerebral blood flow are expected to be negligible; however, effects secondary to changes in autonomic reflexes induced by dobutamine or to autoregulation resulting from global hemodynamic changes evoked by dobutamine cannot be ruled out.

Dopamine

In isolated human pial arteries with induced tone, dopamine produces relaxation via stimulation of dopamine DA_1 receptors.[43] IV infusion of the dopamine agonist piribedil in normal human volunteers significantly increases cerebral blood flow. This response is greater in patients suffering from migraine, suggesting that patients with migraine may have cerebrovascular dopamine DA_1 receptor supersensitivity.[14]

Isoproterenol

Isoproterenol relaxes isolated cerebral blood vessels by stimulating β_1-adrenoceptors. IV administration of isoproterenol increases cerebral blood flow and has been shown to attenuate cerebral vasospasm.[182]

Norepinephrine and Epinephrine

The response most frequently observed following IV or intra-arterial administration of norepinephrine and epinephrine is a decrease in cerebral blood flow, particularly when the cerebral vessels are maximally dilated. However, the vasoconstrictor effects of catecholamines may be masked if these vessels initially have a high degree of tone, such as in severe arterial hypertension.[44]

Vasopressin

In addition to being a potent vasoconstrictor of isolated human pial arteries, vasopressin administered IV produces a dose-dependent reduction in cerebral blood flow in animals.[115]

Calcium Channel Antagonists

Calcium channel antagonists relax isolated cerebral vessels contracted with a variety of endogenous vasospastic substances and reverse experimentally induced cerebral vasospasm in dogs.[173, 183] Studies with verapamil, diltiazem, and nifedipine have demonstrated that cerebral arteries are more susceptible to calcium channel antagonists than are peripheral arteries. These drugs are currently being evaluated in patients for the prevention and treatment of cerebral vasospasm and for the treatment of cerebral ischemia secondary to cardiac arrest (Brain Resuscitation Clinical Trials II, NIH Grant NS15295).

Nitroglycerin and Nitroprusside

These vasodilators are equieffective in relaxing isolated cerebral blood vessels with induced tone,[173] but reports of their effects on cerebral blood flow in humans are conflicting. During anesthesia, cerebral blood flow is constant during nitroprusside-induced hypotension because of autoregulatory mechanisms, whereas in the conscious state, nitroprusside appears to decrease cerebral blood flow before it reduces blood pressure. It has been proposed that nitroprusside reduces cerebral blood flow by impairing autoregulation or by an effect mediated through reflex activation of the sympathetic nervous system in response to arterial vasodilation.[80]

RENAL CIRCULATION

The kidneys are highly vascularized organs that together receive 20%–25% of the cardiac output. The control of renal hemodynamics is intimately tied to glomerular filtration rate (GFR) and the handling of salt and water, and is under the influence of local regulatory mechanisms (autoregulation) as well as extrinsic neuronal and hormonal factors. The kidney also produces a number of vasoactive substances, such as angiotensin II, bradykinin, and the prostanoids, which interact in a complex way to regulate renal vascular resistance. The most important and well characterized of these systems include the adrenergic system, the renin-angiotensin system, and the eicosanoids.

Receptors in the Renal Circulation

α-Adrenoceptors

Morphological and histochemical studies have demonstrated that the kidney has a dense adrenergic innervation.[4] Adrenergic nerve fibers and terminals are associated with all the major blood vessels of the kidney, including the interlobular arteries, the afferent and efferent arterioles, and the cells of the juxtaglomerular apparatus and specific tubule segments.[4] Radioligand binding studies have revealed the existence of α_1-, α_2-, β_1-, and β_2-adrenoceptors in the kidney.[125, 180, 181] However, the number, proportion, and distribution of these receptor subtypes in the kidney appear to vary among different species.[180] Furthermore, the physiologic processes controlled by these receptors are incompletely understood and are presently under intense investigation.

Catecholamines regulate renal hemodynamics primarily by α-adrenoceptor-mediated vasoconstriction, probably via activation of α_1-adrenoceptors.[180] This results in an increase in renal vascular resistance and a decrease in renal blood flow.[33, 94] Micropuncture studies have shown that renal nerve stimulation[105] or infusion of norepinephrine[135] causes an increase in afferent and efferent arteriolar resistance and a decrease in the glomerular ultrafiltration coefficient. These results have been confirmed by a recent study in which norepinephrine caused vasoconstriction in isolated interlobular arteries and afferent and efferent arterioles.[47]

Postsynaptic α_2-adrenoceptors have been identified in the glomerulus and certain segments of the nephron.[109, 125] This receptor subtype inhibits renin release,[148] inhibits vasopressin action in the collecting tubule,[109] and inhibits salt and water absorption in the proximal convoluted tubule.[155] Other nonvascular effects attributable to α-adrenoceptors include stimulation of sodium and water absorption (α_1) and stimulation of gluconeogenesis in the proximal convoluted tubule (α_1).[125]

β-*Adrenoceptors*

Renal vascular β-adrenoceptors mediate vasodilation and consequently a decrease in renal vascular resistance.[94] However, α-adrenoceptors appear to greatly outnumber β-adrenoceptors, and β-adrenoceptor-mediated vasodilation occurs to a lesser degree in the kidney than in other vascular beds.[94] Perhaps the most important known role of β-adrenoceptors in the kidney is in the regulation of renin release from the juxtaglomerular apparatus.[33] Stimulation of renal nerves under conditions that do not affect renal perfusion pressure, renal blood flow, GFR, or sodium excretion causes renin release.[139] This response can be blocked by β_1- but not by β_2-adrenoceptor antagonists.[139] β-Adrenoceptor agonists also stimulate fluid absorption by approximately 60% in the proximal convoluted tubule in vitro and double the rate of net chloride reabsorption in the cortical collecting tubule in vitro.[91]

Dopamine Receptors

Dopamine receptors of both the DA_1 and DA_2 subtypes have been identified in the kidney.[53, 54] Low concentrations of dopamine infused directly into the renal artery induce vasodilation that is inhibited by dopamine receptor antagonists.[67] In addition, dopamine relaxes glomerular arterioles in vitro.[49] The vasodilatory effect of dopamine in the renal circulation is mediated by dopamine DA_1 receptors linked to adenylate cyclase.[134] Although a physiologic role for dopamine in regulating renal hemodynamics is not yet conclusive, evidence suggests there is dopaminergic innervation to the kidney that is capable of mediating renal vasodilation.[33]

Dopamine receptors of the DA_1 subtype have also been found in renal cortical tubules,[53, 54] whereas glomeruli appear to possess dopamine DA_2 receptors.[53] Although the role of dopamine in the glomerulus is unknown, dopamine has been shown to inhibit fluid absorption in the straight portion of the proximal tubule,[99] which may, in part, explain the natriuresis observed following dopamine infusions.

Muscarinic Cholinergic Receptors

There are muscarinic cholinergic receptors in both glomeruli[186] and in the renal vasculature.[49] Acetylcholine dilates the renal circulation in vivo[7] and relaxes glomerular arterioles in vitro.[49] Acetylcholine also increases cAMP levels in glomeruli[186] and decreases the glomerular ultrafiltration coefficient.[7] The existence of a distinct cholinergic innervation of the kidney is controversial,[33] so the physiologic significance of these receptors is unknown.

Angiotensin Receptors

All of the components of the renin-angiotensin system are present in the region of the juxtaglomerular apparatus,[136] which has strengthened the view that locally formed angiotensin II participates in the control of renal vascular resistance, renal blood flow, and GFR.

Infusion of angiotensin II in a number of species elicits a dose-dependent decrease in renal blood flow with smaller and more variable effects on GFR.[136] Since filtration fraction increases, it has been proposed that angiotensin II preferentially increases efferent arteriolar resistance.[78] This notion is supported by in vitro studies in which isolated rabbit afferent arterioles failed to respond to angiotensin II, whereas efferent arterioles were highly sensitive to the vasoconstrictive effect of angiotensin II.[47]

Some studies have shown that under certain conditions, angiotensin II may also increase preglomerular resistance.[136] For example, when angiotensin II is infused during inhibition of prostaglandin synthesis, the vasoconstrictive effects of angiotensin II—especially on preglomerular resistance vessels—are more pronounced.[6]

Therefore, the alteration in renal hemodynamics observed with angiotensin II may depend partly on the status of other intrarenal hormonal systems.[136]

Specific angiotensin II receptors have also been found in glomeruli.[174] Mesangial cells, but not glomerular epithelial cells, display a contractile response to angiotensin II.[108] Thus, angiotensin II, by modulating mesangial cell contractility, may regulate blood flow along the glomerular capillary and/or the surface area available for filtration.[108] This mechanism may account for the decrease in the glomerular ultrafiltration coefficient observed with angiotensin II.[135]

Although the exact role of the renin-angiotensin system in regulating renal hemodynamics is uncertain, current evidence suggests that angiotensin II may maintain GFR during periods of low renal perfusion pressure.[78] Thus, when renal perfusion pressure is reduced to low levels in dogs, autoregulation of renal blood flow and GFR is well maintained.[78] However, when renin is depleted or when angiotensin converting enzyme is inhibited by captopril, regulation of renal blood flow persists, but GFR falls.[78] Similar observations have been made in humans with renal arterial stenosis, a condition in which the renin-angiotensin system is activated. In these patients, captopril causes a marked decrease in GFR,[15] supporting the view that angiotensin II, by increasing efferent arteriolar resistance, helps to maintain glomerular capillary pressure, and hence filtration rate, when renal perfusion is compromised.[78]

Prostaglandin Receptors

The kidney is a major site of prostaglandin synthesis and one of the richest sources of cyclo-oxygenase activity.[201] Many studies have established that PGE_2 and prostacyclin participate in the control of renal blood flow, but a role for other arachidonic acid metabolites, such as TXA_2 and the leukotrienes, remains to be defined.

There is general agreement that prostaglandins do not contribute in a major way to the control of kidney function in the unstressed state.[201] Current evidence suggests that PGE_2 and prostacyclin may play a role in attenuating vasoconstriction produced by renal nerve activity or angiotensin II.[201] In support of this view are the findings that PGE_2 and prostacyclin reduce renal vascular resistance[201] and relax glomerular arterioles in vitro,[48] that cyclo-oxygenase inhibition

enhances the vasoconstrictor effects of norepinephrine and angiotensin II,[6] and that these vasoconstrictors can, in turn, stimulate the synthesis of vasodilatory prostaglandins.[122] Thus, PGE_2 and prostacyclin appear to function in a negative feedback loop that serves to maintain renal blood flow during states in which vasoconstrictor activity in the kidney is high.[201]

In certain pathologic states such as ureteral obstruction[130] and glycerol-induced acute renal failure,[10] and in the spontaneous hypertensive rat,[106] there is increased renal synthesis of TXA_2 accompanied by an increase in renal vascular resistance. Inhibition of TXA_2 synthesis reduces the vasoconstriction seen in the ureter-obstructed kidney,[201] which suggests that TXA_2 may be a causative factor in the increased renal vascular resistance seen in such conditions.

Leukotriene Receptors

The leukotrienes C_4 and D_4 are potent renal vasoconstrictors.[154] Their vascular effects appear to be due to direct activation of specific leukotriene receptors, and not mediated by TXA_2.[154] LTC_4 has also been shown to contract mesangial cells in tissue culture.[38]

Bradykinin Receptors

Bradykinin, a peptide formed in the kidney,[24] is a potent renal vasodilator in vivo[7] and relaxes glomerular arterioles in vitro.[49] This peptide also stimulates the synthesis of prostaglandins, which may partially account for its vasodilatory action.[24, 123] The role of the renal kallikrein-kinin system is unknown, but it has been implicated in the pathogenesis of hypertension, Bartter's syndrome, and certain renal disorders.[24]

Histamine Receptors

Histamine receptors of both the H_1 and H_2 subtypes have been identified in the renal vasculature and glomerulus.[186] Infusion of histamine increases renal blood flow with little change in GFR. Histamine also decreases the glomerular ultrafiltration coefficient and stimulates cAMP formation in the glomerulus,[186] suggesting a direct glomerular action.

Serotonin Receptors

Serotonin causes renal vasoconstriction[31] and has been reported to increase cAMP levels in glomeruli.[170] Both histamine and serotonin may be involved in the pathogenesis of immunologic glomerular diseases.[34]

Effects of Various Drugs on the Renal Circulation

Dobutamine

Dobutamine does not increase renal blood flow in patients with cardiomyopathic heart failure, but it does increase urine flow, sodium excretion, and creatinine clearance in those patients.[114] The improvements in renal function associated with dobutamine are likely secondary to improved cardiac output[178] and not to direct effects of dobutamine on renal hemodynamics.

Dopamine

Dopamine is commonly used to dilate the renal vasculature and maintain renal blood flow.[64] Its mechanism is stimulation of dopamine DA_1 receptors on preglomerular and postglomerular vessels.[66] GFR usually does not increase, despite increases in renal blood flow. At higher doses (76 μg/kg/min), the α-adrenoceptor agonist activity of dopamine predominates, and a net renal vasoconstrictor response is observed, resulting in a decrease in renal blood flow.

Isoproterenol

Isoproterenol dilates the renal vasculature and thereby decreases renal vascular resistance and increases renal blood flow. In patients with cardiogenic or septic shock, in whom renal vascular resistance is high, the vasodilator action of isoproterenol is especially marked, which significantly augments renal blood flow. Isoproterenol also stimulates renin release via a direct action on $β_1$-adrenoceptors in the juxtaglomerular apparatus.

Epinephrine and Norepinephrine

Norepinephrine and epinephrine constrict the renal vasculature and decrease renal blood flow.[65] Epinephrine, at doses that have little effect on systemic arterial blood pressure (up to 0.3 μg/kg/min, IV), consistently increases renal vascular resistance and decreases renal blood flow. Since GFR is only slightly altered, filtration fraction is consistently increased. Secretion of renin is increased as a result of direct stimulation of $β_1$-adrenoceptors in the juxtaglomerular apparatus.[68, 177]

It has recently been recognized that hypokalemia associated with epinephrine infusion or high endogenous epinephrine levels reflects increased cellular potassium uptake from the extracellular fluid.[50] It has subsequently been demonstrated that epinephrine-induced potassium uptake is a $β_2$-adrenoceptor-mediated effect and can be inhibited by $β_2$-adrenoceptor antagonists.[18, 194] The significance of $β_2$-adrenoceptor-mediated potassium uptake in renal tissue is not known.

Propranolol (and other β-blockers)

The effects of β-adrenoceptor antagonists on renal function have been recently reviewed.[51, 200] In general, administration of β-adrenoceptor antagonists is associated with modest decrements in both GFR and renal blood flow in experimental animals and man. Propranolol infusion decreases renal blood flow and concomitantly increases renal vascular resistance.[179] In contrast, infusion of nadolol has been associated with no change or even an increase in renal blood flow.[13, 56, 86] It has been proposed that all β-adrenoceptor antagonists, with the exception of nadolol, compromise renal hemodynamics.[13] The mechanism appears to be unopposed α-adrenoceptor-mediated vasoconstriction that results as the β-adrenoceptor-mediated renal vasodilator system is eliminated. The increase in renal plasma flow associated with nadolol is unique among β-adrenoceptor blockers; the mechanism is currently unknown.

Vasopressin

Vasopressin is used to treat polyurea due to diabetes insipidus, such as that seen after cranial surgery or traumatic head injury. The primary effect of vasopressin (2–5 units given intramuscularly every 2–3 days) is to stimulate renal water absorption and antidiuresis. High doses of vasopressin (75 units) will constrict the renal vasculature; however, this effect is not necessary to achieve antidiuresis. Indeed, the nonpressor vasopressin analogue, desamino 8-D arginine vasopressin, is the drug currently chosen to treat polyuria.[79] It is important to note that in some critical care situations, including postsurgical recovery, trauma, and cardiogenic and septic shock, endogenous vasopressin levels may be elevated 100 to 1,000 times the basal levels, resulting in reduced renal perfusion and anuria.

Nitroglycerin and Nitroprusside

Nitroglycerin and nitroprusside are vasodilators that relax both arterial and venous smooth muscle. Nitroprusside generally maintains renal blood flow and GFR; renin secretion may be stimulated by producing systemic arterial vasodilation and lowering perfusion pressure, or it may directly affect the juxtaglomerular apparatus.[77, 188] Urine volume and sodium excretion are reported to improve rapidly in patients with heart failure following nitroprusside administration.[77] This response is probably secondary to improved cardiac performance.

Calcium Channel Blockers

Calcium channel blockers have important actions in the kidney. Diltiazem maintains renal blood flow and sustains or increases GFR and natriuresis, while lowering systemic arterial blood pressure.[101] Verapamil is reported to lower blood pressure in hypertensive patients without lowering renal blood flow.[55] Verapamil is not associated with clinically significant fluid retention or significant changes in plasma renin activity, aldosterone concentration, or sodium, potassium, bicarbonate, creatinine, or uric acid levels.[32] Nifedipine provides effective vasodilator therapy for hypertension without producing the sodium retention, plasma volume expansion, and effects on renin release associated with traditional vasodilator therapy.[137] Sodium, uric acid, and water excretion are markedly increased by nifedipine. Nifedipine, like verapamil, does not increase plasma renin activity, plasma and urinary aldosterone levels, or plasma volume at effective antihypertensive doses.[55] Nifedipine has been shown to be useful in combination with β-adrenoceptor blockers in hypertensive patients,[26] in whom the combination of antihypertensive therapies maintains renal blood flow and GFR and reduces renal vascular resistance.

Captopril

Captopril inhibits the formation of angiotensin II from angiotensin I and can elevate plasma and tissue kinin levels. The predominant effect of captopril is renal vasodilation. The magnitude of the renal vasodilatory response is proportional to intrarenal angiotensin II–mediated increases in vascular tone. Potentiation of renal vasodilatory kinins cannot be excluded, but the modest vasodilatory effect of captopril in low renin states suggests that even low levels of angiotensin II may contribute significantly to renal vascular tone.[113]

SPLANCHNIC CIRCULATION

A significant number of pharmacologic agents are known to influence the splanchnic circulation. Many of these compounds have been used successfully to investigate and characterize the physiology of this vascular bed, while others are known to have therapeutic utility in cardiovascular and/or gastrointestinal disease. The α- and β-adrenergic, serotonergic, dopaminergic, cholinergic, prostanoid, histaminergic, opiate, and purinergic receptors and their subtypes have been defined in this circulatory bed.

Receptors in the Splanchnic Circulation

α-Adrenoceptors

Norepinephrine constricts the splanchnic circulation in anesthetized animals.[71, 92] Specifically, norepinephrine-induced vasoconstriction is observed in the stomach, small intestine, colon, liver, and pancreas,[25] and this response is mediated by α-adrenoceptors. In the anesthetized cat, prazosin, a selective α_1-adrenoceptor antagonist, only partially attenuates the intestinal vasoconstriction produced by sympathetic nerve stimulation,[142] suggesting that separate populations of α-adrenoceptor subtypes (i.e., α_1 and α_2) coexist in the splanchnic circulation.[70] Phenoxybenzamine, a nonselective α-adrenoceptor antagonist, completely blocks the intestinal vasoconstriction produced by sympathetic nerve stimulation.[142] Hepatic blood volume responses to both sympathetic nerve stimulation and infusions of catecholamines are mediated through postsynaptic vascular α_2-adrenoceptors, whereas portal pressure responses are mediated through both α_1- and α_2-adrenoceptors.[168]

β-Adrenoceptors

Stimulation of β-adrenoceptors with isoproterenol results in a vasodilatory response in all organs supplied by the splanchnic circulation.[25] This response is inhibited by the β-adrenoceptor antagonist, propranolol.[92, 151] However, propranolol alone does not significantly alter blood flow in any of the organs supplied by the splanchnic circulation,[151] suggesting that β-adrenoceptors are not involved in the maintenance of normal vascular tone in this circulatory bed. It appears that the β-adrenoceptor subtype mediating splanchnic vasodilation is β_2.[151]

Serotonin (5-HT) Receptors

The splanchnic vascular responses to serotonin are variable and depend on dose, route of administration, and species.[138, 151] Generally, IV administration of serotonin produces vasodilation in the stomach, small bowel, and colon and vasoconstriction in the liver and pancreas.[25] The problems in assessment of the vascular responses to serotonin are compounded by the fact that serotonin also produces motility responses of visceral smooth muscle that influence local blood flow in the mesenteric circulation.[138] Serotonin is found endogenously throughout most of the gastrointestinal tract. Because of the variability of the responses, it has not been possible to classify serotonin receptors in the splanchnic circulation or to establish a physiologic role of serotonin in this vascular bed.[151]

Dopamine Receptors

The splanchnic circulation contains dopamine receptors which, when stimulated, produce vasodilation.[151, 208] At high doses, dopamine causes vasoconstriction through stimulation of α-adrenoceptors.[144, 208] The hepatic vascular responses are variable. Low doses of dopamine administered directly into the hepatic artery produce vasodilation[153] in experimental animals. Similar doses of dopamine administered into the portal vein cause venoconstriction. Higher doses cause hepatic artery constriction and portal vein vasodilation. It is doubtful whether the actions of dopamine on the splanchnic circulation have physiologic significance.[151]

Muscarinic Cholinergic Receptors

In general, cholinergic agonists administered into the intestinal circulation produce vasodilation.[25] However, this vasodilatory response is dose dependent, and at higher doses, vasoconstriction may be observed in the mesenteric circulation.[25] This vasoconstrictor response appears to be secondary to the vascular compression that results from stimulation of the visceral smooth muscle of the intestine.[57, 151] Acetylcholine also causes vasodilation in the gastric and pancreatic circulations but does not change hepatic blood flow.[25] All vascular responses in the splanchnic circulation to cholinergic agonists can be blocked by atropine, indicating that they are mediated by muscarinic cholinergic receptors.[151]

Prostaglandin Receptors

The prostaglandins have variable effects on the splanchnic circulation. Prostaglandins of the E series are vasodilatory in the stomach and small intestine.[25] $PGF_{2\alpha}$ causes vasoconstriction.[25, 57] Prostacyclin is a potent vasodilator of the mesenteric vascular bed,[58, 60] and because it has a short plasma half-life and it redistributes blood flow to the mucosa, prostacyclin has been proposed as a useful drug for treating nonocclusive mesenteric ischemia.[60] PGD_2 causes splanchnic vasoconstriction when administered as a bolus injection, whereas continuous infusions of this prostanoid result in vasodilation.[60] The effects of the prostaglandins on colonic, hepatic, and pancreatic blood flow have not been studied.

Histamine Receptors

Histamine administration produces vasodilation in all organs supplied by the splanchnic vascular circulation.[25] This effect is more pronounced in the stomach, small bowel, and pancreas than in the colon and liver. In the mesenteric circulation, histamine, besides increasing blood flow, also increases oxygen consumption and decreases vascular resistance even in cases of ischemia produced by hemorrhage.[59] The vasodilatory response involves stimulation of both histamine H_1 and H_2 receptors.[145, 197] Using specific receptor agonists and antagonists, it has been shown that stimulation of the histamine H_1 receptor produces an immediate and transient increase in blood flow, whereas H_2 receptor stimulation causes sustained vasodilation.

Opiate Receptors

Opiates produce vasodilation in the splanchnic circulation. The vasodilatory response produced by morphine and methionine-enkephalin in the stomach and small bowel are blocked by naloxone, an opiate receptor antagonist.[146, 147] The opiates are without effect in the pancreatic circulation and have not been studied in the colonic and hepatic vasculatures.[25]

Purinergic Receptors

In the canine intestinal circulation, adenosine induces a dose-dependent vasodilation and an increase in oxygen consumption.[197] The adenosine antagonist, theophylline, attenuates this response. An adenosine analogue, 2-chloroadenosine, is sixfold more potent than the parent compound in enhancing intestinal blood flow, and this effect is also antagonized by theophylline.[197] Adenosine and 2-chloroadenosine produce mesenteric vasodilation by acting at distinct adenosine receptors in the intestinal vasculature.[197]

Effects of Various Drugs on the Mesenteric Circulation

Dobutamine

In the anesthetized dog, low doses of dobutamine infused IV dramatically increase blood flow to the mucosa of the stomach: increases of more than 200% are consistently observed (unpublished observation). Similar doses of dobutamine do not significantly change blood flow to the colon or small intestine. The effects of dobutamine on pancreatic and hepatic blood flow have not been investigated.

Dopamine

Dopamine is commonly used clinically in the management of congestive heart failure and renal insufficiency and, as discussed earlier, produces splanchnic vasodilation.[151] The response is variable, however, since higher doses of dopamine produce vasoconstriction, probably by stimulation of α-adrenoceptors.

Isoproterenol

Isoproterenol, a β-adrenoceptor agonist, causes splanchnic vasodilation. This response occurs even in the face of a fall in systemic blood pressure,[72] indicating a selectively greater vasodilation in the splanchnic vascular bed than elsewhere.[69] The vasodilatory response of the mesenteric circulation to isoproterenol is inhibited by propranolol. However, propranolol alone produces no significant effect on this vascular bed, indicating the lack of involvement of β-adrenoceptors in the maintenance of resting splanchnic vascular tone.

Norepinephrine and Epinephrine

Norepinephrine and epinephrine produce generalized vasoconstriction of the splanchnic circulation. This effect appears to be mediated by both α_1- and α_2-adrenoceptors, which are known to coexist in this vascular bed.

Vasopressin

Like norepinephrine, vasopressin causes vasoconstriction in all organs supplied by the splanchnic circulation.[25] The gastric, small bowel, and pancreatic blood supplies are most sensitive to vasoconstriction produced by vasopressin.

Calcium Channel Blockers

Nifedipine, diltiazem, and perhexiline have been studied for their effects on the mesenteric circulation. All three agents produce mesenteric vasodilation when infused into the canine superior mesenteric artery.[60, 198] Nifedipine and diltiazem also relax KCl- and norepinephrine-contracted canine mesenteric vascular strips in vitro. The use of calcium channel blockers to treat hypertension may also be associated with vasodilation and pooling of blood in the high-capacitance mesenteric vascular bed.

Nitroprusside

Sodium nitroprusside produces moderate increases in blood flow to the small intestine and the liver.[25] This compound has no apparent effect on gastric blood flow[25] and has not been studied in the colonic, hepatic, and pancreatic arterial supplies. Nitroprusside minimally reduces hepatic venous tone.[69]

Cimetidine

The histamine H_2 receptor antagonist, cimetidine, attenuates the response of the mesenteric circulation to histamine. However, cimetidine alone does not alter splanchnic blood flow indicating that histamine H_2 receptors do not regulate resting vascular tone in the mesenteric circulation.[167] In the rat, cimetidine administered at high doses induces mesenteric vasoconstriction, which suggests that histamine H_2 receptors may play a physiologic role in the control of the splanchnic circulation in this species.[93] Experiments in the canine hepatic circulation indicate that only the histamine H_1 receptor is involved in mediating the histamine response in this vascular bed.[152] This suggests that cimetidine would perhaps not influence this circulation; however, this remains to be examined.

Acknowledgment

The authors are indebted to Ms. Stephany Ruffolo for her assistance in the preparation of this manuscript.

REFERENCES

1. Altura BT, Altura BM, Quirion R: Identification of benzomorphan κ₂-opiate receptors in

cerebral arteries which subserve relaxation. *Br J Pharmacol* 1984; 82:459.

2. Altura BT, Quirion R, Pert CB, et al: Phencyclidine ("angel dust") analogs and σ opiate benzomorphans cause cerebral arterial spasm. *Proc Natl Acad Sci USA* 1983; 80:865.

3. Amenta F, Cavallotti C, DeRossi M, et al: Dopamine-sensitive cAMP generating system in rat extracerebral arteries. *Eur J Pharmacol* 1984; 97:105.

4. Barajas L: Innervation of the renal cortex. *Fed Proc* 1978; 37:1192.

5. Barry DI, Paulson OB, Jarden JO, et al: Effects of captopril on cerebral blood flow in normotensive and hypertensive rats. *Am J Med* 1984; 76:79.

6. Bayliss C, Brenner BM: Modulation by prostaglandin synthesis inhibitors of the action of exogenous angiotensin II on glomerular ultrafiltration in the rat. *Circ Res* 1978; 43:889.

7. Bayliss C, Deen WM, Myers BD, et al: Effects of some vasodilator drugs on transcapillary fluid exchange in renal cortex. *Am J Physiol* 1976; 230:1148.

8. Bello-Reuss E, Higashi Y, Kaneda Y: Dopamine decreases fluid reabsorption in straight portions of rabbit proximal tubule. *Am J Physiol* 1982; 242:F634.

9. Belov YV: Pathogenesis of hemodynamic pulmonary edema. *Patol Fiziol Eksp Ter* 1982; 3:16.

10. Benabe JE, Klahr S, Hoffman MK, et al: Production of thromboxane A by the kidney in glycerol induced acute renal failure. *Prostaglandins* 1980; 19:333.

11. Berne RM: Myocardial blood flow: Metabolic determinants, in Zelis R (ed): *The Peripheral Circulation.* New York, Grune & Stratten, Inc, 1975, pp 117–129.

12. Berne RM, Winn HR, Rubio R: The local regulation of cerebral blood flow. *Prog Cardiovasc Dis* 1981; 24:243.

13. Bernstein K, O'Connor D: Antiadrenergic antihypertensive drugs: Their effects on renal function. *Annu Rev Pharmacol Toxicol* 1984; 24:105.

14. Bes A, Guell A, Victor G, et al: Effects of a dopaminergic agonist on CBF in migraine patients, in Heistad DD, Marcus ML (eds): *Cerebral Blood Flow: Effects of Nerves and Neurotransmitters.* New York, Elsevier North Holland, Inc, 1982, pp 13–168.

15. Blythe WB: Captopril and renal autoregulation. *N Engl J Med* 1983; 308:390.

16. Borowski E, Starke K, Ehrl H, et al: A comparison of pre- and postsynaptic effects of α-adrenolytic drugs in the pulmonary artery of the rabbit. *Neuroscience* 1977; 2:285.

17. Brodde OE: Vascular dopamine receptors: Demonstration and characterization by in vitro studies. *Life Sci* 1982; 31:89.

18. Brown M, Brown D, Murphy M: Hypokalemia from beta-2-receptor stimulation by circulating epinephrine. *N Engl J Med* 1983; 309:1414.

19. Buck SH, Walsh JH, Yamamura HI, et al: Neuropeptides in sensory neurons. *Life Sci* 1982; 30:1857.

20. Burke SE, DiCola G, Lefer AM: Protection of ischemic cat myocardium by CGS-13080, a selective potent thromboxane A_2 synthetase inhibitor. *J Cardiovasc Pharmacol* 1983; 5:842.

21. Burnstock G: Purinergic receptors in the heart. *Circ Res* 1980; 46:I-175.

22. Busija DW, Heistad DD: Effects of cholinergic nerves on cerebral blood flow in cats. *Circ Res* 1981; 48:62.

23. Busija DW, Marcus ML, Heistad DD: Effects of sympathetic nerves on the cerebral circulation in cats, in Heistad DD, Marcus ML, (eds): *Cerebral Blood Flow: Effects of Nerves and Neurotransmitters.* New York, Elsevier North Holland, Inc, 1982, pp 301–308.

24. Carretero OA, Scicli AG: The renal kallikrein-kinin system. *Am J Physiol* 1980; 238:F247.

25. Chou CC, Kvietys PR: Physiological and pharmacological alterations in gastrointestinal blood flow, in Granger DN, Buckley GB (eds): *Measurements of Blood Flow: Application to the Splanchnic Circulation.* Baltimore, Williams & Wilkins Co, 1981, pp 447–509.

26. Christensen M, Pedersen L, Mikkelsen E: Renal effects of acute calcium blockade with nifedipine in hypertensive patients receiving beta-adrenoceptor blocking drugs. *Clin Pharmacol Ther* 1982; 32(5):572.

27. Cocks JM, Angus JA: Endothelium-dependent relaxation of coronary arteries by noradrenaline and serotonin. *Nature* 1983; 305:627.

28. Cohen ML, Mason N, Wiley KS, et al: Further evidence that vascular serotonin receptors

are of the 5HT$_2$ type. *Biochem Pharmacol* 1983; 32:567.

29. Cohen RA, Shepherd JT, Vanhoutte PM: Inhibitory role of the endothelium in the response of isolated coronary arteries to platelets. *Science* 1983; 221:273.

30. Cohen RA, Shepherd JT, Vanhoutte PM: Effects of the adrenergic transmitter on epicardial coronary arteries. *Fed Proc* 1984; 43:2862.

31. Collis MG, Vanhoutte PM: Vascular reactivity of isolated perfused kidneys from male and female spontaneously hypertensive rats. *Circ Res* 1977; 41:759.

32. de Leeuw P, Smout A, Willemse P, et al: Effects of verapamil in hypertensive patients, in Zanchetti A, Kirkler D (eds): *Calcium Antagonists in Cardiovascular Therapy*. Amsterdam, Excerpta Medica, 1981, pp 233–237.

33. DiBona GF: The function of the renal nerves. *Rev Physiol Biochem Pharmacol* 1982; 94:75–181.

34. Dousa TP, Shah SV, Abboud HE: Potential role of cyclic nucleotides in glomerular pathophysiology. *Adv Cyclic Nucleotide Res* 1980; 12:285.

35. Duckles SP: Acetylcholine and vasoactive intestinal polpeptide: Cerebrovascular neurotransmitters, in Heistad DD, Marcus ML (eds): *Cerebral Blood Flow: Effects of Nerves and Neurotransmitters*. New York, Elsevier North Holland, Inc, 1982, pp 441–446.

36. Duckles SP, Said SI: Vasoactive intestinal peptide as a neurotransmitter in the cerebral circulation. *Eur J Pharmacol* 1982; 78:371.

37. Dumont L, Lelorier J, Stanley P, et al: Effect of nitroglycerin on regional myocardial blood flow following an experimental coronary system. *Angiology* 1984; 35:553.

38. Dunn MJ, Simonson M: The effects of leukotriene C$_4$ (LTC$_4$) on rat glomerular mesangial cells in culture. *Kidney Int* 1985; 27:256.

39. Edvinsson L, Birath E, Uddman R, et al: Indoleaminergic mechanisms in brain vessels, localization, concentration, uptake and in vitro responses of 5-hydroxytryptamine. *Acta Physiol Scand* 1984; 121:291.

40. Edvinsson L, Emson P, McCulloch J, et al: Neuropeptide Y: Cerebrovascular innervation and vasomotor effects in the cat. *Neurosci Lett* 1983; 43:79.

41. Edvinsson L, Falck B, Owman C: Possibilities for a cholinergic action on smooth mus-

culature and on sympathetic axons in brain vessels mediated by muscarinic and nicotinic receptors. *J Pharmacol Exp Ther* 1977; 200:117.

42. Edvinsson L, Gross PM, Mohamed A: Characterization of histamine receptors in cat cerebral arteries in vitro and in situ. *J Pharmacol Exp Ther* 1983; 225:168.

43. Edvinsson L, Hardebo JE, McCulloch J, et al: Effects of dopaminergic agonists and antagonists in isolated cerebral blood vessels. *Acta Physiol Scand* 1978; 104:349.

44. Edvinsson L, MacKenzie ET: Amine mechanisms in the cerebral circulation. *Pharmacol Rev* 1977; 28:275.

45. Edvinsson L, McCulloch J, Rosell S, et al: Antagonism by (D-Pro2, D-Trp 7,9)-substance P of the cerebrovascular dilation induced by substance P. *Acta Physiol Scand* 1982; 116:411.

46. Edvinsson L, Owman C, Siesjö B: Physiological role of cerebrovascular sympathetic nerves in the autoregulation of cerebral blood flow. *Brain Res* 1976; 117:519.

47. Edwards RM: Segmental effects of norepinephrine and angiotensin II on isolated renal microvessels. *Am J Physiol* 1983; 244:F526.

48. Edwards RM: Effects of prostaglandins on vasoconstrictor action in isolated renal arterioles. *Am J Physiol* 1985; 248:F779.

49. Edwards RM: Response of isolated renal arterioles to acetylcholine, dopamine and bradykinin. *Am J Physiol* 1985; 248:F183.

50. Epstein F, Rosa R: Adrenergic control of serum potassium. *N Engl J Med* 1983; 309:1450.

51. Epstein M, Oster J: Beta-blockers and the kidney. *Mineral Electrolyte Metab* 1982; 8:237.

52. Feigl EO: Parasympathetic control of coronary blood flow. *Fed Proc* 1984; 43:2881.

53. Felder RA, Blecher M, Calcagno PL, et al: Dopamine receptors in the proximal tubule of the rabbit. *Am J Physiol* 1984; 247:F499.

54. Felder RA, Blecher M, Eisner GM, et al: Cortical tubular and glomerular dopamine receptors in rat kidney. *Am J Physiol* 1984; 246:F557.

55. Fleckenstien A: Use of calcium antagonists in the treatment of hypertension, in *Calcium Antagonists in Heart and Smooth Muscle*. New York, John Wiley & Sons, Inc, 1983, pp 306–311.

56. Foley J, Penner B, Fung H: Short-term renal hemodynamic effects of nadolol and metoprolol in normotensive and hypertensive subjects. *Clin Pharmacol Ther* 1981; 29:245.

57. Fondacaro JD: Intestinal blood flow and motility, in Shepherd AP, Granger DN, (eds): *Physiology of the Mesenteric Circulation.* New York, Raven Press, 1984, pp 107–120.

58. Fondacaro JD, Jacobson ED: The role of prostacyclin (PGI$_2$) in metabolic hyperemia. *Prostaglandins* 1981; 21(suppl):25.

59. Fondacaro JD, Schwaiger M, Jacobson ED: Effects of vasodilators on mesenteric ischemia and hypoxia induced by hemorrhage. *Circ Shock* 1979; 6:255.

60. Fondacaro JD, Walus KM, Schwaiger M, et al: Vasodilation of the normal and ischemic canine mesenteric circulation. *Gastoenterology* 1981; 80:1542.

61. Forster C, Drew GM, Hilditch A, et al: Dopamine receptors in human basilar arteries. *Eur J Pharmacol* 1983; 87:227.

62. Fu LHW, Toda N: Analysis of the contractile response to serotonin and tryptamine of isolated dog cerebral, femoral and mesenteric arteries. *Jpn J Pharmacol* 1983; 33:473.

63. Furchgott RF, Zawadski JV: The obligatory role of endothelial cells in the relaxation of arterial smooth muscle by acetylcholine. *Nature* 1980; 288:375.

64. Goldberg L: Cardiovascular and renal actions of dopamine potential clinical applications. *Pharmacol Rev* 1972; 24:1.

65. Goldberg M, Aranow H, Smith A, et al: Pheochromocytoma and essential hypertensive vascular disease. *Arch Intern Med* 1950; 86:823.

66. Goldberg L, Glock D, Kohli J, et al: Separation of peripheral dopamine receptors by a selective DA-1 antagonist, SCH 23390. *Hypertension* 1984; 6(suppl):I-25.

67. Goldberg L, Volkman PH, Kohli JD: A comparison of the vascular dopamine receptor with other dopamine receptors. *Annu Rev Pharmacol Toxicol* 1978; 18:57.

68. Gombas E, Hulet W, Bopp P, et al: Reactivity of renal and systemic circulation to vasoconstrictor agents in normotensive and hypertensive subjects. *J Clin Invest* 1962; 41:203.

69. Greenway CV: Effects of sodium nitroprusside, isosorbide dinitrate, isoproterenol, phentolamine and prazosin on hepatic venous response to sympathetic nerve stimulation in

the cat. *J Pharmacol Exp Ther* 1979; 209(1):56.

70. Greenway CV: Neural control and autoregulatory escape, in Shepherd AP, Granger DN, (eds): *Physiology of the Intestinal Circulation.* New York, Raven Press, 1984, pp 61–71.

71. Greenway CV, Lawson A: The effects of adrenaline and noradrenaline on venous return and regional blood flow in the anesthetized cat with special reference to intestinal blood flow. *J Physiol (London)* 1966; 187:579.

72. Greenway CV, Stark RD: Hepatic vascular bed. *Physiol Rev* 1971; 51:23.

73. Griffith SG, Lincoln J, Burnstock G: Serotonin as a neurotransmitter in cerebral arteries. *Brain Res* 1982; 247:388.

74. Gross GJ, Feigl EO: Analysis of coronary vascular β-receptors in situ. *Am J Physiol* 1975; 228:1909.

75. Gross PM: Histamine H$_1$- and H$_2$-receptors are differentially and spatially distributed in cerebral vessels. *J Cereb Blood Flow Metab* 1981; 1:441.

76. Gruetter CA, Ignaro LJ, Hyman AL, et al: Contractile effects of 5-hydroxytryptamine in isolated intrapulmonary arteries and veins. *Can J Pharmacol* 1981; 59:157.

77. Guiha N, Cohn J, Mikulic E, et al: Treatment of refractory heart failure with infusion of nitroprusside. *N Engl J Med* 1974; 291:587.

78. Hall JE, Guyton AC, Jackson TE, et al: Control of glomerular filtration rate by renin-angiotensin system. *Am J Physiol* 1977; 233:F366.

79. Hays R: Agents affecting H$_2$ renal conservation of water, in Gilman AG, Goodman L, Gilman A (eds): *The Pharmacological Basis of Therapeutics.* New York, Macmillan Publishing Co, 1980, pp 916–928.

80. Henriksen I, Paulson OB: The effects of sodium nitroprusside on cerebral blood flow and cerebral venous blood gases in man. *Acta Med Scand Suppl* 1983; 678:91.

81. Herliky JT, Bockman EL, Berne RM, et al: Adenosine relaxation of isolated vascular smooth muscle. *Am J Physiol* 1976; 230:1239.

82. Heusch G, Deussen A: The effects of cardiac sympathetic nerve stimulation on perfusion of stenotic coronary arteries in the dog. *Circ Res* 1983; 53:8.

83. Heusch G, Deussen A, Schipke J, et al: α$_1$-

and α_2-adrenoceptor-mediated vasoconstriction of large and small canine coronary arteries in vivo. *J Cardiovasc Pharmacol* 1984; 6:961.

84. Heyndrickx GR, Boettcher DH, Vatner SF: Effects of angiotensin, vasopressin and methoxamine on cardiac function and blood distribution in conscious dog. *Am J Physiol* 1976; 231:1579.

85. Hills LD, Braunwald E: Coronary-artery spasm. *N Engl J Med* 1978; 299:695.

86. Hollenberg N, Adams D, McKinstry D, et al: β-Adrenoceptor-blocking agents and the kidney: Effect of nadolol and propranolol on the renal circulation. *Br J Clin Pharmacol* 1979; 7(suppl 2):219.

87. Hoshida S, Ohmori M, Kuzaya T, et al: Augmented thromboxane A_2 generation and efficacy of its blockade in acute myocardial infarction. *Jpn Circ J* 1983; 47:1026.

88. Hyman AL: The direct effects of vasoactive agents on pulmonary veins: Studies of responses to acetylcholine, serotonin, histamine and isoproterenol in intact dogs. *J Pharmacol Exp Ther* 1969; 168:96.

89. Hyman AL, Kadowitz PJ: Evidence for the existence of postjunctional α_1- and α_2-receptors in the cat pulmonary vascular bed. *Am J Physiol* 1985; 249:891.

90. Hyman AL, Nandiwada P, Knight DS, et al: Pulmonary vasodilator responses to catecholamines and sympathetic nerve stimulation in the cat. *Circ Res* 1981; 48:407.

91. Iino Y, Troy JL, Brenner BM: Effects of catecholamines on electrolyte transport in cortical collecting tubule. *J Membr Biol* 1981; 61:67.

92. Immink WFGA, Beijer HJM, Charbon GA: Hemodynamic effects of norepinephrine and isoprenaline in various regions of the canine splanchnic area. *Pflugers Arch* 1976; 365:107.

93. Impicciatore M, Morini G, Chiavarini M, et al: A possible physiological role of histamine H_2-receptors in rat mesenteric circulation. *Eur J Pharmacol* 1983; 90:231.

94. Insel PA, Snavely MD: Catecholamines and the kidney: Receptors and renal function. *Annu Rev Physiol* 1981; 43:625.

95. Kadowitz PJ: Pulmonary vascular responses to nitrendipine, in Scriabine A, Vanov S, Deck D (eds): *Nitrendipine*. Baltimore, Urban & Schwarzenberg, 1984, pp 361–367.

96. Kadowitz PJ, Gruetter CA, Spanhake FW, et al: Pulmonary vascular responses to prostaglandins. *Fed Proc* 1981; 40(2):1991.

97. Kadowitz PJ, Hyman AL: Hydralazine and the treatment of primary pulmonary hypertension. *N Engl J Med* 1982; 306:1357.

98. Kadowitz PJ, Hyman AL: Pulmonary vascular responses to histamine in sheep. *Am J Physiol* 1983; 224:H423.

99. Kaneda Y, Bello-Reuss E: Effect of dopamine on phosphate reabsorption in isolated perfused rabbit proximal tubule. *Mineral Electrolyte Metab* 1983; 9:147.

100. Kern MJ, Ganz P, Horowitz JD, et al: Potentiation of coronary vasoconstriction by β-adrenergic blockade in patients with coronary artery disease. *Circulation* 1983; 67:1178.

101. Kinoshita M, Kusakawa R, Shimono Y, et al: Effects of diltiazem hydrochloride on renal hemodynamics and urinary electrolyte excretion. *Jpn Circ J* 1978; 42(5):553.

102. Kipshidze NN, Korotkov AA, Marsagishvili LA, et al: Efficacy of various dopamine doses in acute myocardial ischemia complicated by cardiogenic shock experimental study. *Kardiologiia* 1981; 21:80.

103. Kobayashi H, Maoret M, Ferrante M, et al: Subtypes of β-adrenergic receptors in rat cerebral microvessels. *Brain Res* 1981; 220;194.

104. Koike H, Ito K, Miyamoto M, et al: Effects of long-term blockade of angiotensin converting enzyme with captopril (SQ14,225) on hemodynamics and circulating blood volume in SHR. *Hypertension* 1980; 2:299.

105. Kon V, Ichikawa I: Effector loci for renal nerve control of cortical microcirculation. *Am J Physiol* 1983; 245:F545.

106. Konieczkowski M, Dunn MJ, Storke JE, et al: Glomerular synthesis of prostaglandin and thromboxane in spontaneously hypertensive rats. *Hypertension* 1983; 5:446.

107. Kontos HA: Regulation of the cerebral circulation. *Annu Rev Physiol* 1981; 43:397.

108. Kreisberg JI: Contractile properties of the glomerular mesangium. *Fed Proc* 1983; 42:3053.

109. Krothapalli RK, Suki WN: Functional characterization of the alpha adrenergic receptor modulating the hydroosmotic effect of vasopressin in the rabbit cortical collecting tubule. *J Clin Invest* 1984; 73:704.

110. Kukovetz WR, Poch G, Holzmann S, et al: Role of cyclic nucleotides in adenosine-mediated regulation of coronary flow. *Adv Cyclic Nucleotide Res* 1978; 9:397.

111. Lee TJF: Cholinergic mechanism in the large cat cerebral artery. *Circ Res* 1982; 50:870.

112. Lefer AM, Okamatsu S, Smith EF, et al: Beneficial effects of a new thromboxane synthetase inhibitor in arachidonate-induced sudden death. *Thromb Res* 1981; 23:265.

113. Lefer AM, Trachte G: Effects of converting enzyme inhibition in circulatory shock, in Horowitz Z (ed): *Angiotensin Converting Enzyme Inhibitors: Mechanisms of Action and Clinical Implications*. Baltimore, Urban & Schwarzenberg, 1981, pp 273–284.

114. Leier C, Heban P, Huss P, et al: Comparative systemic and regional hemodynamic effects of dopamine and dobutamine in patients with cardiomyopathic heart failure. *Circulation* 1978; 58:466.

115. Lluch S, Conde MV, Diéguez G, et al: Evidence for the direct effect of vasopressin human and goat cerebral arteries. *J Pharmacol Exp Ther* 1984; 228:749.

116. Lock JE, Olley PM, Coceani F: Enhanced β-adrenergic receptor responsiveness in hypoxic neonatal pulmonary circulation. *Am J Physiol* 1981; 240:H697.

117. Loeb HS, Bredakis J, Gunnar RM: Superiority of dobutamine over dopamine for augmentation of cardiac output in patients with chronic low output cardiac failure. *Circulation* 1977; 55:375.

118. Magnoni MS, Kobayashi H, Cazzaniga F, et al: Hypertension reduces the number of beta-adrenergic receptors in rat brain microvessels. *Circulation* 1983; 67:610.

119. Magorien RD, Leier CV, Kolibash AJ, et al: Beneficial effects of nifedipine on rest and exercise myocardial energetics in patients with congestive heart failure. *Circulation* 1984; 70:884.

120. Marco E, Balfagon G, Marin J, et al: Indirect adrenergic effect of histamine in cat cerebral arteries. *Naunyn Schmiedebergs Arch Pharmacol* 1980; 312:239.

121. Maurer P, Moskowitz MA, Levine L, et al: The synthesis of prostaglandins by bovine cerebral microvessels. *Prostaglandins Med* 1980; 4:153.

122. McGiff JC, Growshaw K, Terragno NA, et al: Release of a prostaglandin like substance into renal venous blood in response to angiotensin II. *Circ Res* 1979; 26(suppl I):I121.

123. McGiff JC, Terragno NA, Malik K, et al: Release of a prostaglandin E like substance from canine kidney by bradykinin. *Circ Res* 1972; 31:36.

124. McPherson GA, Summers RJ: A study of α_1-adrenoceptors in rat renal cortex: Comparison of [^{3}H]-prazosin binding with α_1-adrenoceptor modulating gluconeogenesis under physiological conditions. *Br J Pharmacol* 1982; 77:177.

125. McPherson GA, Summers RJ: Evidence from binding studies for α_2-adrenoceptors directly associated with glomeruli from rat kidney. *Eur J Pharmacol* 1983; 90:333.

126. Medgett IC, Langer SZ: Characterization of smooth muscle α-adrenoceptors and of responses to electrical stimulation in the cat isolated perfused middle cerebral artery. *Naunyn Schmiedebergs Arch Pharmacol* 1983; 323:24.

127. Mills MD, Burchell HB, Parker RL, et al: Myocardial infarction and sudden deaths following administration of pitressin: Additional electrocardiographic study of 100 patients given pitressin for cholecystography. *Staff Meet Mayo Clin* 1949; 24:254.

128. Mohrmann DE, Feigl EO: Competition between sympathetic vasoconstriction and metabolic vasodilation in the canine coronary circulation. *Circ Res* 1978; 42:79.

129. Moncada S, Vane JR: *Biochemical Aspects of Prostaglandins and Thromboxanes*. New York, Academic Press, 1977.

130. Morrison AR, Nishikawa K, Needleman P: Unmasking of thromboxane A_2 synthesis by ureteral obstruction in the rabbit kidney. *Nature* 1977; 267:259.

131. Mudge GH, Goldberg S, Gunther S, et al: Comparison of metabolic and vasoconstrictor stimuli on coronary vascular resistance in man. *Circulation* 1979; 59:544.

132. Mueller SM, Rusterholz DB: "Trophic" influence of sympathetic nerves on the peripheral and cerebral vasculature, in Heistad DD, Marcus ML (eds): *Cerebral Blood Flow: Effects of Nerves and Neurotransmitters*. New York, Elsevier North Holland, Inc, 1982, pp 17–325.

133. Muramatsu I, Sakakibara Y, Hong SC, et al: Effects of cinepazide on the purinergic responses in the dog cerebral artery. *Pharmacology* 1984; 28:27.

134. Murthy VV, Gilbert JC, Goldberg LI, et al: Dopamine sensitive adenylate cyclase in canine renal artery. *J Pharm Pharmacol* 1973; 29:567.

135. Myers BD, Deen WM, Brenner BM: Effects of norepinephrine and angiotensin II on the determinants of glomerular ultrafiltration and proximal tubule fluid reabsorption in the rat. *Circ Res* 1975; 37:101.

136. Navar LG, Rosivall L: Contribution of the renin-angiotensin system to the control of intrarenal hemodynamics. *Kidney Int* 1984; 25:857.

137. Oliveri M, Gartorelli C, Polese A, et al: Treatment of hypertension with nifedipine, a calcium antagonist agent. *Circulation* 1979; 59(5):1056.

138. Ormsbee HS III, Fondacaro JD: Action of serotonin on the gastrointestinal tract. *Proc Soc Exp Biol Med* 1985; 178:333.

139. Osborn JL, DiBona GF, Thames MD: Beta-1 receptor mediation of renin secretion elicited by low frequency renal nerve stimulation. *J Pharmacol Exp Ther* 1981; 216:265.

140. Ozaki N, Kawakita S, Toda N: Effects of dobutamine on isolated canine cerebral, coronary, mesenteric and renal arteries. *J Cardiovasc Pharmacol* 1982; 4:1456.

141. Packer M, Medina N, Yushak M, et al: Detrimental effects of verapamil in patients with primary pulmonary hypertension. *Br Heart J* 1984; 52:106.

142. Patel P, Bose D, Greenway C: Effects of prazosin and phenoxybenzamine on α- and β-receptor-mediated responses in intestinal resistance and capacitance vessels. *J Cardiovasc Pharmacol* 1981; 3:1050.

143. Paul KS, Whalley ET, Forster C, et al: Prostacyclin and cerebral vessel relaxation. *J Neurosurg* 1982; 57:334.

144. Pawlik WW, Shepherd AP, Mailman D, et al: Effects of dopamine and epinephrine on intestinal blood flow and oxygen uptake. *Adv Exp Med Biol* 1976; 75:511.

145. Pawlik WW, Tague LL, Tepperman BL, et al: Histamine H$_1$- and H$_2$-receptor vasodilation of canine intestinal circulation. *Am J Physiol* 1977; 223:E219.

146. Pawlik WW, Walus KM, Fondacaro JD: Effects of methionine-enkephalin on intestinal circulation and oxygen consumption. *Proc Soc Exp Biol Med* 1980; 165:26.

147. Pawlik WW, Walus KM, Fondacaro JD, et al: Local gastrointestinal vascular effects of methionine-enkephalin. *Hepatogastroenterology* 1983; 30:66.

148. Pettinger WA, Keeton TK, Campbell WB: Evidence for a renal α-adrenergic receptor inhibiting renin release. *Circ Res* 1976; 38:338.

149. Raskin NH: Pharmacology of migraine. *Annu Rev Pharmacol Toxicol* 1981; 21:463.

150. Rehr RB, Jackson JA, Winniford MD, et al: Mechanism of nitroglycerin-induced coronary dilation: Lack of relation to intracoronary thromboxane concentrations. *Am J Cardiol* 1984; 54:971.

151. Richardson PDI: Pharmacology of intestinal blood flow and oxygen uptake, in Shepherd AP, Granger DN (eds): *Physiology of the Intestinal Circulation*. New York, Raven Press, 1984, pp 393–402.

152. Richardson PDI, Withrington PG: A comparison of the effects of bradykinin, 5-hydroxytryptamine and histamine on the hepatic arterial and portal venous vascular beds of the dog: Histamine H$_1$ and H$_2$ receptor populations. *Br J Pharmacol* 1977; 60:123.

153. Richardson PDI, Withrington PG: Responses of the canine hepatic arterial and portal venous vascular beds to dopamine. *Eur J Pharmacol* 1978; 48:337.

154. Rosenthal A, Pace-Asciak CR: Potent vasoconstriction of the isolated perfused rat kidney by leukotrienes C$_4$ and D$_4$. *Can J Physiol Pharmacol* 1983; 61:325.

155. Rouse D, Suki WN: Alpha$_2$-adrenergic inhibition of fluid absorption in rabbit superficial proximal convoluted tubules. *Kidney Int* (in press).

156. Rousseau MF, Vincent MF, van Hoof F, et al: Effects of nicardipine and nisoldipine on myocardial metabolism, coronary blood flow and oxygen consumption in angina pectoris. *Am J Cardiol* 1984; 54:1189.

157. Ruffolo RR Jr: α-Adrenoceptors. *Monogr Neural Sci* 1984; 10:224.

158. Ruffolo RR Jr: The pharmacology of dobutamine. *Pharmacotherapy* (in press).

159. Ruffolo RR Jr, Messick K: Systemic hemodynamic effects of dopamine (±)-dobutamine and the (+)- and (−)-enantiomers of dobutamine in anesthetized normotensive rats. *Eur J Pharmacol* 1985; 109:173.

160. Ruffolo RR Jr, Messick K, Horng JS: Inter-

actions of three inotropic agents, ASL-7022, dobutamine and dopamine, with α- and β-adrenoceptors in vitro. *Naunyn Schmiedebergs Arch Pharmacol* 1984; 326:317.

161. Ruffolo RR Jr, Yaden EL: Vascular effects of the stereoisomers of dobutamine. *J Pharmacol Exp Ther* 1983; 224:46.

162. Sadoshima S, Busija D, Brody M, et al: Protection against stroke by sympathetic nerves, in Heistad DD, Marcus ML (eds): *Cerebral Blood Flow: Effects of Nerves and Neurotransmitters*. New York, Elsevier North Holland, Inc, 1982, pp 309–315.

163. Saeed M, Holtz J, Elsner D, et al: Sympathetic control of myocardial oxygen balance in dogs mediated by activation of coronary vascular α_2-adrenoceptors. *J Cardiovasc Pharmacol* 1985; 7:167.

164. Schmid PG, Abboud FM, Wendling MG, et al: Regional vascular effects of vasopressin: Plasma levels and circulatory responses. *Am J Physiol* 1974; 227:998.

165. Schnaar RL, Sparks HV: Response of large and small coronary arteries to nitroglycerin, $NaNO_2$ and adenosine. *Am J Physiol* 1972; 223:223.

166. Schwaiger M, Fondacaro JD, Jacobson ED: Effects of glucagon, histamine and perhexiline on the ischemic canine mesenteric circulation. *Gastroenterology* 1979; 77:730.

167. Schwaiger M, Jacobson ED: Peripheral vascular H_2-receptors to histamine. *Circ Shock* 1979; 6:213.

168. Segstro R, Greenway C: α-Receptor subtype mediating sympathetic mobilization of blood from the hepatic venous system in anesthetized cats. *J Pharmacol Exp Ther* 1986; 236:224.

169. Sercombe R, Aubineau P, Edvinsson L, et al: Pharmacological evidence in vitro and in vivo for functional $beta_1$ receptors in the cerebral circulation. *Pflügers Arch* 1977; 368:241.

170. Shah SV, Northrup TE, Hui YSF, et al: Action of serotonin (5-hydroxytryptamine) on cyclic nucleotides in glomeruli of rat renal cortex. *Kidney Int* 1979; 15:463.

171. Shelygina NM, Osychnyuk VI, Mikheeva AI, et al: Pulmonary circulation hemodynamics in patients with chronic nonspecific lung diseases treated with adrenaline. *Ter Arkh* 1980; 52:39.

172. Siegel RJ, Shah PK, Nathan M, et al: Prosta-

glandin E_1 infusion in unstable angina: Effects on anginal frequency and cardiac function. *Am Heart J* 1984; 108:863.

173. Shimizu K, Ohta T, Toda N: Evidence for greater susceptibility of isolated dog cerebral arteries to Ca antagonists than peripheral arteries. *Stroke* 1980; 11:261.

174. Skorecki KL, Ballermann BJ, Rennke HG, et al: Angiotensin II receptor regulation in isolated renal glomeruli. *Fed Proc* 1983; 42:3064.

175. Slotnik IL, Teigland JD: Cardiac accidents following vasopressin injection (pitressin). *JAMA* 1951; 146:1126.

176. Smedegard G, Hedquist P, Dahlen SE, et al: Leukotriene C_4 affects pulmonary cardiovascular dynamics in monkey. *Nature* 1982; 295:327.

177. Smythe C, Nickel J, Bradley S: The effect of epinephrine (USP), L-epinephrine, and L-norepinephrine on glomerular filtration rate renal plasma flow and the urinary excretion of sodium, potassium, and water in normal man. *J Clin Invest* 1952; 31:499.

178. Sonnenblick E, Frishman W, Le Jemtel T: Dobutamine: A new synthetic cardioactive sympathetic amine. *N Engl J Med* 1979; 300:17.

179. Sullivan J, Adams D, Hollenberg N: β-Adrenergic blockade in essential hypertension: Reduced renin release despite renal vasoconstriction. *Circ Res* 1976; 38:532.

180. Summers RJ: Renal α-adrenoceptors. *Fed Proc* 1984; 43:2917.

181. Summers RJ, Kuhar MJ: Autoradiographic localization of β-adrenoceptors in rat kidney. *Eur J Pharmacol* 1983; 91:305.

182. Sundt TM, Onofrio BM: Clinical experience in the management of cerebral vasospasm using intravenous isoproterenol and lidocaine hydrochloride in Langfitt TW, McHenry LC, Reivich M, et al (eds): *Cerebral Circulation and Metabolism*. New York, Springer-Verlag, 1975, pp 343–346.

183. Takagi T, Kamiya K, Fukuoka H, et al: Effect of Ca antagonists on experimental cerebral vasospasm. *Acta Neurol Scand* 1979; 60(suppl. 72):486.

184. Toda N: Actions of bradykinin on isolated cerebral and peripheral arteries. *Am J Physiol* 1977; 232:H267.

185. Toda N: Alpha adrenergic receptor subtypes

in human, monkey and dog cerebral arteries. *J Pharmacol Exp Ther* 1983; 226:861.

186. Torres VE, Northrup TE, Edwards RM, et al: Modulation of cyclic nucleotides in isolated rat glomeruli. *J Clin Invest* 1978; 62:1334.

187. Tuttle RR, Pollock GD, Todd G, et al: The effect of dobutamine on cardiac oxygen balance, regional blood flow, and infarction severity after coronary artery narrowing in dogs. *Circ Res* 1977; 41:357.

188. Tuzel I: Sodium nitroprusside: A review of its clinical effectiveness as a hypotensive agent. *J Clin Pharmacol* 1974; 14:494.

189. Uski TK, Andersson KE: Effects of prostanoids on isolated feline cerebral arteries: I. Characterization of the contraction-mediating receptor. *Acta Physiol Scand* 1984; 120:131.

190. Uski TK, Andersson KE, Brandt L, et al: Characterization of the prostanoid receptors and of the contractile effects of prostaglandin $F_{2\alpha}$ in human pial arteries. *Acta Physiol Scand* 1984; 121:369.

191. Vanhoutte PM: Does 5-hydroxytryptamine play a role in hypertension? *Trends Pharmacol Sci* 1982; 3:370.

192. Vanhoutte PM, Cohen RA: Effects of acetylcholine on the coronary artery. *Fed Proc* 1984; 43:2878.

193. Vatner SF: α-Adrenergic tone in the coronary circulation of the conscious dog. *Fed Proc* 1984; 43:2867.

194. Vincent H, Boomsma F, Man in't Veld A, et al: Effects of selective and nonselective β-agonists on plasma potassium and norepinephrine. *J Cardiovasc Pharmacol* 1984; 6:107.

195. Von Holst H, Granstrom E, Hammarstrom S, et al: Effect of leukotrienes C4, D4, prostacyclin and thromboxane A2 on isolated human cerebral arteries. *Acta Neurochim* 1982; 62:177.

196. Wahl M, Kuschinsky W, Bosse O, et al: Micropuncture evaluation of β-receptors in pial arteries of cats. *Pflügers Arch* 1974; 348:293.

197. Walus KM, Fondacaro JD, Jacobson ED: Effects of adenosine and its derivatives on the canine intestinal vasculature. *Gastroenterology* 1981; 81:327.

198. Walus KM, Fondacaro JD, Jacobson ED: Effects of calcium and its antagonists on the canine mesenteric circulation. *Circ Res* 1981; 48:692.

199. Walus KM, Fondacaro JD, Jacobson ED: Hemodynamic and metabolic changes during stimulation of ileal motility. *Dig Dis Sci* 1981; 26(12):1069.

200. Weber M, Drayer J: Renal effects of beta adrenoceptor blockade. *Kidney Int* 1980; 18:686.

201. Weber PC, Siess W, Scherer B, et al: Prostaglandins and the renal circulation, in Herman AG, Vanhoutte PM, Denolin H, et al (eds): *Cardiovascular Pharmacology of the Prostaglandins*. New York, Raven Press, 1982, pp 267–286.

202. Whalley ET, Fritz H, Geiger R: Kinin receptors and angiotensin converting enzyme in rabbit basilar arteries. *Naunyn Schmiedebergs Arch Pharmacol* 1983; 324:296.

203. White RP, Hagen AA: Cerebrovascular actions of prostaglandins. *Pharmacol Ther* 1982; 18:313.

204. Willerson JT, Hutton I, Watson JT, et al: Influence of dobutamine on regional myocardial blood flow and ventricular performance during acute and chronic myocardial ischemia in dogs. *Circulation* 1976: 53:828.

205. Wilson DA, O'Neill JT, Said SI, et al: Vasoactive intestinal polypeptide and the canine cerebral circulation. *Circ Res* 1981; 48:138.

206. Winn HR, Rubio R, Curnish RR, et al: Changes in regional cerebral blood flow (rCBF) caused by increase in CSF concentration of adenosine and 2-chloroadenosine. *J Cereb Blood Flow Metab* 1981; 1(suppl 1):S401.

207. Winquist RJ, Webb RC, Bohr DE: Relaxation to transmural nerve stimulation and exogenously added norepinephrine in porcine cerebral vessels. *Circ Res* 1982; 51:769.

208. Yeh BK, McNay JL, Goldberg LI: Attenuation of dopamine renal and mesenteric vasodilation of haloperidol: Evidence for a specific receptor. *J Pharmacol Exp Ther* 1969; 168:303.

31

Ventilatory Support of the Failing Circulation: Phasic High Intrathoracic Pressure Support and Cardiac Cycle–Specific Ventilation

Michael R. Pinsky, M.D.

Normal cardiovascular homeostasis depends on the effective interplay of factors that include cardiac pump function, circulating blood volume, and vasomotor tone. The influence of increased airway pressure in reducing venous return is well known. In contrast, it has recently been demonstrated that in patients with cardiac pump failure, specific ventilatory maneuvers in which airway pressure is increased may increase cardiac output. The following discussion of ventilatory support of the failing circulation relates to the setting of cardiac pump failure and accordingly may not be applicable to conditions in which cardiovascular collapse is not due primarily to cardiac pump failure.

OVERVIEW

Cardiovascular function is intimately related to ventilation. As described in chapter 21, "Hemodynamic Effects of Artificial Ventilation," ventilation can affect cardiovascular performance by changing either lung volume or intrathoracic pressure (ITP). Although changes in lung volume independent of changes in ITP may affect ventricular diastolic compliance and induce reflex va-

sodepressor effects, it is primarily the change in ITP that affects cardiac function by altering the pressure gradients for both systemic venous return and left ventricular (LV) ejection.

The heart within the thorax is a pressure chamber within a pressure chamber. It follows that increases in ITP will simultaneously impede venous return and augment LV ejection. Decreases in ITP will increase venous return but, by pulling outward on the LV wall, impair LV ejection. Thus, negative swings in ITP can be conceptualized as mechanically inducing cardiac dysfunction by increasing LV afterload. Buda et al.,[5] in conscious humans, and Summer et al.,[50] in anesthetized dogs, demonstrated that the negative ITP generated by a Mueller maneuver impedes LV ejection. Pinsky[32] demonstrated that such negative swings in ITP augment systemic venous return and right ventricular (RV) output as well. The overall effect is to decrease cardiac output despite an increase in intrathoracic blood volume and LV preload. In an extension of their study, Buda et al.[5] suggested that positive swings in ITP generated by a Valsalva maneuver improved LV ejection. However, cardiac output was not increased. Since venous return falls during a Valsalva maneuver because of the increase in right

is the backpressure to ve-
rax,[35] LV preload decreased
in ejection fraction. Thus,
s in ITP induced by the Val-
l not increase cardiac output
tions, primarily because intra-
ume decreases, decreasing LV

not equal to atmospheric pres-
olic pressure load is more accu-
as transmural LV pressure,[5] that
ary pressure minus extracavitary
Thus for a constant LV intracav-
negative swings in ITP will in-
systolic pressure load, and positive
will increase LV contraction by
LV. Both positive and negative
during ventilation and ventilatory
n be clinically important.

Stalcup and Mellins[46] demonstrated that during an asthmatic attack, a child's breathing pattern may generate profoundly negative swings in
ITP that may precipitate acute pulmonary edema.
Similarly, obstructive sleep apnea can be thought
of as a series of Mueller maneuvers, which may
contribute to LV failure. Finally, since patients
with pulmonary edema of any cause develop stiff
lungs owing to alveolar collapse, their spontaneous respiratory efforts significantly decrease
the ITP necessary to generate a tidal breath and
therefore may not only increase venous return but
also increase LV afterload, both of which increase pulmonary capillary hydrostatic pressure
and worsen the pulmonary edema. In all these
conditions, efforts directed at preventing the normal or exaggerated fall in ITP during inspiration
will decrease intrathoracic blood volume and may
remove the additional LV afterload.

Positive swings in ITP, by unloading the
LV, may augment LV ejection and increase cardiac output in heart failure states despite the
obligatory fall in intrathoracic blood volume.
This concept has been dramatically illustrated in
the cardiopulmonary resuscitation (CPR) literature. Rudikoff et al.[41] have demonstrated that the
rise in ITP created by active chest compression
during CPR creates a pressure gradient between
the thoracic and systemic vascular systems generating forward blood flow. Criley et al.[8] further
demonstrated that increased ITP produced by
coughing could sustain arterial blood pressure
and prolong consciousness in asystolic patients.
Furthermore, in patients with depressed LV func-

tion and volume overload, cardiac output does
not decline with the application of positive end-
expiratory pressure (PEEP),[6] and in some cases it
may be greater than during intermittent positive
pressure breathing (IPPB) alone.[11] Similarly,
spontaneous expiratory Valsalva maneuvers, or
grunting, have been shown to augment the failing
circulation in patients with severe LV dysfunction.[36]

THEORETICAL CONSIDERATIONS

To understand better how increased ITP can augment the failing circulation, a conceptual framework is needed that directly relates ITP to blood
flow. Since the intrathoracic vascular structures
are pliable and easily acted on by changes in ITP,
such changes in ITP will affect the perceived intrathoracic vascular pressures when measured relative to atmospheric pressure. Changes in ITP independent of changes in lung volume will have
no effect on blood flow from the right ventricle
(RV) through the pulmonary circulation to the
left atrium (LA), because all these vascular structures will be equally affected by ITP, and thus
the pressure gradient from the pulmonary artery
(PA) to LA will not change. All changes in ITP,
however, will affect the pressure gradients for
both systemic venous return and LV ejection.

Systemic Venous Return

As originally described by Starling[48] and characterized by Guyton et al.,[14] venous blood flow
back to the RA can be thought of as draining
down a pressure gradient from the systemic venous reservoirs to the heart. The force generated
by LV ejection into the arterial circulation is almost spent by the time the blood has reached the
systemic venous reservoirs, so that the major determinants of hydrostatic pressure are blood volume and vasomotor tone. In a supine paralyzed
dog with a normal intravascular blood volume,
this pressure is between 5 and 15 torr. Since the
resistance to venous blood flow is very small
compared with arterial vascular resistance, the
venous pressure gradient—venous reservoir pressure minus RA pressure (RAP)—is adequate to
maintain the normal venous return. Since the RA
and intrathoracic venae cavae are pliable and easily acted on by ITP, increases in ITP will increase RAP measured relative to atmospheric
pressure. Therefore, increases in RAP from in-

creased ITP will decrease the pressure gradient for venous return, whereas decreases in RAP from decreased ITP will increase the pressure gradient for venous return. Thus, any maneuver that decreases ITP will increase venous return, and any maneuver that increases ITP will impede venous return.[35]

Left Ventricular Ejection: The Concept of Afterload

LV ejection or systolic performance is determined by intrinsic LV myocardial contractility, heart rate, end-diastolic volume, and afterload.[41] LV afterload can be defined as maximal LV wall stress.[20] By the Laplace equation, wall stress of a sphere is equal to the radius of the sphere and the pressure difference across the wall of the sphere from the inside out. If the volume of the sphere increases, the radius of the sphere also increases and thus for the same pressure gradient the wall stress increases. Similarly, for the same volume, if the pressure gradient increases, the wall stress will increase as well. Although the LV resembles not a sphere, but rather an elongated ellipsoid, systolic wall stress (afterload) is usually equated with the maximum volume and pressure gradient during systole. In practice, this condition occurs at the end of isometric contraction prior to LV ejection, when both LV volume (end-diastolic volume, LVEDV) and pressure (now equal to aortic diastolic pressure) are elevated. LV stroke volume varies directly with LVEDV (Starling's law of the heart) and inversely with afterload. Since end-diastolic volume is a determinant of both preload and afterload, LV afterload is often equated with only LV ejection pressure, whereas end-diastolic volume is equated with LV preload. Although this analysis of preload and afterload is clinically attractive, it may misrepresent actual changes in afterload if end-diastolic volumes change significantly. For example, nitroprusside infusion induces a nonspecific vasodilation. This decreases both LV systolic pressure and venous return. Since end-diastolic volumes fall, for a given LV systolic pressure LV afterload will be less. If LV output is limited by afterload factors, such as would occur in severe LV failure states, the decrease in afterload may result in an increase in stroke volume despite a decrease in end-diastolic volume. Thus, in severe heart failure states, nitroprusside may increase cardiac output and decrease LV filling pressure while aortic pressure stays constant.

Left Ventricular Afterload: The Concept of Transmural Pressure

LV afterload, or wall stress, is a function of both LVEDV and the pressure generated by the LV during systole. The pressure generated by the LV is equal to the intracavitary pressure minus the extracavitary pressure, here called transmural pressure. By convention, intracavitary pressure or LV pressure (LVP) is measured relative to atmospheric pressure. Extracavitary pressure is pericardial pressure (PCP). When pericardial disease is present or biventricular end-diastolic volume exceeds the unstressed pericardial volume, PCP will rise relative to ITP. However, under most other conditions PCP equals juxtacardiac ITP. Therefore, transmural LVP can be defined as LVP minus ITP. Under normal conditions of spontaneous or positive pressure ventilation, ITP changes minimally because of the high compliance of the lung and the low resistance of the airways. Thus, the small changes in ITP (usually less than 5 torr) can be ignored and transmural LVP can be approximated as aortic pressure.[5, 50] However, when the changes in ITP are exaggerated, as they are during various disease states, and with the use of large tidal volumes and high PEEP, the effect of ITP on LV ejection can be significant.[5]

Let us consider how changes in ITP may affect LV afterload. Clinically, a reduction in LV afterload is usually achieved by reducing arterial pressure. This would reduce systolic ventricular pressure and wall stress for a given ventricular end-diastolic volume. This decrease in afterload is mechanically identical to increasing the pressure surrounding the heart, ITP, while keeping arterial pressure constant. Thus, identical reductions in LV afterload can be achieved by either reducing the pressure within the ventricle or increasing the pressure surrounding it. This concept is illustrated in Figure 31–1, in which positive ITP is compared with nitroprusside infusion.

This phenomenon can also be viewed from the standpoint of the systemic circulation. The LV ejects its stroke into the aorta, a structure that has both intrathoracic and extrathoracic components. The aorta drains most of its blood into extrathoracic tissues whose surrounding pressure is close to atmospheric pressure. Changes that primarily affect ITP do not affect the pressures surrounding these extrathoracic vessels as much, if at all. If LV stroke volume is constant, the in-

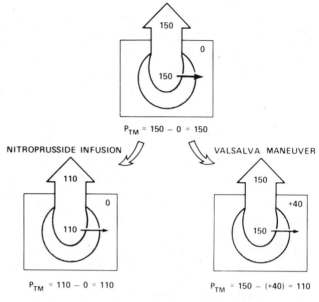

FIG 31–1.

Schematic representation of the left ventricular wall *(crescent)*, thoracic cavity *(box)*, and aorta *(arrow)*, showing that similar changes in left ventricular transmural pressure (P_{TM}) can be induced by decreasing aortic pressure (nitroprusside infusion) or raising intrathoracic pressure (Valsalva maneuver).

creases in ITP will not increase transmural LVP, but it will increase extrathoracic aortic pressure. The extrathoracic arterial bed, however, does not sense ITP as its surrounding pressure. Accordingly, there will be an initial increase in intraluminal pressure equal to the increase in ITP. This phenomenon can be demonstrated in any patient in whom continual arterial pressure recordings are made. If such a patient were to perform a Valsalva maneuver, arterial pressure and ITP would increase equally.[43] If increases in ITP were transmitted to the peripheral circulation without changing systemic vascular resistance, then arterial pressure would rise and tissue blood flow would increase. However, LV afterload measured by transmural LVP would remain constant.[28] Normally, reflex mechanisms in the steady state maintain a constant arterial pressure, despite variation in blood flow, by altering autonomic tone. Increases in arterial pressure generated by increased ITP induce a reflex vasodilation, to return arterial pressure toward its original value. This vasodilation decreases transmural LVP, allowing the LV to eject more completely during systole. Thus, for a given end-diastolic volume, increases in ITP will induce a fall in transmural LVP, increasing LV stroke volume while arterial pressure relative to atmosphere will remain constant.[28] Negative swings in ITP have the opposite effect: a decrease in arterial pressure causes a reflex increase in arterial tone, which in turn in-

creases transmural LVP and impedes LV ejection. This decreases stroke volume and induces LV dilation.[5] In summary, increases in ITP unload the LV, improving ejection; decreases in ITP increase LV afterload, impeding LV ejection.

Cardiac Output as a Balance Between Venous Return and Left Ventricular Ejection

In the steady state, total blood flow is a balance between cardiac output and venous return. As described by Guyton et al.,[13] this balance defines a given RAP and blood flow for any level of cardiac contractility, blood volume, and vasomotor tone. The point of equilibrium is shown graphically in Figures 31–2 and 31–3 for normal and failing hearts, respectively, as the intersection of the venous return and LV function curves at point *A*. Intravascular volume loading can be represented in this analysis by a parallel shift of the venous return curve to the right, such that for the same RAP venous blood flow will be greater, because the venous reservoir pressure will be increased *(dotted venous return curves)*. As can be seen from these illustrations, this volume loading will manifest itself as an increase in LV preload (point *B*). When cardiac function is normal (see Fig 31–2), increasing preload will increase cardiac output by the Frank-Starling mechanism (preload dependent). When cardiac function is

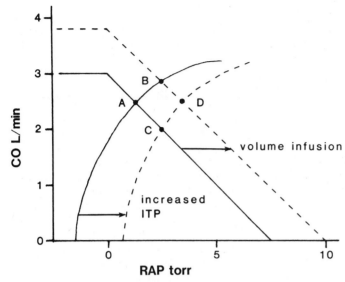

FIG 31–2.

Graphic analysis of the relationship between venous blood flow to right atrial pressure (venous return curve) and cardiac output to right atrial pressure (cardiac function curve) when cardiac function is normal. Venous return curves lie on points *A–C* for normovolemia and on points *B–D* for volume infusion, with cardiac function curves initially on line *A–B*, shifting to line *C–D* with increased ITP. Note that volume infusion increases blood flow by inducing a parallel shift of the venous return curve, whereas increased ITP reduces cardiac output by a parallel shift of the cardiac function curve. See text for discussion.

depressed (see Fig 31–3), similar increases in preload may not significantly increase cardiac output (preload independent), and indeed the decreasing venous return as induced clinically by diuretics usually does not decrease cardiac output. Increases in ITP from increases in RAP decrease the pressure gradient for venous return. In the Guyton analysis this is represented by a shift to the right of the LV function curve on the RAP axis *(dotted LV function curves)* without any change in its shape (contractility). If nothing else occurs in the system, then cardiac output will decrease and RAP will rise to a new equilibrium point, *C*, from point *A*. This shift of the LV function curve on the venous return curve is believed

to be the major mechanism in the decreasing cardiac output seen when patients are first placed on positive pressure ventilation. In this setting, cardiac output can be returned to point *A* values only by increasing venous return. In practice this can occur by either intravascular volume infusion or increased sympathetic tone, both of which can generate the rightward shift of the venous return curve represented by the dotted venous return curve intersection at point *D*. If the increase in ITP also decreases transmural LVP, as described in the previous section, then cardiac function should be improved.[28] This is graphically represented by the dotted cardiac function curve in Figure 31–3 whose slope is greater (increased

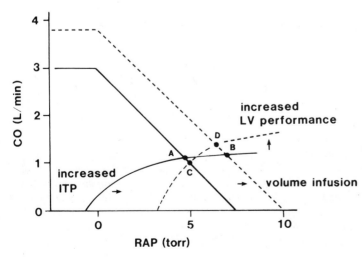

FIG 31–3.

Graphic analysis of the relation between venous blood flow to right atrial pressure (venous return curve) and cardiac output to right atrial pressure (cardiac function curve) when cardiac function is impaired. Curve shifts in response to volume loading and increased ITP are similar to those shown in Figure 31–2, except that improved cardiac performance also improves with increased ITP, the slope of the increased ITP cardiac function curve. See text for discussion.

performance) than the original function curves *(solid curves)*. As can be seen from this analysis, increasing cardiac performance by decreasing LV afterload will significantly increase cardiac output only in the failing heart (see Fig 31–3). Improving LV performance when cardiac function is normal usually does not increase cardiac output because the venous return curve at equilibrium is already near its maximal flow (point *A*).

This analysis is analogous to the effects of vasodilators like nitroprusside on cardiac output in normal and in failing hearts. When cardiac function is normal, cardiac output depends primarily on determinants of venous return,[37] and thus vasodilators like nitroprusside frequently induce a fall in cardiac output due to peripheral pooling of blood (decreased venous return), despite decreased LV afterload (increased LV performance). However, in congestive heart failure states, in which LV contractility is reduced and minimally responsive to changes in diastolic volume (preload independent), decreasing LV afterload improves cardiac output. It therefore follows that increasing ITP may increase cardiac output in congestive heart failure states by decreasing LV afterload if cardiac function remains preload independent.

METHODS OF INCREASING INTRATHORACIC PRESSURE

From the preceding discussion, one might predict that increasing ITP would always improve LV ejection. The degree to which LV ejection and cardiac output are augmented by increases in ITP is related not only to how venous return is affected, but also to the method by which ITP is increased. ITP can be elevated above atmospheric pressure by applying positive pressure to the airways, the thorax, or both.

During mechanical ventilation, positive pressure is delivered to the airway and expands the lungs. As the lungs expand, they push against the thoracic walls. It is this deformational pressure on the walls of the thoracic cavity induced by lung expansion that increases ITP, and not the lung expansion itself. For example, if there were a pneumothorax open to the outside, such that the lungs did not touch the chest wall, then positive pressure inspiration would increase lung volume but would not increase ITP. If, on the other hand, the thoracic cavity was intact and its compliance

reduced, as may occur with tense ascites elevating the diaphragm, then positive pressure inspiration would require a greater airway pressure to generate a given tidal volume; however, all of this increase in driving pressure would be transferred to the pleural space to overcome the decreased thoracic compliance.

Under most clinically relevant conditions, increasing ITP is accomplished usually by positive pressure breathing and further by the application of PEEP. Studies demonstrating that in heart failure states PEEP increases cardiac output more than positive pressure breathing alone were cited in the first section of this chapter. Unfortunately, as lung volume increases, pulmonary vascular resistance also increases,[52] as the alveolar vessels are constricted by the expanding alveoli. Therefore, acute RV failure or cor pulmonale may develop with excessive lung inflation. Acute RV dilation associated with the sudden application of continuous positive airway pressure (CPAP) has recently been described in a human,[19] and may explain some of the hemodynamic deterioration seen when CPAP or PEEP is added to a respiratory circuit.

ITP can also be increased by applying positive pressure to the chest wall and diaphragm. In practice, conventional manual chest compression during CPR increases ITP in this manner.[41] ITP has also been increased during CPR by simultaneous ventilation and chest compression.[7] By simultaneously decreasing thoracic compliance, this form of CPR generates a much greater increase in ITP for a given tidal volume. Since lung volumes do not increase beyond what would occur with a normal tidal breath, this form of CPR does not increase pulmonary vascular resistance more than similar tidal volume breathing does, although the increase in ITP is much greater. This modification of "conventional" CPR technique is presently thought to generate improved blood flow compared with sequential ventilation and chest compression techniques.[21, 23] In practice, however, it is more difficult to accomplish.

On the basis of these considerations, Pinsky et al.[28] used positive pressure breathing with static chest wall and abdominal binding to increase ITP in an animal model of acute heart failure. The chest and abdominal binders were fixed, limiting thoracic expansion during ventilation. However, since positive pressure inspiration increased lung volume and therefore thoracic volume, the binders became tight during inspiration, decreasing chest wall expansion. To increase ITP further, large tidal volume breaths were delivered (Vt = 25 ml/kg) and a rapid respiratory rate (40/min) was used. Using this system, mean ITP throughout the respiratory cycle could be increased from unbound values of approximately 1 torr to binder values of approximately 12 torr. Since at end-expiration the binders were loose and did not affect chest wall or diaphragmatic compliance, end-expiratory ITP was unchanged (approximately -3 torr). Presumably, allowing ITP to fall to its normal end-expiratory level did not compromise venous return as much as might have occurred with continually increased ITP. This method of increasing ITP, by combining positive pressure ventilation with chest and abdominal binding, has also been used in humans,[29] and is referred to in the literature as phasic high intrathoracic pressure support (PHIPS).

Thus, ITP can be increased by increasing lung volume during positive pressure ventilation, compressing the chest, or combining both. The combined approach, although more complicated, should minimize both the overdistention of the lung and the trauma to the chest wall and abdomen associated with vigorous chest wall compression.[33]

THE EFFECT OF INCREASES IN INTRATHORACIC PRESSURE ON CARDIAC PERFORMANCE

Methods of Estimating LV Performance

It is difficult to assess LV performance serially during a respiratory maneuver in humans, primarily because most clinical methods require stable steady-state conditions or hemodynamic equilibrium, precluding repeated analysis. Two-dimensional echocardiography can measure LV volume, ventricular septal shift, and velocity of circumferential fiber shortening (V_{cf}),[47] all of which are important indices of LV systolic performance. However, changing lung volume or cardiac rotation may make serial measurements of LV performance invalid. Radiocontrast cineradiography with LV injections of contrast material can assess LV systolic function, wall dysynergy, and valve function. Unfortunately, the hyperosmolar radiocontrast material induces significant hemodynamic effects, including vasodilation and arrhythmias,[40] which preclude its use in evaluating serial change in LV performance. Radionu-

clide gated blood pool imaging can accurately measure LV ejection fraction (LVEF)[47] but requires a finite acquisition time that exceeds measurement of sudden changes in LV ejection. Gated blood pool imaging is useful, however, in comparing different steady-state hemodynamic conditions. If patients are undergoing cardiac surgery, various marker devices can be placed on the heart to measure cardiac dimensions intraoperatively and postoperatively. Rankin et al.[39] placed temporary ultrasonic crystals along the minor axes of the LV in patients to measure the effect of increases in ITP on LV performance. Similarly, Ingels et al.[18] implanted tantalum intramyocardial markers around the LV that could be permanently used to assess LV function in such patients. These two techniques have the disadvantages of necessitating a thoracotomy and pericardiotomy, and having limited dimensional analyses. The intramyocardial marker technique is superior in that it can be quantitated in the stable postoperative period by standard left ventriculograms.[17]

Many indicators of LV performance can be measured. Most are affected to some degree by all of the determinants of cardiac performance: that is, preload (end-diastolic volumes), afterload (peak systolic wall stress), heart rate, and intrinsic myocardial contractility. For example, if LVEF is the indicator followed, it can be seen to increase as preload, heart rate, or contractility increases and to fall as afterload increases. This effect is also true for such parameters as stroke volume, V_{cf}, an estimate of fiber shortening velocity, and maximum LV dp/dt. The only LV systolic function index that appears to be preload independent is LV end-systolic volume.[49] Independent of LVEDV, as afterload changes, parallel changes in end-systolic volume occur. For a given level of contractility there is only one end-systolic volume that the LV can obtain for a given end-systolic pressure. As end-systolic pressure rises, the LV is unable to empty as completely as when the pressure was less. Likewise, as end-systolic pressure falls, the LV ejects to a lower end-systolic volume. This end-systolic pressure-volume relationship describes a line whose slope is proportional to the LV contractility. The relation is mechanically defined as end-systolic elastance (E_{ES}). As contractility increases, the slope of the end-systolic pressure-volume curve, E_{ES}, also increases. If contractility is unchanged, end-systolic volume will be determined only by end-systolic pressure (afterload). E_{ES} is independent of preload and relatively independent of afterload.[44] These points are illustrated in Figure 31–4, where the *x*-axis is LV volume and the *y*-axis is LV pressure. The bottom line represents the passive filling curve during diastole (diastolic compliance curve). The upper straight line, labeled E_{ES}, represents the end-systolic pressure-volume relationship determined by ventricular contractility. The pressure-volume history described through points *ABCD* represents a normal cardiac cycle. During diastole *(DAB)* the LV passively fills. Point *B* on the LV diastolic compliance curve represents the end-diastolic volume generated by a given LV filling pressure. The ventricle contracts, generating pressure until the aortic valve opens at point *C;* contraction then continues until a point is reached on its E_{ES} curve *(D)*. The end-systolic volume so achieved will now be determined solely by end-systolic pressure. Increases in LV filling pressure will increase LV stroke volume and LVEF (not shown). Increases in LV stroke volume can also occur at a constant LV filling pressure and contractility if ejection is augmented. Such augmentation can occur by either an increase in pleural pressure or a decrease in systemic vascular resistance. Both these mechanisms are diagramed in Figure 31–4. With the first beat after a 10-torr increase in pleural pressure, central aortic pressure is increased by the same amount as pleural

pressure (point *E*). The higher pleural pressure also augments systole, resulting in a higher stroke volume (to point *F*). If the extrathoracic vessels respond by reflexly dilating to keep aortic pressure constant, then the aortic valve will open at its original pressure *(C)* and ejection will be slightly greater (point *G*).

The same changes can be diagramed relative to transmural pressure (see Fig 31–4,B). Using transmural pressure, the pressure-volume history described through points *ABCD* represents one baseline ventricular cycle that is similar to that shown in Figure 31–4,A. During the first contraction after pleural pressure is increased, ejection from the ventricle (and thoracic aorta) is assisted by the raised pleural pressure. Because the (extrathoracic vascular) pressure that the ventricle "sees" is less elevated by the increase in pleural pressure, ejection is increased *(C–F)*. If the extrathoracic vessels respond by reflexly dilating to keep pressure constant, then the aortic valve opens at a lower (transmural) pressure (point *E*) and ejection is further increased (point *G*) without any change in the position or slope of the E_{ES} curve.

The effect of ITP on LV systolic performance can also be considered from the standpoint of LV systolic wall stress. Since LV systolic wall stress is a function of both transmural LV systolic pressure and LVEDV, as venous return is reduced by higher ITP, LV systolic wall stress will

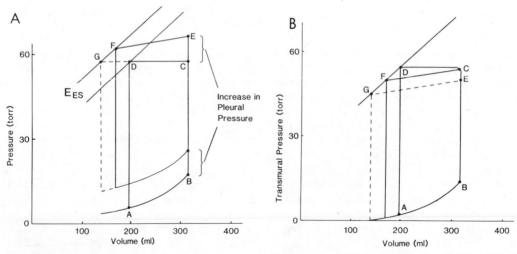

FIG 31–4.
Effect of increased ITP on LV pressure-volume during ejection in a heart with a fixed diastolic compliance and contractility state. The effect of augmented ejection and systemic vasodilation are shown for ventricular pressure relative to atmospheric pressure **(A)** and relative to pleural pressure **(B)**. See text for discussion.

be less and LV ejection may be improved. This effect of end-diastolic volume on wall stress and afterload, and therefore on LV ejection, is diagramed in Figure 15–17 in chapter 15, "Technical Problems in Data Acquisition." Because the work the LV must perform during ejection will be less for the same stroke volume, myocardial oxygen demand may be decreased.

Cardiac output can increase without a change in contractility either by an increase in preload or by an augmentation of systole or by a decrease in afterload. Therefore, studies that define improved cardiac performance without considering these three factors cannot clarify the mechanism by which cardiac performance is improved.

Observations in Humans

Buda et al.[5] studied the effects of sustained increases in ITP on LV performance in five subjects with implanted tantalum intramyocardial markers. The markers were implanted at the time of coronary artery bypass graft surgery or cardiac transplantation. All subjects were functionally asymptomatic, were clinically free of congestive heart failure, and had no dyssynergy on previous left ventriculography. No subject was taking propranolol. The markers were inserted in the mid-LV wall outlining the LV cavity as seen in the 30-degree right anterior oblique projection. The markers were visualized by single plane cardiac fluoroscopy. Also recorded were radial arterial pressure and airway pressure from a mouthpiece. LV end-diastolic and end-systolic volumes and V_{cf} were derived for each heartbeat. V_{cf}, an estimate of ventricular fiber shortening velocity, is thought to change in parallel to changes in contractility. From the ventricular volumes, ejection fraction and stroke volume were derived. The study compared quiet spontaneous respiration with a 7-second Valsalva maneuver of 20 cm H_2O. The strain phase was further divided into the initial three heartbeats (early) and the final three heartbeats (late) to ascertain sequential changes in LV performance throughout the Valsalva maneuver.

Figure 31–5 summarizes the results of this Valsalva maneuver for all five patients, expressed as percent of control (quiet spontaneous respiration). Both end-diastolic and end-systolic volumes fell precipitously during the strain phase, with a concomitant decline in cardiac output. Systolic arterial pressure rose early in the strain phase but fell later as stroke volume progres-

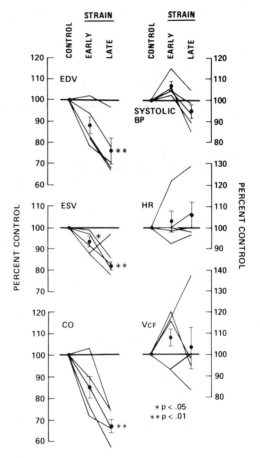

FIG 31–5.
Valsalva maneuver. Each line represents the average of three beats for each subject as a percent change from the respective baseline values for the measurements listed. The increase in V_{cf} despite a decreasing preload suggests that increased ITP unloads the LV. *Closed circles* and *I bars* denote the mean change ± SEM. *EDV*, end-diastolic volume; *ESV*, end-systolic volume; *CO*, cardiac output; *BP*, blood pressure; *HR*, heart rate; V_{cf}, velocity of circumferential fiber shortening. (From Buda et al: *N Engl J Med* 1979; 301:453–549. Reproduced by permission of the *New England Journal of Medicine*.)

sively fell. V_{cf} rose in three of five subjects early in the strain phase at a time when end-diastolic volume was falling and heart rates were relatively constant.

The observation that a Valsalva maneuver decreases LVEDV, stroke volume, and cardiac output agrees with the results of previous work.[3] From these changes one would predict a fall in V_{cf} by the Frank-Starling mechanism. However, if one considers that transmural LV systolic pressure (LVP − pleural pressure) decreases during the Valsalva maneuver, it appears that by unloading the LV, the increased ITP allows the LV to maintain its V_{cf} despite a decreasing preload.

Rankin et al.[39] studied the effect of combined increased ITP and lung volume as induced by the application of PEEP in patients during the immediate postoperative period, using sonomicrometer crystals to assess LV volumes and catheters in the left atrium and pericardial space. They also found that steady-state increases in ITP decrease LV dimensions associated with decreased LV filling pressure. Although they were able to document that the observed fall in LV dimensions are due to a decrease in LV filling pressure, presumably due to a decrease in venous return, they were unable to estimate systolic LV function.

From these studies it is clear that when LV function is normal, sustained increases in ITP generated by either a Valsalva maneuver or PEEP result in a decrease in cardiac output primarily due to the associated precipitous decrease in venous return, despite minimal improvements in LV performance. Viquerat et al.[51] studied the effect of 12 cm H_2O PEEP on ventricular volumes and cardiac output in 11 patients with the adult respiratory distress syndrome using multiple gated equilibrium cardiac blood pool scintigraphy and thermodilution techniques. They found that RV and LV end-diastolic volumes and stroke volumes decrease in a parallel fashion with the application of 12 cm H_2O PEEP, suggesting that when LV contractility is normal, even in the setting of stiff lungs, increases in ITP will induce a hemodynamically significant decrease in venous return and intrathoracic blood volume. This fall in venous return with PEEP is analogous to phase 2 of the Valsalva maneuver, where with sustained increased ITP, cardiac output and the aortic pulse pressure decline. However, in congestive heart failure this "normal" aortic pressure response is not seen. In congestive heart failure, sustained increases in ITP increase aortic pressure and pulse pressure and keep them elevated until release of the strain phase.[43, 53] This "square wave" response is thought to be due to several factors. First, with vascular congestion, increases in ITP will not greatly diminish LV preload. Second, with heart failure slight decreases in preload do not significantly decrease LV stroke volume, since the ventricular function (Frank-Starling) curve is relatively flat and small changes in pre-

load in either direction do not alter LV stroke volume. Finally, increases in ITP, by decreasing LVEDV, might improve LV ejection by decreasing peak LV systolic wall stress.

On the basis of the observation that increases in ITP affect the failing cardiovascular system differently from the normal one, it is interesting to examine studies done to assess the hemodynamic effects of PEEP (sustained increased ITP) on the failing circulation. Grace and Greenbaum[11] demonstrated that in the setting of LV dysfunction and circulatory volume overload, PEEP did not decrease cardiac output, and in those with severe dysfunction cardiac output was actually increased. In 12 of 13 patients with pulmonary artery occlusion pressures (wedge pressure, WP) greater than or equal to 19 torr, cardiac output increased by a mean of 500 ml/min with the application of 5 cm H_2O PEEP. Mathru et al.[24] studied the effect of different forms of ventilatory support in 20 patients after aortocoronary bypass surgery. In 12 patients WP was 17 torr or greater, and in all 20 patients LV stroke volume and cardiac output increased with application of 5 cm H_2O PEEP. Although PEEP can augment cardiac output, higher levels of airway pressure also can impair cardiac output by increasing pulmonary vascular resistance.

Rasanen et al.[38] compared the effect of three levels of ITP on cardiovascular function and myocardial ischemia in 12 patients with acute myocardial infarction complicated by respiratory failure. The three levels of ITP were created by three levels of ventilatory support: no support, or spontaneous ventilation; 50% support, or intermittent mandatory ventilation (IMV) for half the breaths; and 100% support with IPPB. They observed that maximal ischemia developed with no support and decreased with both IMV and IPPB. With all three modes, WP decreased progressively from no support to 100% support (20 ± 2 torr to 15 ± 2 torr; $P < .05$) and systolic arterial pressure also fell, consistent with a decrease in both intrathoracic blood volume and LV systolic work induced by a decrease in LV afterload.

If any conclusions can be drawn from these clinical studies it is that sustained increased ITP may improve LV function, but the effects are minimal primarily because of the obligatory fall in venous return associated with such sustained increases in ITP. That cardiac output may not fall in congestive heart failure states despite the application of PEEP has clinical relevance. In patients with combined cardiac dysfunction and hypoxemic respiratory failure, PEEP may be more aggressively given to improve oxygen delivery to the tissues, since the anticipated fall in cardiac output may not occur or may not be as great as when cardiac function is normal. However, as with any potentially detrimental therapy, appropriate hemodynamic monitoring is imperative.

THE EFFECT OF PHASIC INCREASES IN INTRATHORACIC PRESSURE ON LEFT VENTRICULAR PERFORMANCE

At this point we move from clinical practice to explore physiologic research with some potential for clinical application. Although the studies presented in this section appear valid and specific aspects have been duplicated in different research laboratories and intensive care units, they do not belong in the subset of studies that are accepted for general clinical application. They do, however, point to an exciting beneficial interaction between increases in ITP and LV function.

As was illustrated in the studies by Rankin et al.[38] and Viquerat et al.,[51] sustained increases in ITP induced by PEEP decrease biventricular end-diastolic blood volume and thus cardiac output by the Frank-Starling mechanism. Although this phenomenon may be due to mechanical restriction of the heart within the cardiac fossa as lung volume increases, simple decreases in venous return can explain the fall in cardiac output. Braunwald et al.[1] demonstrated that PEEP decreased not only cardiac output but intrathoracic blood volume as well, and therefore caused pooling of blood in the periphery. When this pooling effect was counteracted by a peripheral vasoconstrictor (metaraminol), returning intrathoracic blood volume to pre-PEEP levels, cardiac output also returned to normal despite an increase in vascular resistance and the continued application of PEEP. Thus, it is the decrease in intrathoracic blood volume and not the increase in ITP induced by PEEP that impairs cardiac output. Presumably, if intrathoracic blood volume can be maintained, increasing ITP should augment LV ejection.

The most dramatic example of an increase in ITP inducing an increase in steady-state forward blood flow comes from the CPR literature. Rudi-

koff et al.[41] demonstrated that most of the forward blood flow observed during CPR in dogs occurs secondary to an increase in ITP, such that simultaneous ventilation-compression induces a greater increase in ITP and forward blood flow than either ventilation or chest compression alone. They also demonstrated that active chest compression creates a pressure gradient between the thoracic and extrathoracic vascular system, thus generating forward blood flow.[7] The effect of ITP on cerebral blood flow during ventricular fibrillation was elegantly illustrated by Criley and co-workers.[8, 26] By having patients perform a series of forceful coughs, Criley et al. were able to maintain consciousness in their patients for more than 60 seconds. They point out that the interspersed negative swings in ITP during the rapid voluntary inspiration phase of the cough are just as important as the strain phase (positive swing in ITP), since they accelerate venous blood flow back to the thoracic reservoir.[26] Without such augmented venous blood flow, the forward arterial blood flow would quickly cease as intrathoracic blood volume diminished in a fashion analogous to the fall in LVEDV and cardiac output seen with sustained Valsalva maneuvers, described above.[5, 39] Although "cough CPR" has interesting physiologic implications regarding the determinants of blood flow during CPR, like standard CPR it represents only a very temporary means of maintaining forward blood flow. It appears, however, that potentially important cardiac augmentation can be given for longer periods by similar respiratory maneuvers that are similar in effect to "cough CPR" in the setting of severe cardiac failure.

Phasic Increases in ITP Induced by Spontaneous Respiration

Acute hypotension induces reflex tachypnea and hyperpnea[12] and has been demonstrated in a chronically instrumented dog model to result not only in an increase in the ITP swings during respiration but in a decrease in mean ITP as well.[10] This reflex ventilatory response to hypotension and pulmonary vascular congestion, although apparently induced by increased lung stiffness, may augment cardiac function. Increased respiratory drive can increase functional residual capacity (FRC) and lower ITP because of sustained inspiratory muscle tone, or it may increase ITP if accompanied by expiratory grunting. Pinsky et al.[36] described a 28-year-old patient with severe congestive cardiomyopathy who involuntarily generated increases in ITP during spontaneous ventilation by expiratory grunting. This patient's respiration during the initial 36 hours of his hospitalization resembled repetitive Valsalva maneuvers superimposed on Kussmaul's breathing. This respiratory pattern was presumably involuntary since it also occurred during sleep. The aortic and pulmonary arterial pulse pressure increased with each expiratory grunt. Cardiac index was 2.4 L/min/m^2, esophageal pressure was 12 torr, and WP was 26 torr during spontaneous ventilation with grunting. When 20 cm H_2O mask CPAP was applied, the grunting ceased, but cardiac index, WP, and esophageal pressure were unchanged. Removing the CPAP support immediately resulted in a generalized hemodynamic deterioration with a cardiac index of 1.6 L/min/m^2, an esophageal pressure of 6 torr, and no change in WP. Institution of IPPB with 20 cm H_2O PEEP returned this patient to his previous improved, hemodynamic condition. Thus, it appears that spontaneous respiratory straining, like "cough CPR," can augment forward blood flow. In a beating (albeit poorly functioning) heart, however, the mechanism of augmentation is a reduction in LV afterload associated with improvement in LV stroke volume, without change in systemic vascular resistance. Although the stimulus for this expiratory grunting is unknown, it is seen in other conditions when pulmonary edema is present.[15]

MECHANICAL AUGMENTATION OF THE CIRCULATION

Phasic High Intrathoracic Pressure Support of the Failing Circulation

Mechanically generated increases in ITP augment LV ejection[5] and impede venous return.[35] When systemic vascular resistance (SVR) decreases in response, as it usually does, increasing ITP is analogous to the infusion of vasodilators like nitroprusside. When cardiac function is normal, vasodilators decrease cardiac output by causing peripheral pooling of blood, despite the decrease in LV afterload. In congestive heart failure, decreasing LV afterload by vasodilators improves cardiac output.[19] Thus IPPB, by improving LV ejection, may augment cardiac output if its effect on LV ejection is more pronounced than its effect on venous return. Accordingly, Pinsky et al.[28]

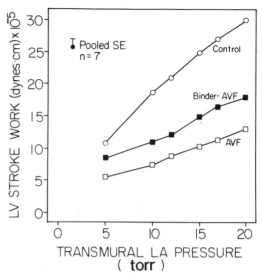

FIG 31–6.
Relation between left ventricular *(LV)* stroke work and transmural left atrial *(LA)* pressure (LV filling pressure). Mean values and slopes of acute ventricular failure *(AVF)* and binder-AVF curves are significantly less than control ($P < .01$). Mean values for binder-AVF are significantly greater than AVF ($P < .05$), although slopes are similar. (From Pinsky, et al.[28] Reproduced by permission of *Journal of Applied Physiology*.)

studied the effects of phasic increases in ITP on LV performance in a canine model of acute ventricular failure (AVF) induced by β-blockade. Increased ITP was induced without overdistension of the lungs by applying chest and abdominal binders that decreased thoracic cage compliance during inspiration but did not elevate ITP at end-expiration. Large tidal volume (30 ml/kg) IPPB at a rapid respiratory rate (40/min) was also used to increase ITP from 1.1 ± 1 torr in an unbound AVF state to 12.3 ± 2.3 torr in a bound state. Frank-Starling curves were constructed for normal (control) pre-AVF conditions and then AVF and AVF plus binder restriction (AVF-binder) conditions (Fig 31–6). Increasing ITP (binder-AVF) resulted in an increase in LV stroke work, as well as stroke volume and cardiac output, at any LV filling pressure during AVF conditions ($P < .05$). This increase in flow appeared to occur without a significant change in the aortic pressure-flow relation (Fig 31–7), suggesting that there is no change in arterial tone. (A lack of change in the pressure-flow relation in the autoregulatory range suggests no change in arterial tone.) However, the systolic pressure load of the

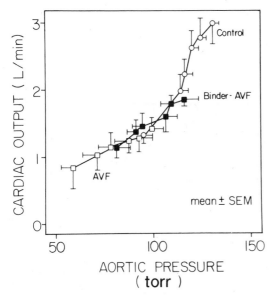

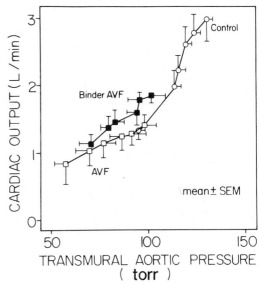

FIG 31–7.
Relation between cardiac output and aortic pressure (aortic pressure-flow curve). (From Pinsky et al.[28] Reproduced by permission of *Journal of Applied Physiology*.)

FIG 31–8.
Relationship between cardiac output and transmural aortic pressure (left ventricular outflow pressure). (From Pinsky et al.[28] Reproduced by permission of *Journal of Applied Physiology*.)

LV can be defined as transmural mean arterial pressure (MAP), which, owing to the increase in ITP during AVF-binder conditions, is less for a given cardiac output for AVF-binder than for AVF alone (Fig. 31–8). Thus, positive ITP improves LV performance in AVF conditions by reducing LV afterload. Presumably, this effect is associated with reflex vasodilation, because after bilateral carotid nerve sectioning the shift of the pressure-flow curve shown in Figure 31–7 was abolished.

In a related clinical trial patients in cardiogenic shock on IPPB were studied both with and without chest and abdominal binders by Pinsky and Summer.[29] They found that in humans, as in the canine preparation, cardiac outputs increased without a change in LV filling pressure (Fig 31–9). In this study, the patients' transmural MAP did not change, whereas MAP relative to atmospheric pressure increased (Fig 31–10), suggesting that peripheral vasodilation was not as important in these patients as in the canine study. This is not surprising, since the seven patients in this study were all on high-dosage infusion of vasopressor agents (dopamine and/or norepinephrine). This suggests that a major effect of increased ITP is to augment systole, in addition to any decrease in afterload that may occur.

Although these two studies demonstrate that phasic high intrathoracic pressure support (PHIPS) can augment and maintain steady-state cardiac output in severe ventricular failure states, the studies are limited in that the effects of increased ITP during AVF and ITP were increased using relatively large tidal volumes (30 ml/kg). Thus, in a subsequent study, Pinsky et al.[31] analyzed the independent effects of altering mean ITP, ITP swings during IPPB, respiratory rate, and tidal volume on cardiac function under normal (control) and AVF conditions. Consistent with the Braunwald et al. study,[1] they found that increasing mean ITP decreases both LV filling pressure and intrathoracic blood volume (Fig 31–11). This decrease occurs independently of the method by which mean ITP is increased. Similarly, the magnitude of the ITP swings only minimally affects this relation.[31] When ventricular function is normal, increases in ITP can decrease cardiac output by decreasing LV filling pressure. In AVF, increases in ITP improve LV performance, defined as a shift of the Frank-Starling relation to the left. That is, cardiac output can be increased despite a decrease in LV filling pressure. This effect is not unlimited, however, in that if LV filling pressure falls below some critical value, further increases in ITP will not further

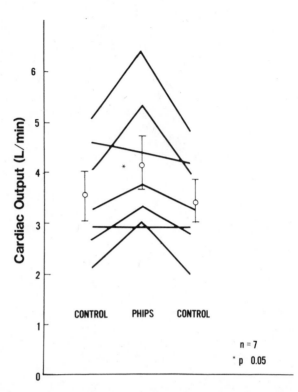

FIG 31–9.
Effect of phasic high intrathoracic pressure support *(PHIPS)* on cardiac output for all subjects in study by Pinsky and Summer.[29] Circles are mean values for group (*bars* denote SE). Cardiac output increases significantly with PHIPS from initial control values (*P* < .05). (From Pinsky and Summer.[29] Reproduced by permission of *Chest.*)

increase cardiac output. In essence, the heart once again becomes preload dependent. These points are illustrated in Figure 31–12, which is a trend recording of some of the observed variables for one animal during AVF-binder conditions, in which mean ITP was sequentially increased by increasing airway pressure using high-frequency jet ventilation. Note that when compared with the preceding and following apneic periods, sequential increases in mean pleural pressure are associated with reciprocal decreases in all intrathoracic vascular pressures (transmural RAP, transmural PAP, and transmural LAP). Despite this fall in ventricular filling pressures, biventric-

Fig 31–10.
A, effect of PHIPS on mean arterial pressure *(MAP)* for all subjects. *Circles* denote mean values for group (*bars* denote SE). MAP increased significantly with PHIPS from initial control values (*P* < .01). *B,* effect of PHIPS on transmural MAP (MAP minus esophageal pressure) for all subjects. *Circles* denote mean values for group (*bars* denote SE). *Asterisk* indicates estimated transmural MAP using same P_{es} as initial control step. There is no significant difference in mean values among three steps. (From Pinsky and Summer.[29] Reproduced by permission of *Chest.*)

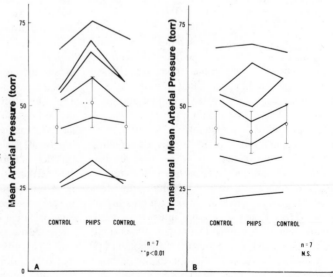

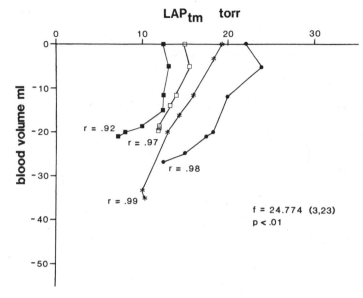

FIG 31–11.
Relation between transmural left atrial pressure *(LAP)* and blood volume shifts out of the thorax in response to increasing ventilator driving pressure in four close-chested dogs. Each data point represents resultant change in blood volume and transmural LAP to stepwise increases in ventilator driving pressure during high-frequency jet ventilation at a ventilatory frequency of 100 min^{-1} and a duty cycle of 20%. Although not a true measure of vascular compliance, these similar curves suggest a "dynamic" intrathoracic vascular compliance of approximately 4 ml/torr. (From Pinsky et al.[31] Reproduced by permission.)

ular stroke volume and aortic pressure initially increase with the first four increases in airway and pleural pressures. In this example the increase in cardiac output is limited when transmural LAP falls below 14 torr, such that further increases in mean pleural pressure decrease transmural LAP but do not further augment blood flow. This suggests that in AVF, once the LV preload has fallen below a limiting minimal threshold, the LV again becomes preload dependent for changes in stroke volume.

To summarize the results of these studies, LV performance is affected by changes in ITP primarily by the degree to which LV ejection is responsive to changes in LV filling pressure and afterload. Increasing ITP invariably decreases LV filling pressure and intrathoracic blood volume. To the extent that LV ejection is dependent on

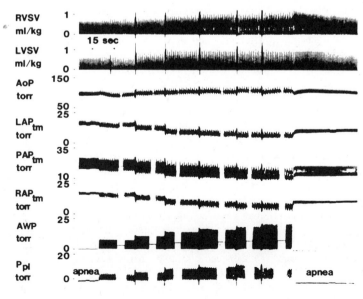

FIG 31–12.
Sequential trend recording of right ventricular stroke volume *(RVSV)*, left ventricular stroke volume *(LVSV)*, aortic pressure *(AoP)*, transmural left atrial pressure *(LAP_{tm})*, transmural pulmonary arterial pressure *(PAP_{tm})*, transmural right atrial pressure *(RAP_{tm})*, airway pressure *(AWP)*, and juxtacardiac pleural pressure *(P_{pl})* as ventilator driving pressure is increased in a stepwise fashion. Time between each interval shown is approximately 60 sec. The high-frequency jet ventilation is both preceded and followed by 15 seconds of apnea for comparison. See text for discussion. (From Pinsky et al.[31] Reproduced by permission.)

LV filling pressure (preload), increases in ITP will decrease LV ejection by the Frank-Starling mechanisms. To the extent that LV ejection is dependent on the pressure gradient between the LV and the extrathoracic vessels for LV ejection, increases in ITP will improve LV ejection by decreasing this pressure gradient. Further increase in LV ejection may occur if arterial tone is reflexly lowered. There is a spectrum of response to increased ITP that depends on both the contractile state of the LV and the level of intravascular volume, such that maximal augmentation of LV performance by elevation in ITP occurs when initial LV function is compromised and intravascular volume is expanded. Analyzed within this framework, the results of the clinical studies described in chapter 21, "Hemodynamic Effects of Artificial Ventilation," and in this chapter appear less contradictory.

Potential Positive Heart-Lung Interactions in Both the Normal and the Failing Heart: Cardiac Cycle–Specific Jet Ventilation—A Modest Proposal

From the preceding sections, it should be clear that changes in ITP independent of changes in lung volume can affect cardiac output by altering the pressure gradients for systemic venous return and LV ejection. Both systemic venous blood flow and LV ejection are not constant throughout the cardiac cycle but show a marked variation in flow. This is obviously true for ejection because it occurs only during systole; however, systemic venous return also shows profound cardiac cycle–specific flow variation.[2] Thus, the effects of increasing ITP at specific points within the cardiac cycle may differentially affect systemic venous return, LV ejection, or both, despite similar mean ITP and ventilation. This concept is intriguing in that some of the heretofore accepted hemodynamic complications of artificial ventilation (see chapter 21, "Hemodynamic Effects of Artificial Ventilation") may be avoidable at the same time as oxygen delivery to the tissues is improved.

The effects of cardiac cycle–specific increases in ITP may be difficult to predict beforehand because ventilation has many opposing and interrelated consequences. As ITP increases, the pressure gradient between intrathoracic and extrathoracic venous structures decreases. Thus, flow into the intrathoracic venae cavae will decrease. However, the pressure gradients between intrathoracic venae cavae, RA, and RV will be unchanged. Only to the extent that increases in lung volume differentially compress the intrathoracic vascular structures and decrease venous inflow by decreasing vena caval volume will RV filling be affected. By constricting the cardiac fossa, increases in lung volume limit absolute cardiac blood volume. Recently, Hoffman and Ritman suggested that total heart blood volume (atria plus ventricles) is constant throughout the cardiac cycle.[16] Using measurements derived from scanning via the Dynamic Spacial Reconstructor,[9] they found that absolute heart volume varied by less than 1% from end-systole to end-diastole. It would appear from these observations that increases in lung volume during systole may impair atrial filling and thus ventricular preload during the next diastole. Likewise, diastolic increases in lung volume would primarily impair ventricular filling.

Ventricular ejection may also be differentially affected by cardiac-specific ventilation. As lung volume increases above FRC, alveolar vascular capacitance falls, while extra-alveolar vascular capacitance increases.[27] From isolated heart-lung preparation studies it appears that when the lungs are relatively oligemic, such as in hypovolemic states, the increase in extra-alveolar vascular capacitance predominates. This would tend to decrease the systolic pressure load to the RV as well as decrease pulmonary venous blood flow. In hypervolemic states, the extra-alveolar vessels are already engorged and the decreased alveolar vascular capacitance predominates, which increases PA pressure and thus RV afterload[4] and may augment LV filling pressure as well. Therefore, jet ventilation during systole might increase RV afterload in hypovolemia, but decrease RV afterload in volume-loaded subjects. For the ejecting LV, the situation may be just as complicated. Increasing ITP prior to ejection may transfer aortic blood from intrathoracic to extrathoracic vessels. This will have the effect of decreasing both transmural aortic pressure and intrathoracic aortic blood volume, so that LV ejection will occur against a decreased transmural aortic pressure. If ITP is lower during ejection, then vascular capacitance will be increased. Both of these factors may improve LV systolic performance. If the diastolic increase in ITP continues into isometric systole, then ejection will be associated with an ITP-initiated forward aortic blood flow prior to actual LV ejection. By initiating forward blood flow prior to ejection the inertial force necessary for LV ejection will be reduced.

This reduction may be important, since in LV failure states overcoming inertial forces may account for 15% of the energy expenditure of ejection.[45] Increasing ITP during LV ejection should augment the pressure difference between the LV and extrathoracic vessels without decreasing LV afterload. Stroke volume should be increased for a given preload and afterload. This would result in an increase in mean aortic pressure and aortic pulse pressure, which may induce secondary reflex vasodilation via baroreceptors. The increase in stroke volume will tend to maintain aortic pressure and therefore coronary perfusion in spite of the peripheral vasodilation. Also, myocardial work may be less even when coronary perfusion is unchanged. Either of these effects would increase coronary sinus oxygen saturation.

On the basis of this logic, Pinsky et al., in preliminary reports,[34, 38] characterized the effects of cardiac cycle–specific increases in ITP in a canine model. They analyzed the effects of cardiac cycle–specific increases in ITP in three hemodynamically different conditions: normal heart function and circulatory blood volume (control), normal heart with severe hemorrhage-induced hypovolemia (hypovolemia), and AVF induced by β-blockade and volume infusion.

Cardiac cycle–specific increases in ITP were generated by synchronizing inspiratory jet pulses from a high-frequency jet ventilator (HFJV) relative to the QRS on the electrocardiogram (ECG). A variable delay circuit placed between the ECG signal and the ventilator allowed selective timing of the jet pulses within the cardiac cycle of every heartbeat. HFJV is ideally suited for this task for various reasons. First, HFJV by itself induces minimal hemodynamic variations, primarily because the tidal volumes used are small. HFJV can ventilate effectively at a frequency similar to the normal heart rate. Also, inspiratory jet pulses are of an adjustable duration that can be brief enough to occur selectively during only specific intervals in the cardiac cycle.

In these studies the cardiac cycle was partitioned into four discrete intervals by reference to the ECG signal and the aortic pressure profile. From the R wave to the dicrotic notch was defined as systole, and from the dicrotic notch to the next R wave as diastole. Systole was further divided into early and late components by the upstroke of the aortic pressure signal, with late systole comprising ejection and early systole comprising electrical and isometric mechanical systole. Diastole was divided in half, with early

diastole starting from the dicrotic notch and late diastole consisting of approximately the mid-part of the aortic pressure decay. Timing of the jet pulses within the cardiac cycle was determined by the position of the peak of the airway pressure pulse measured at the distal end of the endotracheal tube within the above-defined four intervals. As in the previous studies, to further increase ITP without further increasing lung volume, chest and abdominal binders were also applied during the control and AVF runs.

The most dramatic effects occurred during the AVF plus binder condition. Synchronous HFJV increased cardiac output and decreased LV filling pressure, compared with steady-state apneic values ($P < .01$), and systolic jet pulses improved cardiac output more than diastolic jet pulses ($P < .05$), apparently because LV filling pressures were higher with systolic jet pulses (not significant). Although early and late systolic pulses increase LV stroke volume, their effect on aortic pulse pressure is dissimilar. Early systolic jet pulses decreased the aortic pulse pressure, while late systolic jet pulses increased aortic pulse pressure by an amount equal to the increase in ITP. Since aortic pulse pressure is primarily determined by stroke volume and the pressure-volume characteristics of the central arterial tree, decreases in pulse pressure will occur if either stroke volume decreases or central arterial blood volume decreases or arterial compliance increases. Since early systolic jet pulses increase stroke volume, the observed decrease in pulse pressure must be due to a decrease in central arterial blood volume prior to ejection. This is consistent with the hypothesis that early systolic jet pulses evacuate the thoracic aortic blood prior to LV ejection. Late systolic jet pulses, on the other hand, mechanically augment ejection. When compared with either apnea or IPPB alone (similar increase in ITP), systolic synchronous HFJV was associated with a higher cardiac output in all three conditions. This comparison is shown for AVF in Figure 31–13, where the effect of IPPB, apnea, and both early systolic and early diastolic jet pulses on various hemodynamic variables is illustrated. In contrast to the response to PHIPS, the effect appears to be primarily mechanical with minimal reflex interaction, in that it is not abolished by ganglionic (hexamethonium) or α-adrenergic (phentolamine) blockage.

During control conditions both IPPB and HFJV decrease cardiac output by decreasing intrathoracic blood volume. This effect is mini-

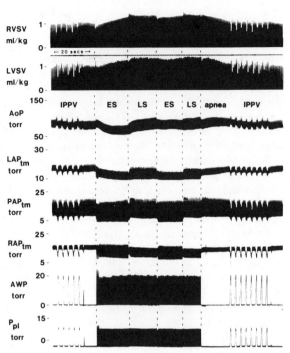

FIG 31–13.
Sequential trend recordings of hemodynamic effects of various forms of artificial ventilation and apnea during acute ventricular failure for a canine model. Abbreviations are as in Figure 31–12. Note that IPPB results in ever-changing hemodynamic condition. Synchronous high-frequency jet ventilation occurring in either early systole or late systole results in a reproducible and different hemodynamic response, although both improve cardiac output and decrease LV filling pressures. See text for discussion.

mized by synchronous jet pulses occurring in early systole or late diastole and maximized by jet pulses occurring around the dicrotic notch (early diastole). These effects are shown for the control condition in Figure 31–14, which has a format similar to Figure 31–13. Although not shown in Figure 31–14, jet pulses occurring in late diastole also minimize the decrease in venous return to an amount similar to early systole. With hypovolemia, this sparing of cardiac output is

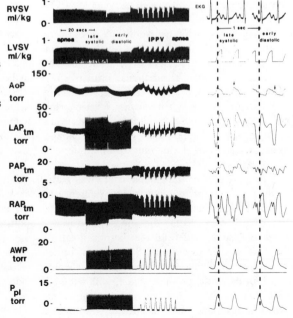

FIG 31–14.
On the left side is a continuous trend recording of the hemodynamic effects of late systolic and early diastolic jet pulses as compared with apnea and intermittent positive pressure breathing *(IPPB)* in the control-binder condition. On the right side is an accelerated trend recording of these specific jet pulses, with RVSV replaced by the electrocardiogram (ECG) for illustration. Abbreviations are as in Figure 31–12. Note the instantaneous effect of changing the jet pulse timing on all observed hemodynamic variables *(left)*, despite an identical airway and pleural pressure tracing *(right)*. Arrows indicate changes in venous return to (and stroke volume of) the RV; these changes always precede changes on the left side. This is typical of normal ventricular function because cardiac output is preload dependent.

maintained only by limiting jet pulses to late diastole.

Since late systolic jet pulses increase aortic pressure, unlike other cardiac cycle–specific jet pulses, the effect of such timed jet pulses on coronary blood flow may not be similar to that in other organs. In control conditions, ventilation in late systole increased coronary sinus oxygen saturation 40% above apneic levels, while other timed jet pulses did not increase either mean aortic pressure or coronary sinus oxygen saturation.

Cardiac cycle–specific increases in ITP during AVF appear to act on the cardiovascular system in a fashion analogous to aortic balloon counterpulsation. As usually performed, counterpulsation has two separate functions. First, balloon inflation in early diastole increases diastolic aortic pressure, increasing the pressure gradient for coronary blood flow. Second, rapid balloon deflation immediately prior to systole depletes the thoracic aorta of volume, which decreases systolic aortic pressure and augments LV ejection.[26] Since, under normal conditions, coronary blood flow is dependent on perfusion pressure, increases in transmural diastolic aortic pressure would be expected to increase coronary arterial blood flow.[22] To the extent that myocardial work is decreased or coronary flow is increased, coronary sinus oxygen saturation will increase. Thus, late systolic jet pulses may aid in LV ejection not only by mechanically augmenting ejection but also by increasing the pressure gradient for coronary blood flow in a manner analogous to aortic balloon inflation in diastole or by decreasing the work the LV performs, and thus decreasing myocardial oxygen consumption. Similarly, early systolic and diastolic jet pulses are associated with either a constant or a reduced aortic pulse pressure despite an increase in LV stroke volume, suggesting that the LV is emptying its stroke into a relatively depleted thoracic aorta. Thus, jet pulses occurring in diastole or early systole may aid LV ejection by depleting the thoracic aorta of volume prior to ejection in a fashion analogous to aortic balloon deflation prior to systole.

From the theoretical analysis and these preliminary studies, it appears that cardiac cycle–specific increases in ITP may have different hemodynamic effects, depending on where in the cardiac cycle the increase in ITP occurs and whether LV contractility is normal or reduced. When LV contractility is normal, synchronizing

HFJV to occur at the end of diastole is associated with the least impairment of venous return and thus of cardiac output, compared with similar mean airway pressure IPPB. Likewise, when cardiac contractility is reduced, synchronizing HFJV to occur during electrical or mechanical systole is associated with the greatest increase in cardiac output. These results suggest that it may be possible to obtain positive heart-lung interactions in all patients requiring artificial ventilatory support, and that in severe heart failure states these interactions may function to sustain the circulation, optimizing oxygen transport.

Acknowledgments

Work was supported in part by a Veterans Administration and by National Research Service Award IF32HL-06238-01. Dr. Pinsky is the recipient of a VA Career Development Award.

REFERENCES

1. Braunwald E, Binion JT, Morgan WL, et al: Alterations in central blood volume and cardiac output induced by positive pressure breathing and counteracted by metaraminol (Aramine). *Circ Res* 1957; 5:670–675.
2. Brecher GA, Hubay CA: Pulmonary blood flow and venous return during spontaneous respiration. *Circ Res* 1955; 3:210–214.
3. Brooker JZ, Alderman EL, Harrison DC: Alterations in left ventricular volumes induced by Valsalva maneuver. *Br Heart J* 1974; 36:713–718.
4. Brower R, Wise RA, Hassapoyannes C, et al: The effect of lung inflation on lung blood volume and pulmonary venous flow. *J Appl Physiol* 1985; 58:954–963.
5. Buda AJ, Pinsky MR, Ingels NB, et al: Effect of intrathoracic pressure on left ventricular performance. *N Engl J Med* 1979; 301:453–459.
6. Calvin JE, Driedgen AA, Sibbald WJ: Positive end-expiratory pressure (PEEP) does not depress left ventricular function in patients with pulmonary edema. *Am Rev Respir Dis* 1981; 124:121–128.
7. Chandra N, Rudikoff M, Weisfeldt ML: Simultaneous chest compression and ventilation at high airway pressure during cardiopulmonary resuscitation. *Lancet* 1980; 1:176–178.
8. Criley JM, Bloufuss AII, Kissell GL: Cough-induced cardiac compression. *JAMA* 1976; 263:1246–1250.

9. Dynamic Spacial Reconstructor. *Science* 1980; 210:273–280.

10. Fisher J, Wise RA, Pinsky MR, et al: Respiratory pattern changes accompanying acute falls in cardiac output. *Physiologist* 1980; 22:181.

11. Grace MP, Breenbaum DM: Cardiac performance in response to PEEP in patients with cardiac dysfunction. *Crit Care Med* 1982; 10:358–360.

12. Grunstein MM, Derenne JP, Milic-Emili J: Control of depth and frequency of breathing during baroreceptor stimulation. *J Appl Physiol* 1975; 39:395–494.

13. Guyton AC, Jones CF, Coleman TE: Graphic analysis of cardiac output regulation, in Guyton AC, Jones CF (eds): *Circulatory Physiology: Cardiac Output and Its Regulation*. Philadelphia, WB Saunders Co, 1963, pp 237–262.

14. Guyton AC, Lindsey AW, Abernathy B, et al: Venous return at various right atrial pressures and the normal venous return curve. *Am J Physiol* 1957; 189:690–715.

15. Harrison VC, Heese H, Klein M, et al: The significance of grunting in hyalane membrane disease. *Pediatrics* 1968; 41:549–559.

16. Hoffman EA, Ritman EL: Constancy of total heart volume throughout cardiac cycle and role of lung inflation: A computer tomographic measurement with DSR. *Fed Proc* 1984; 43(3):509.

17. Ingels NB Jr, Ricci LR, Daughters GT II, et al: Effect of heart rate augmentation on left ventricular volume and cardiac output on the transplanted human heart. *Circulation* 1977; 53 (suppl II):32–37.

18. Ingels NB Jr, Daughters GT II, Stinson EB, et al: Measurement of mid-wall dynamics in intact man by radiography of surgically implanted markers. *Circulation* 1975; 52:859–867.

19. Jardin FF, Fercot J-C, Gueret P, et al: Echocardiographic evaluation of ventricles during continuous positive pressure breathing. *J Appl Physiol* 1984; 56:619–627.

20. Katz LN: The performance of the heart. *Circulation* 1960; 21:483–498.

21. Koehler RC, Chandra N, Guerci AD, et al: Augmentation of cerebral perfusion by simultaneous chest compression and lung inflation with abdominal binding after cardiac arrest in dogs. *Circulation* 1983; 67:266–275.

22. Lefemine AA, Low HBC, Cohen ML, et al: Assisted circulation: III. The effect of synchronized arterial counterpulsation on myocardial oxygen consumption and coronary flow. *Am Heart J* 1962; 64:789–795.

23. Luce JM, Ross BK, O'Quin RJ, et al: Regional blood flow during cardiopulmonary resuscitation in dogs using simultaneous and non-simultaneous compression and ventilation. *Circulation* 1983; 67:258–265.

24. Mathru M, Rao RLK, Eletr AA, et al: Hemodynamic response to changes in ventilatory patterns in patients with normal and poor left ventricular reserve. *Crit Care Med* 1982; 10:423–426.

25. Mullins CB, Sugga WL, Kennelly BM, et al: Effect of arterial counterpulsation on left ventricular volume and pressure. *Am J Physiol* 1971; 220:694–698.

26. Niemann JT, Rosborough J, Hausknecht M, et al: Documentation of systemic perfusion in man and in an experimental model: A "window" to the mechanism of blood flow in external CPR. *Crit Care Med* 1980; 8:141–146.

27. Permutt S, Howell JBL, Proctor DF, et al: Effect of lung inflation on static pressure-volume characteristics of pulmonary vessels. *J Appl Physiol* 1961; 16:64–70.

28. Pinsky MR, Summer WR, Wise RA, et al: Augmentation of cardiac function by elevation of intrathoracic pressure. *J Appl Physiol* 1983; 54:950–955.

29. Pinsky MR, Summer WR: Cardiac augmentation by phasic high intrathoracic pressure support in man. *Chest* 1983; 84:370–375.

30. Pinsky MR: Cause-specific management of shock. *Postgrad Med* 1983; 73:127–148.

31. Pinsky MR, Matuschak GM, Klain M: Determinants of cardiac augmentation by elevations in intrathoracic pressure. *J Appl Physiol* 1985; 58:1189.

32. Pinsky MR: Determinants of pulmonary arterial blood flow variation during respiration. *J Appl Physiol* 1984; 56:1237–1243.

33. Pinsky MR, Matuschak GM, Bernardi L, et al: Hemodynamic effects of cardiac cycle-specific increases in intrathoracic pressure. *J Appl Physiol* 1986; 60:604–612.

34. Pinsky MR, Matuschak GM, Rogers RM, et al: Hemodynamic effect of cardiac cycle–specific increases in intrathoracic pressure in normo- and hypovolemia. *J Appl Physiol* 1986; 61:44–53.

35. Pinsky MR: Instantaneous venous return

curves in an intact canine preparation. *J Appl Physiol* 1984; 56:756–771.

36. Pinsky MR, Matuschak GM, Itzkoff JM: Respiratory augmentation of left ventricular function during spontaneous ventilation in severe left ventricular failure by grunting: An auto-EPAP effect. *Chest* 1984; 86:267–269.

37. Pouleur H, Corell JW, Ross J Jr: Effects of nitroprusside on venous return and central blood volume in the absence and presence of acute heart failure. *Circulation* 1980; 61:328–337.

38. Rasanen J, Nikki P, Heikkila J: Acute myocardial infarction complicated by respiratory failure: The effects of mechanical ventilation. *Chest* 1984; 85:21–28.

39. Rankin JS, Olsen CO, Arentzen CE, et al: The effects of airway pressure on cardiac function in intact dogs and man. *Circulation* 1982; 66:108–120.

40. Read RC, Johnson JH, Vich JA: Vascular effects of hypertonic solution. *Circ Res* 1960; 8:538–548.

41. Rudikoff MT, Maughan WL, Elfron M, et al: Mechanisms of blood flow during cardiopulmonary resuscitation. *Circulation* 1980; 61:345–352.

42. Sarnoff SJ: Myocardial contractility as described by ventricular function curves: Observations on Starling's law of the heart. *Physiol Rev* 1955; 35:107–122.

43. Sharpey-Schafer EP: Effects of Valsalva's maneuver on the normal and failing circulation. *Br Med J* 1955; 1:693–695.

44. Sodums MT, Badke FR, Starling MR, et al: Evaluation of left ventricular contractile performance utilizing end-systolic pressure-volume relationships in a conscious dog. *Circ Res* 1984; 54:731–739.

45. Spencer MP, Greiss FC: Dynamics of ventricular ejection. *Circ Res* 1962; 10:274–279.

46. Stalcup SA, Mellins RB: Mechanical forces producing pulmonary edema in acute asthma. *N Engl J Med* 1977; 297:592–596.

47. Starling MR, Crawford MH, Sorensen SG, et al: Comparative accuracy of apical biplane cross-sectional echocardiography and gated equilibrium radionuclide angiography for estimating left ventricular size and performance. *Circulation* 1981; 63:1075–1084.

48. Starling EH: The effects of heart failure on the circulation. *Lancet* 1897; 1:652–655.

49. Suga H, Sagawa K: Instantaneous pressure-volume relationships and their ratio in the excised, supported canine left ventricle. *Circ Res* 1974; 35:117–126.

50. Summer WR, Permutt S, Sagawa K, et al: Effects of spontaneous respiration on canine left ventricular function. *Circ Res* 1979; 45:719–728.

51. Viquerat CE, Righetti A, Suter PM: Biventricular volumes and function in patients with adult respiratory distress syndrome ventilated with PEEP. *Chest* 1983; 83:509–514.

52. Whittenberger JL, McGregor M, Berglund E, et al: Influence of state of inflation of the lung on pulmonary vascular resistance. *J Appl Physiol* 1960; 15:878–882.

53. Zeema MJ, Masters AP, Margouleff D: Dyspnea: The heart or the lungs? Differentiation at bedside by use of the simple Valsalva maneuver. *Chest* 1984; 85:59.

32 _____ Mechanical Circulatory Assistance

Peter F. Ferson, M.D.

Robert L. Hardesty, M.D.

Bartley P. Griffith, M.D.

Alfredo Trento, M.D.

Adequate oxygen delivery to the various organs depends not only on gas exchange within the pulmonary circuit, but also on the ability of the circulatory system to effectively deliver the oxygenated blood. When cardiac failure prevents adequate oxygen delivery, standard methods of hemodynamic support with appropriate volume management and pharmacologic manipulation will often correct the underlying defect. If such efforts fail and resulting tissue hypoxia persists, further support can occasionally be provided by mechanical circulatory assistance. Improved hemodynamic status may in turn improve ventilatory status and thus diminish demand on the circulatory system.

The clinical applications for mechanical circulatory support include a spectrum of circumstances from acute reversible cardiac or cardiorespiratory failure to chronic end-stage myocardial disease. In the latter instance, circulatory assist devices or total artificial hearts are used to support candidates for cardiac transplantation pending location of an organ donor.

There are several methods available for mechanical circulatory support. Those commonly used are diastolic counterpulsation, left ventricular (LV) assistance, and prolonged total circulatory bypass. These methods have varying capacity to assist or to replace entirely the function of a failing heart or heart and lungs.

DIASTOLIC COUNTERPULSATION

The object of diastolic counterpulsation, or augmentation, is to improve myocardial function, and thus systemic perfusion, by producing a biphasic alteration in the arterial pressure. If the arterial pressure can be lowered during systole, then the myocardial work and oxygen demand can be diminished. Concurrently elevating the diastolic pressure will increase coronary perfusion and increase myocardial oxygen supply.

Three methods or devices have been used for diastolic augmentation: the arterial counterpulsation pump, the intra-aortic balloon pump (IABP), and external counterpulsation.

Arterial Counterpulsation Pump

Use of the arterial counterpulsation pump was described by Clauss and associates[8] in 1961. With this device a prosthetic graft is attached to one or both femoral arteries, and through these conduits a volume of blood is rapidly withdrawn and reinjected into the arterial circuit. Withdrawing blood just prior to ventricular systole will lower the aortic pressure and allow ejection against a decreased resistance. If the same volume of blood is rapidly reinfused after the aortic valve is closed the diastolic pressure will rise and diastolic perfusion of the coronary and peripheral circulation will increase.

Timing of the removal and reinfusion of the blood volume is important since infusing blood into the arterial circuit while the ventricle is ejecting would increase the workload on the heart. Conversely, removing blood too early would lower the diastolic pressure and decrease coronary perfusion. The triggering mechanism can be coordinated with the arterial pressure as read from a transducer, or with the R wave on the electrocardiogram (ECG). Appropriate timing of the counterpulsation will result in the desired changes in arterial pressure (lowered systolic pressure and elevated diastolic pressure), as shown in Figure 32–1.

Use of the arterial counterpulsation pump met with some experimental and clinical success but was limited by problems with hemolysis and thrombosis.

Intra-aortic Balloon Pump

The IABP was developed to minimize the problems seen with the arterial counterpulsation pump. Moulopoulos and co-workers[30] reported experimental success with this device in 1962, and since then IABP support has become the most widely used method of circulatory support. Instead of withdrawing and infusing a volume of blood, in IABP the arterial pressure and resistance are changed by inflating and deflating a cylindric balloon within the aorta (Fig 32–2). Inflating the balloon displaces a volume of blood and achieves similar results as infusing the same volume by the counterpulsation pump. Rapidly deflating the balloon lowers the aortic pressure and is comparable to withdrawing volume with the counterpulsation pump. As with the counterpulsation pump, timing is critical. Too early an inflation will increase the resistance during ventricular ejection and increase myocardial workload, while overly delayed inflation will not achieve maximal diastolic augmentation. Conversely, early deflation will minimize the period of augmentation and diminish coronary blood flow. It will also allow the aortic pressure to rise again prior to ventricular ejection, and the systolic unloading effect will be lost. If the balloon is left inflated too long, the result will be elevated resistance during early systole and increased ventricular tension. Triggering of the inflation and deflation can be coordinated with the arterial waveform, or more commonly with the ECG.

Timing of IABP use depends first on receiving the appropriate triggering signal (usually the R wave). This signal is used to initiate either inflation or deflation of the device, and the duration of the inflation or deflation is then also adjusted. Both inflation and deflation can be manually advanced or delayed to achieve the optimal result, as reflected in the arterial waveform (Fig 32–3). Since the anticipated duration of the inflation or deflation mode is programmed in this fashion, optimal augmentation will be achieved if the heart rate remains constant and the rhythm remains stable. Changes in the heart rate will alter

Arterial Counterpulsation Pump Function

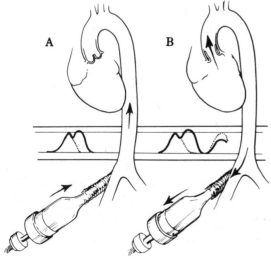

FIG 32–1.
Arterial counterpulsation pump function. **A,** during diastole a volume of blood is injected into the femoral artery. *Dotted line* in the arterial pressure wave represents the expected normal waveform; *solid line* represents the increased arterial pressure with diastolic augmentation. **B,** during ventricular systole blood is rapidly withdrawn from the femoral artery. This decreases the arterial systolic pressure, as represented by the solid waveform.

IABP Function

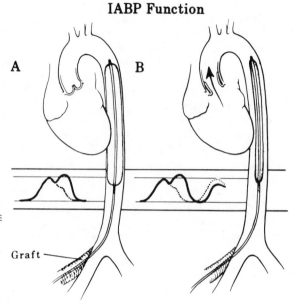

FIG 32–2.
Intra-aortic balloon pump function. **A,** the balloon is inserted through a graft on the femoral artery. Rapid inflation of the balloon during diastole will displace a volume of blood within the aorta and elevate the diastolic pressure. This is reflected in the solid arterial waveform as compared with the normal waveform *(dotted line)*. **B,** during systole the balloon is deflated, emptying the aorta and thus lowering the systolic pressure. Again, the *dotted line* arterial wave represents the unassisted, normal waveform.

the length of diastole and require readjusting the timing, whereas an irregular rhythm will result in erratic periods of augmentation.

Technical Considerations

Insertion of the IABP was previously always performed through a side-arm prosthetic graft sutured to the common femoral artery. More recently techniques have been described for inserting balloons through a sheath placed in the femoral artery by the Seldinger technique. The tip of the balloon should be placed in the distal arch of the aorta, just at the origin of the subclavian artery. Fluoroscopic guidance will enhance rapid correct placement. Without fluoroscopy the catheter length can be measured so that the balloon tip may be placed at the level of the angle of Louis; placement is confirmed with a still ra-

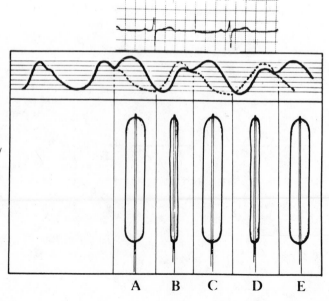

FIG 32–3.
Arterial pressure effect of IABP. Initial inflation of the balloon *(A)* results in an augmented diastolic pressure. The peak systolic pressure is reduced *(B)* by emptying of the balloon immediately prior to ventricular ejection. Subsequent cycles repeat the diastolic augmentation and the systolic unloading effect.

A   B   C   D   E

diograph. Either method requires a patent aorto-iliac system for insertion. This often limits the ability to insert a balloon in patients with extensive peripheral vascular disease. If the ascending aorta is exposed, as during open heart surgery, and an IABP cannot be advanced through a diseased aortoiliac arterial system, insertion through a side graft placed on the ascending aorta can be performed. Insertion through the subclavian artery has also been described.[26] Aside from a patent aortoiliac system, the patient must also have a competent aortic valve to avoid the increased retrograde flow and ventricular distention from elevated diastolic pressures. Since timing of the balloon inflation and deflation is crucial, it is preferable, although not essential, that the cardiac rhythm be regular.

Both carbon dioxide and helium have been used to inflate the balloon. Carbon dioxide has the theoretical advantage of being safer if rupture of the balloon should occur; however, balloon rupture is rare. Helium, with its lower molecular weight, has the distinct advantage of providing less resistance to flow and allows more rapid inflation and deflation.

Hemodynamics

The hemodynamic effects of the IABP have been extensively studied. The IABP can lower the systolic pressure and elevate the diastolic pressure.[3, 5, 7, 33, 35] Its ability to favorably alter other parameters such as the cardiac output or the coronary artery blood flow is not so clearly supported. Scheidt et al.[33] and Bregman et al.[7] demonstrated a measured rise in the cardiac output when the IABP was used in patients with shock following myocardial infarction, and in patients who could not be weaned from cardiopulmonary bypass after cardiac surgery. However, Steele et al.[35] and Aroesty et al.[3] did not demonstrate an elevation of the cardiac output from the IABP in patients with unstable angina without ventricular dysfunction. These differences may reflect an interaction between the IABP and the body's autoregulatory mechanism, such that if the cardiac output is adequate (as in a patient with angina without shock), the addition of the IABP will not further increase it.

It is most likely that the ability of the IABP to improve cardiac output in patients with ventricular dysfunction is related to its ability to improve the oxygen supply/demand ratio in the myocardium and thus improve the ability of the

ventricle to provide forward flow. This assumption presumes that the IABP can improve coronary flow and/or diminish myocardial oxygen demand, but again, these changes have not been uniformly demonstrated. The response may vary according to myocardial needs. Yahr et al.[42] measured a rise in the coronary blood flow, and Bregman et al.[7] noted an increased flow in coronary vein grafts with the IABP. Leinbach et al.[22] failed to demonstrate increased coronary flow when IABP assist was used in patients with post-myocardial infarction shock, and Williams and associates[41] showed no increase in regional blood flow after IABP insertion for unstable angina. Williams et al.[41] did note a reduction in myocardial oxygen consumption, and Scheidt et al.[33] found a decrease in coronary sinus lactate levels.

This variability in the observations of coronary blood flow is probably due to the differing circumstances at the time of observation. The increased coronary vein graft flow with IABP, for instance, was detected in patients following cardiac surgery. In this condition, they could be presumed to be experiencing global ischemia, without major obstructing lesions.[7] Under these circumstances, and with a well-vascularized myocardium, any increase in the perfusion pressure should result in increased flow to an ischemic myocardium. Those studies in which the IABP failed to improve coronary blood flow, on the other hand, were conducted in patients with fixed obstructions in the coronary arteries.[22, 41] These obstructions may limit flow to the infarcted or ischemic areas in spite of IABP elevation of the diastolic pressure. Both Williams and Scheidt, however, do suggest that there is an alteration in the myocardial oxygen supply/demand ratio that is probably not related to localized ischemia.

Clinical Applications

The use of the IABP has been proposed for several clinical applications, listed in Table 32–1. In some applications the use of the IABP has

TABLE 32–1.

Application of IABP

Post-Myocardial Infarction Shock
Acute myocardial infarction to limit infarct size
Unstable angina
Post-cardiac surgery to wean from bypass
Hemodynamic support prior to cardiac
   transplantation

---

been generally accepted as beneficial, while in other applications the clinical and experimental evidence does not support initial enthusiasm.

Post-Myocardial Infarction Shock. The initial concept of diastolic counterpulsation and thus of the IABP centered on the belief that more patients with shock after myocardial infarction would survive if the ischemic zone of myocardium adjacent to the infarct could be protected while collateral vessels developed.

Reported series have varied in their definition of shock, and have lacked adequate controls. In an early experience Kantrowitz et al.[19] reported survival in one of three patients treated with the IABP for post-myocardial infarction shock. A larger cooperative clinical trial, for which Kantrowitz served as chairman, was reported by Scheidt et al. in 1973.[33] In this series of 87 patients, 15 (17%) survived the hospital stay, and 8 patients (9%) survived for more than 1 year. Scheidt et al. defined shock as systolic pressure less than 80 torr with oliguria despite measured adequate filling pressures and the application of "standard" medical therapy. Despite its clear definition of shock, this study lacked controls, and therefore did not indicate anticipated survival without treatment. The study is also rather dated, and the alternative therapy would not have included currently available pressor agents or vasodilators. Willerson et al.[40] reported similar results in 1975 in a series of 27 patients in cardiogenic shock, 3 (11%) of whom survived with IABP support and left the hospital. Willerson et al.[40] included patients without shock but with severe LV failure and with ventricular tachycardia.

Hagemeijer and co-workers[13] in 1977 reported markedly better results, with 60% 1-month survival in 25 patients treated for post-myocardial infarction shock. This series excluded patients over 65 years old and patients who had had ischemic episodes less than 36 hours before IABP, thus selecting patients with a higher probability of survival. In 1978 McEnany and co-workers[28] reported a study of 728 patients supported by IABP. Of these, there were 145 patients with post-myocardial infarction shock, of whom 32% survived the immediate hospitalization. Again there were no controls and the criteria for diagnosing shock are unclear. Also, the management of these patients was not restricted to the use of the IABP, since selected patients underwent car-

diac catheterization and repair of correctable lesions.

It is accepted practice to use the IABP to maintain preoperative stability in patients with correctable lesions (such as mitral insufficiency or ventricular septal defect following infarct), or to support patients being evaluated for the presence of such lesions. Without operative intervention, however, survival of such patients with IABP support is poor.[33]

Limiting Infarct Size. A justification for the use of the IABP to treat shock following myocardial infarction is the concept that there is a zone of injured myocardium next to an infarct that can be saved if it is supported until perfusion is reestablished by collateral vessels. Expanding this concept has resulted in the use of the IABP after uncomplicated infarction to limit the infarct size. Neither the experimental nor the clinical experience with this application has been rewarding. In 1978 Leinbach and co-workers[23] treated 11 patients with an anterior myocardial infarction less than 6 hours old with the IABP. The patients were all free of signs of shock or pulmonary edema. Although the ECG findings improved in five patients, in six patients they did not. Coronary angiography indicated that those patients who showed ECG improvement had a patent left anterior descending artery. A major limitation of clinical studies is inability to clearly measure infarct size. Haston et al.[15] and Takanashi et al.[38] ligated the anterior descending artery in baboons and in pigs, respectively. They used myocardial staining techniques to compare infarct size in animals supported with IABP with infarct size in control animals. In both studies there was no difference in the histologically measured infarct size between the IABP-supported subjects and the controls.

Unstable Angina. Another common application of the IABP is in the management of unstable angina. Here its greatest benefit seems to be in maintaining cardiac stability pending surgical intervention. Steele et al.[35] reported in 1976 on a series of 18 patients who were selectively treated for unstable angina with IABP support and coronary artery bypass. Survival in this small series was 100%. Levine and co-workers[24] described a series of 93 patients with medically refractory angina who were treated with a combination of IABP support and coronary bypass; 89

survived. Weintraub et al.[39] reported that 59 of 60 patients treated in a similar manner for unstable angina survived.

As with the previous clinical applications, the specific benefit of the IABP with respect to survival in patients with unstable angina is difficult to determine. In all of these studies there were no adequate controls. The standard nonsurgical therapy consisted of oral propranolol and sublingual nitrates. None of these series mentions the use of pulmonary artery catheters to assess the preload, and there was no use of intravenous vasodilators. It is clear, however, that use of IABP was helpful in relieving the uncontrolled anginal episodes. Levine et al. noted partial or complete relief from angina after IABP support in all patients in their series, and Weintraub et al. saw partial or total relief in 95% of their patients.

Post-Cardiac Surgery. The IABP is most widely used after cardiac surgery to support patients who cannot be weaned from cardiopulmonary bypass with volume loading and catecholamine therapy. Successful results in such patients are very gratifying, particularly if one considers the anticipated lack of survival. Bregman et al.,[7] in a study of 15 such patients, reported an in-hospital survival of 73%. McEnany et al.[28] reported 54% immediate survival in 225 patients, and Golding et al.[11] reported 73% in-hospital survival and 67% long-term survival in 99 patients followed up for an average of 18 months. These reports also mention associated groups of patients in whom the IABP was inserted preoperatively to prevent anticipated myocardial ischemia in high-risk patients. While such prophylactic use of the IABP may be appropriate, the circumstances of the studies are so variable that comparison among them is difficult.

The success of the IABP when used in patients after cardiac surgery may be a result of the nature of the myocardial injury. After a myocardial infarction there appears to be a localized area of irreversible injury (and a surrounding zone of potentially salvageable myocardium that is still poorly perfused). After cardiopulmonary bypass, however, the heart may have global but reversible cellular injury. In that case, when the myocardial blood flow has been restored by coronary bypass or has been adequate in the absence of coronary disease, cellular injury can be reversed by transiently improving the oxygen supply/demand ratio.

Pretransplantation Support. The previously described applications of the IABP are for acute, short-term problems. The usual duration of IABP support is from less than 24 hours to 2–3 weeks. Occasionally a patient with cardiomyopathy awaiting cardiac transplantation will be assisted with the IABP for a longer period. Ashar and Turcotte[4] described such a patient who was successfully assisted for 327 days with an IABP unit while awaiting transplantation. In our experience with cardiac transplantation, 70% of 14 patients who had IABP support prior to transplantation survived 1 year after transplantation compared with 78% of 42 patients who did not need pretransplantation support.

Complications of IABP Support

Problems can occur both at the time of IABP insertion and during prolonged support. Thrombocytopenia almost always occurs, although it is rarely of clinical significance. About 20% of attempts at insertion will fail because of occluded iliac arteries. Thrombosis or embolization can cause leg ischemia while the balloon is in place, and thrombus being stripped from the catheter during removal can occlude the femoral or distal arteries. The most disastrous complication of IABP insertion is aortic dissection, although its incidence is clinically apparent in less than 10% of insertions. Newer catheters with a central lumen, allowing the device to be inserted over a previously placed guide wire, can reduce this risk. The presence of an abdominal aortic aneurysm is a relative contraindication to insertion. Paraplegia is a very rare but devastating consequence of IABP. Isner et al.[18] reported findings in a series of 45 patients who died after IABP support. Sixteen patients (36%) had complications related to the IABP, and nine (20%) of the 45 who died were found to have unsuspected arterial dissection.

External Counterpulsation

External counterpulsation uses an inflatable pants-like garment that is placed on the patient's lower extremities and is inflated and deflated synchronously with the heartbeat. Its function thus is quite similar to the IABP, but the technique has the distinct advantage of being less invasive and associated with fewer risks. However, patient intolerance due to discomfort often limits the use of the device. The hemodynamic effects of external counterpulsation have not been studied as thoroughly as those of the IABP, but it is clear that external counterpulsation can elevate the diastolic pressure. It is also evident that the ability to unload the ventricle by lowering systolic pressure is poor.[2, 31] Whether the increased diastolic pressure obtained with external counterpulsation increases coronary blood flow has not been adequately studied. Clinical experience is also less than with the IABP. A large randomized trial treating patients with acute myocardial infarction with external counterpulsation was reported by Amsterdam et al. in 1980.[2] In a group of 258 patients they noted no difference in survival of patients treated with external counterpulsation compared with controls. They did identify a subgroup of patients who were over 46 years old and able to tolerate the device for more than 3 hours. In this subgroup the survival in the treated patients was statistically better than in the controls. Defining a subset of the entire series that shows statistical difference from the controls may be a misleading manipulation of the data; however, the number in the subset is large (206 patients) and the conclusions may be valid.

LEFT VENTRICULAR ASSISTANCE

In spite of appropriate pharmacologic support and diastolic augmentation, a few patients will continue to have inadequate cardiac output because of ventricular failure. In these patients partial cardiopulmonary bypass to partially or totally replace LV function can successfully perfuse other organs while reversible myocardial dysfunction improves or while a donor heart is obtained for appropriate candidates.

The LV assist device (LVAD) diverts blood away from the left heart and actively returns it to the arterial circuit. Inflow to the pump is usually established by cannulating the left atrium or the apex of the LV. Drainage from the left atrium may not totally decompress the LV, but it is easier to achieve than transapical drainage, is safer for decannulation, and is less damaging to the ventricle.[32] The blood flow is then typically diverted to an external centrifugal pump. Alternatively, a pneumatically powered compression pump is placed in the abdominal cavity and driven by pneumatic tubing from an outside source. The blood is returned through a cannula or a graft sutured onto the ascending aorta or to the abdominal aorta or iliac arteries (Fig 32–4).

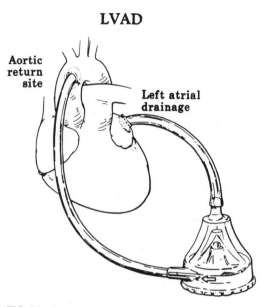

FIG 32–4.
Left ventricular assist device.

The concept of using a bypass pump to support circulation in patients with cardiac failure was proposed by Stuckey and co-workers in 1957.[36] Three patients with shock following myocardial infarction were placed on cardiopulmonary bypass. All three patients were weaned from bypass and one survived to leave the hospital. Takanashi et al.[38] compared the hemodynamic effects of transapical LV bypass with those of IABP in swine that had experimentally induced infarction. The LVAD circuit was superior to the IABP in diminishing myocardial oxygen consumption and limiting the infarct size. As with diastolic augmentation, most experience with the LVAD has been after cardiac surgery, in patients who could not be weaned from cardiopulmonary bypass with IABP support. The immediate survival is typically about 10%,[10, 17] but 50% early survival has been reported.[32] In some instances the right ventricle or both ventricles have been assisted.[32] While the LVAD has not been used as frequently as the IABP, McGee et al.[29] estimated that it would have been beneficial in 3% of 14,168 cardiac surgical procedures.

As with the IABP, patients may become totally dependent on the LVAD and may put the clinician in a moral and ethical dilemma regarding withdrawal of support. Sweet et al.[37] reported a bedside technique of multiple-gated radionuclide imaging of LV function that may help predict the ultimate survival of patients receiving LVAD support.

A major disadvantage of the LVAD is the need to return a critically ill patient to the operating room for removal of the cannulas. Litwak and co-workers[25] designed Silastic cannulas with Dacron cuffs that can be sutured to the appropriate structures. Each cannula is prefitted with an obturator that completely occludes the lumen with a flush surface at the inflow end. To decannulate a patient only the distal end of these cannulas in a subcutaneous location needs to be exposed. After the connectors are separated the obturators are inserted and the incision is closed over the cannulas, leaving the prosthetic material in place. However, McCormick and co-workers[27] reported that two of four survivors of LVAD support suffered serious infectious complications from the retained graft material. These authors recommended the removal of all prosthetic material in survivors.

Hematologic abnormalities have been associated with the LVAD. Al-Mondhiry et al. saw thrombocytopenia in all patients treated with LVAD support when they could not be weaned from cardiopulmonary bypass.[1] They also noted disseminated intravascular coagulation in 12 of 24 such patients; this correlated with the time on cardiopulmonary bypass prior to weaning with the LVAD.

PROLONGED CARDIOPULMONARY BYPASS

Occasionally patient survival will be jeopardized by combined cardiac and pulmonary insufficiency. If injury is reversible in both systems, prolonged cardiopulmonary bypass, or extracorporeal membrane oxygenation (ECMO), may be considered. Lande et al.[21] demonstrated its feasibility in 18 patients who had suffered cardiac arrest and could not be resuscitated, or who had refractory cardiogenic shock. Although there were no survivors, there were objective signs of improvement, and three patients were weaned from bypass. Bartlett et al.[6] reported experience with 28 patients supported with ECMO for cardiopulmonary failure. There were five survivors, and the authors had best results in children with postoperative cardiac failure. We have had most success with children, particularly infants with

persistent fetal circulation following initial repair of congenital diaphragmatic hernias.[14]

ECMO uses various methods of cannulation, and a membrane oxygenator with or without a perfusion pump. The cannulation sites and appropriate pump are selected according to the clinical circumstances. If combined cardiac and pulmonary support is necessary, a perfusion pump is added to the circuit and bypass initiated in a venoarterial mode. That is, blood is withdrawn from a central vein, passed through a membrane oxygenator, and actively returned to the arterial circuit. Cannulation can be of the femoral vein and artery or of the jugular vein and the subclavian or carotid artery. We have used the jugular-carotid method in infants with no apparent neurologic defects (Fig 32–5).[14] It is essential to return the oxygenated blood as proximally as possible to ensure cerebral and coronary oxygenation. Even with cannulation of the ascending aorta, Secker-Walker et al.[34] noted that when flow rates through the bypass circuit were less than 85% of the cardiac output, the coronary flow was supplied by the poorly oxygenated blood ejected from the ventricle.

In certain instances of isolated pulmonary insufficiency, particularly in neonates, arteriovenous or venovenous modes may have value. We

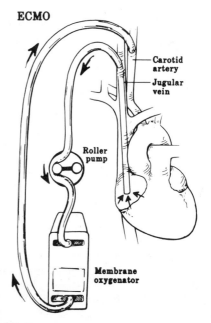

ECMO

FIG 32–5.
Venoarterial extracorporeal membrane oxygenation.

have been able to adequately oxygenate prematurely delivered fetal lambs with respiratory distress by placing a membrane oxygenator in a circuit connecting the umbilical artery and vein. A perfusion pump was unnecessary since the increase in cardiac output required by the arteriovenous fistula was easily tolerated. Returning the oxygenated blood directly to the pulmonary circuit in this fashion increases oxygen content in the pulmonary arteries and decreases pulmonary vascular resistance.[12]

Gattinoni et al.[9] have described a variation of ECMO. They used a low-flow venovenous circuit with a membrane lung to remove carbon dioxide and maintain oxygenation by low-frequency, continuous-flow oxygen ventilation. This system of extracorporeal carbon dioxide removal (ECCO-R) and low-frequency positive-pressure ventilation (LFPPV) resulted in the survival of 11 of 18 patients with severe adult respiratory distress syndrome.

Minimizing the flow through the extracorporeal circuit may minimize the hazards of ECMO. Hematologic problems similar to those with prolonged cardiopulmonary bypass are likely. Heiden and associates noted a "foreign-surface coagulopathy" in 28 patients treated with ECMO.[16] They noted marked thrombocytopenia while using the oxygenating circuit and at autopsy found evidence of focal emboli and hemorrhage in the various organs. Cardiopulmonary bypass circuits also alter the serum complement levels.[20] Prolonged use of such circuits in patients with respiratory distress syndrome caused by sepsis may therefore alter resistance to infection.

TRANSPLANTATION

Total replacement of a failing heart or heart and lungs is the ultimate mechanical circulatory support. Unlike patients with chronic renal failure, who can be maintained on hemodialysis, individuals with end-stage cardiac or respiratory failure have no option other than transplantation. As noted earlier, patients with acute cardiac failure and patients with chronic cardiomyopathy are equally acceptable candidates for transplantation. Survival at 1 year in our series has been 80%, both for patients who were morbidly ill and received pressors or IABP support, and for those who were hemodynamically stable. Patients with

cardiac failure that does not respond to mechanical methods of circulatory support should be considered as candidates for transplantation. Ideally they are less than 55 years old and free of systemic disease such as diabetes mellitus. Active infection, recent pulmonary emboli, and malignancy are contraindications to cardiac transplantation.

The use of an artificial heart to chronically sustain circulatory function has not yet been shown to be practical. Several centers have used artificial hearts to support patients pending cardiac transplantation. The cardiac surgery service at the University Health Center of Pittsburgh has used the Jarvik-7 artificial heart in four moribund patients as a bridge to transplantation. Three of these patients survived to receive transplanted hearts. We encourage further investigation in the use of such devices.

Patients with increased pulmonary resistance ($>$ 6 Wood units) are also excluded as candidates for orthotopic cardiac transplantation since acute right ventricular failure can occur if a nonhypertrophied right ventricle is implanted. Such patients may be considered for heterotopic cardiac transplantation, which leaves the recipient heart in place and allows the hypertrophied right ventricle to pump against the pulmonary circuit. Another alternative when cardiac failure is complicated by pulmonary hypertension is combined heart-lung transplantation. This procedure is also considered for young ($<$ 45 years old) patients with irreversible pulmonary failure from nonmalignant diseases, primary pulmonary hypertension, pulmonary hypertension secondary to congenital heart disease, and emphysema. Whether rejection of the lung can be followed by endomyocardial biopsy is unclear. Combined heart-lung transplantation entails the benefit of removing all diseased lung tissue, compared with isolated lung transplantation, but additional clinical experience is required to show other comparative advantages.

ETHICAL CONSIDERATIONS

It is practical to recognize that while the application of cardiopulmonary assist devices will allow some patients to recover, others will remain dependent on machines for their existence, and on the health care team for assistance in related ethical decision-making.

While the latter circumstance presents the practitioner, the patient, and the family with difficult moral and ethical decisions, we support the use of assist devices to maintain unstable patients until evaluation can be completed. If an untreatable condition is then found to exist, the support can be removed after proper discussion with all parties involved. We find no moral distinction between initially withholding treatment and later terminating that treatment if it has been found to be of no benefit to the patient.

REFERENCES

1. Al-Mondhiry A, Pierce WS, Richenbacher W: Hemostatic abnormalities associated with prolonged ventricular assist pumping: Analysis of 24 patients. *Am J Cardiol* 1984; 53:1344.
2. Amsterdam EA, Banas J, Criley JM, et al: Clinical assessment of external pressure circulatory assistance in acute myocardial infarction. *Am J Cardiol* 1980; 45:349–356.
3. Aroesty JM, Weintraub RM, Paulin S, et al: Medically refractory unstable angina pectoris: II. Hemodynamic and angiographic effects of intraaortic balloon counterpulsation. *Am J Cardiol* 1979; 43:883–888.
4. Ashar B, Turcotte LR: Analyses of longest IAB implant in human patient (327 days). *Trans Am Soc Artif Intern Organs* 1981; 27:372–374.
5. Bardet J, Rigaud M, Kahn JC, et al: Treatment of post-myocardial infarction angina by intra-aortic balloon pumping and emergency revascularization. *J Thorac Cardiovasc Surg* 1977; 74:299–306.
6. Bartlett RH, Gazzaniga AB, Fong SW, et al: Extracorporeal membrane oxygenator support for cardiopulmonary failure. *J Thorac Cardiovasc Surg* 1977; 73:375–385.
7. Bregman D, Parodi EN, Edie RN, et al: Intraoperative unidirectional intra-aortic balloon pumping in the management of left ventricular power failure. *J Thorac Cardiovasc Surg* 1975; 70:1010–1023.
8. Clauss RH, Birtwell C, Albertal G, et al: Assisted circulation: I. The arterial counterpulsator. *J Thorac Cardiovasc Surg* 1961; 41:447–458.
9. Gattinoni L, Pesenti A, Kolobow T: A new look at therapy of the adult respiratory distress syndrome: Motionless lungs. *Int Anesthesiol Clin* 1983; 21(2):97.
10. Golding LR, Jacobs G, Groves LK, et al: Clinical results of mechanical support of the failing left ventricle. *J Thorac Cardiovasc Surg* 1982; 83:597–601.
11. Golding LR, Loop FD, Peter M, et al: Late survival following use of intraaortic balloon pump in revascularization operations. *Ann Thorac Surg* 1980; 30:48–51.
12. Griffith BP, Borovetz HS, Hardesty RL, et al: Arteriovenous ECMO for neonatal respiratory support. *J Thorac Cardiovasc Surg* 1979; 77:595–601.
13. Hagemeijer F, Laird JD, Haalebos MM, et al: Effectiveness of intraaortic balloon pumping without cardiac surgery for patients with severe heart failure secondary to a recent myocardial infarction. *Am J Cardiol* 1977; 40:951–956.
14. Hardesty RL, Griffith BP, Debski RF, et al: Extracorporeal membrane oxygenation. *J Thorac Cardiovasc Surg* 1981; 81:556–563.
15. Haston HH, McNamarra JJ: The effects of intraaortic balloon counterpulsation on myocardial infarct size. *Ann Thorac Surg* 1979; 28:335–341.
16. Heiden D, Mielke CH, Rodvien R: Platelets, hemostasis, and thromboembolism during treatment of acute respiratory insufficiency with extracorporeal membrane oxygenation. *J Thorac Cardiovasc Surg* 1975; 70:644.
17. Holub DA, Hibbs CW, Sturm JT, et al: Clinical trials of the abdominal left ventricular assist device (ALVAD): Progress report. *Cardiovasc Dis* 1979; 6:359–372.
18. Isner JM, Cohen SR, Virmani R, et al: Complications of the intraaortic balloon counterpulsation device: Clinical and morphologic observations in 45 necropsy patients. *Am J Cardiol* 1980; 45:260–268.
19. Kantrowitz A, Tjonneland S, Freed P, et al: Initial clinical experience with intaaortic balloon pumping in cardiogenic shock. *JAMA* 1968; 203:135–140.
20. Kirklin JK, Westaby S, Blackstone EH, et al: Complement and the damaging effects of cardiopulmonary bypass. *J Thorac Cardiovasc Surg* 1983; 86:845–857.
21. Lande AJ, Edwards L, Bloch JH, et al: Clinical experience with emergency use of prolonged cardiopulmonary bypass with a membrane pump-oxygenator. *Ann Thorac Surg* 1970; 10:409–421.

22. Leinbach RC, Buckley MJ, Austen WG, et al: Effects of intra-aortic balloon pumping on coronary flow and metabolism in man. *Circulation* 1971; 43(suppl I):I77–I81.

23. Leinbach RC, Gold HK, Harper RW, et al: Early intraaortic balloon pumping for anterior myocardial infarction without shock. *Circulation* 1978; 58:204–210.

24. Levine FH, Gold HK, Leinbach RC, et al: Management of acute myocardial ischemia with intraaortic balloon pumping and coronary bypass surgery. *Circulation* 1978; 58(suppl I):I69–I72.

25. Litwak RS, Koffskky RM, Lukban SB, et al: Implanted heart assist device after intracardiac surgery. *N Engl J Med* 1974; 291:1341–1343.

26. Mayer JH: Subclavian artery approach for insertion of intra-aortic balloon. *J Thorac Cardiovasc Surg* 1978; 76:61–63.

27. McCormick JR, Berger RL, Davis Z, et al: Infection in remnant of left ventricular assist device after successful separation from assisted circulation. *J Thorac Cardiovasc Surg* 1981; 81:727–731.

28. McEnany MT, Kay HR, Buckley MJ, et al: Clinical experience with intraaortic balloon pump support in 728 patients. *Circulation* 1978; 58(suppl I):I124–I132.

29. McGee MG, Zillgitt SL, Trono R, et al: Retrospective analyses of the need for mechanical circulatory support (intraaortic balloon pump/abdominal left ventricular assist device or partial artificial heart) after cardiopulmonary bypass. *Am J Cardiol* 1980; 46:135–141.

30. Moulopoulos SD, Topaz S, Kolff WJ: Diastolic balloon pumping (with carbon dioxide) in the aorta: A mechanical assistance to the failing circulation. *Am Heart J* 1962; 63:669–675.

31. Parmley WW, Chatterjee K, Charuzi Y, et al: Hemodynamic effects of noninvasive systolic unloading (nitroprusside) and diastolic augmentation (external counterpulsation) in patients with acute myocardial infarction. *Am J Cardiol* 1974; 33:819–825.

32. Pierce WS, Parr GVS, Myers JL, et al: Ventricular-assist pumping in patients with cardiogenic shock after cardiac operations. *N Engl J Med* 1981; 305:1606–1610.

33. Scheidt S, Wilner G, Mueller G, et al: Intra-aortic balloon counterpulsation in cardiogenic shock. *N Engl J Med* 1973; 288:979–984.

34. Secker-Walker JS, Edmonds JF, Spratt EH, et al: The source of coronary perfusion during partial bypass for extracorporeal membrane oxygenation (ECMO). *Ann Thorac Surg* 1976; 21:138–143.

35. Steele P, Pappas G, Vogel R, et al: Isosorbide dinitrate and intra-aortic balloon pumping in preinfarctional angina. *Chest* 1976; 69:712–717.

36. Stuckey JH, Newman MM, Dennis C, et al: The use of the heart-lung machine in selected cases of acute myocardial infarction. *Surg Forum* 1957; 8:342–344.

37. Sweet SE, Sussman HA, Ryan TJ, et al: Sequential radionuclide imaging during paracorporeal left ventricular support. *Chest* 1980; 78:423.

38. Takanashi Y, Campbell CD, Laas J, et al: Reduction of myocardial infarct size in swine: A comparative study of intraaortic balloon pumping and transapical left ventricular bypass. *Ann Thorac Surg* 1981; 32:475–485.

39. Weintraub RM, Aroesty JM, Paulin S, et al: Medically refractory unstable angina pectoris: I. Long-term follow-up of patients undergoing intraaortic balloon counterpulsation and operation. *Am J Cardiol* 1979; 43:877–882.

40. Willerson JT, Curry GC, Watson JT, et al: Intra-aortic balloon counterpulsation in patients in cardiogenic shock, medically refractory left ventricular failure and/or recurrent ventricular tachycardia. *Am J Med* 1975; 58:183–191.

41. Williams DO, Korr KS, Gewirtz H, et al: The effect of intraaortic balloon counterpulsation on regional myocardial blood flow and oxygen consumption in the presence of coronary artery stenosis in patients with unstable angina. *Circulation* 1982; 66:593–597.

42. Yahr WZ, Butner AN, Krakauer JS, et al: Cardiogenic shock: Dynamics of coronary blood flow with intraaortic phase-shift balloon pumping. *Surg Forum* 1968; 19:122.

Index